Textbook of Microbiology for Dental Students

Other Books by Dr. D.R. Arora

- Textbook of Microbiology, 5/e
- Exam-Oriented Microbiology (Questions & Answers)
- Medical Parasitology, 4/e
- Medical Mycology
- Essentials of Microbiology for B.Sc. Nursing Students
- Practical Microbiology
- Practical Microbiology for Dental Students
- MCQs in Microbiology — with explanation (In Press)

Textbook of Microbiology for Dental Students

Fourth Edition

Dr. D.R. Arora M.D., Ph.D., M.N.A.M.S.

Dean, Faculty of Allied Health Sciences, SGT University, Budhera, Gurgaon

Lead Assessor & Member, Core Accreditation Committee, National Accreditation Board
for Testing and Calibration Laboratories (NABL), Gurgaon; Principal Assessor,
National Accreditation Board for Hospitals & Healthcare Providers (NABH), New Delhi;
Assessor, National Accreditation Board for Education and Training (NABET), New Delhi;
Member, Technical Resource Group on Laboratory Services,
National AIDS Control Organization (NACO), New Delhi

Formerly
Professor & Head, Department of Microbiology,
Postgraduate Institute of Medical Sciences, Rohtak (Haryana);
Professor & Head, Department of Microbiology,
Maharaja Agarsen Medical College, Agroha, Hisar (Haryana);
Medical Superintendent & Professor of Microbiology,
SGT Medical College, Hospital & Research Institute, Budhera, Gurgaon;
W.H.O. Fellow; and Visiting Professor, University of Mauritius

Dr. Brij Bala Arora M.D.

Ex-Senior Professor & Head, Department of Pathology,
Postgraduate Institute of Medical Sciences, Rohtak, Haryana; and
SGT Medical College, Budhera, Gurgaon

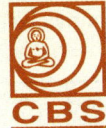

CBS

CBS Publishers & Distributors Pvt. Ltd.

New Delhi • Bengaluru • Chennai • Kochi • Kolkata • Mumbai
Hyderabad • Nagpur • Patna • Pune • Vijayawada

ISBN: 978-81-239-2786-2

First Edition: 1999
Reprint: 2001
Second Edition: 2006
Reprint: 2007
Third Edition: 2009
Reprint: 2011, 2012
Fourth Edition: 2015
Reprint: 2017

Published by **Satish Kumar Jain** and produced by **Varun Jain** for
CBS Publishers & Distributors Pvt. Ltd.,
4819/XI Prahlad Street, 24 Ansari Road, Daryaganj, New Delhi - 110002
delhi@cbspd.com, cbspubs@airtelmail.in • www.cbspd.com
Ph.: 23289259, 23266861, 23266867 • Fax: 011-23243014

Corporate Office: 204 FIE, Industrial Area, Patparganj, Delhi - 110 092
Ph: 49344934 • Fax: 011-49344935
E-mail: publishing@cbspd.com • publicity@cbspd.com

Branches:
• *Bengaluru:* 2975, 17th Cross, K.R. Road, Bansankari 2nd Stage,
  Bengaluru - 70 • Ph: +91-80-26771678/79 • Fax: +91-80-26771680
  E-mail: cbsbng@gmail.com, bangalore@cbspd.com
• *Chennai:* No. 7, Subbaraya Street, Shenoy Nagar, Chennai - 600030
  Ph: +91-44-26681266, 26680620 • Fax: +91-44-42032115
  E-mail: chennai@cbspd.com
• *Kochi:* Ashana House, 39/1904, A.M. Thomas Road, Valanjambalam,
  Ernakulum, Kochi • Ph: +91-484-4059061-65
  Fax: +91-484-4059065 • E-mail: cochin@cbspd.com
• *Kolkata:* 6-B, Ground Floor, Rameshwar Shaw Road, Kolkata - 700014
  Ph: +91-33-22891126/7/8 • E-mail: kolkata@cbspd.com
• *Mumbai:* 83-C, Dr. E. Moses Road, Worli, Mumbai - 400018
  Ph: +91-9833017933, 022-24902340/41 • E-mail: mumbai@cbspd.com

Representatives:

• Hyderabad: 0-9885175004   • Nagpur: 0-9021734563
• Patna: 0-9334159340   • Pune: 0-9623451994
• Vijayawada: 0-9000660880

Printed at:
Neekunj Print Process, Delhi (India)

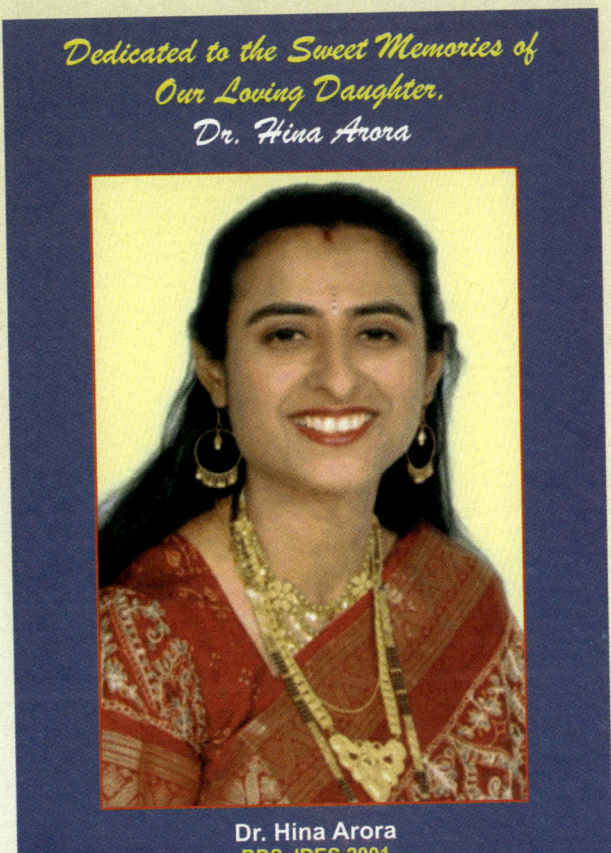

Dedicated to the Sweet Memories of
Our Loving Daughter,
Dr. Hina Arora

Dr. Hina Arora
BDS, IDES 2001
09-04-1976 to 02-11-2009

Syllabus in Microbiology for Dental Students
As per DENTAL COUNCIL OF INDIA

A. GENERAL MICROBIOLOGY:

- History, introduction, scope, aims and objectives.
- Morphology and physiology of bacteria.
- Detailed account of sterilization and disinfection.
- Brief account of culture media and culture techniques.
- Basic knowledge of selection, collection, transport, processing of clinical specimens and identification of bacteria.
- Bacterial genetics and drug resistance in bacteria.

B. IMMUNOLOGY:

- Infection – definition, classification, source, mode of transmission and types of infectious disease.
- Immunity.
- Structure and functions of immune system.
- The complement system.
- Antigen.
- Immunoglobulins – antibodies – general structure and the role played in defence mechanism of the body.
- Immune response.
- Antigen-antibody reactions with reference to clinical utility.
- Immunodeficiency disorders – a brief knowledge of various types of immunodeficiency disorders – a sound knowledge of immunodeficiency disorders relevant to dentistry.
- Hypersensitivity reactions.
- Autoimmune disorders – basic knowledge of various types – sound knowledge of autoimmune disorders of oral cavity and related strucutres.
- Immunology of transplantation and malignancy.
- Immunohaematology.

C. SYSTEMATIC BACTERIOLOGY:

- Pyogenic cocci – *Staphylococcus*, *Streptococcus*, pneumococcus, gonococcus, meningococcus – brief account of each coccus – detailed account of mode of laboratory diagnosis, chemotherapy and prevention – detailed account of cariogenic streptococci.
- *Corynebacterium diphtheriae* – mode of spread, important clinical features, laboratory diagnosis, chemotherapy and active immunization.
- Mycobacteria – tuberculosis and leprosy.
- *Clostridium* – gas gangrene, food poisoning and tetanus.
- Non-sporing anaerobes – in brief about classification and morphology, in detail about dental pathogens – mechanism of disease production and prevention.
- Spirochaetes – *Treponema pallidum* – detailed account of oral lesions of syphilis, *Borrelia vincenti*.
- Actinomycetes.

D. VIROLOGY:

- Introduction.
- General properties, cultivation, host-virus interaction with special reference to interferon.
- Brief account of laboratory diagnosis, chemotherapy and immunoprophylaxis in general.
- A few viruses of relevance to dentistry.
- Herpes virus.
- Hepatitis B virus – brief about other types.
- Human immunodeficiency virus (HIV).
- Mumps virus.
- Brief – measles and rubella virus.
- Bacteriophage – structure and significance.

E. MYCOLOGY:

- Brief introduction.
- Candidiasis – in detail.
- Briefly on oral lesions of systemic mycoses.

F. PARASITOLOGY:

- Brief introduction – protozoans and helminths.
- Brief knowledge about the mode of transmission and prevention of commonly seen parasitic infections in the region.

Preface to the Fourth Edition

The fourth edition of the **Textbook of Microbiology for Dental Students** has been written as per the syllabus prescribed by Dental Council of India. Keeping in mind the requirements of dental students emphasis has been on the oral manifestations of various microorganisms.

The text has been written in a straightforward manner. Details are summarized in a tabular format and there are coloured illustrations. Each chapter has been carefully updated and expanded to include new, medically relevant discoveries. Laboratory diagnosis of various microbial infections has been summarized with the help of flowcharts. The book has been divided into eight sections. These include general microbiology, immunology, systemic bacteriology, virology, mycology, parasitology, oral microbiology, and clinical microbiology. Each chapter ends with key facts and important questions. The former summarize the whole chapter and help the student for last minute revision for theory, practical and viva voce examination, and the latter help the student to know the type of questions asked in the examination.

In oral microbiology, emphasis has been on normal flora of mouth and respiratory tract, dental plaque, dental caries, periodontal diseases and dentoalveolar abscess. In the chapter on hepatitis viruses, emphasis has been on various hepatitis viruses and dentistry. The book will be highly useful to graduate (BDS) and postgraduate (MDS) students of dentistry, and students of other paramedical courses. It is also hoped that it will serve as a useful resource for teachers of dental microbiology.

We are deeply indebted to Dr. P.S. Gill, Professor of Microbiology, Postgraduate Institute of Medical Sciences, Rohtak for computer work, drawings and extensive proof-reading. We honestly acknowledge the most sincere and dedicated professional help, encouragement and support provided by Mr. Dharmvir. Thanks are also due to Mr. B.M. Singh and M/s CBS Publishers & Distributors Pvt. Ltd. for their cooperation and keen interest in the publication of this book. We also wish to thank many students and professional colleagues who have offered their advice and constructive criticism throughout the development of the fourth edition of the book.

D.R. Arora
Brij Bala Arora
draroradr@rediffmail.com

Preface to the First Edition *(Excerpts)*

At present, BDS students and their teachers have to rely on the books written for MBBS students. The syllabus prescribed by Dental Council of India is quite old and ambiguous. Therefore, the topics covered in microbiology by different dental colleges are different. The books for MBBS students do not emphasize the relevance of microbiology applied to dental sciences and the oral manifestations of various microbial diseases. Keeping in view the above problems, a simple and comprehensive book including parasitology has been devised. The text has been presented in a simple language and it has been illustrated with figures, colour plates and tables.

The book is divided into six sections that include general bacteriology, systemic bacteriology, virology, medical mycology, medical parasitology, and oral and clinical microbiology. Each section briefly deals with the essential features of the appropriate topics in each chapter and is supplemented with suitable illustrations and examples. Section on general bacteriology includes immunology. Section on systemic bacteriology deals with all the important pathogens for dental students. Section on virology has been briefly discussed in three chapters, and sections on medical mycology and medical parasitology in one chapter each. Finally chapter VI deals with oral and clinical microbiology.

New nomenclature of various pathogens has been followed throughout the book. Finally adding colour to the textbook are the colour plates that show the exact picture of the pathogens. Throughout the book effort has been made to restrict the volume of the book keeping in view the need of dental students and the syllabus prescribed by Dental Council of India. The authors hope that with the launching of this book a uniformity of teaching in various dental colleges will be initiated. The readers are requested to write any shortcoming and give us suggestions for the improvement of the book in subsequent editions.

D.R. Arora
Brij Bala Arora

Contents

SECTION C

Systemic Bacteriology   157–252

SECTION D

Virology   253–308

SECTION E

Mycology   309–327

SECTION F

Parasitology   329–368

SECTION G

Oral Microbiology   369–378

SECTION H

Clinical Microbiology   379–384

SECTION A
General Microbiology

1. Microbiology (A Brief History)
2. Morphology and Physiology of Bacteria
3. Culture Media and Culture Techniques
4. Selection, Collection, Transport and Processing of Clinical Specimens, and Identification of Bacteria
5. Sterilization and Disinfection
6. Chemotherapy
7. Bacterial Genetics and Drug Resistance in Bacteria
8. Infection

Chapter 1

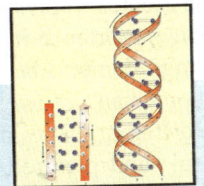

Microbiology
A Brief History

Microbiology is the study of living organisms of microscopic size. This term was introduced by French chemist Louis Pasteur (1822–95), who demonstrated that fermentation was caused by the growth of bacteria and yeasts. **Medical microbiology** is the study of microbes that infect humans, the diseases they cause, and their diagnosis, prevention and treatment. It also deals with the response of the human host to microbial infection. The term **microbe** was first used by Sedillot in 1878, but it has now been replaced by **microorganism**. Microbes were probably the first living things to appear on the earth, and the study of fossil remains indicates that microbial infections and epidemic diseases existed thousands of years ago.

Infectious diseases have been the bane of mankind for centuries and continue to cause high morbidity and sufferings worldwide. Disease and death have always attracted the attention of the human mind. The emergence of acquired immunodeficiency syndrome (AIDS) as a major modern day scourge with tremendous public health importance has brought into limelight even those diseases which were considered rare in the past.

The construction and use of the compound microscope (*micro*, small; and *skop*, to look, to see) was an essential prerequisite to study the microbial forms. To **Antonie van Leeuwenhoek** (1632–1723) (Fig. 1.1) must be ascribed the credit of placing the science of microbiology on the firm basis of direct observation. This Dutch maker of lenses from Holland devised an apparatus and technique which enabled him to observe and describe various microbial forms with accuracy and care. He observed, drew and measured a large number of minute living organisms including bacteria and protozoa and communicated them to Royal Society of London in 1683.

The significance of these observations was not realized then and to Leeuwenhoek the world of 'little

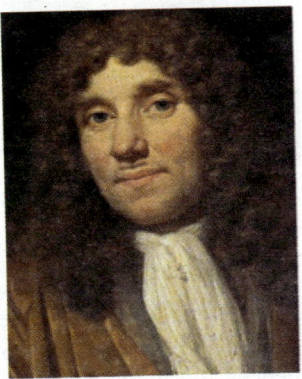

Fig. 1.1. Antonie van Leeuwenhoek (1632–1723).

animalcules' represented only a curiosity of nature. Their importance in medicine and in other areas of biology came to be recognized two centuries later. Antonie van Leeuwenhoek first accurately described the different shapes of bacteria (coccal, bacillary and spiral) and pictured their arrangement in infected material (in 1683).

ORIGIN OF MICROBIAL LIFE

In 1856, **Louis Pasteur** (1822–1895) (Fig. 1.2) was commissioned by an industrialist of Lille to investigate the problem which had arisen in manufacture of alcohol. The beet juice, from which alcohol was derived, was contaminated with a grey material which interfered with alcohol production. During the course of investigation his attention was abruptly focused on the role of microorganisms in alcohol fermentation and spoilage. Undesirable forms of life could be destroyed at temperatures of 50°–60°C in a short period of time. Subsequently this modified process of heating came to be known as **pasteurization**. Pasteur established that different types of fermentations were due to the activity of different kinds of microbes.

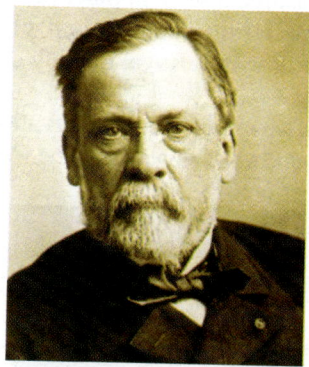

Fig. 1.2. Louis Pasteur (1822–1895).

Joseph Lister (1827–1912), an English surgeon and contemporary of Pasteur, was among the first to appreciate the ramifications of the emerging **germ theory** of disease. He attributed the frequent disastrous consequences following repair of compound fractures to invasions by airborne microorganisms. Lister introduced antiseptics in surgery. By spraying carbolic acid on surgical instruments, wounds and dressings, he reduced surgical mortality due to bacterial infection considerably. He established the guiding principle of antisepsis for good surgical practice upon which the present day specialists depend. For this work he is known as '**father of antiseptic surgery**'.

THE DEVELOPING SCIENCE OF MICROBIOLOGY

In the course of studies, Pasteur introduced the techniques of sterilization and developed steam-sterilizer, hot air oven and autoclave. **Robert Koch** (1843–1910) (Fig. 1.3), a German physician, perfected the bacteriological techniques, staining procedures and methods of obtaining bacteria in pure culture using solid media during his studies on the culture and characters of anthrax bacillus.

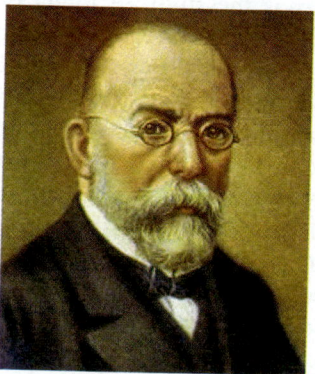

Fig. 1.3. Robert Koch (1843–1910).

The causative agents of various diseases were reported rapidly by different investigators. Robert Koch discovered the bacillus of anthrax (1876), bacillus of tuberculosis (1882) and cholera vibrio (1883); Hansen described the leprosy bacillus in 1874; Neisser discovered the gonococcus in the pus discharge from urethra in 1879; Alexander Ogston in 1880 described the staphylococci in abscesses and suppurative lesions; Eberth observed the typhoid bacillus in 1880; Klebs (1883) and Loeffler (1884) observed and described the diphtheria bacillus; Rosenbach (1886) demonstrated the tetanus bacillus with round terminal spore; Weichselbaum (1887) described and isolated the meningococcus from the spinal fluid of a patient; Bruce (1887) identified the causative agent of malta fever in 1905 and Schaudinn and Hoffmann described the spirochaete of syphilis.

As the agents were being reported in such profusion it became necessary to introduce criteria for proving the claims that a microorganism isolated from a disease was indeed causally related to it. **Henle** indicated such criteria but were enunciated by Koch which consisted of guidelines for the association of particular microorganisms with specific infectious diseases.

Koch observed thread-like organisms in the blood of animals that had died of anthrax, a disease that was a serious threat to farmers, killing their sheep and cattle herds periodically. He cultivated anthrax bacteria in pure culture in clear sterile vitreous humor of an ox's eye. He then injected pure cultures of the bacilli into mice and showed that the bacilli invariably caused anthrax. On autopsy, the blood was swarming with the thread-like bacteria and re-isolated them in the vitreous humor. The cycle was now complete.

Koch's postulates

A microorganism can be accepted as the causative agent of an infectious disease only if following postulates, known as Koch's postulates, are satisfied (Fig. 1.4):

1. The organism must be present in the lesions in every case of the infectious disease.
2. It should be possible to isolate the organism in pure culture from the lesions.
3. Inoculation of the pure culture into suitable laboratory animals should produce a similar disease.
4. It should again be possible to re-isolate the organism in pure culture from the lesions produced in the experimental animals.

A fifth criterion introduced subsequently states that specific antibodies to the organism should be demonstrable in the serum of the patient suffering from the disease. These postulates have proved extremely useful in confirming the authenticity of doubtful claims made regarding the causative agents of infectious diseases.

Koch's postulates have remained a mainstay of microbiology; however, many microorganisms that do not meet the criteria of postulates have been shown to cause disease. For example, *Treponema pallidum* and *Mycobacterium leprae*, causative agents of syphilis and leprosy respectively, cannot be grown *in vitro*; however, there are animal models of infection with these agents. In another example, *Neisseria gonorrhoeae*, which causes gonorrhoea, there is no animal model even though the bacteria can readily be cultured *in vitro*.

THE BEGINNING OF VIROLOGY

For many years the term virus was used to describe any poison or microbial agent capable of causing an infection. In a large number of diseases such as smallpox, chickenpox, measles, influenza, poliomyelitis and the common cold, no bacterial cause could be established. Pasteur had suspected that rabies in dogs could be caused by a microbe too small to be seen under the microscope.

The first man to describe a filtered extract capable of causing disease in plants was Dmitri Iwanowski (1864–1920), a Russian scientist, who started his studies on diseases of tobacco while he was still a student. He reproduced mosaic disease in tobacco plant by applying juice from diseased plants to

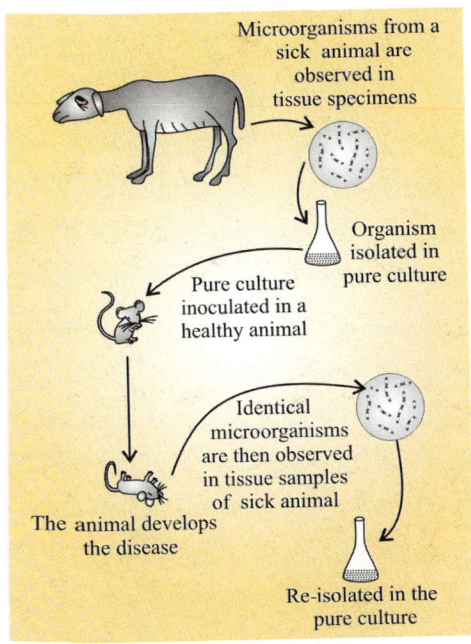

Microorganisms from a sick animal are observed in tissue specimens

Organism isolated in pure culture

Pure culture inoculated in a healthy animal

Identical microorganisms are then observed in tissue samples of sick animal

The animal develops the disease

Re-isolated in the pure culture

Fig. 1.4. Koch's postulates.

healthy leaves from which all bacteria had been removed by passage through fine filters (1892). In 1898, Martinus Beijerinck, unaware of Iwanowski's work, attributed the cause of tobacco-mosaic disease to *Contagium vivum fluidum*, a living liquid virus.

In 1898, Loeffler and Paul Frosch from Germany reported that the causative agent of foot-and-mouth disease in cattle would pass through a bacterial filter. Walter Reed (1902) in Cuba proved that the causative agent of yellow fever was not only a filterable virus but also transmitted through the bite of infected mosquitoes. The term 'filterable' was dropped in time and the tiny infectious agents were merely called viruses. Larger viruses could be seen under light microscope after appropriate staining but their detailed morphology could only be studied by electron microscope introduced by Ruska (1934). The technique of growing them on chick embryos developed by Goodpasture in 1930s and the application of tissue culture in virology expanded the scope of virological techniques considerably.

Ellerman and Bang (1908) suggested the possibility that virus infection could lead to malignancy. Peyton Rous (1911) isolated a virus causing sarcoma in fowls. Several viruses have been blamed to cause natural and experimental tumours in birds and animals. Experimentally, viruses can cause malignant transformation of infected cells in tissue cultures. The discovery of viral and cellular oncogenes have put forth the possible mechanisms of viral oncogenesis.

KEY FACTS

- Microbiology is the biology of *microscopic organisms*, its subjects being microorganisms
- Microorganism is an organism that *cannot be seen without the use of a microscope*
- *Medical microbiology* deals with those *organisms which are responsible for infectious diseases of humans*
- A microorganism can be accepted as the causative agent of an infectious disease if it satisfies *Koch's postulates*
- *Treponema pallidum, Mycobacterium leprae* and *Neisseria gonorrhoeae* do not fulfil all the criteria of Koch's postulates; the first two cannot be *grown in vitro* and for the third there is *no animal model*

IMPORTANT QUESTION

Write short note on Koch's postulates.

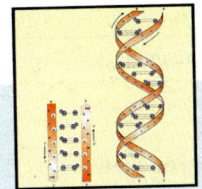

Chapter 2

Morphology and Physiology of Bacteria

Bacteria are free-living, microscopic, unicellular organisms capable of performing all the essential functions of life, e.g., growth, metabolism and reproduction. They possess both deoxyribonucleic acid (DNA) and ribonucleic acid (RNA) and lack chlorophyll. Bacteria have been placed in a kingdom separate from the animal and plant kingdoms, **Protista**.

The kingdom Protista includes unicellular organisms such as bacteria, fungi, protozoa and algae. Based on differences in cellular organization and biochemistry the kingdom Protista has been divided into three groups – prokaryotes, eukaryotes and archaebacteria. The latter are more closely related to eukaryotes than prokaryotes. Archaebacteria do not include any human pathogen.

Cells that have a well-defined nucleus are called *eukaryotes* (*eu*, true; and *karyon*, nucleus), whereas cells that lack a well-defined nucleus are called *prokaryotes* (*pro*, primitive; and *karyon*, nucleus). Bacteria and blue-green algae are prokaryotes, while fungi, other algae, slime molds and protozoa are eukaryotes. In general, the interior organization of eukaryotic cells is more complex than that of prokaryotic cells. The comparison of prokaryotes and eukaryotes is given in Table 2.1.

Bacteria do not contain a membrane-bound nucleus. Their DNA consists of a single circular chromosome, which is attached to a mesosome, a saclike structure in the cell membrane. Bacterial ribosomes are found free in the cytoplasm and attached to the cytoplasmic membrane. They are 70S in size and dissociate into two subunits, 50S and 30S in `size. The cell envelope, in bacteria, consists of cytoplasmic (cell) membrane and cell wall. Some species also produce capsules and slime layers.

SIZE OF BACTERIA

Bacteria are very small in size. The unit of measurement of bacteria is called micrometre (μm). One μm is a millionth part of a metre or a thousandth part of a millimetre (mm). One nanometre (nm) is a billionth part of a metre or a thousandth part of a μm, and one Angstrom unit (Å) is one tenth of a nanometre. The diameter of the smallest body that can be resolved and seen clearly with naked eye is about 200 μm.

Medically important bacteria generally measure 0.2–1.5 μm in diameter and 3–5 μm in length. Therefore, to visualize most bacteria one must use the higher powers of magnification of a good light microscope and enlarge them about 1000 times. To visualize their surfaces distinctly, it is usually necessary to stain them. Electron microscopy is essential for clear visualization of internal structures of the bacteria.

Table 2.1. Comparison of prokaryotes and eukaryotes

Characteristic	Prokaryotes	Eukaryotes
Major groups	Bacteria and blue-green algae	Other algae, fungi, protozoa, plants and animals
Genetic material		
Location	Free in the cytoplasm attached to a structure called a mesosome located in the cell membrane	Contained within a membrane-bound nucleus inside the cell
Form	A single circular piece of DNA	Multiple chromosomes, which are surrounded by basic proteins called histones
Nucleolus	Absent	Present
Replication	By binary fission	By mitosis and meiosis
Extrachromosomal DNA	Plasmids – small circular pieces of DNA containing accessory information, present in the cytoplasm	In mitochondria
Protein production site	No endoplasmic reticulum; ribosomes free in the cytoplasm or attached to the cell membrane	• Rough endoplasmic reticulum, a membrane covered with ribosomes, where protein is made. • Smooth endoplasmic reticulum or Golgi complex, where secreted proteins are packaged and transported to the cell surface.
Ribosomes	70S in size, consisting of a 50S and 30S subunits	80S in size, consisting of a 60S and 40S subunits
Energy production site	Electron transport chain located in the cell membrane; no mitochondria present	Within membrane-bound mitochondria
Intracellular organelles (lysosomes)	Absent	Contain hydrolytic enzymes
Cytoplasmic membrane	With the exception of *Mycoplasma*, bacterial cytoplasmic membrane lacks sterols	Does contain sterols
Cell wall	Present; is a complex structure containing peptidoglycans, proteins, and lipids	Usually absent except in fungi, which contain chitin in the cell wall

SHAPE OF BACTERIA

Bacteria exist in different shapes as under (Fig. 2.1):

1. **Cocci** (from *kokkos* meaning berry) are round or oval cells.
2. **Bacilli** (from *bacillus* meaning rod) are rod- or stick-shaped. In some of the bacilli the length of the cells may be equal to width. Such bacillary forms are known as **coccobacilli**. The latter have to be carefully differentiated from cocci.
3. **Vibrios** are curved or comma-shaped rods.
4. **Spirilla** are non-flexuous spiral forms with one to three fixed curves in their rigid bodies.
5. **Spirochaetes** (from *spira* meaning coil; and *chaite* meaning hair) are slender and flexuous spiral forms.
6. **Mycoplasmas** are cell wall deficient organisms. Therefore, they do not possess stable morphology. They occur as round or oval bodies or as interlacing filaments.

GROUP PATTERNS

The most frequent method of reproduction among bacteria is asexual binary fission, that is, each cell splits in half, forming two new cells. As they increase in number they form distinct groups. Cocci that split along one plane only tend to arrange themselves in pairs (**diplococci**) or in chains (**streptococci**). When the division occurs alternatively in each of two planes, groups of four (**tetrads**) or eight (**octads**) are formed. Haphazard splitting in several planes results in the formation of clusters of cocci (Fig. 2.1).

Bacilli split only across their short axes, therefore, the patterns formed by them are limited. They may appear as end to end pairs (**diplobacilli**), or chains (**streptobacilli**) (Fig. 2.1). In some instances, there occurs incomplete separation of the daughter cells after binary fission. The bacilli remain attached to each other at various angles, resembling the letters V or L. This is called **Chinese letter arrangement** and is characteristic of *Corynebacterium diphtheriae*.

ANATOMY OF A BACTERIAL CELL

The principal structure of a bacterial cell is shown in Fig. 2.2. The interior of the cell, the protoplast, is

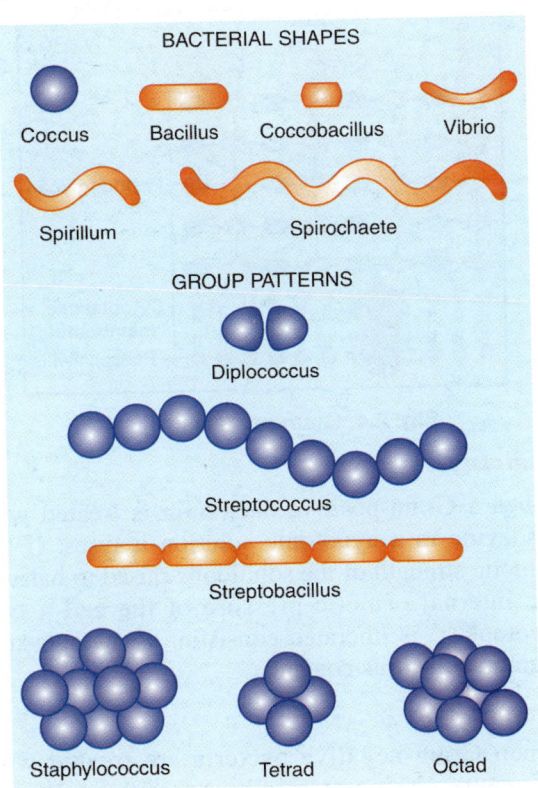

Fig. 2.1. Shape and group patterns of bacteria.

differentiated into cytoplasm and nuclear material. Cytoplasm is bounded by a thin, elastic and semipermeable cytoplasmic membrane. Outside this lies cell wall, which gives the bacterium its shape and rigidity. Cell wall, in many bacteria, is enclosed by a protective gelatinous covering layer called capsule. If the capsule is too thin to be seen with light microscope, it is called **microcapsule**. If it is viscid and diffuses out into the medium it is called **slime layer**. Many bacteria also possess flagella which are the organelles of motility and some species have fimbriae (pili) too.

Bacterial cell wall

- It is a complex rigid structure which gives bacteria their definite shape.
- It is permeable to passage of liquid nutrient material into the cell and to outward passage of substances produced within the cell.
- It is about 10–20 nm in thickness and constitutes 20–30% of dry weight of the cell.
- The cell walls of Gram-positive bacteria are generally thicker than those of Gram-negative bacteria.
- The strength of the bacterial cell wall is due to the presence in it of a substance referred to as peptido-glycan, mucopeptide or murein.

Peptidoglycan consists of three parts – a backbone, composed of alternating N-acetylglucosamine and N-acetylmuramic acid; a set of identical tetrapeptide side chains attached to N-acetylmuramic acid and a set of identical pentapeptide cross-bridges (Fig. 2.3). In all bacterial species the backbone is the same, however, tetrapeptide side chains and pentapeptide cross-bridges vary from species to species.

Peptidoglycan is the major constituent of the cell walls of Gram-positive bacteria constituting 50–90% of the wall. In Gram-negative bacteria it constitutes only 5–10% of the wall. In addition to peptidoglycan, Gram-positive cell walls also contain teichoic acids and polysaccharides (Fig. 2.4). Gram-negative cell walls are more complex (Fig. 2.5). Peptidoglycan in them occurs as an inner layer, outside this lies lipoprotein layer, followed by outer membrane which is made up of outer membrane protein (OMP), porins (pore proteins), phospholipid and the outermost layer

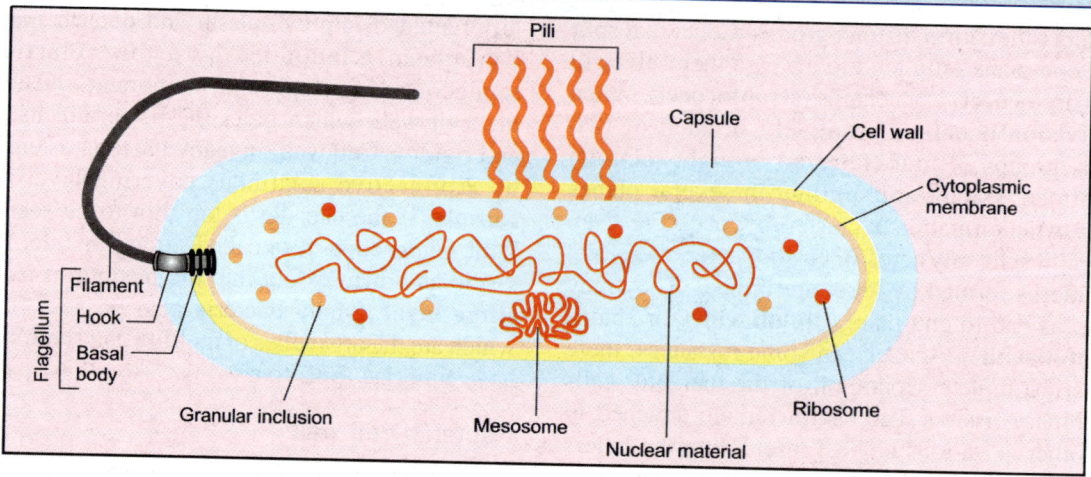

Fig. 2.2. Anatomy of a bacterial cell.

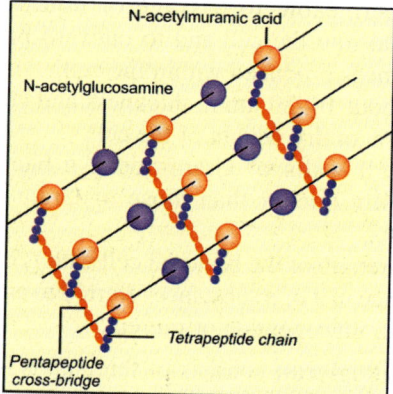

Fig. 2.3. Chemical structure of peptidoglycan.

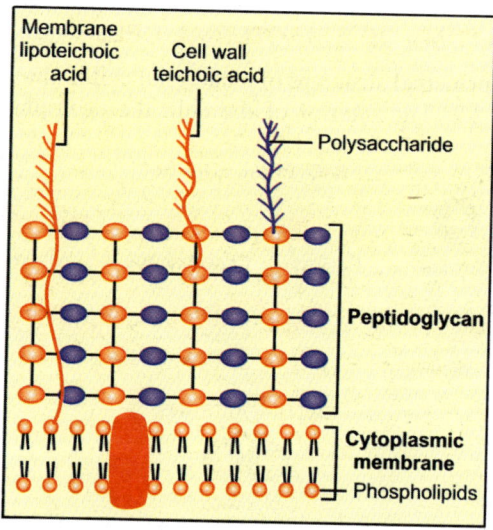

Fig. 2.4. Gram-positive cell wall.

of lipopolysaccharide (LPS). The latter consists of lipid A and core polysaccharide made up of a core and a terminal series of repeat unit. From the core polysaccharide extends outward O polysaccharide. It represents a major surface antigen of the bacterial cell. It is known as O antigen. LPS is firmly bound to the cell surface and is released only when the cells are lysed. It is, therefore, called **endotoxin** and is extremely toxic to animals. All the toxicity of the endotoxin is due to lipid A.

Protoplasts and spheroplasts

The cell wall may be removed by treating the bacteria with lysozyme. It acts by hydrolyzing linkages of the peptidoglycan backbone.

Protoplast

When a Gram-positive bacterium is treated with lysozyme in a hypotonic solution it lyses. If the osmotic strength of the solution is raised to balance the internal osmotic pressure of the cell a free 'protoplast' is liberated consisting of cytoplasmic membrane and its contents.

Spheroplast

When Gram-negative bacteria are treated with lysozyme, the outer membrane of the cell wall prevents access of lysozyme unless disrupted by an

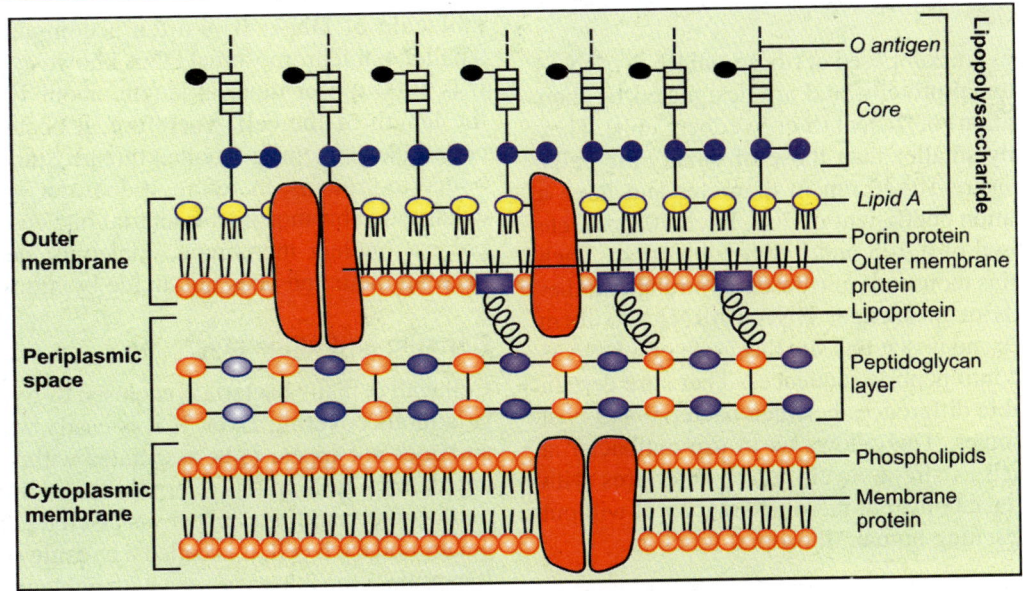

Fig. 2.5. Gram-negative cell wall.

agent such as ethylenediamine tetraacetic acid (EDTA). Lysozyme-EDTA treated bacteria result in the formation of 'spheroplasts' which still possess remnants of the complex Gram-negative cell wall.

Removal of the bacterial cell wall may also be accomplished by growing the organisms in the presence of a substance such as penicillin, bacitracin or cycloserine that block peptidoglycan biosynthesis. A similar result may be obtained by growing the organisms on a medium lacking nutrients like diaminopimelic acid, lysine or hexosamine which are essential for cell wall synthesis. If maintained on osmotically protective medium, protoplasts metabolize and grow in size but they do not multiply. Spheroplasts, on the other hand, when kept on osmotically protective agar medium containing cell wall inhibitor such as penicillin, may multiply by fission or budding and reproduce through many serial subcultures. Because spheroplasts retain a residual cell wall, therefore, they are osmotically less sensitive than protoplasts and are often capable of growing on an ordinary agar medium.

Cytoplasmic membrane

Bacterial cytoplasmic membrane, also called cell membrane, limits the bacterial protoplast externally. It is thin (5–10 nm), elastic and consists of a phospholipid bilayer in which various constituent proteins are embedded (Figs. 2.4 and 2.5). With the exception of *Mycoplasma*, bacterial cytoplasmic membrane lacks sterols. It acts as a semipermeable membrane controlling the inflow and outflow of metabolites to and from the protoplasm. It permits the passive diffusion inward and outward of water and other small molecular substances, but it actively effects the selective transport of specific nutrients into the cell and that of waste products out of it. This is mediated through specific enzymes (permeases) present in the cytoplasmic membrane.

Cytoplasm

Cytoplasm of the bacterial cell is a viscous watery solution of soft gel, containing a variety of organic and inorganic solutes. It contains all the biosynthetic components required by the bacterium for the growth and cell division together with genetic material. The cytoplasm of bacteria differs from that of higher eukaryotic organisms in not containing endoplasmic reticulum, Golgi apparatus, mitochondria, lysosomes and in not showing signs of internal mobility, e.g., cytoplasmic streaming, the formation, migration and disappearance of vacuoles and amoeboid movement. Cytoplasm contains ribosomes, mesosomes and intracytoplasmic inclusion bodies (Fig. 2.2):

Ribosomes

Ribosomes are composed of ribosomal RNA (rRNA) and ribosomal proteins and are designated by their sedimentation coefficient (S or Svedberg unit). They are slightly smaller than those of eukaryotic cells. They measure 10–20 nm in diameter and have a sedimentation coefficient of 70S. Each 70S particle is composed of a 30S and a 50S subparticle. Each cell contains thousands of ribosomes strung together on strands of messenger RNA (mRNA) to form polysomes and it is at this site that code of mRNA is translated into peptide sequences. There are certain considerable differences between bacterial and host cell ribosomes. This allows us to use antibacterial agents such as streptomycin which interferes with bacterial metabolism at the ribosomal level without unduly upsetting human ribosomal function.

Mesosomes

These are convoluted or multilaminated membranous bodies which develop by invagination of cytoplasmic membrane into the cytoplasm (Fig. 2.2). They provide increased membrane surface and are principal sites of respiratory enzymes in bacteria. They are analogous to mitochondria of eukaryotes and are more prominent in Gram-positive bacteria. They are often seen in relation to the nuclear body and the site of synthesis of cross-wall septa, suggesting that they coordinate nuclear and cytoplasmic division during binary fission.

Intracytoplasmic inclusions

Many species of bacteria produce cytoplasmic inclusion bodies which appear as round granules. They are not permanent or essential structures and may be absent under certain conditions of growth. They are large polymeric complexes consisting of volutin (polyphosphates), lipid, glycogen, starch or sulphur. Generally they are present in larger number when bacteria have access to an abundance of energy-yielding nutrients and diminish or disappear under conditions of energy source starvation.

Bacterial nucleus

The genetic information of a bacterial cell is contained in a single, circular, double-stranded molecule of DNA. It is often accompanied by a smaller extrachromosomal DNA known as **plasmid**. It is 1000 μm or more in length, about 1000 times the length of the cell. Therefore, it occurs tightly coiled like a skein of woollen thread. Since it is not bound to proteins, therefore, it does not stain like a eukaryotic chromosome. Bacterial nucleus does not possess nuclear membrane, nucleolus, deoxyribonucleoprotein and does not divide by mitosis.

Capsule and slime layer

Cell wall in many bacteria is enclosed by a protective gelatinous covering layer. If it is easily washed off and does not appear to be associated with the cell in any definite fashion it is referred to as a **slime layer**, on the other hand if it appears as discrete, thickened gel around each cell, it is called a **capsule** (Fig. 2.6). If capsule is too thin to be seen with light microscope, it is called **microcapsule.** In most species it is made up of a complex polysaccharide (e.g., pneumo-

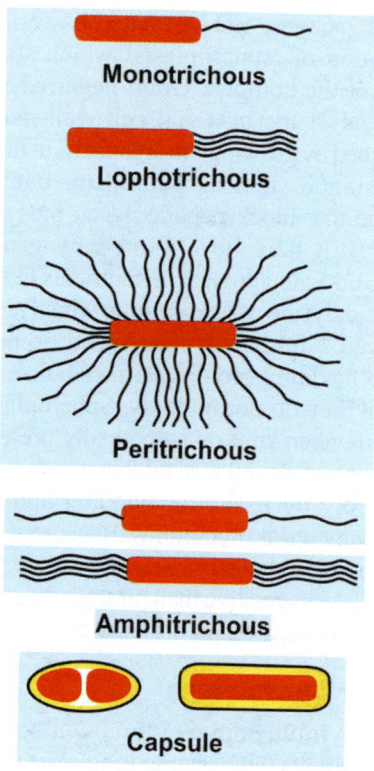

Fig. 2.6. Arrangement of flagella and capsule.

coccus), though in some species its main constituent is polypeptide (e.g., anthrax bacillus). When slime-forming bacteria are grown on a solid culture medium, the slime remains around the bacteria as a matrix in which they are embedded and its presence confers on growth a mucoid character. Slime is freely soluble in water and when the bacteria are grown or suspended in a liquid medium, it passes away from them and disperses through the medium.

Demonstration of capsule

Capsule cannot be stained with ordinary stains like Gram staining.

- It can be visualized by suspending the organisms in India ink and observing microscopically the exclusion of the colloidal ink particles from the area around the cell that is occupied by the capsule.
- It may also be visualized by reaction with specific antibody which causes a characteristic swelling of the capsule. It is known as **Quellung reaction**.

Functions

- Capsules protect the bacteria from antibacterial agents such as lytic enzymes found in nature.
- They inhibit phagocytosis thus contributing to the virulence of the bacteria.

   Loss of capsule by mutation may render the bacterium avirulent. Bacteria tend to lose capsules on repeated subcultures *in vitro*.

Flagella

A large number of bacteria including a few coccal forms, about one half of bacilli and almost all of the spirilla and vibrios are motile by means of flagella. Flagella are long, hollow, helical filaments usually several times the length of the cell. They are 10–20 nm in diameter, 3–20 μm in length and are found on both Gram-positive and Gram-negative bacteria.

Arrangement

There are four types of arrangement of flagella (Fig. 2.6).

1. **Monotrichous:** These organisms have a single polar flagellum.
2. **Lophotrichous:** They have a tuft of flagella at one pole.

3. **Amphitrichous:** They have single polar flagella or tuft of flagella at both poles.
4. **Peritrichous:** Flagella are distributed all round the cell.

   The motility in spirochaetes is due to one or more pairs of **axial filaments** which run between outer membrane and peptidoglycan layer of the cell wall, and are anchored by knobs at both poles.

   Flagella consist mainly of a protein called flagellin which belongs to the same chemical group as myosin – the contractile protein of muscle. Though flagella of different genera of bacteria have the same chemical composition, they are antigenically different. Flagellar antigens induce specific anti-bodies in high titres. These antibodies are not protective but are useful in serodiagnosis.

Demonstration

- Flagella can be demonstrated by ordinary light microscope by special staining techniques in which their thickness is increased by mordanting.
- In some instances, they can be seen with dark ground microscopy.
- However, they can be easily visualized under electron microscope.
- In routine, their presence is inferred by the motility of the bacteria. The latter may be observed either microscopically or by the occurrence of spreading growth in semisolid agar medium.

Structure of flagellum

The flagellum consists of three parts – the **filament**, the **hook** and the **basal body**. The basal body, anchored in the cytoplasmic membrane, comprises a rod and two or more sets of encircling rings. In Gram-negative bacteria four types of rings (M, S, P and L) are seen. Through ring M it attaches to the cytoplasmic membrane, ring S is located just above cytoplasmic membrane and through rings P and L it is attached to peptidoglycan and outer lipopoly-saccharide membrane respectively (Fig. 2.7). Rings P and L are absent in Gram-positive bacteria.

Fimbriae or pili

They are hair-like microfibrils 1–1.5 μm in length and 4–8 nm in diameter. They are straighter, thinner

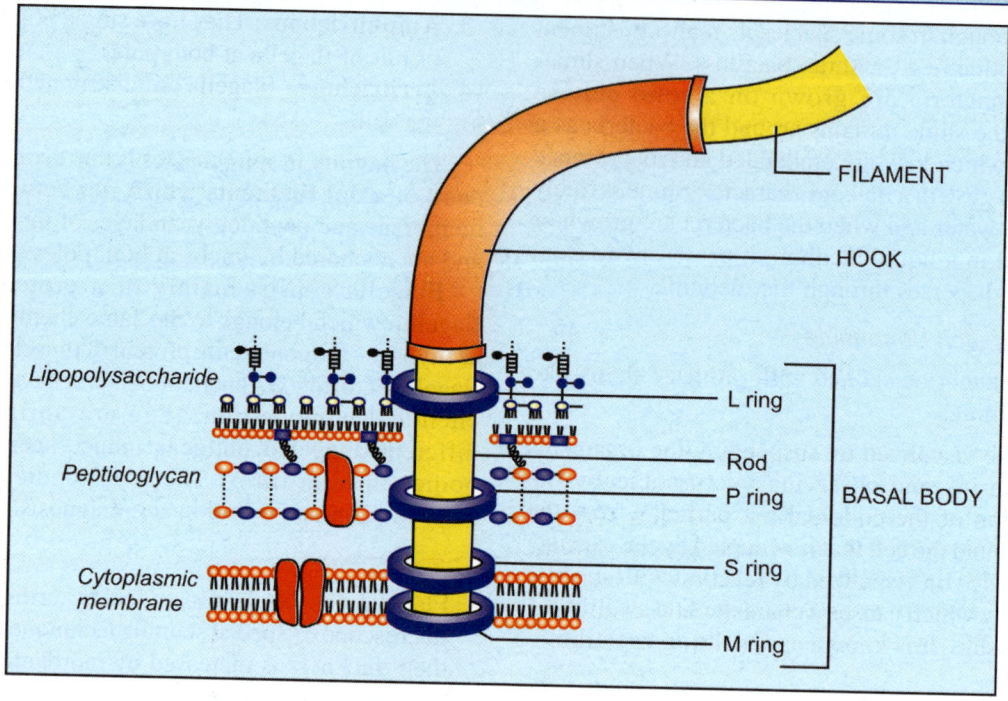

Fig. 2.7. Structure of flagellum.

and shorter than flagella (Fig. 2.2). They are present on many Gram-negative cells and provide a means for adherence to other cells, either bacterial or animal. They are an example of a class of surface structures termed **adhesins** that allow attachment of bacterial cell to cell surfaces (organelles of adhesion). Therefore, they are very important for bacterial survival in an animal host. They occur in both flagellated and non-flagellated bacteria and are far more numerous than flagella. Each bacterium possesses 100–200 peritrichously-borne fimbriae. They can be seen by electron microscopy. They originate in the cytoplasmic membrane and are composed of self-aggregating protein monomers.

In stagnant liquid medium the fimbriate bacteria grow attached together in the form of a pellicle that floats on the surface of the medium where the growth is greatly enhanced by the free supply of oxygen.

Certain bacteria possess specialized fimbriae or pili which are longer and thinner than the common type. These appear to be hollow and constitute conjugation tubes through which DNA is transferred from one organism to another during conjugation.

They are determined by sex factors and are referred to as **sex pili**.

Bacterial spore

Some species of bacteria (Gram-positive only), particularly those of the genera *Bacillus* and *Clostridium*, are capable of forming endospores inside the original cell. These endospores can be released from the original cell as free **spores**. Each bacterium forms one spore which on germination forms a single vegetative cell. Sporulation in bacteria, therefore, is a method of preservation and not of reproduction.

Spores are small, highly resistant, metabolically dormant structures which develop as a response to starvation. They are not formed as long as conditions continue to favour maximal vegetative growth. Formation of spore occurs over a period of 4–8 hours after the cells stop growing upon depletion of their carbohydrate supply.

Sporulation

It develops from a portion of protoplasm near one end of the cell. This part of the bacterial cell is known

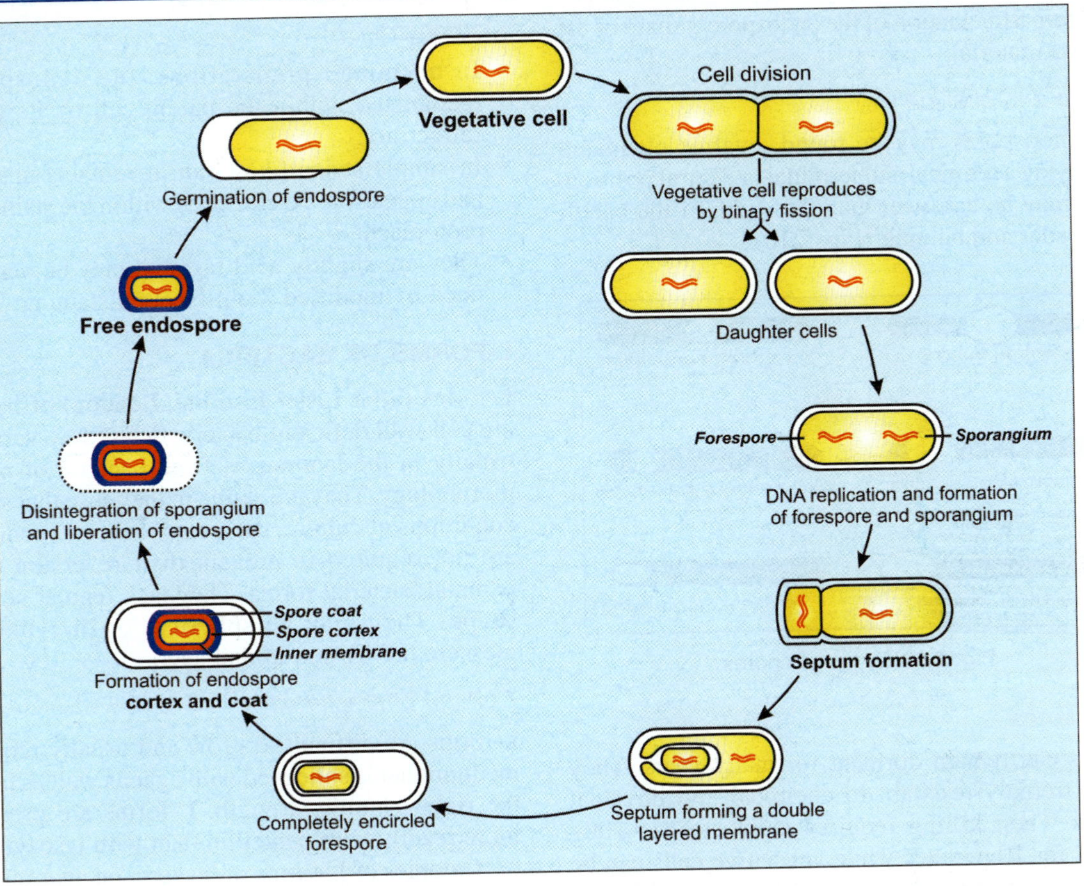

Fig. 2.8. Morphological events in sporulation.

Figure labels (clockwise from top):

Cell division

Vegetative cell

Vegetative cell reproduces by binary fission

Daughter cells

Forespore — Sporangium

DNA replication and formation of forespore and sporangium

Septum formation

Septum forming a double layered membrane

Completely encircled forespore

Formation of endospore cortex and coat — Spore coat, Spore cortex, Inner membrane

Disintegration of sporangium and liberation of endospore

Free endospore

Germination of endospore

as **forespore** and the remaining part as **sporangium** (Fig. 2.8). Bacterial DNA replicates and partitions into two halves and one of them, which is equivalent to one genome of the cell, is incorporated into fore-spore. A transverse septum derived from the cyto-plasmic membrane is then formed by a process of invagination which divides forespore and sporan-gium. The forespore is subsequently completely encircled by dividing septum as a double layered membrane.

The two spore membranes now engage in active synthesis of various layers of the spore. The inner layer becomes the **inner membrane**. Between the two layers is laid **spore cortex** and outer layer is transformed into **spore coat** which consists of several layers. In some species from outer layer also develops **exosporium** which bears ridges and folds (Fig. 2.9).

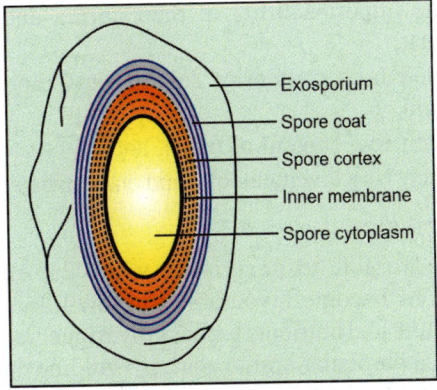

Fig. 2.9. Bacterial spore.

Figure labels: Exosporium, Spore coat, Spore cortex, Inner membrane, Spore cytoplasm

Finally exosporium disintegrates, releasing free spore. Mesosomes appear to play a role in the development of endospore and may be involved in the compartmentation of the endospore's share of the nuclear material.

Shape and position

The endospores may be round, oval or elongated occupying a terminal, subterminal or central position. They may be narrower than the width of the bacilli or broader and bulging (Fig. 2.10).

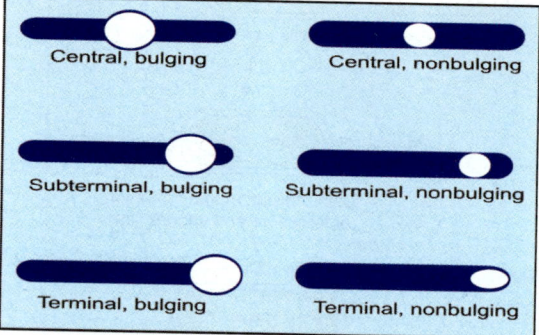

Central, bulging	Central, nonbulging
Subterminal, bulging	Subterminal, nonbulging
Terminal, bulging	Terminal, nonbulging

Fig. 2.10. Types of spores.

Resistance

Spores can remain dormant for many years. They are extremely resistant to chemical and physical agents. Their killing requires moist heat at 100–120°C for 10 minutes while vegetative cells can be killed by heating at 60°C for 10 minutes. Marked resistance of the spores is due to:

- the impermeability of their cortex and outer coat,
- their high content of calcium and dipicolinic acid,
- their low content of water, and
- their very low metabolic and enzymatic activity.

Germination

Spores are able to **germinate** when the external conditions become favourable to growth by access to moisture and nutrients particularly trigger nutrients such as a particular amino acid, pyrimidine or sugar in a suitable aqueous environment. Within a short period of time spore loses its heat resistance, refractility, dipicolinic acid and calcium. It then swells and absorbs water, after which the spore coat ruptures, and a new vegetative cell grows out.

Demonstration

- In unstained preparations, the endospore is recognized within the parent cell by its greater refractility.
- In simple stains like Gram it remains unstained and appears as a clear space within the stained cell protoplasm.
- They are slightly acid-fast and may be demonstrated by modified Ziehl-Neelsen staining.

L-FORMS OF BACTERIA

L-forms (after Lister Institute, London) of bacteria are cell wall deficient bacteria derived by variation, usually in the laboratory, from bacteria of normal morphology. They are stable in the sense that special conditions of culture, such as presence of penicillin, are not required to prevent their reversion to the parental bacterial forms. They lack regular size and shape. They may be spherical or disc-like and measure 0.1–20 µm in diameter.

Cultural characteristics

L-forms are difficult to grow and usually require a medium that is solidified with agar as well as having the right osmotic strength. L-forms are produced more readily with penicillin than with lysozyme.

Colonies of L-forms of bacteria on agar medium show a characteristic '**fried-egg**' appearance with a dark thick centre, where many of the organisms embed themselves and grow within the agar, and a lighter periphery consisting of organisms lying on the surface of the agar. In liquid medium they grow in the form of clumps. Some L-forms are capable of reverting to normal bacillary forms upon removal of the inducing stimulus. Other L-forms are, however, stable and never revert. Presence of residual peptidoglycan is essential for reversion. It acts as a primer in its own biosynthesis.

KEY FACTS

- All living cells are either *prokaryotes* or *eukaryotes*
- Prokaryotes such as *bacteria are simple cells* with no internal membranes or organelles
- *Eukaryotes have a nucleus and organelles* such as mitochondria, and complex *internal membranes* (e.g., fungi, human cells)

- *Structures external* to cell wall of bacteria are *flagella, pili* or fimbriae, *capsule* and *slime layer*
- Flagella are used for movement, pili for adhesion, and capsules protect the bacteria from antibacterial agents such as lytic enzymes and inhibit phagocytosis thus contributing to the virulence of bacteria
- *Peptidoglycan is present in the cell wall of both Gram-positive and Gram-negative bacteria*, but it is thicker in the former and gives rigidity and shape to the organism
- Peptidoglycan comprises long chains of N-acetyl-glucosamine and N-acetylmuramic acid; a set of identical tetrapeptide side chains attached to N-acetylmuramic acid and a set of identical penta-peptide cross-bridges
- Lipopolysaccharide (LPS) is the outermost layer of outer membrane of Gram-negative (but not Gram-positive) bacteria; LPS is endotoxin and, therefore, Gram-positive bacteria do not produce endotoxin
- *Bacterial cytoplasm contains* chromosomal nuclear material, ribosomes, mesosomes and inclusions/storage granules
- *Sporulation* is a response to starvation in *Bacillus* spp. and *Clostridium* spp.

IMPORTANT QUESTIONS

1. Differentiate in a tabulated form between:
   (a) Prokaryotes and eukaryotes
   (b) Bacterial flagella and fimbria
2. Write short notes on:
   (a) Bacterial capsule
   (b) Bacterial cell wall
   (c) Bacterial spore
   (d) Bacterial flagella
   (e) Bacterial fimbria
   (f) Bacterial nucleus

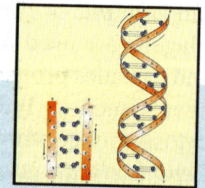

Chapter 3

Culture Media and Culture Techniques

Bacteria reproduce by a process called binary fission, in which a parent cell divides to form a progeny of two cells. This results in a logarithmic growth rate – one bacterium will produce 16 bacteria after four generations.

Generation time

The time required for a bacterium to give rise to two daughter cells is known as generation time. In *Escherichia coli* it is 20 minutes, in tubercle bacilli it is 20 hours and in lepra bacilli it is 20 days.

Batch culture and continuous culture

When bacteria are grown in liquid medium, multiplication is arrested after a few cell divisions due to depletion of nutrients and/or accumulation of toxic products. This is known as batch culture. By use of special devices like chemostat or turbidistat in which nutrients are replaced and bacteria are removed continuously it is possible to maintain continuous culture of bacteria for industrial and research purposes.

When pathogenic bacteria multiply in the host tissues the situation is intermediate between batch culture and continuous culture because they get inexhaustible source of nutrients but they have to face host defence mechanisms.

In liquid media, growth of bacteria is diffuse and on solid media they form colonies. Each colony consists of a clone of cells derived from a single parent cell. Bacteria in a culture medium or clinical specimen can be counted by two methods:

1. Total count

This is total number of bacteria present in a specimen irrespective of whether they are living or dead. This is done by counting the bacteria under microscope using counting chamber and by comparing the growth with standard opacity tubes.

2. Viable count

This measures only viable (living) cells which are capable of growing and producing colonies on a suitable medium.

BACTERIAL GROWTH CURVE

When a bacterium is inoculated into a suitable culture medium and incubated, its growth follows a characteristic course. If both total and viable counts are made at different intervals and plotted in relation to time, then a characteristic growth curve is obtained. A typical growth curve contains four major phases (Fig. 3.1).

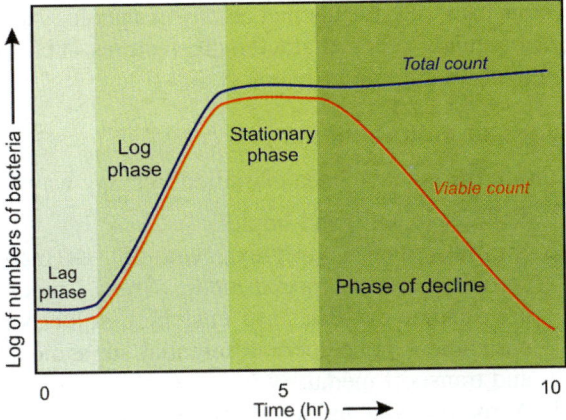

Fig. 3.1. Bacterial growth curves.

Lag phase

When bacteria are seeded into fresh medium, multiplication usually does not begin immediately. The period between inoculation and beginning of multiplication is known as lag phase. During this period the organisms adapt themselves to growth in fresh medium and increase in size and metabolic activity. Therefore, *lag phase is regarded as a period not of rest but of intense metabolic activity*. The duration of lag phase varies with the species, nature of culture medium, temperature of incubation, etc. It is generally shorter in a nutrient-rich than in a minimal medium.

Log or exponential growth phase

During this phase the bacteria are multiplying at their maximum rate and their number increases exponentially or by geometric progression with time. If logarithm of bacterial count is plotted against time a straight line is obtained. In the log phase, the bacterial cells are small and uniformly stained. Exponential phase is of limited duration because of:
- exhaustion of nutrients,
- accumulation of toxic metabolic end products,
- rise in cell density,
- change in pH, and
- decrease in oxygen tension (in case of aerobic organisms).

Stationary phase

Due to above reasons exponential growth slows down and the bacterial population enters the stationary phase in which the number of viable cells remains constant. There is almost a balance between the bacterial reproduction and bacterial death. During this phase, bacteria become Gram-variable, show irregular staining and spores start forming in spore-forming bacteria.

Phase of decline

Stationary phase is followed eventually by the phase of decline because rate of death exceeds the rate of reproduction and the number of viable cells declines. Finally, after a variable period, all the cells die and culture becomes sterile.

CULTURE MEDIA

Numerous culture media have been devised. The original media used by Louis Pasteur were liquids such as urine or meat broth. Liquid media have many disadvantages. Bacteria growing in these media may not exhibit specific characteristics for their identification. With liquid media it is difficult to isolate different types of bacteria from mixed populations. However, liquid media are used for obtaining bacterial growth from blood or water when large volumes have to be used as inoculum, for preparing bulk cultures for antigens and vaccines, and for preparation of inoculum for biochemical reactions and antibiotic susceptibility testing.

In 1881, Robert Koch described means of cultivating bacteria on solid media. First he used as his growth medium pieces of potato, then 2.5–5.0% gelatin to prepare solid media fortifying them with 1% meat extract as an essential ingredient. But gelatin is not satisfactory as it liquefies at 24°C (incubation temperature for most pathogenic bacteria is 37°C) and also by many proteolytic bacteria. At the suggestion of Anglina Hesse, the American wife of his assistant, he substituted agar-agar in place of gelatin as solidifying agent for the media. She had used it to solidify broths in her kitchen.

Agar-agar or '**agar**' for short is prepared from a variety of seaweeds. It does not add to the nutritive properties of medium and is not affected by the growth of bacteria. The exact concentration to be used may require some adjustment according to the batch of agar. A concentration of 1–2% usually yields a suitable gel. In preparing agar media, the appropriate amount of agar powder is added to the liquid medium and dissolved by placing the mixture in a steamer at 100°C for 1 hour or longer. Most agars dissolve to give a clear solution but sometimes it is necessary to filter off particulate impurities.

The melting and solidifying points of agar solutions are not the same. At the concentrations normally used, most bacteriological agars melt at about 95°C and solidify only when cooled to about 42°C. Agar can be added to any nutrient liquid medium if the advantages of a solid medium are desired. Most of the culture media are sterilized by autoclaving at 121°C for 15 minutes. Nutrients that are damaged by autoclaving are sterilized separately by filtration, etc. The sterilized agar base is then melted in the steamer and cooled to about 45–50°C followed by addition of heat-labile ingredients, but once these are added the medium must at once be poured into petri dishes because it cannot be remelted without damaging the heat-sensitive ingredients.

If heated at a low pH, agar is hydrolysed to products that do not solidify on cooling. Agar usually does not alter the pH of the medium to which it is added but if it contains free acid this must be neutralized before it is autoclaved.

Another important ingredient of common media is **peptone**. It consists of water-soluble products obtained from lean meat or other protein material such as heart muscle, casein, fibrin or soya flour, usually by digestion with the proteolytic enzymes pepsin, trypsin or papain. Its constituents are peptones, proteoses, amino acids, a variety of inorganic salts including phosphates, potassium and magnesium, and certain accessory growth factors such as nicotinic acid and riboflavin. Special brands of peptone such as neopeptone and proteose peptone are available for special use.

Other common ingredients of the culture media include casein hydrolysate, meat extract, yeast extract, malt extract, blood and serum.

While bacteria grow diffusely in liquid media, they produce discrete visible growth on solid media in petri dishes. If a mixed culture is inoculated in suitable dilution on solid medium, different bacteria form well-separated colonies, which are clones of cells originating from a single bacterial cell. On solid media, bacteria have distinct colony morphology and exhibit many other characteristic features such as pigment production or haemolysis.

Types of culture media

Culture media have been classified in many ways:

1. Solid, semisolid and liquid.
2. Simple (basal), complex, synthetic, defined, semidefined and special media. Special media are further divided into enriched, selective, enrichment, indicator or differential, sugar media and transport media.
3. Aerobic media and anaerobic media.

Basal media

These include peptone water and nutrient broths which form the basis of most media used in the study of the common pathogenic bacteria. There are three types of nutrient broth:

1. **Meat infusion broth** consisting of a watery extract of lean meat to which peptone is added.
2. **Meat extract broth** prepared as a mixture of commercial peptone and meat extract.
3. **Digest broth** consisting of a watery extract of lean meat that has been digested with a proteolytic enzyme so that additional peptone need not be added.

Meat extract broth is most commonly used. It can be made solid by addition of 1–2% agar. If the concentration of agar is reduced to 0.2–0.5%, it is called **semisolid agar**. If its concentration is raised to 6%, it is called **hard agar**. In semisolid agar the motile organisms show growth in entire medium, and on surface of hard agar swarming of *Proteus* is inhibited.

Enriched media

These are prepared to meet the nutritional requirements of fastidious organisms by addition of substances such as blood, serum and egg to a basal medium. Important examples of enriched media are blood agar for isolation of *Streptococcus*, chocolate agar for isolation of *Neisseria* and Loeffler's serum slope for the isolation of *Corynebacterium diphtheriae*.

Selective media

When a substance is added to a solid medium which inhibits the growth of unwanted bacteria but permits the growth of wanted bacteria in the form of colonies it is known as selective medium. Important examples of this type of media are Lowenstein-Jensen medium for isolation of *Mycobacterium tuberculosis* and blood tellurite agar medium for isolation of *C. diphtheriae*.

Enrichment media

When a substance is added to a liquid medium which inhibits the growth of unwanted bacteria and favours the growth of wanted bacteria it is known as enrichment medium. Important examples of this type of media are tetrathionate and selenite broth for *Salmonella* and *Shigella*, and alkaline peptone water for *Vibrio cholerae*.

Indicator media or differential media

When a substance is added into a medium which would produce a visible change in the medium following the growth of a particular organism, it is designated as indicator or differential medium. For example, MacConkey medium contains lactose and neutral red. Lactose-fermenting organisms after growth on this medium produce acid and in acidic pH neutral red becomes red in colour. Thus *Escherichia coli* which is lactose fermenter produces red or pink colonies on this medium.

Transport media

When the clinical sample is being transported from the hospital to the laboratory, delicate organisms like *Neisseria gonorrhoeae* may not survive or the normal flora (*E. coli*) may overgrow pathogenic flora. To avoid this, media have been devised to maintain the viability of the pathogen. Transport media maintain the viability of microorganisms present in a specimen without supporting the growth of any organism. These maintain the organisms in a state of suspended animation so that no organism overgrows another or dies out. These media typically contain only buffers and salts. They lack carbon, nitrogen and organic growth factors; hence do not facilitate microbial multiplication. Stuart's transport medium and Amies transport medium are examples of transport media.

Storage media

Bacteria are best preserved and stored by lyophilization. But for preservation and storage for a few months or so, they can be stab inoculated on semi-solid agar or on Dorset egg medium followed by incubation. When growth appears they can be stored in refrigerator.

Defined synthetic media

These media are prepared from pure chemical substances, therefore, their exact composition is known. These are used for research purposes.

Sugar media

For the identification of most of the organisms, sugar fermentation reactions are carried out. The term sugar denotes any fermentable substance such as:

- Monosaccharides like pentoses (arabinose and xylose) and hexoses (dextrose and mannose).
- Disaccharides like saccharose and lactose.
- Polysaccharides like starch and inulin.
- Trisaccharides like raffinose.
- Alcohols like glycerol and sorbitol.
- Glucosides like salicin and aesculin.
- Noncarbohydrate substances like inositol.

For the preparation of sugar media, 1% of the concerned sugar is added to peptone water with a suitable indicator. Durham's tube (a small tube) is kept inverted in the tube containing this medium to detect gas production. For fastidious organisms like *C. diphtheriae* and pneumococci, Hiss's serum sugar is used.

Anaerobic media

For the growth of anaerobes, the media used contain reducing substances. These include thioglycollate broth and cooked meat broth. Sterile muscle tissue, in cooked meat broth, contains reducing substances, particularly glutathione, which permit the growth of many strict anaerobes. In addition to its reducing effect, the meat provides a variety of nutritional substances for bacterial growth.

AEROBIC CULTURE

For cultivation of aerobes the incubation is done in an incubator under normal atmospheric condition.

The temperature of incubation for most of the human pathogenic bacteria is 37°C. For cultivation of many fungi incubation of the inoculated media should be carried out at 26–28°C. To prevent drying of the medium when prolonged incubation is necessary, as in the cultivation of the tubercle bacilli, screw-capped bottles should be used instead of test tubes or plates.

CULTURE IN AN ATMOSPHERE WITH ADDED CARBON DIOXIDE

Some organisms such as capnophilic streptococci, require extra CO_2 in the air in which they are grown and others, such as the pneumococcus and gono-coccus grow better in air supplemented with 5–10% CO_2. For this CO_2 jars are used. The required amount of air is withdrawn with a vacuum pump and replaced with CO_2 from a cylinder. CO_2 incubators which provide a predetermined and regulated amount of CO_2 in a suitably humid atmosphere are commercially available. Screw caps on containers of liquid media must not be tight and should preferably be replaced by a closure that allows entry of CO_2.

CULTURE IN MICROAEROPHILIC ATMOSPHERE

Microorganisms like *Actinomyces israelii* are microaerophilic. Culture of such organisms is done by an evacuation replacement method with 5% O_2, 10% CO_2 and 85% N_2.

ANAEROBIC CULTURE

A variety of methods are available for the culture of anaerobic organisms in the clinical laboratory. Exclusion of oxygen from the medium is the simplest method, and is effected by growing the organisms within the culture medium such as freshly steamed liquid media and deep nutrient agar with 0.5% glucose and minimal shaking and solidified rapidly by placing the tube in cold water.

Liquid media soon become aerobic unless a reducing agent such as glucose 0.5–1.0%, ascorbic acid 0.1%, cysteine 0.1%, sodium thioglycollate 0.1%, or particles of meat in cooked meat broth are added. Liquid media should be prereduced by holding in a boiling water bath for 10 minutes to drive off dissolved oxygen, then quickly cooled to 37°C just before use.

Cooked meat broth, CMB (original medium known as 'Robertson's bullock-heart medium') has a special place in anaerobic bacteriology; and thioglycollate broth and its modifications are also very useful. CMB is suitable for growing anaerobes in air and also for the preservation of stock cultures of aerobic organisms. The inoculum is introduced deep in the medium in contact with the meat. Meat particles are placed in 30 ml bottles to a depth of about 2.5 cm and covered with about 15 ml broth.

Anaerobes have special nutritional requirements for vitamin K, haemin and yeast extract, and all primary isolation media for anaerobes should contain these three ingredients.

Anaerobic Jars

When an oxygen-free or anaerobic atmosphere is required for obtaining surface growths of anaerobes, anaerobic jars provide the method of choice. The most reliable and widely used anaerobic jar is the **McIntosh-Fildes' anaerobic jar**. It is a cylindrical vessel made of glass or metal with a metal lid which is held firmly in place by a clamp (Fig. 3.2). The lid has two tubes with taps, one acting as gas inlet and the other as the outlet. On its undersurface it carries a gauze sachet carrying alumina pellets coated with palladium. It acts as a room temperature catalyst for

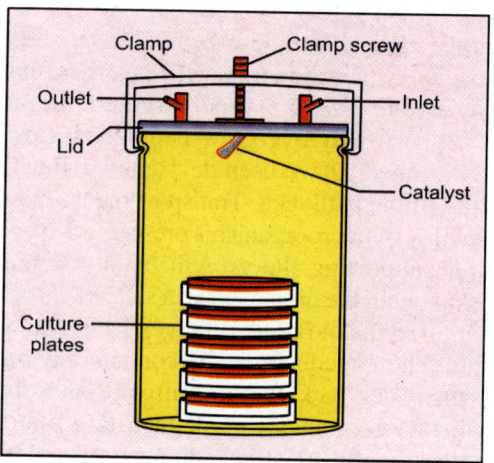

Fig. 3.2. Anaerobic jar.

the conversion of hydrogen and oxygen into water. It acts as a catalyst, as long as the sachet is kept dry.

Inoculated culture plates are placed inside the jar and the lid clamped tight. The outlet tube is connected to a vacuum pump and the air inside is evacuated. The outlet tap is then closed and the inlet tube connected to a hydrogen supply. Hydrogen is drawn in rapidly. As soon as this inrush of gas has ceased the inlet tap is also closed. After about 5 minutes inlet tap is again opened. There occurs again an immediate inrush of hydrogen since the catalyst creates a reduced pressure within the jar due to the conversion of hydrogen and leftover oxygen into water. If there is no inrush of hydrogen, it means the catalyst is inactive and must be replaced. The jar is left connected to the hydrogen supply for about 5 minutes, then the inlet tap is closed and the jar is placed in the incubator, catalysis will continue until all the oxygen in the jar has been used up.

The **GasPak** is now the method of choice for preparing anaerobic jar. The GasPak is commercially available as a disposable envelope containing chemicals which generate hydrogen and carbon dioxide on the addition of water. After the inoculated plates are kept in the jar, the GasPak envelope with water added, is placed inside and the lid screwed tight. Hydrogen and carbon dioxide are liberated and the presence of a cold catalyst in the envelope permits the combination of hydrogen and oxygen to produce an anaerobic environment. The outstanding feature of the GasPak system is the disposable gas generator envelope, which does away with the need for a vacuum pump and cylinders of compressed gas; the operation of the jar is consequently very quick and simple. As the standard GasPak jar is not evacuated before use a relatively large volume of water is formed during catalysis.

An **indicator** should be used for verifying the anaerobic condition in the jar. Methylene blue is generally used for this purpose. When it is placed in an anaerobic environment it is reduced from its coloured oxidized form to a colourless reduced leuco-compound.

In addition to, or instead of, using a chemical indicator, some workers include in the jar a plate inoculated with a known strict anaerobe such as

Clostridium tetani or *Bacteroides fragilis*, and a strict aerobe, such as *Pseudomonas aeruginosa*. This method is quite reliable if the indicator anaerobe grows and the aerobe does not.

The major disadvantage of any anaerobic jar system is that the plates have to be removed from the jar to be examined. This, of course, exposes the colonies to oxygen, which is especially hazardous to the anaerobes during their first 48 hours of growth. For this reason, a suitable holding system should always be used in conjunction with anaerobic jars, placed in an oxygen-free holding system, removed one by one for rapid microscopic examination of colonies, and then quickly returned to the holding system. Plates should never remain in room air on the open bench.

Anaerobic chamber

This is an ideal anaerobic incubation system, which provides oxygen-free environment for inoculating media and incubating cultures. Identification and susceptibility tests can also be performed in anaerobic chambers.

Anaerobic chambers may be fitted with airtight rubber gloves to insert hands and manipulate specimens, plates, tubes or they may be gloveless where airtight rubber sleeves fit tightly against user's bare forearms. All anaerobic chambers contain a catalyst, dessicant, H_2 gas (5–10%), CO_2 gas (5–10%), N_2 gas (80–90%) and an indicator.

Anaerobic bags or pouches

These bags are available commercially and one or two inoculated plates are placed into a bag and an oxygen removal system is activated and the bag is sealed and incubated. Plates can be examined for growth without removing the plates from bag, thus without exposing the colonies to oxygen. But as with anaerobic jar, plates must be removed from the bags in order to work with the colonies at the bench. These bags are also useful in transport of biopsy specimen for anaerobic cultures.

INCUBATION

Inoculated plates should be incubated at 37°C for at least 48 hours, and reincubated for another 2–4 days to allow slow-growing organisms (certain species of *Actinomyces*) to form colonies. If clostridial myonecrosis is suspected clinically, plates can be inspected as early as 6–12 hours after inoculation. In such emergency situations, duplicate sets of plating media can be incubated in two different jars, one set incubated for 18–24 hours and the other for 3–5 days for slow growers.

CARBON DIOXIDE

Some organisms such as pneumococci and gonococci grow better in air supplemented with 5–10% CO_2.

TEMPERATURE

Each bacterium multiplies best within a restricted temperature range. For most of the pathogenic bacteria optimum temperature for growth is 37°C (our body temperature) with upper and lower temperature limits of 40–50°C and 15–20°C respectively. The organisms with optimum temperatures of 37°C, less than 20°C and 55–80°C are known as mesophiles, psychrophiles and thermophiles respectively.

MOISTURE AND DESICCATION

Moisture is very essential for the growth of bacteria because 80% of their body weight is made up of water. However, the effect of drying varies in different organisms. For example *Treponema pallidum*, gonococci and human immunodeficiency virus die quickly after drying while tubercle bacilli and staphylococci may survive drying for several weeks. However, bacterial spores can survive for several years and drying in cold and vacuum (lyophilization) is a method for preservation of bacteria and viruses.

pH

Like other living organisms, microorganisms are very susceptible to changes in the acidity or alkalinity of the surrounding medium. Most of the medically important bacteria can grow at neutral or slightly alkaline pH (7.2 – 7.6). Some bacteria like lactobacilli and cholera vibrio grow at acidic and alkaline pH respectively.

LIGHT AND OTHER RADIATIONS

Darkness provides a favourable condition for growth and viability of bacteria. Ultraviolet rays from direct sunlight or a mercury lamp are bactericidal. Bacteria are also killed by ionizing radiations. Photochromogenic mycobacteria form pigment only on exposure to light.

OSMOTIC EFFECT

Because of the mechanical strength of the cell wall, bacteria are more tolerant to osmotic variation, therefore, they can grow in media with widely varying contents of salt, sugar and other solutes. Sudden exposure of bacteria to solutions of high salt concentration may cause **plasmolysis**. This is due to osmotic withdrawal of water leading to shrinkage of protoplast and its retraction from the cell wall. This occurs more readily in Gram-negative than Gram-positive bacteria. On the other hand, sudden transfer of bacteria from concentrated solution to distilled water may cause **plasmoptysis** due to excessive osmotic imbibition of water leading to swelling and bursting of cell.

MECHANICAL AND SONIC STRESSES

In spite of the mechanical strength of the cell wall, bacteria can be ruptured and killed by vigorous shaking with glass beads and ultrasonic vibrations.

KEY FACTS

- Bacteria *reproduce* by *binary fission* leading to logarithmic growth of cell numbers; generation time of bacteria varies from minutes to hours or days
- Bacterial *growth* in laboratory media can be divided into a **lag phase**, *log* phase, *stationary* **phase** and *decline* phase
- Depending on their oxygen requirements, bacteria can be divided into *obligate aerobes, facultative anaerobes, obligate anaerobes* and *micro-aerophiles*
- For *cultivation* and *identification* of bacteria, basal media, enriched media, selective media, enrichment media, differential media, etc. are used

- Depending upon the expected organisms, the inoculated media are incubated in *aerobic culture, culture in an atmosphere with added carbon dioxide, culture in microaerophilic atmosphere* and *anaerobic culture*

IMPORTANT QUESTIONS

1. Describe:
   (a) Bacterial growth curve
   (b) Anaerobic culture methods

2. Write short notes on:
   (a) Selective media
   (b) Enrichment media
   (c) Differential media
   (d) Transport media

Chapter 4

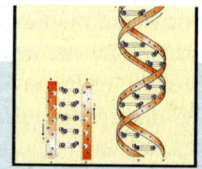

Selection, Collection, Transport and Processing of Clinical Specimens, and Identification of Bacteria

The laboratory diagnosis of an infectious disease begins with the collection of a clinical specimen. Proper collection of an appropriate clinical specimen is the first step in obtaining an accurate laboratory diagnosis of an infectious disease. A poorly collected specimen not only may result in failure to recover important microorganisms, but may also lead to incorrect or even harmful therapy if treatment is directed towards a commensal or contaminant.

The quality of a clinical microbiological report is directly related to the quality of the specimen on which it is based. Care in obtaining a proper specimen and its prompt submission to the laboratory are essential. In general, specimens of frank pus, wound exudate or excised tissue sent in sterile container are preferable to swabs, which are relatively inefficient sampling device.

General rules for collection and transportation of specimen

- Apply strict aseptic techniques throughout the procedure.
- Wash hands before and after the collection.
- Collect the specimen before the administration of antimicrobial agents.
- Prevent contamination of the specimen with externally present organisms or normal flora of the body.

- Collect the specimen at the appropriate phase of disease.
- Collect the specimen from the actual infection site.
- Collect adequate quantity for the desired tests.
- Collect the specimen aseptically in a sterile and appropriate container.
- Close the container tightly so that its contents do not leak during transportation.
- Ensure that the outside of the specimen container is clean and uncontaminated.
- Label the container appropriately and complete the requisition form.
- Immediately transport the specimen to the laboratory.

Criteria for rejection of specimens

- Missing or inadequate identifications.
- Incomplete forms.
- Leaking container or blood stained containers.
- Specimens collected in an inappropriate container.
- Haemolysed blood sample.
- Insufficient quantity.
- Dried up specimen.
- Contamination suspected.
- Specimen collected in formalin.
- Inappropriate transport or storage.

Collection and transportation of specimens

Blood for culture

- Using a pressure cuff, locate a suitable vein in the arm. Deflate the cuff while disinfecting the venepuncture site.
- Wearing sterile gloves thoroughly disinfect the venepuncture site as follows:
  - Using 70% ethanol, cleanse an area about 50 mm in diameter. Allow to air-dry.
  - Using 2% tincture of iodine and a circular action, swab the area beginning at the point where the needle will enter the vein. Allow the iodine to dry on the skin for at least 1 minute.
- Lift the tape or remove the protective cover from the top of culture bottle. Wipe the top of the bottle using an ethanol-ether swab.
- Using a sterile syringe and needle withdraw 5 ml of blood from an adult and 1 ml from a young child.
- Insert the needle through a hole in the cap and through rubber or plastic liner of the bottle cap, and dispense 5 ml of blood from an adult and 1 ml from a young child into the culture medium bottles (Fig. 4.1a) respectively. Cap must not be removed for introduction of the blood. In adults large quantity (5 ml) of blood is required since the number of organisms in the blood particularly in mild and recovering cases may be quite small, even as few as one per ml. As blood's natural bactericidal or bacteriostatic action may interfere with the growth of any bacteria present, this effect is annulled by diluting (inoculating) 5 ml of blood in an adult and 1 ml of blood in a young child in 50 ml and 10 ml of the medium (10-fold dilution) respectively. *Organisms causing bacteraemia in young children are usually present in sufficient concentration to be detected in small volume (1 ml) of blood.*

- Using a fresh ethanol-ether swab wipe the top of the culture bottle and replace the tape or protective cover. Without delay, mix the blood with the broth. Blood must not be allowed to clot in the culture medium because any bacteria will become trapped in the clot.
- Clearly label the bottle with the name and number of the patient, and the date and time of collection.
- As soon as possible, incubate the inoculated medium.
- Collect blood during early stage of disease since the number of bacteria is higher in acute and early stage of disease.
- Collect blood during paroxysm of fever since the number of bacteria is higher at high temperature in patients with fever.
- In the absence of antibiotic administration, 99% culture positivity can be seen with three blood cultures.
- Transport the specimen to the laboratory. If not possible keep in incubator or at room temperature. *Do not refrigerate.*

Blood for serological tests

For serological tests collect about 5 ml of blood to ensure there will be enough serum for all the tests that may be required. Immediately transfer the blood from the syringe into a dry stoppered sterile tube or bottle (without anticoagulant) and allow to clot. When the serum has separated, pipette it off into a sterile tube.

Urine

- Midstream urine sample is collected after giving proper instructions to the patient.

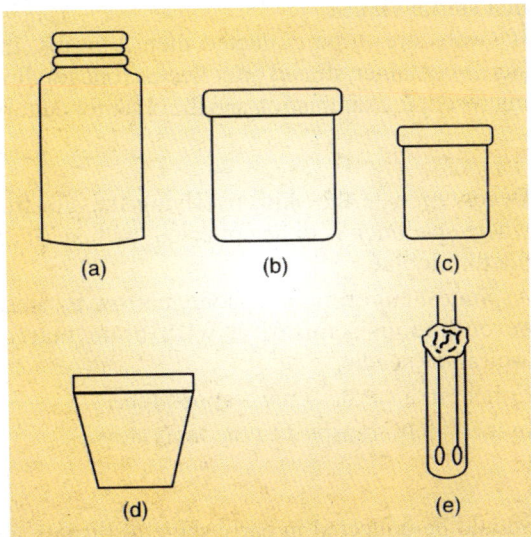

Fig. 4.1. (A) McCartney bottle, (B) Urine/stool container, (C) CSF container, (D) Sputum container, (E) Throat swabs.

(a) Clean the genitalia properly. (In case of male, retract the prepuce, clean it with sterile normal saline. In case of female, wash perineum and periurethral area with soap and water. Separate apart labia with fingers of one hand).

(b) Collect a "clean-catch" midstream urine sample in a sterile container (Fig. 4.1b).

- Transport immediately to the laboratory. If a delay of more than 1–2 hours is unavoidable, refrigerate at 4°C.
- In catheterized patients, do not collect urine from collection bag or after opening the closed drainage. Clean the area over the collecting tubes and puncture with the help of a sterile needle and syringe and draw out the sample.
- Suprapubic aspiration under aseptic condition may be done in infants.

Cerebrospinal fluid (CSF)

Cerebrospinal fluid must be collected by an experienced physician. Rigorous aseptic precautions must be observed to prevent the introduction of infection into the central nervous system. The fluid is usually collected from the arachnoid space.

- A sterile wide-bore needle is inserted between fourth and fifth lumber vertebrae and the CSF is allowed to drip into a sterile dry container (Fig. 4.1c).
- Only 3–5 ml of fluid should be collected, because the removal of a larger volume may lead to headache.
- Immediately deliver the sample with a request form to the laboratory.
- CSF must be examined without delay and the results of the tests reported to the medical officer as soon as they become available. If delay in processing is inevitable then store it at 37° C. *Do not refrigerate.*
- The fluid should be handled with special care because a lumber puncture is required to collect the specimen.

Sputum

- Collect the sputum in a wide-mouthed container, which is preferably disposable, made up of transparent thin plastic, unbreakable and leak-proof (Fig. 4.1d).

- Ask the patient to rinse the mouth with plain water and then inhale deeply 2–3 times, cough up deeply and spit in the sputum container by bringing it close to the mouth. If the patient has difficulty in coughing sputum, postural drainage, and appropriate physiotherapy often cause exudate to move in the bronchi and stimulate productive coughing.
- Make sure the sputum sample is of good quality and not just the saliva. A good sputum sample is thick, purulent and sufficient in amount (2–3 ml).
- Sputum sample may be refrigerated up to 3–4 hours.

Throat swab

- Two swabs should be collected (Fig. 4.1e).
- Depress the tongue with a tongue blade.
- Swab the inflamed area of the throat, pharynx or tonsils with a sterile swab taking care to collect the pus or piece of membrane.
- Take care not to contaminate the swab with saliva.

Pus and other discharge

- Do not apply antiseptic before collection.
- Clean with normal saline.
- In case of discharge, 1–2 ml of sample is collected in a sterile vial.
- If swabs are to be collected then 2 swabs, in a sterile container, should be collected (one for direct microscopic examination and the other for culture).

Bone marrow

- Decontaminate the skin, overlying the site from where specimen is to be collected, with spirit and tincture iodine.
- Aspirate 1 ml or more of bone marrow by sterile percutaneous aspiration with bone marrow aspiration needle.
- Collect in a sterile screw-capped tube.
- Immediately transport to the laboratory.

Stool

- Should be collected in early stage of disease and prior to treatment with antimicrobials.
- Do not collect the specimen from bed pan.
- Should not be contaminated with urine.

- Collect about a spoonful of the specimen, especially that which contains mucus, pus or blood, into a clean, dry, leak-proof container (Fig. 4.1b).
- If possible, submit more than one specimen on different days.
- The fresh stool specimen must be processed within 1–2 hours of passage.
- If delay is unavoidable then store it at 2–8°C.

Rectal swab

- Collect the swab only if stool collection is not possible.
- Insert swab at least 2.5 cm beyond the anal sphincter so that it enters the rectum.
- Rotate it once before withdrawing.
- Transport in Cary-Blair or other transport medium.

IDENTIFICATION OF BACTERIA

Most important duty of a medical microbiologist is isolation and accurate identification of disease causing microorganism from morbid material and its antibiotic susceptibility. Identification of the isolate is carried out by examination of stained and unstained smears of the morbid material, isolation in pure culture on appropriate culture media, study of macroscopic (colonial characters) and microscopic morphology of the isolate and biochemical characters. Finally antibiotic susceptibility of the isolate is carried out and specific chemotherapy initiated.

An unstained wet film or **hanging drop preparation** is examined under light microscope for observation of motility and an unstained wet film may be examined under **dark-ground microscope** for demonstration of motility of spirochaetes. Presence of *Treponema pallidum*, with characteristic spiral shape and motility, in exudate from a chancre is sufficient for presumptive diagnosis of syphilis.

A number of staining techniques for the identification of bacteria are available. Of these, Gram stain and Ziehl-Neelsen are most important. A Gram-stained smear shows the Gram reaction, size, shape and grouping pattern of bacteria, absence or presence of spores, their shape, size and intracellular position. Presence of Gram-negative diplococci inside the polymorphs in cerebrospinal fluid (CSF) and urethral discharge gives the provisional diagnosis

of meningococcal meningitis and gonorrhoea respectively. With Ziehl-Neelsen staining, it is possible to identify tubercle bacilli and atypical mycobacteria, lepra bacilli, and *Nocardia*. They resist decolorization with 20%, 5% and 0.5% sulphuric acid respectively.

Gram stain

The Gram stain is named after Hans Christian Gram, a bacteriologist from Denmark, who developed the technique in 1880s. This staining method is most frequently used in diagnostic bacteriology.

Method

- Heat-fixed smear of specimen or bacterial culture is first stained with one of the basic pararosaniline dyes such as crystal violet, methyl violet, or gentian violet which is a mixture of the two preceding dyes for one minute.
- Pour Gram's iodine over the slide for two minutes.
- Decolorize with alcohol or acetone for 10–30 seconds.
- Counterstain with dilute carbol fuchsin or safranin for 30 seconds.
- Wash thoroughly in water, blot and dry in air.
- Examine under oil-immersion lens.

On the basis of their reaction to the Gram stain, bacteria can be divided into two groups, i.e., Gram-positive and Gram-negative. Both Gram-positive and Gram-negative bacteria take up violet colour with pararosaniline dyes. After treatment with decolorizing agent, Gram-positive bacteria retain this dye and violet colour while Gram-negative lose the dye and become colourless. They then take up counterstain and appear red in colour.

Mechanism of Gram staining

The exact mechanism of Gram reaction is not known. It may, however, be attributed to the following factors:

- Gram-positive bacteria have a more acidic protoplasm, which may account for their retaining the basic primary dye more strongly than Gram-negative bacteria.
- The violet basic dye and the iodine form a dye-iodine complex inside both Gram-positive and

Gram-negative bacteria but during alcohol or acetone wash, cell membranes (outer membrane of cell wall and cytoplasmic membrane) are dissolved. However, dye-iodine complex is retained in Gram-positive cells by the thick peptidoglycan mesh, whereas it is readily washed out through the very thin peptidoglycan layer remaining in Gram-negative cells after both membranes have been dissolved.

- Gram-negative bacteria do not retain the stain, but Gram-positive may fail to do so when overdecolorization is done or the smears are made from old cultures. This appears to be due to the fact that such cultures consist largely of dead, dying or degenerated cells, the physical and chemical properties of which are altered. Some species are Gram-variable because they are extremely sensitive to small changes in the technique.

Albert's stain

- Prepare the film, dry in air and fix by heat.
- Cover slide with Albert's stain and allow to act for 3–5 minutes.
- Wash in water and blot dry.
- Cover the slide with Albert's iodine, allow to act for one minute.
- Wash in water and blot dry.

By this method granules stain bluish-black, the protoplasm green and other organisms mostly light green.

Ziehl-Neelsen stain

Next to Gram stain, this is the method most frequently used in diagnostic bacteriology. It is of value in distinguishing a few bacterial species, e.g., tubercle bacilli, atypical mycobacteria, lepra bacilli and *Nocardia* from all others. Tubercle bacilli, atypical mycobacteria and lepra bacilli are relatively impermeable to simple stains but when stained with hot concentrated carbol fuchsin, subsequently resist decolorization by 20%, 20% and 5% sulphuric acid respectively. Decolorized non-acid-fast organisms are counterstained with methylene blue. *Nocardia* which resists decolorization with 0.5% sulphuric acid, can also be stained with Gram stain and is Gram-positive.

Method

- Cover the slide with filtered carbol fuchsin and heat until steam rises. Allow the preparation to stain for 5 minutes, heat being applied at intervals to keep the stain hot. The stain must not be allowed to evaporate and dry on the slide, if necessary, pour more carbol fuchsin to keep the whole slide covered with carbol fuchsin.
- Wash with water.
- Decolorize the stained smear with 20% sulphuric acid and wash with water. The step is repeated till the film is only very faintly pink.
- Wash the slide well with water.
- Counterstain it with 2% methylene blue for 15–20 seconds.
- Wash, blot, dry and examine smear under oil-immersion lens.

Acid-fast bacilli stain bright red, while the tissue, cells and other organisms are stained blue.

Principle of acid-fastness

Acid-fastness has been attributed to the high content of lipids, fatty acids and higher alcohols found in acid-fast bacteria. Of the lipids, mycolic acid, a high molecular weight hydroxy acid wax containing carboxyl groups, is most important because it is acid-fast even in free state.

Other stains

A number of other staining procedures are available. They include simple stains such as methylene blue or basic fuchsin. They impart same colour to all organisms and are used only for colour contrast. Too thin bacteria may be rendered visible by light microscope by **silver impregnation method** which thickens the bacteria. This method is used for demonstration of spirochaetes and flagella. In case of **negative staining**, bacteria (spirochaetes) or fungi (*Cryptococcus*) are mixed with India ink or nigrosin that provide a uniform coloured background against which the unstained organisms can be seen. Bacterial capsules which do not take simple stains can be seen by negative staining. Special staining techniques for demonstration of spores, flagella, cell walls and capsule of bacteria are also available.

Differential identification characteristics

Accurate identification can be accomplished by isolation of bacteria in pure form followed by study of colonial morphology, examination of stained smear, biochemical reactions, antigenic structure, serotyping, biotyping, bacteriocin typing, phage typing, animal pathogenicity and antibiotic susceptibility determination.

Clinical material is inoculated onto a solid medium (nutrient agar, blood agar or MacConkey agar) in such a way so as to ensure isolated discrete colonies. Enriched, enrichment, selective and differential media, depending upon the organism suspected, are employed. Selective growth conditions, i.e., presence or absence of oxygen and presence of CO_2, etc. are also employed keeping in view the organisms suspected. The culture plates are incubated at optimum temperature. Most of the pathogenic bacteria grow best at 37°C.

Biochemical reactions

A large number of biochemical tests can be employed for the identification of different bacteria. These include:

1. **Indole production:** Certain bacteria which possess enzyme tryptophanase, degrade amino acid tryptophan to indole, pyruvic acid and ammonia. Indole production is detected by inoculating the test organism into peptone water and incubating it at 37°C for 48–96 hours. Then add 0.5 ml of Kovac's reagent and shake gently. A red colour in the alcohol layer indicates a positive reaction. Kovac's reagent consists of:

Paradimethylaminobenzaldehyde	10 g
Amyl or isoamyl alcohol	150 ml
Conc. hydrochloric acid	50 ml

Dissolve aldehyde in alcohol and slowly add the acid and store in refrigerator. Shake gently before use. Indole is extracted from the medium by amyl or isoamyl alcohol and forms **red colour ring** by forming a red coloured complex with paradimethyl-aminobenzaldehyde. Negative test will show yellow coloured ring (colour of Kovac's reagent).

2. **Methyl red (MR) test:** This test detects the production of sufficient acid by fermentation of glucose so that pH of the medium falls and it is maintained below 4.5. Inoculate the test organism in glucose phosphate broth and incubate at 37°C for 2–5 days. Then add five drops of 0.04% solution of methyl red, mix well and read the result immediately. Positive tests are **bright red** and negative are yellow. If the test is negative after 2 days repeat it after 5 days.

3. **Voges-Proskauer (VP) test for acetoin production:** Many bacteria ferment carbohydrates with the production of acetyl methyl carbinol (acetoin). In the presence of potassium hydroxide and atmospheric oxygen, acetoin is converted to diacetyl, and α-naphthol serves as a catalyst to form a pink complex. This test is usually done in conjunction with the methyl red test.

Inoculate test organism in glucose phosphate broth and incubate at 37°C for 48 hours. Then add 1 ml potassium hydroxide and 3 ml of 5% solution of α-naphthol in absolute alcohol. A positive reaction is indicated by the development of **pink colour** in 2–5 minutes and crimson in 30 minutes.

4. **Citrate utilization:** This test is used to study the ability of an organism to utilize citrate as sole source of carbon for the growth. Liquid (Koser's) and solid (Simmon's) media containing citrate as sole source of carbon can be used. A part of colony is picked up by a straight wire and inoculated into either of these media. The ability of an organism to utilize citrate as a sole source of carbon is detected by the **production of turbidity** (due to growth) in liquid medium. Solid medium also contains bromothymol blue as indicator, therefore, on the solid medium the **appearance of growth and blue colour** is positive and original green colour and no growth is negative.

Indole, MR, VP and citrate tests are done in routine for the classification of Gram-negative enteric bacteria. They are commonly referred to as **IMViC tests**.

5. **Sugar fermentation:** The ability of an organism to ferment various sugars is tested by inoculation of the test organism in different sugar media containing Andrade's indicator. A small inverted tube (**Durham's tube**) completely filled with liquid and containing no air bubbles is usually included in each culture tube. Production of acid is

indicated by the change of the colour of the medium to red or pink, and the gas, if produced, collects in Durham's tube.

6. **Nitrate reduction:** This test detects the production of enzyme nitrate reductase which reduces nitrate to nitrite. *All the organisms of the family Enterobacteriaceae are positive for this test.* Inoculate test organism in 5 ml medium containing potassium nitrate, peptone and distilled water. Incubate it at 37°C for 96 hours. Then add 0.1 ml test reagent which consists of equal volumes of sulphanilic acid and α-naphthylamine in 5 N acetic acid mixed just before use. A **red colour** developing within a few minutes indicates the presence of nitrite and hence the ability of test organism to reduce nitrate to nitrite.

7. **Urease test:** This test detects the ability of an organism to produce urease enzyme. The test organism is inoculated on the entire slope of Christensen's medium which contains urea and phenol red indicator in addition to other constituents including agar. It is incubated at 37°C and examined after 4 hours and after overnight incubation. Development of **purple-pink** colour indicates production of urease. The latter in the presence of water converts urea into ammonia and carbon dioxide. Ammonia makes the medium alkaline and phenol red indicator changes to purple-pink in colour.

8. **Hydrogen sulphide production:** Some organisms produce hydrogen sulphide from sulphur-containing amino acids. It may be detected by suspending strips of filter paper impregnated with lead acetate between the cotton plug and the tube. It has variable sensitivity. When cultured in media containing lead acetate or ferric ammonium citrate or ferrous acetate they turn them **black or brown**. This method is more sensitive than lead acetate strip method.

9. **Potassium cyanide test:** This tests the ability of an organism to grow in the presence of potassium cyanide. Inoculate buffered peptone water medium, containing 1 in 13,000 concentration of potassium cyanide, with test organism. Incubate at 37°C for 24–48 hours. Development of **turbidity** in the medium indicates the ability of the organism to grow in the presence of potassium cyanide.

10. **Catalase production:** Put a loopful of 10% hydrogen peroxide on colonies of the test organism on nutrient agar. Alternatively, pick up a few colonies of the test organism with platinum loop from nutrient agar plate and dip it in a drop of 10% hydrogen peroxide on a clean glass slide. The production of **gas bubbles** from the culture indicates a positive reaction. A false positive result may be obtained if the growth is picked up from medium containing catalase, e.g., blood agar or if an iron wire loop is used.

11. **Oxidase test:** This test depends on the presence, in bacteria, of certain oxidases that catalyse the oxidation of reduced tetramethyl-*p*-phenylene-diamine dihydrochloride (oxidase reagent) by molecular oxygen. Put a drop of freshly prepared 1% solution of oxidase reagent on a piece of filter paper. Then rub a few colonies of test organism on it. If it is oxidase-positive, it will produce a **deep purple colour** within 10 seconds. Alternatively, pour oxidase reagent over the colonies of the test organism on the culture plate. The colonies of oxidase-positive organisms rapidly develop a deep purple colour.

Bacteriocin, bacteriophage and serotyping

Each species of an organism contains a number of different strains. These epidemiological markers are useful for intraspecies differentiation of various strains.

Animal pathogenicity

Various experimental models used in diagnostic microbiology laboratory are mouse, rat, guinea pig, rabbit, nine-banded armadillo and monkey. Various routes of inoculation are intradermal, subcutaneous, intramuscular, intraperitoneal, intracerebral and intravenous. Oral and nasal routes can also be used. The identification of the organism is carried out on the basis of clinical and postmortem findings, and cultural characteristics.

KEY FACTS

- Bacteria are divided into two major classes according to staining characteristics – *Gram-positive* (violet) and *Gram-negative* (red)

- Cell walls of some bacteria such as the *mycobacteria* contain lipids (mycolic acids); they are relatively impermeable to simple stains but when treated with hot concentrated carbol fuchsin, subsequently resist decolourization by 20% sulphuric acid, these bacteria are called ***acid-fast organisms***

- Isolated organisms are identified by *biochemical reactions, bacteriocin, bacteriophage and serotyping*, and *animal pathogenicity tests*

IMPORTANT QUESTION

Outline general rules for collection and transportation of various clinical specimens.

Chapter 5

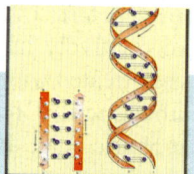

Sterilization and Disinfection

STERILIZATION AND DISINFECTION

Sterilization is defined as the process by which an article, a surface or a medium is freed of all micro-organisms including viruses, bacteria, their spores and fungi, both pathogenic and nonpathogenic.

Disinfection is a process of destruction or removal of organisms capable of giving rise to infection. A **disinfectant** is a chemical or physical agent that is applied to inanimate objects to kill microbes. Disinfectants are capable of killing vegetative bacteria, fungi, viruses and rarely bacterial spores.

Antisepsis is the destruction or inhibition of microorganisms in living tissues thereby limiting or preventing the harmful effects of infection. A disinfectant that is applied to living tissue, to kill microbes, is referred to as an **antiseptic**. Note that not all disinfectants are antiseptics because an antiseptic additionally must not be so harsh that it damages living tissue.

Various agents used in sterilization and disinfection may be divided into:

A. Physical agents
1. Sunlight
2. Drying
3. Heat
4. Filtration
5. Radiations

B. Chemical agents
1. Phenols and cresols
2. Halogens
3. Metallic salts
4. Aldehydes
5. Alcohols
6. Dyes
7. Vapour-phase disinfectants
8. Surface active disinfectants

A. PHYSICAL AGENTS

1. Sunlight

Sunlight possesses ultraviolet rays which along with heat rays are responsible for appreciable germicidal activity. These rays, however, cannot penetrate through glass, i.e., window panes. This is one of the natural methods of sterilization of water in tanks, rivers and lakes.

2. Drying

Water constitutes 80% of the weight of the bacteria and is also essential for the growth of bacteria. Therefore, drying has deleterious effect on many bacteria. However, spores are unaffected by drying.

3. Heat

Heat is the most reliable, certain and rapid method of sterilization. It can be easily controlled and unlike chemical disinfection, leaves no potentially harmful residue. Unless the material to be sterilized is heat-sensitive, this method should be preferred. There are two types of heat – dry heat and wet heat.

Dry heat

It is believed to kill microorganisms by causing destructive oxidation of essential cell constituents. Dry heat at 100°C for 60 minutes and 115°C for 60 minutes can kill all vegetative bacteria and fungal spores respectively. Bacterial spores can be killed by dry heat at 160°C for one hour or 180°C for 20 minutes. On the whole dry heat is less efficient sterilization process than moist heat.

Moist heat

It causes denaturation and coagulation of proteins. When steam condenses on cooler surface, it releases its latent heat and raises the temperature of its surface. If spores are present, steam condenses on them and increases their water content leading to hydrolysis and breakdown of bacterial proteins.

I. Sterilization by dry heat

(A) Red heat

Inoculating wires and *loops, points of forceps* and *spatulas* are sterilized by holding them almost vertical in a bunsen burner flame until red hot (Table 5.1).

(B) Flaming

Scalpel blades, needles, mouths of culture tubes and bottles, glass slides and *cover slips* are sterilized by passing the article through the bunsen flame without allowing them to become red hot.

(C) Incineration

This is an efficient method for rapidly destroying contaminated materials such as *soiled dressings* and *pathological materials*, etc.

(D) Hot air oven

It is a method of choice for sterilization of glassware such as assembled *all glass syringes*, *test tubes*, *petri dishes*, *pipettes* and *flasks*; *metal instruments* such as *forceps*, *scissors* and *scalpels*; sealed materials such as *oils*, *greases* and *dry powder* which are impervious to steam and *swab sticks* packed in test tubes. It is not suitable for materials like fabrics which may be damaged by heat.

Hot air oven is electrically heated and is fitted with a thermostat that maintains the chamber air at a chosen temperature and a fan that distributes hot air in the chamber (Fig. 5.1). It must not be overloaded and spaces must be left for circulation of air through the load. Holding time for sterilization in hot air oven is **one hour at 160°C** or **20 minutes at 180°C**. It is timed as beginning when the thermometer first shows 160°C or 180°C respectively.

Sterilization controls: Two types of controls are available.

A. Biological control: An envelope containing a filter paper strip impregnated with 10^6 spores of *Bacillus subtilis* subsp. *niger* (NCTC 10075 or ATCC 9372) is placed within the load (Table 5.2). After sterilization is over, the strip is removed and inoculated into tryptone soy broth and incubated aerobically at 37°C for five days. No growth of *B. subtilis* subsp. *niger* indicates proper sterilization.

Table 5.1. Sterilization by dry heat

Mode of sterilization	Instrument	Temperature and time	Sterilization of	Advantages/ disadvantages
Red heat	Bunsen burner	Till red hot	Inoculating wires and loops, points of forceps and spatulas	Sterilization is rapid and thorough
Flaming	Bunsen burner	Waving through the flame	Scalpel blades, needles, mouths of culture tubes and bottles, glass slides and cover slips	1. Surface sterilization is possible 2. Rapid method
Hot air	Hot air oven	160°C for 1 hour or 180°C for 20 minutes	Glassware, metal instruments, sealed materials such as oils, greases, dry powder, etc.	Can be used for loads that cannot be penetrated by steam.

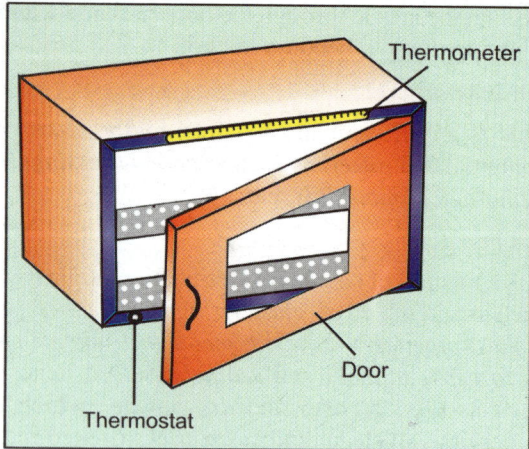

Fig. 5.1. Hot air oven.

Table 5.2. Biological controls of different sterilization methods

Method of sterilization	Biological control
Hot air oven	*Bacillus subtilis* subsp. *niger*
Autoclave	*Bacillus stearothermophilus*
Ethylene oxide	*Bacillus globigi* (a red-pigmented variant of *Bacillus subtilis*)
Filtration	*Serratia marcescens, Pseudomonas diminuta*
Ionizing radiations	*Bacillus pumilis*

B. Chemical control: A Browne's tube containing red solution is placed within the load. A change of colour of the solution from **red to green** indicates proper sterilization.

II. Sterilization by moist heat

Sterilization by moist heat means killing of the microorganisms with hot water or steam. Moist heat is divided into 3 forms (Table 5.3):

A. *At temperatures below 100°C.*
B. *At a temperature of 100°C.*
  (a) Boiling water
  (b) Free steam
C. *At temperature above 100°C.*

(A) Moist heat at temperatures below 100°C

Heat-labile fluids may be disinfected (not sterilized) by heating at temperatures below 100°C. Such treatment is sufficient to kill mesophilic vegetative bacteria. This includes:

- **Pasteurization** of milk and butter. The temperature employed is either **63°C for 30 minutes** (holder method) or **72°C for 20 seconds** (flash method) followed by rapid cooling to 13°C or lower. By this method non-sporing organisms such as mycobacteria *Brucella* and salmonellae are destroyed. However, *Coxiella burnetii*, causative agent of Q fever, may survive pasteurization by holder method.

Table 5.3. Sterilization by moist heat

Mode of sterilization	Instrument	Temperature and time	Sterilization of	Advantages/ disadvantages
Below 100°C	Water bath	56°C for 1 hour or 65–75°C for 10 minutes	Serum, body fluids, vaccines and spatulas	May be used for disinfection. Most vegetative mesophilic bacteria are killed.
At 100°C	Boiling water bath	100°C for 10–20 min.	Glass, metal and rubber items	Kills all vegetative bacteria and some spores.
Steaming at 100°C	Arnold steamer	100°C for 20 minutes on 3 successive days	Culture media containing sugar and gelatin	Prevents decomposition of media. *Spores of thermophilic bacteria may escape killing.*
Above 100°C	Autoclave	121°C for 15–20 minutes	Culture media and other aqueous solutions, dressing material, linen, gloves, etc.	Most reliable method of sterilization.

The flash method is preferable for pasteurization of milk because it is less likely to change the flavour and nutrient content, and it is more effective against resistant pathogens such as *C. burnetii*. Although pasteurization inactivates most viruses and vegetative stages of 97–99% of bacteria and fungi, they do not kill endospores and thermoresistant species (mostly nonpathogenic lactobacilli, micrococci and yeasts). Therefore, milk is not sterile after regular pasteurization, which explains why even an unopened carton of milk will eventually spoil on prolonged storage. Newer techniques have now been used to produce sterile milk that has storage period of 3 months. In this method, the milk is processed with **ultrahigh temperature** of **134°C for 1–2 seconds**.

- **Heat-labile fluids** such as serum may be disinfected by heating at 56°C for one hour. If temperature rises above 59°C it will coagulate.
- **Vaccines** prepared from nonsporing bacteria may be inactivated in a water bath at 60°C for one hour.
- **Household utensils and patient's clothing** may be disinfected by washing in water at 70–80°C for several minutes. Media such as Lowenstein–Jensen and Loeffler's serum slope are rendered sterile by heating at 80–85°C for half an hour on three successive days in an inspissator. Items which cannot withstand heat at 100°C may be disinfected by steam at sub-atmospheric pressure at a temperature of 75°C with formaldehyde vapour. This is known as **low temperature steam-formaldehyde (LTSF) sterilization**.

(B) Moist heat at a temperature of 100°C

(a) **Boiling at 100°C:** Boiling at **100°C for 10–30 minutes** kills all vegetative bacteria and some bacterial spores. Therefore, it is not recommended for sterilization of instruments for surgical procedures.

(b) **Free steam at 100°C:** Steam at normal atmospheric pressure is at 100°C. But, in addition, it has latent heat which on condensing on the article to be sterilized releases its latent heat. A **Koch** or **Arnold steam sterilizer** consists of a vertical metal cylinder with a removable conical lid having a small opening for the escaping steam. Water is added on the bottom and there is a perforated shelf above water

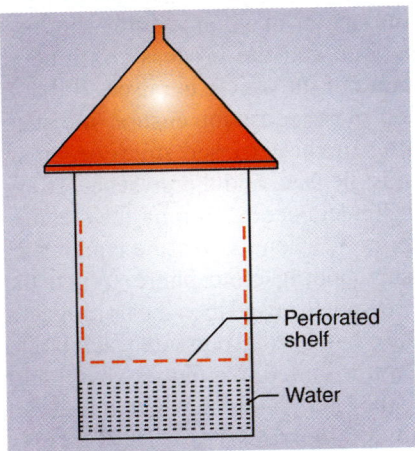

Fig. 5.2. Steam sterilizer.

level (Fig. 5.2). On this shelf articles to be sterilized are placed.

One single exposure to steam for 90 minutes ensures complete sterilization but for media containing *sugar* and *gelatin*, which may get decomposed on long heating, an exposure of **100°C for 20 minutes on three consecutive days** is employed. This is known as **tyndallization** or **intermittent sterilization**. First exposure to steam kills all vegetative bacteria, and any spores present, being in a favourable medium, will germinate and will be killed on the subsequent occasions. Therefore, non-nutrient media cannot be sterilized by this method.

(C) Moist heat at temperature above 100°C

Steam above 100°C or saturated steam is a more efficient sterilizing agent than hot air because:

- it provides greater lethal action of moist heat;
- it is quicker in heating up the exposed articles; and
- it can penetrate easily porous material such as cotton wool stoppers, paper and cloth wrappers, bundles of surgical linen, and hollow apparatus.

When the steam meets the cooler surface of the article, it condenses into a small volume of water and liberates its considerable latent heat to that surface, for example, 1600 ml of steam at 100°C, i.e., at atmospheric pressure condenses into 1 ml of water at 100°C liberating 518 calories of heat. The large contraction in volume brings more steam to the same site and the process continues until the temperature of the article is raised to that of steam. The water of condensation ensures moist conditions for killing of the exposed microorganisms. Pure steam must be used and the presence of air avoided since air hinders penetration by the steam.

Water boils when its pressure equals the pressure of the surrounding atmosphere. When the atmospheric pressure is raised then the boiling temperature is also raised. At normal pressure water boils at 100°C but when it is boiled in a closed vessel at increased pressure the temperature at which it boils and that of the steam it forms rises above 100°C. This principle has been exploited in autoclave and pressure cooker.

Sterilization by **steam under pressure (autoclaving)** is suitable for *culture media* and *aqueous solutions* (since atmosphere of steam prevents evaporation during heating), *dressing material, linen, gloves*, etc. Satisfactory sterilization can be achieved at **15 pounds per square inch** (psi) pressure equivalent to **121°C in 15–20 minutes**. In fact the only practical and dependable method of sterilization is steam under pressure using different types of autoclaves. *However, the autoclave is ineffective for sterilizing substances that repel moisture (oils, waxes or powders).*

All the air must be removed from the autoclave chamber and the articles to be sterilized so that the latter are exposed to pure steam. There are three reasons for this:

1. The admixture of air with steam results in lower temperature being achieved.
2. Air hinders penetration of steam into the interstices of porous materials, surgical dressings, syringes, etc.
3. The air being denser forms a separate and cooler layer in the lower part of the autoclave, so it prevents adequate heating of articles there.

Several types of steam sterilizers are available. The **laboratory autoclave** or **pressure cooker type autoclave** (Fig. 5.3) consists of a vertical or horizontal cylinder of gun metal or stainless steel in a supporting frame or case. The lid is fastened by screw clamp and rendered air tight by asbestos gasket. Lid bears a pressure gauge and a steam release

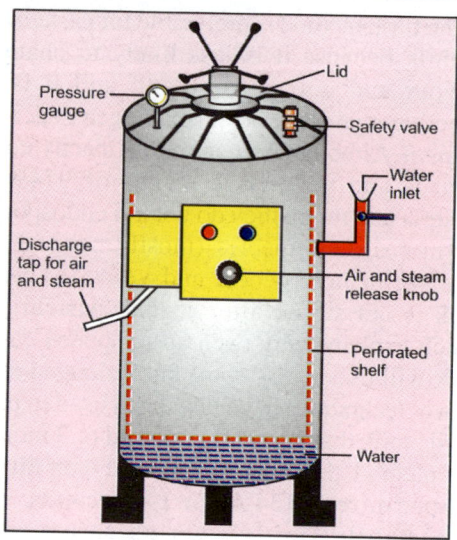

Fig. 5.3. Autoclave.

valve or safety valve. The latter opens and closes when the steam pressure rises or falls the desired level respectively. On its upper part of the side, the autoclave has a discharge tap for air and steam, and an air and steam release knob. Heating is done by electricity. Water is added on the bottom of the autoclave. Above this is a perforated shelf on which articles to be sterilized are placed.

The lid is closed, discharge tap is opened and safety valve is adjusted to the required pressure. As heating continues, the steam and air mixture escapes. To know when all the air inside the autoclave has escaped the discharge tap is connected with one end of a rubber tube and the other end of it is placed in water. When the air bubbles stop coming it indicates that all the air from inside the autoclave has been removed. The discharge tap is now closed. Steam pressure rises inside and when it reaches the desired set level (15 psi) the safety valve opens and excess steam escapes. From this point the **holding time** (15 minutes) is counted.

When the holding time is over, the heating is stopped and autoclave allowed to cool till pressure gauze indicates that inside pressure has reached to the atmospheric pressure. The discharge tap is now opened and air is allowed to enter the autoclave. The lid is now opened and the sterilized articles removed. If the tap or lid is opened when the pressure inside is high, the liquid media boil violently and may explode. On the other hand, if the articles are not removed for a long time after the normal atmospheric pressure has reached inside the autoclave, an excessive amount of water will be evaporated and lost from the media.

Sterilization controls: Two types of controls are available:

(A) Biological control: An envelope containing a filter paper strip impregnated with 10^6 spores of *Bacillus stearothermophilus* (NCTC 10003 or ATCC 7953) is placed with the load in the coolest and least accessible part of the autoclave chamber (Table 5.2). After sterilization is over the strip is removed and inoculated into tryptone soy broth and incubated aerobically at 56°C for 5 days. No growth of *B. stearothermophilus* indicates proper sterilization. Spores of this organism withstand 121°C for up to 12 minutes and this has made the organism ideal for testing autoclaves.

(B) Chemical control: A Browne's tube containing red solution is placed within the load. A change of colour of the solution from **red to green** indicates proper sterilization.

4. Filtration

Liquids such as sera and solutions of heat-labile substances such as *sugars* and *urea*, used for preparation of media, can be sterilized by filtration. This method is also useful for:

- sterilization of pharmaceutical products;
- separation of bacteriophages and bacterial toxins from bacteria; and
- for the isolation of organisms which are scanty in fluids.

The filter disc retains the organisms which can then be cultured.

Limitations

Mycoplasma and viruses, which are very small, cannot be kept back by the bacterial filters, therefore, serum sterilized by filtration cannot be employed for clinical use. *Serratia marcescens* and *Pseudomonas diminuta* have been used to test the efficacy of different filters (Table 5.2). Several types of filters are now available. These include earthenware filters, asbestos (Seitz) filters, sintered glass filters, membrane filters, syringe filters, and air filters.

5. Radiations

Two types of radiations are used:

- Non-ionizing.
- Ionizing.

Non-ionizing radiations

These include infrared and ultraviolet radiations:

Infrared rays bring about sterilization by generation of heat. Articles to be sterilized are placed in a moving conveyor belt and passed through a tunnel that is heated by infrared radiations to a temperature of 180°C. The articles are exposed to that temperature for a period of 7.5 minutes. Articles sterilized include metallic instruments and glassware. It is mainly used in central sterile supply department. Efficiency can be checked by using Brown's tube No. 4 (blue spot).

Ultraviolet (UV) radiations in the range of 250 to 260 nm wavelength are highly effective. Low pressure mercury vapour lamps emit over 95% of radiations with the wavelength of 253.7 nm. Most vegetative bacteria are susceptible to UV radiations. Spores are highly resistant and susceptibility of viruses is variable. Human immunodeficiency virus is not inactivated by UV radiations. UV radiations induce thymine dimers in DNA and this interferes with DNA replication. They can penetrate only a few mm into liquids and not at all into solids. Therefore, their use is best restricted to disinfection of clean surfaces like *inoculation hoods*, *laboratories*, *wards*, and *operation theatres*. Source of UV radiations must be shielded to prevent the radiations falling on eyes and skin because it may damage them.

Ionizing radiations

These include *X-rays*, *gamma rays* and *cosmic rays*. These have very high penetrative power and are highly lethal to all cells including bacteria. They damage DNA by various mechanisms. Spores are more resistant than vegetative bacteria. Large commercial plants use gamma radiations for sterilization of prepacked disposable items such as *plastic syringes, transfusion sets, catheters, cannulas, culture plates*, etc. that are unable to withstand heat because there is no appreciable increase in the temperature. Therefore, this method is known as **cold sterilization**. *Bacillus pumilis* has been used to test the efficacy of ionizing radiations (Table 5.2).

B. CHEMICAL AGENTS

1. Phenols

These are obtained by distillation of coal tar and have a powerful microbicidal action. They cause cell membrane damage thus releasing cell contents and causing cell lysis. They are resistant to inactivation by organic matter and are active against Gram-positive and Gram-negative bacteria, moderately active against mycobacteria, and have little activity against spores and viruses. They are used mainly for *discarded cultures, contaminated pipettes and other infected material.* Phenol is bactericidal at a concentration of 1%. At a concentration of 0.5% it is used for preservation of sera and vaccines.

Phenol derivatives

Certain phenol derivatives like cresols, chlorhexidine, chloroxylenol and hexachlorophane are commonly used as antiseptics.

- **Cresols:** Cresols are obtained by distillation of coal tar, are emulsified with green-soap and sold under the trade names of Lysol and Creolin. They are active against a wide range of organisms. They are most commonly used for sterilisation of infected glassware, cleaning floors and disinfection of excreta. They are not inactivated by the presence of organic matter.
- **Chlorhexidine (Hibtane):** It is a relatively non-toxic skin disinfectant. It is most active against Gram-positive organisms, and fairly effective against Gram-negative ones. Aqueous solutions are used in the treatment of wounds.
- **Chloroxylenol (Dettol):** It is less toxic and less irritant, and is also less active. It is readily inactivated by organic matter. It is inactive against *Pseudomonas*.
- **Hexachlorophane:** It is more active against Gram-positive than Gram-negative bacteria. It is applied on skin as prophylaxis against staphylococcal infections. It is bacteriostatic at very high dilutions. It is potentially toxic and should be used with care.

2. Halogens

Halogens are oxidizing agents and cause damage by oxidation of essential sulfhydryl groups of enzymes. Chlorine and iodine are the halogens which are used as disinfectants. They are bactericidal and sporicidal. They are active in very high dilutions and their action is very rapid. In addition to chlorine itself there are three types of chlorine compounds, the hypochlorites, and the inorganic and organic chloramines. **The disinfectant action of all the chlorine compounds is due to release of free chlorine.** When elemental chlorine or hypochlorites are added to water, the chlorine reacts with water to form hypochlorous acid. It is a strong oxidising agent and effective disinfectant. The activity of chlorine is markedly influenced by the presence of organic matter.

Sodium hypochlorite, chloramine and bleaching powder are most widely used for disinfection of HIV infected material. Hypochlorite solution decays rapidly, therefore, it should be prepared daily.

- **Chlorine** has a special place in the *treatment of water supply* and combinations of hypochlorite and detergents are useful for cleansing and disinfection in food and dairy industry. Hypochlorites have a wide spectrum of activity against viruses and very little activity against tubercle bacilli. They are available in liquid or powder form as salts of calcium, lithium and sodium.
- **Iodine** in alcoholic and aqueous solutions is used almost exclusively as a *skin disinfectant* (antiseptic). Like chlorine, it is also inactivated by organic matter. It is also active against tubercle bacilli and a number of viruses. Mixtures of iodine with various surface active agents that act as carriers for iodine are known as **iodophores**, an example of this is **betadine**. It can be used as a *bactericidal antiseptic for intact skin* and for *disinfection of superficial wounds.* It is also active against fungi and *Trichomonas*.

3. Metallic salts

All metallic salts have some degree of toxicity for bacteria. The most toxic are those of mercury and silver and the least toxic are those of sodium and potassium. Mercury compounds act on bacteria by combining with sulfhydryl (SH) groups of bacterial proteins and other essential intracellular compounds. Merthiolate (sodium ethylmercurithiosalicylate) is used in a dilution of 1 in 10,000 for the preservation of sera. In the past, 1% solution of silver nitrate was instilled in the eye in newborn babies for the prophylaxis of gonococcal ophthalmia.

4. Aldehydes

Two aldehydes (formaldehyde and glutaraldehyde) are currently of considerable importance, although others also possess antimicrobial activity.

- **Formaldehyde** is an irritant, water soluble gas. It is highly lethal to bacteria and their spores, fungi and viruses. However, it is not active against prions. It is cheap and can be used for *sterilization of rooms*, *furniture* and a wide variety of articles liable to be damaged by heat, such as *clothing, woollen blankets, mattresses, respirators, heat-sensitive instruments*, etc. It may be used in gaseous form or an aqueous solution. It combines readily with proteins and is less effective in the presence of organic matter. Irritant residues of formaldehyde may be removed by exposure of the disinfected articles to ammonia vapour. *Form-aldehyde is a suspected carcinogen. It must, therefore, be used and stored in a flame-hood or well-ventilated area.*
- **Glutaraldehyde** is more effective and less irritant than formaldehyde. It possesses high microbicidal activity against bacteria and their spores, mycelial and spore forms of fungi and various types of viruses, including human immunodeficiency viruses and enteroviruses. Two per cent alkaline buffered solution is used for sterilization of heat-sensitive instruments like *cystoscopes, broncho-scopes, thermometers*, etc. *Gluteraldehyde is toxic and irritant to skin and mucous membrane, there-fore, contact with it must be avoided. It must be used in a flame-hood or well-ventilated area.*

5. Alcohols

Several alcohols possess antimicrobial activity. The antimicrobial activity of alcohol can be attributed to their ability to denature proteins. They are active against vegetative bacteria including tubercle bacilli, fungi and lipid-containing viruses but not against spores. Their action on nonlipid viruses is variable. They are most frequently used as skin disinfectants. They must be used at a concentration of 60–70% in water because the presence of water is essential for the antimicrobial activity.

- **Isopropyl alcohol** is preferred over ethyl alcohol as it is a better fat solvent, more bactericidal and less volatile. It is commonly used for *disinfection of clinical thermometers.*
- **Methyl alcohol** is effective against fungal spores.
- **Alcohol-based hand-rubs** are recommended for the decontamination of highly soiled hands in situations where proper hand-washing is inconvenient or not possible. However, it must be remembered that alcohol is ineffective against spores and may not kill all types of nonlipid viruses.

  Alcohols are volatile and flammable and must not be used near open flames. Working solutions should be stored in proper containers to avoid evaporation of alcohols.

6. Dyes

Two groups of dyes, the aniline dyes and the acridines have been used extensively as skin and wound anti-septics. Both groups are bacteriostatic in high dilution but have low bactericidal activity. They are much more active against Gram-positive than Gram-negative bacteria.

Aniline dyes include brilliant green, malachite green and crystal violet. Their activity is inhibited by the presence of organic matter like pus. They have no activity against tubercle bacilli, therefore, addition of malachite green to Lowenstein-Jensen medium makes it selective for the isolation of tubercle bacilli. They interfere with the synthesis of the peptidoglycan component of the cell wall.

Acridine dyes include acriflavine, proflavine, euflavine and aminacrine. They are little, if at all, affected by the presence of organic matter. Acridine dyes interfere with the synthesis of nucleic acids and proteins in both bacterial and mammalian cells.

7. Vapour-phase disinfectants

Two most important vapour-phase agents are ethylene oxide and formaldehyde.

Ethylene oxide is a colourless gas soluble in water. It is highly lethal to all kinds of microbes including spores and tubercle bacilli. It is useful for sterilization of articles liable to be damaged by heat, e.g., *plastic and rubber articles, blankets, pharmaceutical products* (*crude drugs and powders*) and *complex apparatus* such as *heart-lung machines.*

It is highly effective sterilizing agent because it rapidly penetrates packing materials, even plastic wraps. It forms explosive mixture when more than 3% is present in air. This hazard can be overcome by using a mixture of 10% ethylene oxide in carbon dioxide. It has an alkylating action on proteins. Inhibition produced by it is irreversible, resulting in enzyme modification and inhibition of enzyme activity. *Bacillus globigi*, a red-pigmented variant of *B. subtilis*, has been used to test ethylene oxide sterilizers (Table 5.2).

Formaldehyde gas is liberated by spraying or heating of formalin, by addition of formalin to potassium permanganate or by volatilization of paraformaldehyde. Its antimicrobial activity depends upon several factors. The atmosphere must have a high relative humidity (more than 60% and preferably 80–90%) and a temperature of at least 18°C.

It is used for fumigation of operation theatres, wards and laboratories. After sealing the windows and other outlets formaldehyde gas is generated by adding 150 g of potassium permanganate to 280 ml of formalin for every 1000 cubic feet of room volume. Rooms are left unopened for 48 hours. Then open the doors and windows to allow vapours to disperse and neutralize any residual formaldehyde with ammonia by exposing 250 ml of SG 880 ammonia per litre of formalin used.

Beta-propiolactone (BPL) is a condensation product of ketone and formaldehyde. It is active against all microorganisms including viruses. In liquid form it is used to sterilize vaccines and sera. It is more efficient than formaldehyde for fumigation purpose. BPL destroys microorganisms more readily than ethylene oxide but does not penetrate materials well and may be **carcinogenic**. For these reasons, BPL has not been used as extensively as ethylene oxide.

8. Surface active disinfectants

Substances that alter the energy relationships at interfaces leading to reduction of surface or interfacial tension, are known as **surface active agents** or **surfactants**. They possess both hydrophobic (water-repelling) and hydrophilic (water-attracting) groups. On the basis of charge or the absence of ionization of the hydrophilic group, these surfactants are classified into anionic, cationic, non-ionic and amphoteric compounds. **Non-ionic surfactants** do not have antimicrobial activity.

Cationic compounds such as quarternary ammonium compounds are the most important surfactants. These act on phosphate groups of cell membrane phospholipids and also enter the cell. This leads to loss of membrane semipermeability and leakage from the cell of nitrogen and phosphorus containing compounds. The agent which enters the cell, denatures its proteins. They possess strong bactericidal but weak detergent properties. They are essentially bacteriostatic and are more active against Gram-positive than Gram-negative bacteria.

They are also fungistatic and active against viruses with lipid envelopes (e.g., herpes and influenza) and much less against nonenveloped viruses (e.g., enteroviruses). Commercially available preparations of cationic compounds include cetrimide (cetavalon), benzalkonium chloride and laurodin. These compounds are most active in alkaline pH. Antimicrobial activity is affected greatly by acidic pH, organic matter and anionic surface active agents such as ordinary soaps.

Anionic surfactants such as common soaps usually have strong detergent but weak antimicrobial properties. These agents are most active at acid pH and effective against Gram-positive organisms but are relatively ineffective against Gram-negative organisms. These compounds cause gross disruption of lipoprotein framework of the cell membrane.

Amphoteric agents such as tego compounds possess detergent properties of anionic and antimicrobial activity of cationic compounds. They are active over a wide range of pH but their activity is markedly reduced by organic matter. At a concentration of 1% in water they are effective against a wide range of Gram-positive and Gram-negative organisms and some viruses.

Table 5.4 gives a list and the recommended concentration of disinfectants commonly used in the hospitals.

Table 5.4. List and the recommended concentrations of disinfectants commonly used in the hospitals

Disinfectant	Recommended concentration
Ethanol	70% (700 g/litre)
Methylated spirit	70% (700 g/litre)
Glutaraldehyde	2% activated (available commercially as cidex)
Bleaching powder (calcium hypochlorite)	14 g/litre of water
Sodium hypochlorite	1% solution, 0.1% solution
Hydrogen peroxide	3% solution
Lysol	2.5% solution
Savlon®	2.0%, 5.0%
Dettol®	4.0%
Betadine	2.0%

DISPOSAL OF BIOMEDICAL WASTE

Hospitals generate various kinds of wastes from wards, operation theatres and outpatient areas. These wastes include bandages, cotton, soiled linen, body parts, sharps (needles, syringes, etc.), medicines (discarded or expired), laboratory wastes, etc. Wastes which carry infective organisms should be properly collected, segregated, stored, transported, treated and disposed to prevent nosocomial infection. According to the Ministry of Environment and Forests (MoEF) gross generation of biomedical waste (BMW) in India is 4,05,702 kg/day of which only 2,91,983 kg/day is disposed, which means that almost 28% of the wastes is left untreated and not disposed finding its way in dumps or water bodies and re-enters our system.

Biomedical waste (BMW)

It is a broader term applied to waste generated in the diagnosis, treatment or immunization of human beings or animals, in research or in the production or testing of biological products. It also includes waste coming out of medical treatment given at home.

Infectious wastes include all those medical wastes, which have the potential to transmit viral, bacterial or parasitic diseases. It includes both human and animal infectious waste and waste generated in laboratories, and veterinary practice. Infectious waste is hazardous in nature.

Hazardous waste is a waste which has a potential to pose a threat to human health and life. The persons most at risk are the staff of hospitals particularly nurses and waste handlers. In countries such as India, scavengers and ragpickers are at serious risk.

It is important to note that not all hospital waste has the potential to transmit infection. It is estimated that 80% is noninfectious general waste, 15% is infectious and 5% other hazardous waste (Table 5.5). However, if the infectious component gets mixed with the general noninfectious waste, the entire bulk of waste becomes potentially infectious.

Table 5.5. Classification of hospital waste

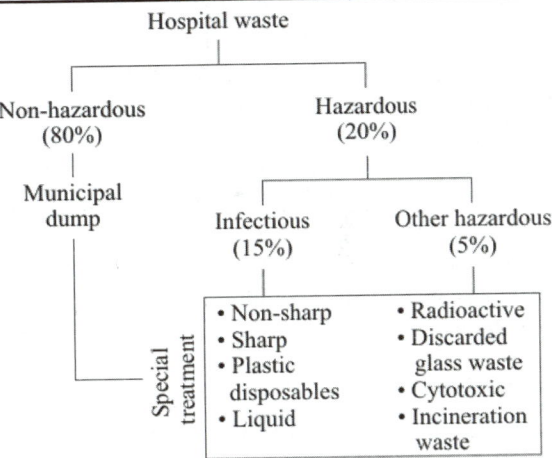

Ministry of Environment and Forests (MoEF), Government of India under the provision of the Environment Protection Act, 1986, notified the Biomedical Waste (Management and Handling) Rules, 1998 (Second and third amendments 2000 and 2003). Subsequently, MoEF notified the new draft Biomedical Waste (Management and Handling) Rules, 2011 under the Environment (Protection) Act, 1986 to replace the earlier Biomedical Waste (Management and Handling) Rules, 1998 and the amendments thereof.

Salient features of the draft Rules

1. Every occupier of the healthcare establishment (HCE) generating biomedical waste, irrespective of the quantum of wastes comes under BMW Rules and requires to obtain authorization from the prescribed authority.
2. BMW shall be segregated and kept in the colour-coded containers or bags at the point of generation prior to its storage, transportation, treatment and disposal.
3. There are eight categories of BMW now (Table 5.6).

Disposal of biomedical waste by deep burial shall be prohibited in towns and cities. Disposal by deep burial is permitted only in rural areas where there is no access to common biomedical waste treatment facility, with prior approval from the prescribed authority. The deep burial facility shall be located as per provisions and guidelines issued by Central Pollution Control Board from time to time.

Liquid waste generated from laboratory, washing, cleaning, housekeeping and disinfecting activities shall be treated so as to meet the discharge standards stipulated under these rules.

Incineration ash (ash from incineration of any biomedical waste) shall be disposed through secured landfill, if toxic or hazardous constituents are present beyond the prescribed limits as given in Hazardous Waste (Management, Handling and Transboundary Movement) Rules, 2008.

Waste segregation

Waste should be segregated at source, since 80% of the waste is non-hazardous and can be disposed of easily into the municipal bin. It is important that hazardous waste component is separated from non-hazardous waste. Mixing of waste will render the entire waste potentially hazardous. Waste should be segregated in bags of different colours to facilitate appropriate treatment and disposal (Table 5.7).

KEY FACTS

- *Sterilization* is a process that *kills* or *removes all* organisms (and their spores) in a material or an object

- *Disinfection* is a process that *kills* or *removes pathogenic organisms* in a material or an object
- *Antisepsis* is the application of a chemical agent externally on a *live surface* (skin or mucosa) to destroy organisms or to inhibit their growth (all antiseptics are disinfectants but not vice versa)
- Important agents used in sterilization and disinfection are physical agents (dry and moist heat), and chemical agents (phenols and cresols, halogens, aldehydes, alcohols, vapour-phase disinfectants and surface active disinfectants)
- **In dentistry**, sterilization is usually achieved by *moist heat* (steam under pressure in an autoclave; most popular), *dry heat* (hot air oven) or *gaseous chemicals*
- The sterilization cycle (either in an autoclave or a hot air oven) can be divided into the *heating-up period*, the *holding period* and the *cooling period*
- The indicators that must be routinely used for checking sterility are *mechanical indicators* (i.e., temperature and pressure gauges of the autoclave), *chemical indicators* and *biological indicators*
- **Hospital waste** should be *segregated at source*, since 80% of the waste is non-hazardous and can be disposed of easily into the municipal bin; waste should be segregated in bags of different colours to facilitate appropriate treatment and disposal

IMPORTANT QUESTIONS

1. Define terms sterilization, disinfection and antisepsis. Tabulate various methods used for sterilization and disinfection.
2. Describe:
   (a) Physical methods of destruction of microorganisms
   (b) Chemical methods of destruction of microorganisms
3. Write short notes on:
   (a) Hot air oven
   (b) Autoclave
   (c) Tyndallization
   (d) Pasteurization
   (e) Vapour-phase disinfectants
   (f) Disposal of hospital waste

Table 5.6. Categories of biomedical waste

Category	Waste category (Type)	Treatment and disposal option
Category No. 1	**Human anatomical waste** (human tissues, organs, body parts)	Incineration@@
Category No. 2	**Animal waste** (animal tissues, organs, body parts, carcasses, bleeding parts, fluid, blood and experimental animals used in research, waste generated by veterinary hospitals/ colleges, discharge from hospitals, animal houses)	Incineration@@
Category No. 3	**Microbiology and biotechnology waste and other laboratory waste** (wastes from clinical samples, pathology, biochemistry, haematology, blood bank, laboratory cultures, stocks of microorganisms, live or attenuated vaccines, human and animal cell culture used in research and industrial laboratories, wastes from production of biologicals, toxins, petri dishes and devices used for transfer of cultures)	Disinfection at source by chemical treatment@ or by autoclaving/microwaving followed by mutilation/shredding## and after treatment final disposal in secured landfill or disposal of recyclable wastes (plastics or glass) through registered or authorized recyclers
Category No. 4	**Waste sharps** (needles, glass syringes or syringes with fixed needles, scalpels, blades, glass, etc. that may cause puncture and cuts. This includes both used and unused sharps)	Disinfection by chemical treatment@ or destruction by needle and tip cutters, autoclaving or microwaving followed by mutilation or shredding##, whichever is applicable and final disposal through authorized CBWTF or disposal in secured landfill or designated concrete waste sharp pit
Category No. 5	**Discarded medicines and cytotoxic drugs** (wastes comprising of outdated, contaminated and discarded medicines)	Disposal in secured landfill or incineration@@
Category No. 6	**Soiled waste** (items contaminated with blood, and body fluids including cotton, dressings, soiled plaster casts, linen, beddings, other material contaminated with blood	Incineration@@
Category No. 7	**Infectious solid waste** (wastes generated from disposable items other than the waste sharps such as tubings, hand gloves, saline bottles with IV tubes, catheters, glass, intravenous sets, etc.	Disinfection by chemical treatment@ or autoclaving or microwaving followed by mutilation or shredding## and after treatment final disposal through registered or authorized recyclers
Category No. 8	**Chemical waste** (chemicals used in production of biologicals, chemicals used in disinfection, as insecticides, etc.)	Chemical treatment@ and discharge into drains meeting the norms notified under these Rules and solids disposal in secured landfill

Notes:

@ Chemical treatment using at least 1% hypochlorite solution or any other equivalent chemical reagent. It must be ensured that chemical treatment ensures disinfection.

Mutilation/shredding must be such that it prevents unauthorized reuse.

@@ There will be no chemical pretreatment before incineration. Chlorinated plastics/bags shall not be incinerated.

Table 5.7. Colour coding and type of container for disposal of biomedical waste

Colour coding	Type of container to be used	Waste category number	Treatment options as per schedule I
Yellow	Non-chlorinated plastic bags	Categories 1, 2, 5, 6	As per Table 5.6
Red	Non-chlorinated plastic bags/puncture-proof container for sharps	Categories 3, 4, 7 (4 – Waste sharps) (In the earlier Rules, soiled wastes are for Red colour)	As per Table 5.6
Blue	Non-chlorinated plastic bags container	Category 8 (chemical waste)	As per Table 5.6
Black	Non-chlorinated plastic bags	Municipal waste	Disposal in Municipal dump sites

Notes:

1. Waste collection bags for waste types needing incineration shall not be made of chlorinated plastics.
2. Category 3 if disinfected locally need not be put in containers/non-chlorinated plastic bags.
3. The municipal waste such as office waste (like paper waste), kitchen waste, food waste and other non-infectious waste shall be stored in black-coloured containers/bags and shall be disposed of in accordance with Municipal Solid Waste (Management and Handling) Rules, 2000.
4. No untreated BMW of categories 1, 2, 3 and 6 shall be kept beyond a period of 48 hours.

Chapter 6

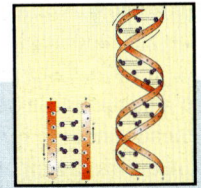

Chemotherapy*

Chemotherapy may be defined as the treatment of infectious diseases with specific drugs that selectively inhibit/kill the infecting microorganisms with no/minimal effect on the recipient. Due to analogy between the malignant cell and the pathogenic microbes, treatment of neoplastic diseases with drugs is also called chemotherapy. The year 1935 was an important one for the chemotherapy of systemic bacterial infections. The dye prontosil was shown to protect mice against systemic streptococcal infection and to be curative in patients suffering from such infections. It was soon found that prontosil was cleaved in the body to release *p*-aminobenzene sulphonamide (sulphanilamide), which was shown to have antibacterial activity.

Compounds produced by microorganisms (antibiotics) were eventually discovered to inhibit the growth of other microorganisms. For example, Alexander Fleming was the first to realize that the mold *Penicillium* prevented the multiplication of staphylococci. A concentrate from a culture of this mold was prepared, and the remarkable antibacterial activity and lack of toxicity of the first antibiotic, penicillin, were demonstrated.

With the advent of penicillin, the search was on for other normally occurring antimicrobials. Thus came streptomycin (1944), chloramphenicol (1947), chlortetracycline (1948), the cephalosporins (1948, though not used clinically until early 1960s), and neomycin (1949). Other aminoglycosides such as kanamycin appeared in 1950s, and gentamicin, tobramycin and amikacin in the subsequent 20 years. In the present decade we are seeing new cephalosporins and quinolones.

Antimicrobial agents exploit the structural and metabolic differences between bacterial and eukaryotic cells to provide selectivity necessary for good antimicrobial therapy. Penicillin, for example, interferes with the synthesis of the bacterial cell wall and human cells do not possess cell wall. There are fewer antifungal and antiprotozoal agents because the eukaryotic cells of the host and those of parasites have close metabolic and structural similarities. *Nevertheless, hosts, and parasitic and fungal cells do have some significant differences, and effective therapeutic agents have been discovered or developed to exploit them.*

Specific therapeutic attack on viral diseases has posed more complex problems, because of the

---

* This chapter has been contributed by Dr. Seema Gupta, MD, Assistant Professor of Pharmacology, Government Medical College, Jammu (J&K).

intimate involvement of viral replication with the metabolic and replicative activity of the host cell. Thus, most substances that inhibit viral replication have unacceptable toxicity to host cells. However, recent advances in molecular virology have identified specific viral agents that can be attacked.

Antimicrobial agent is a chemical substance inhibiting the growth or causing the death of a microorganism. Many chemicals have this property if sufficiently high concentrations are used. **Chemotherapeutic agents** are the chemical substances used to kill or inhibit the growth of microorganisms already established in the tissues of the body.

The term **antibiotic** is defined as a substance produced by a microorganism or a similar substance produced wholly or partially by chemical synthesis that is capable of inhibiting the growth or causing death of other microorganisms in low concentrations. For example, chloramphenicol was originally obtained from *Streptomyces venezuelae* but now it is produced completely by a synthetic process. Penicillins and cephalosporins are prime examples where the core nucleus has been chemically modified so as to alter their antibacterial spectrum, resistance to inactivating enzymes and pharmacokinetics. Commonly used antibiotics have been derived from *Streptomyces, Cephalosporium, Micromonospora* and *Bacillus.*

ANTIMICROBIAL AGENTS

The principal types of antimicrobial agents are listed in Table 6.1. These have been grouped according to their site of action. Antibacterial agents (drugs) may be bactericidal or bacteriostatic. Bactericidal drugs (penicillins, cephalosporins, aminoglycosides, fluoroquinolones, vancomycin, bacitracin, poly-myxin B, isoniazid, rifampin) kill bacteria, whereas bacteriostatic drugs (sulphonamides, trimethoprim, tetracyclines, macrolides, linezolid, clindamycin, chloramphenicol, cycloserine) inhibit the growth of bacteria. The bacteriostatic drugs depend on the host defence mechanisms such as phagocytes to kill the bacteria. Therefore, these drugs are not used in patients with neutropenia.

While most antimicrobial agents are effective when administered alone, sometimes a combination of antimicrobial agents provides a synergistic effect. Penicillin with gentamicin is used to treat strepto-coccal endocarditis. Sometimes another compound may be tagged to the primary antimicrobial agent to nullify antibiotic degrading enzymes, e.g., clavunic acid is used to protect amoxicillin from degradation by beta-lactamase enzyme produced by bacteria.

Antimicrobial agents may also be grouped according to the type of organisms against which they are primarily active (Table 6.2).

Mechanisms of action

Since bacterial metabolism is different in many ways from the human metabolism, their metabolic pathways are chosen as targets for inhibition by antimicrobial agents. Penicillin and related compounds inhibit peptidoglycan synthesis, but since such a metabolic pathway is non-existent in humans, antibiotic agents possess no toxicity (excluding hypersensitivity and other drug reactions). Mechanisms of action of antimicrobial agents can be placed under four headings:

Table 6.1. Antimicrobial agents

Inhibitors of cell wall synthesis	Inhibitors of cytoplasmic membrane function	Inhibitors of nucleic acid synthesis	Inhibitors of protein synthesis
Penicillins	Polymyxin B	Sulfonamides	Aminoglycosides
Cephalosporins	Amphotericin B	Trimethoprim	Chloramphenicol
Vancomycin	Azoles	Quinolones	Tetracyclines
Bacitracin		Rifampin	Macrolides
Cycloserine			Clindamycin
Caspofungin			Fusidic acid
Isoniazid			

Table 6.2. Antibacterial, antifungal and antiviral antimicrobial agents

Type	Antimicrobial agents
1. Antibacterial	Penicillins, cephalosporins, aminoglycosides, macrolides, sulphonamides, trimethoprim, quinolones, chloramphenicol, tetracyclines, vancomycin, bacitracin, polymyxin B, isoniazid, rifampin, cycloserine, clindamycin, fusidic acid, linezolid
2. Antifungal	Amphotericin B, azoles, griseofulvin
3. Antiviral	Acyclovir, famciclovir, zidovudine, lamivudine, navirapine, amantadine, ribavirin

1. Inhibition of cell wall synthesis.
2. Inhibition of cytoplasmic membrane function.
3. Inhibition of nucleic acid synthesis.
4. Inhibition of protein synthesis.

1. Inhibition of cell wall synthesis

Bacteria are surrounded by a rigid cell wall. It maintains the shape of the microorganisms and protects them from osmotic and mechanical trauma. Injury to the cell wall (e.g., by lysozyme) or inhibition of its formation may lead to lysis of the cell. The antibiotics which inhibit cell wall synthesis are β-lactam antibiotics (penicillins and cephalosporins), vancomycin, bacitracin, cycloserine, caspofungin and isoniazid.

Penicillins and cephalosporins are called β-lactam antibiotics because they possess an intact β-lactam ring, essential for antimicrobial activity. β-lactam antibiotics are inactive against organisms devoid of peptidoglycan cell wall such as *Mycoplasma*, protozoa, fungi and viruses. Penicillins and cephalosporins are usually bactericidal. Cephalosporins tend to be more resistant than the penicillin to inactivation by β-lactamases produced by some bacteria.

2. Inhibition of cytoplasmic membrane function

A group of polypeptide antibiotics act on the cytoplasmic membrane, the best example being polymyxin B, which acts essentially as a cationic detergent binding specifically to the membrane. As a result of this, the property of semipermeability is lost and essential low molecular weight intermediates and coenzymes pass into environment causing cell death. Because polymyxin will also combine with the membranes of eukaryotic cells, its selective toxicity is not great and it has to be used with caution.

Amphotericin B and azoles such as ketoconazole, fluconazole, itraconazole and clotrimazole are frequently used antifungal drugs. They show selective toxicity against fungi because cell membrane of fungi contains ergosterol, whereas human cell membrane has cholesterol. Bacteria with the exception of *Mycoplasma* do not have sterols in their cell membranes, hence they are resistant to the action of these drugs. Amphotericin B acts against the fungi by disrupting the cell membrane by binding at the site of ergosterol in the membrane. Azole inhibits synthesis of ergosterol.

3. Inhibition of nucleic acid synthesis

Sulphonamides, trimethoprim, quinolones and rifampin inhibit nucleic acid synthesis (Table 6.1).

4. Inhibition of protein synthesis

Bacteria have 70S ribosomes, whereas mammalian cells have 80S ribosomes. The subunits of each type of ribosomes, their chemical composition, and their functional specificities are sufficiently different to explain why antimicrobial drugs (Table 6.1) can inhibit protein synthesis in bacterial ribosomes without having a major effect on mammalian ribosomes. They interfere with different stages of the process of protein synthesis.

Each 70S bacterial ribosome is composed of a 30S and a 50S ribosomal subunits. Aminoglycosides and tetracyclines act at the level of 30S ribosomal subunits, whereas macrolides (erythromycin, roxithromycin and oleandomycin), chloramphenicol and clindamycin act at the level of 50S ribosomal subunits.

KEY FACTS

- *Penicillins* and *cephalosporins* (β-lactum antibiotics) selectively *interfere with the synthesis of bacterial cell walls*; they are inactive against organisms devoid of peptidoglycan cell wall such as *Mycoplasma*, protozoa, fungi and viruses.

- Penicillins and cephalosporins are usually *bactericidal*.
- Cephalosporins tend to be *more resistant* than the penicillins to inactivation by β-lactamases produced by some bacteria.
- *Tetracyclines*, *aminoglycosides*, and *macrolides* exert their antimicrobial effects *by targeting the bacterial ribosomes*.
- *Sulphonamides* inhibit bacterial nucleic acid synthesis.

IMPORTANT QUESTIONS

1. Define the terms antimicrobial agent, chemotherapeutic agent and antibiotic. Name various mechanisms of action of antimicrobial agents giving examples.
2. Describe the structure and functions of bacterial cell wall. Name various antimicrobial agents which affect cell wall synthesis.

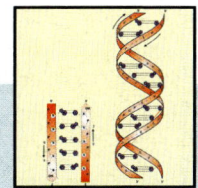

Chapter 7

Bacterial Genetics and Drug Resistance in Bacteria

Genetics is the study of genes, their structure and function, heredity and variation. Like other organisms, bacteria too obey the laws of genetics and breed true. However, a small proportion of their progeny exhibits variations in some properties. The genetic information in bacteria, as in other cells, is contained in the specific sequence of nucleotides in the cell's deoxyribonucleic acid (DNA). The DNA acts as a template for its own replication so that at the time of cell division two copies are available. It also acts as a template (Fig. 7.1) for transcription of messenger RNA (mRNA) which is then translated, by ribosomes into particular polypeptide (DNA → RNA → polypeptide). This is the **central dogma of molecular biology**. DNA is the storehouse of all information for protein synthesis. However, RNA viruses are an important exception in which the genetic material is RNA instead of DNA.

Structure of DNA

DNA molecule is composed of two chains of nucleotides wound together in the form of double helix (Fig. 7.2). Each chain has a backbone of alternatively arranged molecules of deoxyribose sugar and phosphates. To each deoxyribose sugar is attached one of the four nitrogenous bases, i.e., pyrimidines (thymine and cytosine) and purines

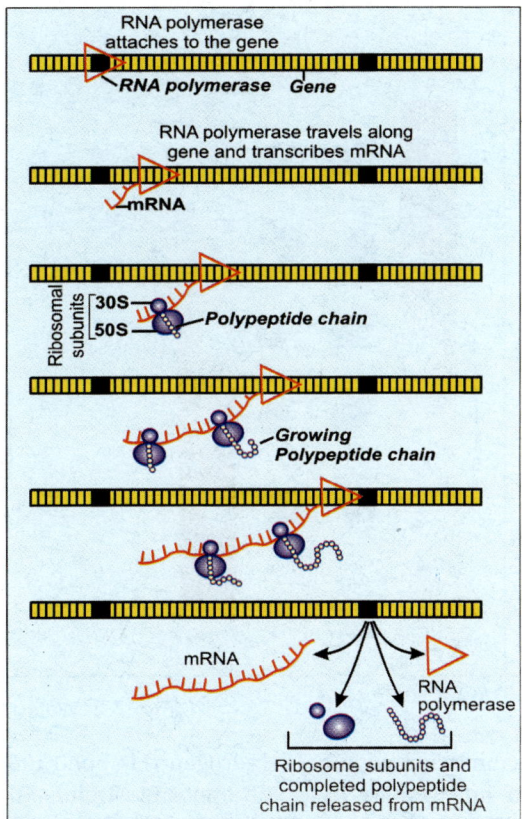

Fig. 7.1. Synthesis of polypeptide.

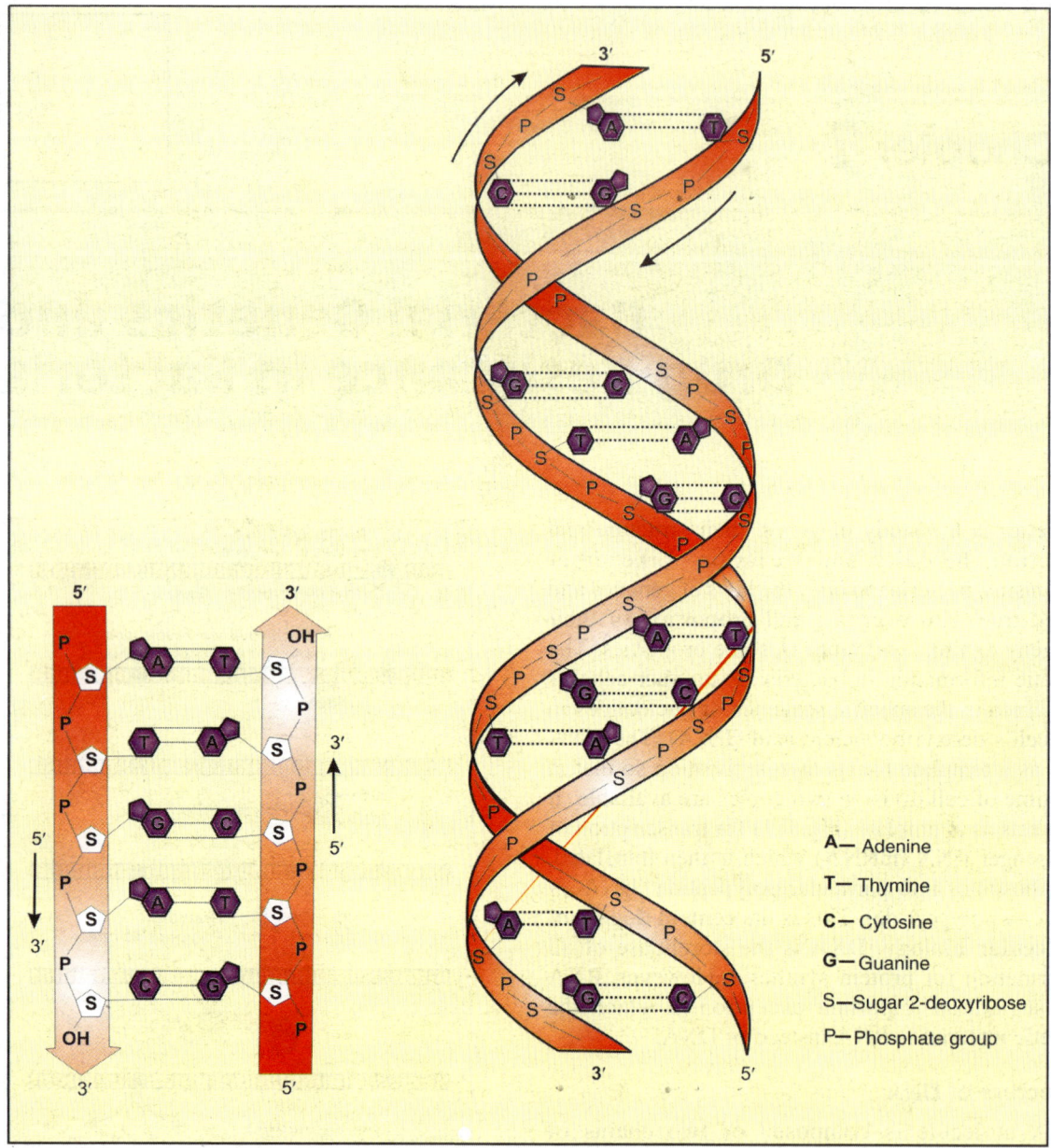

Fig. 7.2. Watson and Crick model of DNA.

(guanine and adenine). Hydrogen (H) bond unites two nitrogenous bases of opposite strands, thus making it double-stranded. Adenine always binds to thymine and guanine to cytosine. Therefore, adenine is complementary to thymine and guanine to cytosine.

Structure of RNA

Structure of RNA is similar to that of DNA with two differences:

1. It has sugar ribose instead of deoxyribose.
2. It has nitrogenous base uracil in place of thymine in DNA.

On the basis of structure and function RNA is of three types:

1. Ribosomal RNA (rRNA): This is RNA of ribosomes. It plays a basic role in the synthesis of proteins by providing a place for the specific selection, arrangement and joining of amino acids.

2. Transfer RNA (tRNA): This RNA has a specific terminal nucleotide sequence that enables it to accept a single molecule of an activated amino acid and transfer it to a ribosome.

3. Messenger RNA (mRNA): This RNA is formed by an enzyme RNA polymerase under the direct influence of DNA. Since DNA acts as a template for synthesis of mRNA, therefore, the bases in the two will be complementary to each other. Adenine, guanine, cytosine and uracil in mRNA will be complementary to thymine, cytosine, guanine and adenine respectively in DNA.

Codon

Genetic information is stored in DNA as a code. The unit of code is known as codon. It consists of a sequence of three bases. Therefore, code is triplet. Each codon specifies or codes for a single amino acid, but more than one codon may exist for a single amino acid. Thus, codon AGA codes for arginine but the codons AGG, CGU, CGC, CGA and CGG also code for the same amino acid. Therefore, code is **degenerate**. Three codons UAA, UAG and UGA do not code for any amino acid and are known as **nonsense codons**. They act as punctuation marks, terminating the message for synthesis of a polypeptide.

A segment of DNA carrying a number of codons specifying for a particular polypeptide is known as **cistron** or **gene**. A large number of genes constitute a **locus** and a large number of loci constitute cell **genome**. Therefore, DNA can be compared with a book of information. Letters represent nucleotides, words represent codons, sentences represent genes, paragraphs represent loci and entire book as DNA molecule or **cell genome**.

Most bacteria contain enough DNA to code for 1,000–3,000 different types of polypeptide chains, i.e., 1,000–3,000 genes. DNA molecule of *Escherichia coli* is 1,000–3,000 μm long. Since it is

much longer than the length of the bacteria, therefore, it is coiled and tightly packed up in a bundle resembling a skein of woollen thread. The length of DNA is usually expressed as kilobases (1 kb = 1,000 base pairs).

EXTRACHROMOSOMAL GENETIC ELEMENTS

Plasmid

In addition to chromosomal DNA, bacteria may also possess extrachromosomal genetic material known as plasmid. It may be defined as a small extrachromosomal piece of genetic material that can replicate autonomously and can maintain in the cytoplasm of a bacterium for many generations. It consists of a circular piece of double-stranded DNA. It is not essential for the normal life and function of the host bacterium though it may confer on it additional properties such as drug resistance, bacteriocin production, toxigenicity, etc. which may confer on the host bacterium survival advantage under appropriate conditions. In addition, it may contain genetic information for controlling its own replication and ensuring segregation of one copy into each daughter cell at cell division. Plasmid contains 50–100 genes. By their ability to transfer genes from one cell to another, plasmids have become important vectors in genetic engineering.

Episome

Plasmid DNA (extrachromosomal) may get integrated into host cell genome. In this state it is often known as episome. But both these terms are frequently used synonymously. Some plasmids confer on the host cell maleness or ability to conjugate (bacterial equivalent of sexual mating in higher organisms). Following conjugation, the recipient acquires the plasmid and in turn becomes male or donor cell.

F plasmid

The plasmid conferring maleness is known as F plasmid. It codes for the production of **sex pilus** through which it establishes contact with the recipient bacterium and transfers a copy of F plasmid into the recipient. Such plasmid that contains the information for self transfer to another cell by conjugation is known as **conjugative** or **self-transmissible plasmid**. Those plasmids which do not possess information for self transfer to another cell are known as **non-conjugative** or **nonself-transmissible plasmids**. They can, however, be transferred with the help of transfer factor such as colicin plasmid (Col I) and through the agency of bacteriophages (transduction).

GENOTYPIC AND PHENOTYPIC VARIATIONS

The characteristics expressed by a cell in a given environment are referred to as its **phenotype** (*phaeno*; display) and the collection of genes encoding these characteristics, the **genotype**. Bacteria, in general, are very adaptable and may alter their phenotype in response to environmental change while the genotype remains unchanged. Not all the genes of the bacterial cell are expressed all the time. For example, typhoid bacillus is normally flagellated but when grown in phenol agar, the flagella are not synthesized, but when subcultured from phenol agar into nutrient broth flagellated cells appear.

Another example of environmental influence is the synthesis of an enzyme β-galactosidase, necessary for lactose fermentation to its constituent sugars – glucose and galactose, in *Escherichia coli*. This organism possesses genetic information for synthesis of the enzyme, but it is produced by the bacteria only when lactose is present in the growth medium. This enzyme is not synthesized if *E. coli* is grown in medium containing glucose only. Such enzymes, which are synthesized only when induced by substrate, are called **induced enzymes**, while those enzymes, which are synthesized both in the presence or absence of the substrate, are known as **constitutive enzymes**. Regulation of enzyme induction illustrates the economy of nature, the enzyme being produced only when appropriate substrates are present.

LAC OPERON (GENE REGULATION)

Operon concept was proposed by Jacob and Monod. Lactose fermentation requires three enzymes – β-galactosidase, galactoside permease and transacetylase coded by structural genes *Lac-z*, *Lac-y* and *Lac-a* of *Lac* operon respectively (Fig. 7.3). Regulatory gene in this case is *Lac-i* which codes for a repressor. It is a protein molecule which can combine with either operator region on the chromosome or with the inducer (lactose). Between *Lac-i* and structural *Lac* genes lie promoter and operator regions. For transcription of mRNA for enzyme synthesis, the RNA polymerase has to attach to promoter region and travel along structural genes sequence. Operator region lies between the promoter and structural genes.

In resting stage when lactose (inducer) is not present in the medium, repressor molecule is bound to the operator, preventing the passage of RNA polymerase from promoter to the structural genes. The repressor molecule has an affinity for lactose, in the presence of which it leaves the operator region free enabling the transcription to take place. Lactose thus acts both as an inducer and the substrate for β-galactosidase. When lactose present is completely metabolized, the repressor again attaches to the operator, switching off transcription.

Phenotypic variations are influenced by environment, are temporary and are not heritable. **Genotypic variations** are stable, heritable and are not influenced by the environment. These are due to mutation or by any of the methods of genetic transfer such as transformation, transduction, lysogenic conversion and conjugation.

MUTATION

It is a random, undirected, heritable variation caused by an alteration in the nucleotide sequence at some point of the DNA of the cell, which may be due to addition, deletion or substitution of one or more bases. Mutations occur spontaneously at fairly constant rate, usually in the range of one per 10^2–10^{10} cell divisions. A large colony of bacteria contains about 10^9 cells, all derived from a single organism by repeated cell divisions. It may be realized that after 10^9 cell divisions, many thousands of different mutations will have occurred, affecting many of the genes in the cell. Similarly, in every infected patient, a variety of mutants arise spontaneously.

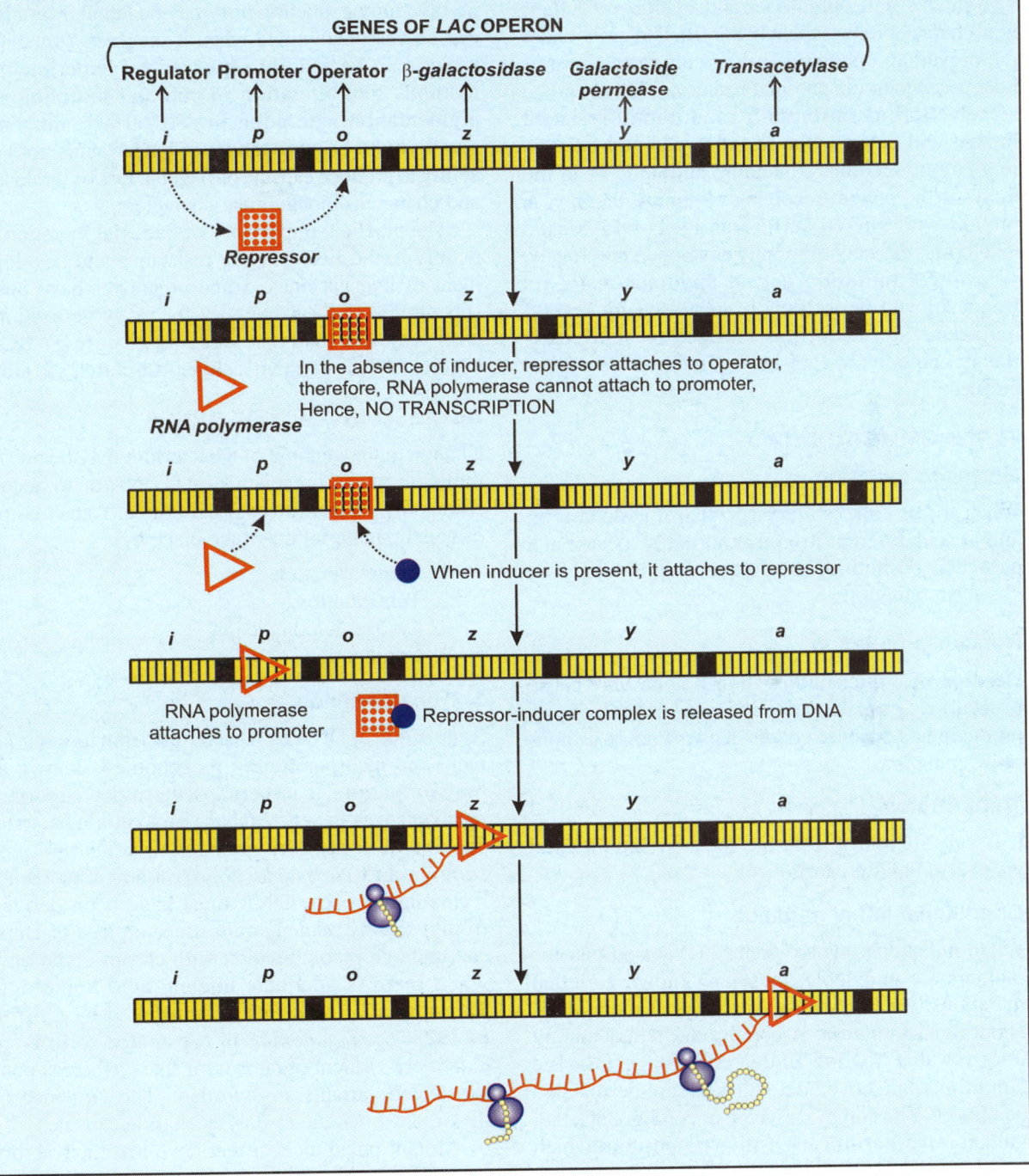

Fig. 7.3. The lac operon of *Escherichia coli*.

Mutants will outnumber and overgrow, if their new character makes them better fitted to grow under the prevailing conditions in the culture medium or host tissue than the parental bacteria. This is known as **selection of mutants**. An antibiotic resistant mutant will outgrow the sensitive parental bacteria in a culture medium containing antibiotic or in the body of the patient receiving antibiotic therapy. A mutant with altered surface antigens will escape deleterious effect of immunity developed previously.

Though mutation occurs spontaneously, its frequency can be artificially increased by several mutagenic agents such as nitrogen mustard, acriflavine, mitomycin-C, 5-bromouracil and 2-aminopurine.

TYPES OF MUTATION

Missense mutation

When triplet code is altered so that it codes for an amino acid different from that normally located at a particular position in the protein, this is known as missense mutation.

Nonsense mutation

Deletion of a nucleotide within a gene may cause premature polypeptide chain termination by producing a nonsense codon. This is known as nonsense mutation.

Transversion

It is substitution of a purine for a pyrimidine and vice versa in base pairing.

Conditional lethal mutation

When mutations involve vital functions so that the mutants are nonviable, these are known as lethal mutations. An important type of lethal mutation is conditional mutation. A conditional lethal mutant may be able to live under certain permissive conditions but not under other or nonpermissive conditions. The commonest type of conditional lethal mutant is **temperature-sensitive (ts) mutant** which is able to live at 35°C (permissive temperature) but not at 39°C (restrictive temperature).

Though mutations are taking place all the time, most mutants go unrecognized as the mutation may involve minor function or it may be lethal. Mutation can be best recognized when it involves a function which can be readily observed by experimental methods like alteration in colonial morphology, pigmentation, alteration in cell surface antigens, sensitivity to bacteriophages or bacteriocins, loss of ability to produce capsule or flagella, loss of virulence and change in biochemical characters.

The practical importance of bacterial mutation is mainly in the field of drug resistance and development of live vaccines. Some organisms have been subcultured in the laboratory for many generations until they lost their virulence for man (e.g., BCG vaccine). This is known as **live attenuated vaccine.**

ACQUISITION OF NEW GENES

Change in the genome of a bacterium may be due to mutation in the organism's own DNA or to acquisition of DNA from an external source. Transmission of genetic material may take place by:

1. Transformation
2. Transduction
3. Lysogenic conversion
4. Conjugation

1. Transformation

Acquisition of DNA by a bacterium from its environment and incorporation in its genome is known as transformation. It is perhaps the most important mechanism of genetic exchange for certain bacterial species, notably *Streptococcus pneumoniae*, *S. sanguis* and *Neisseria gonorrhoeae*. For transformation to occur DNA must have been derived from a closely related strain, since a piece of DNA can undergo recombination with chromosome only when there is adequate nucleic acid homology. Transformation was first demonstrated by Griffith in 1928. *S. pneumoniae* in capsulated form is an extremely virulent organism for mice, whereas noncapsulated variants are avirulent. The virulence of the organism is due to polysaccharide capsule.

Mutant pneumococci that have lost their ability to synthesize this capsule arise spontaneously. These show rough (R) colonies on blood agar as compared to smooth (S) colonies of capsulated form of pneumococcus. Griffith mixed live non-capsulated cells that had originally produced a capsule of one antigenic type with heat-killed smooth cells of a different capsular type. Neither preparation alone caused disease in mice, but mixture of the two preparations was lethal and Griffith was able to isolate from blood of the mice live pneumococci having a capsule of the same antigenic type as that of heat-killed cells. It was later shown that **DNA was the transforming principle** that was released from the heat-killed bacteria and was able to confer upon a live recipient cell the ability to produce a new type of capsule. The DNA that was taken up by the rough cells supplied the genetic information needed to make the missing enzyme needed for capsule synthesis.

2. Transduction

Transfer of a portion of DNA from one bacterium to another by bacteriophages (phages) is known as transduction. It may be generalized when it involves any segment of donor DNA or it may be restricted when a specific bacteriophage transduces only a particular portion of DNA.

Generalized transduction

Phages are viruses that multiply in bacteria. They carry their genetic information inside a protein coat. During assembly each phage head is normally filled with a phage genome, but sometimes an occasional phage particle is formed at a frequency of 1 in 10^6 whose head has been accidentally filled with a similar length of host cell DNA. This is known as '**packing error**'. When such a particle attaches to a second cell the DNA that enters the cell is not phage DNA capable of replicating and lysing the cell but a short segment of chromosome from first host, thus bacterial genes have been transduced by the phage into a second cell.

Since these phages pick up any portion of the host chromosome, they can transduce any gene. Each transducing phage can pick up a piece of bacterial DNA about the same size as its normal phage genome. Genes can be transduced only between fairly closely related strains because bacteriophage attacks a limited range of organisms with the same surface receptors. Transduction is not confined to transfer of chromosomal DNA. Plasmids or episomes may also

be transduced. **The plasmid determining penicillin resistance in staphylococci is transferred from cell to cell by transduction.**

Restricted transduction

Bacteriophages that lyse the host cell are known as virulent phages, however, temperate phage may get incorporated into the host genome and divide with it. These cells are known as **lysogenic**. Molecular basis of lysogeny has been extensively studied in λ phage of *Escherichia coli*. When infected with this phage majority of the cells go into lytic cycle while in a small proportion of them, they get incorporated into host cell genome (**lysogeny**). In some lysogenic cells lytic cycle is resumed. The **prophage** (integrated phage DNA) is excised and codes for viral proteins and DNA. In a small proportion of cells prophage is excised inaccurately so that a neighbouring portion of bacterial DNA is also removed.

Since phage head can contain only a standard amount of DNA, a transducing phage contains a few bacterial genes at one end of its DNA and lacks a few phage genes at the other end, i.e., **phage genome is defective**. When such a piece of DNA is transduced into a second cell the defective phage can still integrate into its normal site on the chromosome. The added bacterial genes are reproduced in the progeny of the recipient bacterium. Since the temperate phage has a specific insertion site it can pick up and transduce only a short length of DNA containing a few genes on either side of this site. This is known as restricted transduction. λ phage is always inserted between the genes for galactose utilization (*gal*) and biotin synthesis (*bio*) and thus can transduce either *gal* or *bio* genes.

3. Lysogenic conversion

In the lysogenic bacteria the prophage behaves as an additional segment of the bacterial chromosome, coding for new characters. This process by which prophage DNA confers additional genetic information to the host cell is known as **lysogenic or phage conversion**. An important example of lysogenic conversion is of *Corynebacterium diphtheriae* by β phage. Only those organisms which are lysogenic produce diphtheria toxin because *tox* gene coding for the production of **diphtheria toxin** is present on the phage DNA. The cells that lose the phage, lose toxin production. Another example of lysogenic conversion is the production of **dick toxin** by *Streptococcus pyogenes*.

Abortive transduction

Sometimes transduced DNA fragment does not integrate into the recipient chromosome, perhaps because of the presence of only a limited degree of homology. However, the transduced fragment can express its genetic information but cannot replicate. They remain only in one progeny cells following division. This process is known as abortive transduction.

4. Conjugation

It is the transfer of DNA that occurs during contact between bacterial cells. This mechanism is much more efficient than transformation or transduction. Transfer of DNA by conjugation is very common among Gram-negative bacteria, but it is rare in Gram-positive bacteria. **It is a major mechanism of transfer of drug resistance and can occur among unrelated genera.**

Conjugation was first described by Lederberg and Tatum in 1946 in *E. coli* K12 strain and has been most extensively studied in this strain. The donor status of a bacterial cell is determined by the presence of a plasmid which codes for **sex pilus**. It is 1–2 μm in length. The tip of the pilus attaches to the surface of a recipient cell and holds the two cells together. Two strands of plasmid separate. One strand enters recipient bacterium while one strand remains in the donor. Each strand then makes a complementary copy (Fig. 7.4). Along with the plasmid DNA a portion of host DNA may also be transferred to the recipient. The donor DNA then combines with recipient DNA leading to **genetic recombination.**

Stability of inheritance of plasmids varies from one plasmid to another. Some are lost very easily while others are very stable indeed and rarely, if ever, lost. Some plasmids can be eliminated from the host cell artificially (cured) by treatment with one of a variety of chemical agents (**curing agents**). These include acridine orange, sodium dodecyl sulphate and ethidium bromide.

Fertility (F) factor

F factor or F plasmid is a transfer factor that contains the genetic information necessary for the synthesis of the sex pilus and for self transfer but it does not possess other identifiable genetic markers such as drug resistance. Cells that possess one or more copies of the F plasmid are called **F⁺** and the cells lacking the F plasmid are called **F⁻**. F⁺ cells have no distinguishing features other than their ability to mate with F⁻ cells and render them F⁺.

Certain *E. coli* strains contain an F plasmid that has become permanently integrated into the cell's chromosome. Such cells are able to transfer chromosomal genes to recipient cell with high frequency and are known as **Hfr (high frequency recombinant)** cells. F plasmid may revert from Hfr state to free state. Sometimes it may carry with it some chromosomal genes from near the site of its attachment leaving a part of its own DNA from other end

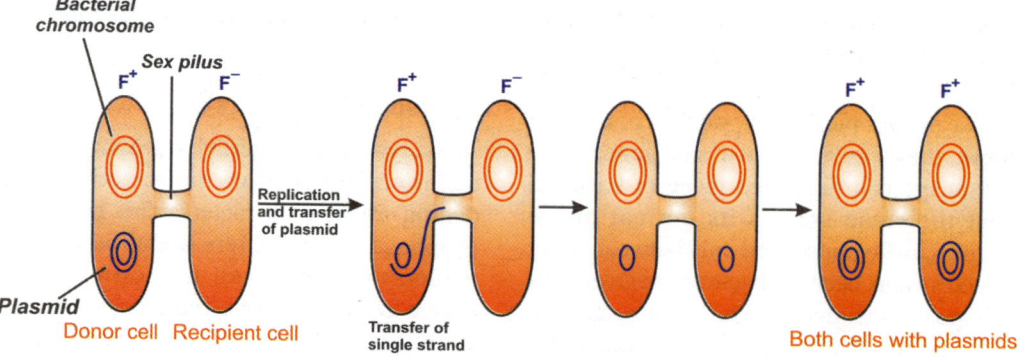

Fig. 7.4. Process of conjugation.

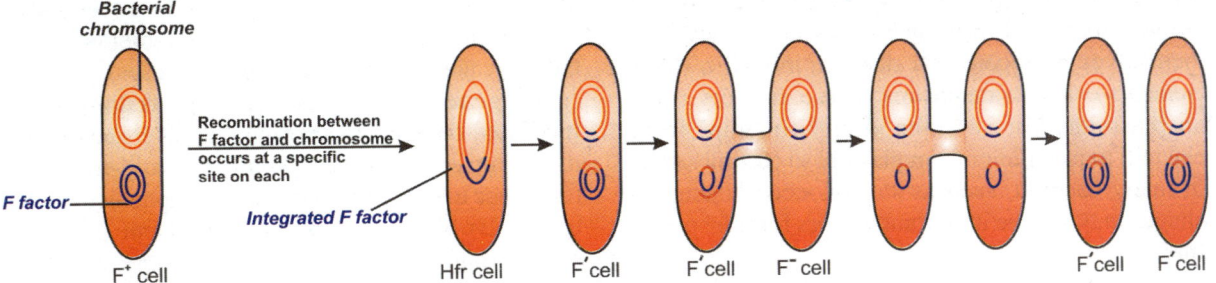

Fig. 7.5. Process of sexduction.

in the donor chromosome (Fig. 7.5). Such F factor possessing chromosomal genes is known as **F´ (F prime)** factor. When an F´ cell mates with a recipient cell, it transfers, along with the F factor, the host genes incorporated with it. This process of transfer of host genes through F factor resembles transduction and is known as **sexduction**.

Resistance plasmid or R plasmid or R factor

It consists of two parts – **resistance transfer factor** and **resistance determinants** (RTF + r). RTF is responsible for conjugal transfer and r determinants code for resistance against various drugs. As many as eight or more r determinants may be carried on each plasmid. Therefore, resistance to eight or more drugs may be transferred simultaneously. Sometimes RTF dissociates from r determinants. Those plasmids which lack RTF, i.e., possess only r determinants are known as **non-conjugative** or **nonself-transmissible plasmids** but they still code for drug resistance. Those plasmids which possess both RTF and r determinants are known as **conjugative** or **self-transmissible plasmids**. Non-conjugative plasmids can, however, be transferred by adding another strain possessing transfer factor like colicin plasmid (Col I) or by bacteriophages.

ANTIBIOTIC RESISTANCE

With antibiotics, as previously with sulphonamides, resistance began to arise. At first, organisms were encountered with low-level resistance to penicillin, and infections caused by these could be treated with larger doses of the antibiotics, because the low-level resistance was due to mutation which decreases the cell permeability to the antimicrobial agent and if larger doses are given then effective concentration of the drug can enter the bacterial cell. In time, however, highly resistant strains emerged which could not be therapeutically controlled.

Genetic basis of resistance

The initial low-level resistant microbial strains carried genes for resistance on the **chromosome**. These were soon replaced by higher-level resistant types, principally harbouring **plasmids**. Plasmid-mediated drug resistance is seen in various pathogenic and commensal bacteria of man and animals. Transfer of drug resistance occurs readily *in vitro*. It also occurs *in vivo* but in normal intestines it is inhibited by several factors like anaerobic conditions, bile salts, alkaline pH and abundance of anaerobic Gram-positive bacteria minimising the chances of contact between donor cells and suitable recipient cells. But in intestines of persons on oral antibiotic therapy, transfer occurs readily due to the destruction of the sensitive normal flora and the selection pressure provided by the drug.

Transferable drug resistance involves all antibiotics in common use. Bacteria containing R plasmid can spread from animal to man. Therefore, indiscriminate use of antibiotics in man and animals or in animal feed can increase the spread of plasmid-mediated drug resistance in the community. Because of the misuse and overuse of antibiotics in the hospitals it is said *'hospital is the heaven for drug resistant bacteria'*.

Some chromosomal-mediated resistances remain a therapeutic problem, namely, those responsible for resistance to methicillin, rifampin, nalidixic acid and isoniazid. However, most resistances of concern are associated with R plasmids. While plasmids may be the vectors of the resistance genes, the genes may themselves be located on discrete movable DNA elements called **transposons**. These are very often on plasmids, but have the ability to 'hop' from plasmid to plasmid or from plasmid to chromosome. In many bacteria, such as staphylococci, bacteriophages may also be important vectors for transposon spread.

Transposons may carry single or multiple resistances. The transposon can enter and remain stable in different species even if its entry vector (e.g., plasmid or phage) is lost, since the resistance transposon can be incorporated in a stable resident plasmid or the chromosome of the new host. The discovery of transposable resistance provided the basis for understanding the rapid spread of resistance markers throughout the bacterial kingdom and helped to explain why different genera seemed to have 'evolved' similar genes of resistance.

Bacteria resist antimicrobial agents by various mechanisms. **Chromosomal resistance**, except when resulting from transposon insertions, is generally mediated by a single low-level, non-enzymatic mechanism. In many organisms, these resistances seem related to decreased permeability, e.g., resistance in meningococci, mycobacteria, pneumococci and methicillin resistance in *Staphylococcus aureus*. Exceptions are the chromosomally located degradative enzymes for the β-lactam antibiotics and the chromosomal-mediated resistance to rifampin (via resistant RNA polymerases) and nalidixic acid (via resistant DNA gyrases).

In general, the **plasmid- or transposon-mediated resistances** are of higher level and involve more active processes. Some plasmid-mediated resistance to penicillin and to chloramphenicol seems to involve decreased permeability, but the exact mechanism is not yet defined. Many plasmid-mediated resistances involve extracellular inactivation of the drug by enzymatic modification or degradation of its active element. In this category are the enzymes (β-lactamases) which destroy the β-lactam ring of the penicillins and cephalosporins, and those which inactivate chloramphenicol.

In clinical practice, resistance acquired by mutation is very important in tuberculosis. If a patient is put on streptomycin alone then initially organisms die in large numbers but soon resistant mutants appear which multiply in number while sensitive parents may be eliminated. If two or more drugs are used and if a mutant appears which is resistant to one of the drugs then it will be killed by other drug/s. **The chance of a mutant developing resistance to more than one drug at one time is remote.** This is the rationale of combined therapy in tuberculosis.

R plasmid-mediated resistance is usually to multiple drugs, therefore, there is no use of combined therapy. Table 7.1 shows important differences

Table 7.1. Mutational and plasmid-mediated drug resistance	
Mutational drug resistance	**Plasmid-mediated drug resistance**
1. It is due to decreased permeability to drug, development of alternate metabolic pathways and development of enzymes inactivating the drug.	It is due to the development of degrading enzymes.
2. Involves resistance to one drug at one time.	Involves many drugs at one time.
3. Degree of resistance is usually low, therefore, infection may be treated by giving higher doses of the antibiotics.	Degree of resistance is usually high, therefore, higher doses of antibiotics do not help.
4. Development of drug resistance can be prevented by treatment with combination of drugs.	Development of drug resistance cannot be prevented by treatment with combination of drugs.
5. Resistance is not transferable to other organisms.	Resistance is transferable to other organisms.
6. Resistant mutants are usually metabolically defective.	They are metabolically normal.
7. Virulence of resistant mutants may be lowered.	Virulence usually not decreased. It may rather be increased by acquisition of virulence plasmids.

between mutational drug resistance and plasmid-mediated drug resistance. Acquisition of resistance by transduction is common in staphylococci. The penicillinase plasmids, which are transmitted by transduction, may also carry determinants of resistance to mercuric chloride and erythromycin.

Transposable genetic elements

Lederberg, in 1960, described an unusual class of *Gal*-mutants in *E. coli* caused by insertion of extra pieces of DNA called **insertion sequences** or **IS elements** at the point of mutation. Since then a large number of IS elements have been described in a wide variety of bacteria. They are common in bacterial plasmids and are common components of many, if not all, bacterial chromosomes. They are also **cryptic** in the sense that they do not confer on the host bacterium a predictable phenotype. Their presence is usually indicated by mutation. IS elements possess ability to transpose, i.e., they can insert into different sites on the same or on different DNA molecules.

In 1974, the discovery of a new type of transposable element that encoded a recognizable gene product (β-lactam antibiotic resistance) was reported. It was termed a **transposon (tn)**. Since then many others carrying a variety of resistance and other genes have been identified. Because of the ability of transposable elements to move from one plasmid to another or to a phage or to the bacterial chromosome they have assumed the popular name of **jumping genes. Unlike plasmids, transposons do not contain genetic information necessary for their own replication**, and their replication, therefore, depends on their physical integration with a bacterial replicon.

IS elements are small (1–2 kb) and cryptic, whereas transposons are larger (4–25 kb) and encode at least one function that alters cell phenotype. Therefore, **transposon may be defined as a segment of DNA with one or more genes in the centre and the two ends carrying inverted repeat sequences of nucleotides – nucleotide sequences complementary to each other but in the reverse order.** Because of this feature each strand of the transposon can form a single-stranded loop carrying the gene/genes and a double-stranded stem formed by

hydrogen bonding between the inverted repeat sequences (Fig. 7.6).

The transfer of genetic material from one DNA molecule to another is known as **transposition**. It does not need genetic homology between transposable element and its site of insertion. It is, therefore, different from recombination. Insertion of transposon leads to the acquisition of new characteristics by the DNA molecule. **It has been suggested that R plasmids may have evolved as collections of transposons each carrying a gene that confers resistance to one or more antibiotics.**

Genetic engineering (Recombinant DNA technology)

Insertion of a foreign DNA molecule into DNA of a vector, which can replicate autonomously in a suitable host, is known as recombinant DNA (rDNA) technology or genetic engineering. This technique makes it possible to isolate any gene coding for any desired protein from microorganisms or from cells of higher form of life including human beings, and their introduction into suitable microorganisms in which genes would be functional, directing the production of the specific protein. Such cloning of genes in microorganisms enables the preparation of the desired protein in pure form, in large quantities and at a reasonable cost.

Applications of genetic engineering

Genetic engineering is a useful tool for the **production of vaccines** (for prevention of disease) **and antigens** (for the diagnosis of disease). Yeast derived recombinant vaccine against hepatitis B is now commercially available. Genes coding for gp120 of human immunodeficiency virus (HIV) have been inserted into vaccinia virus. Inoculation of this hybrid-live virus (gp120/vaccinia hybrid vaccine) elicits both antibody-mediated and cell-mediated immunity against HIV. Vaccinia virus has also been used for the development of hybrid live vaccine against hepatitis B.

Recombinant DNA technology has also been used for the **production of proteins** of therapeutic interest. These include human growth hormone, human insulin, erythropoietin, factor VIII, tissue plasmino-

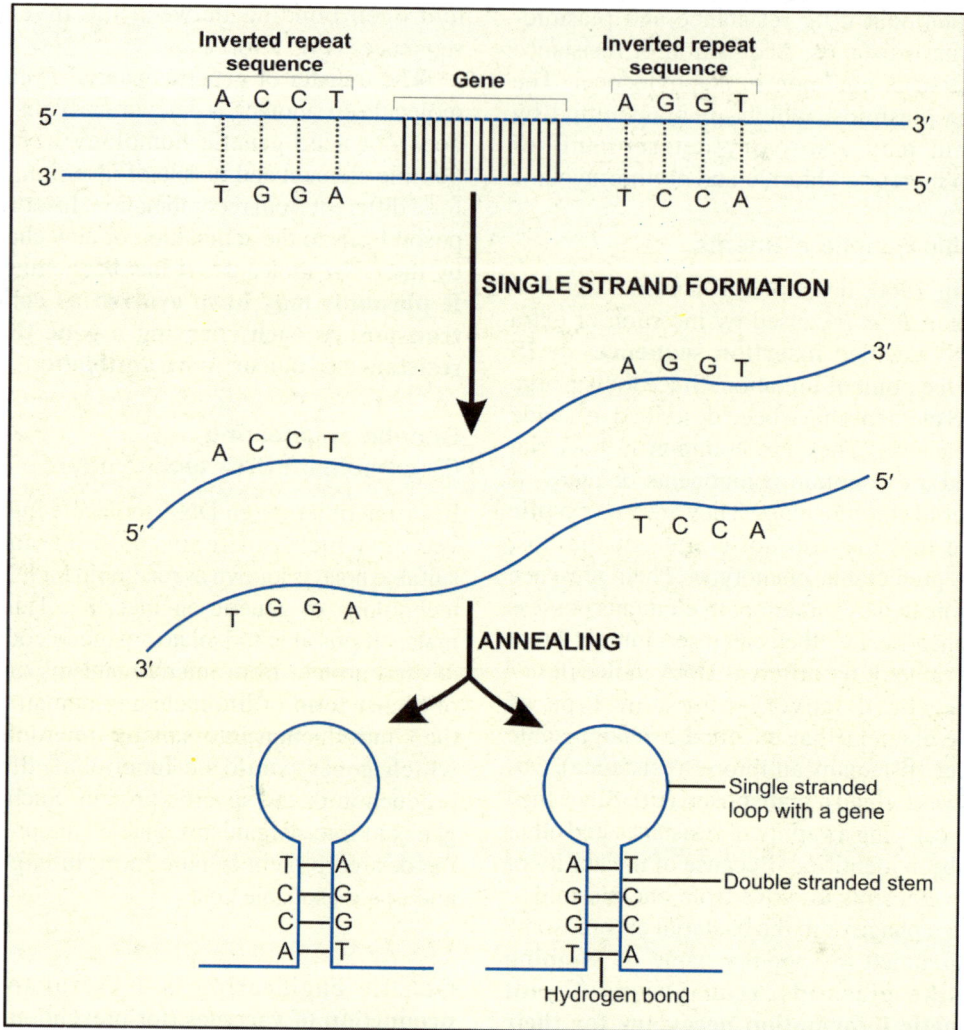

Fig. 7.6. Structure of transposon.

gen activator, interferons, tumour necrosis factor, interleukin-2, granulocyte colony stimulating factor, epidermal growth factor and fibroblast growth factor.

An important application of recombinant technology is gene therapy. Normal genes can be introduced into the patient so that genetic diseases may be cured.

DNA probes

DNA probes are radiolabelled or chromogenically labelled pieces of single-stranded DNA which can be used for the detection of homologous DNA by hybridization.

Development of DNA probe

All microorganisms, simple or complex, contain some unique sequences of nucleic acid within their genome that distinguish them from all other organisms. The method of developing a DNA probe is to cut or isolate those sequences from the nucleic acid of the cell using a set of enzymes known as restriction endonucleases, reproduce them in large quantities and attach a reporter molecule to them so that they can be incorporated into a hybridization reaction. **Hybridization** is the process whereby two single strands of nucleic acid come together to form a stable double-stranded molecule. However, they will bind and stay together only if the sequences of bases along each stretch of nucleic acid are complementary (adenine opposite thymine and cytosine opposite guanine).

Hybridizations are accomplished in tubes or by spotting the unknown organisms on a filter paper such as nitrocellulose paper, lysing them to release the DNA, and denaturing in mild alkali to single strands. The probe can then be added and after thorough washing to remove any unbound probe, the tube or probe is examined for evidence of hybridization. Formalin-fixed, paraffin-embedded tissues can also be probed particularly for viral DNA sequences. DNA probes can also be designed that bind to RNA and this procedure has been used particularly to locate ribosomal RNA.

Applications of DNA probes

- In the diagnostic laboratory, DNA probes are being used for culture confirmation as an alternative to conventional, time-consuming or labour-intensive methods. For example, DNA hybridization makes it possible to rapidly identify *Mycobacterium tuberculosis*, *M. kansasii*, *M. avium* complex, and *M. gordonae* isolated in culture, significantly reducing the time for reporting of the species of the isolate.
- Probe technology may also be used for detection of fastidious organisms directly in clinical specimens. Examples are *Neisseria gonorrhoeae* and *Chlamydia trachomatis*.

Polymerase chain reaction (PCR)

It is a primer-mediated, temperature dependent technique for the enzymatic amplification of a specific sequence (target sequence) to such an extent that it can be detected. The technique can be used to detect very small amounts of specific nucleic acid material in clinical specimens where bacterial, viral or fungal agents are thought to play a causative role. The fundamental basis of this technology is that each pathogenic organism possesses a unique 'signature sequence' in its DNA or RNA composition by which it can be identified. It is based on repeated cycles of high temperature template denaturation, oligonucleotide primer annealing, and polymerase mediated extension (Fig. 7.7).

To multiply a strip of genetic material, four ingredients are combined in a test tube:

1. Target DNA.
2. Short strands of DNA called primers which tag the section to be copied.
3. Polymerase – an enzyme that promotes gene replication in all living cells.
4. Nucleotides – the building blocks for making DNA.

PCR is carried out in three steps:

1. Heat at 94°C is applied to the target DNA, breaking the bonds that hold the strands together. This is known as **denaturation**.
2. The temperature is then reduced to 55°C, promoting the primers to attach themselves to either end of the target strip. This is known as **annealing of primers**.
3. Then polymerase enzyme triggers the formation of new DNA strand from the nucleotides. This is known as **primer extension**. When the temperature is again raised the new strands separate and the process begins again.

These three steps are repeated again and again by manipulating the temperature, a process that is automated by the PCR machine. A cycle takes about 3–5 minutes and after 30 cycles, taking about 3 hours, a single copy of DNA can be increased up to 1,000,000 copies, a sharp contrast to the days required by conventional amplification methods (culture).

Amplified sequences of target DNA can be detected by a variety of methods. If enough amplified DNA is present, it can be visualized by:

1. Gel electrophoresis and ethidium bromide staining.
2. Southern blot and dot-blot analysis with either radioactive or nonradioactive probes.
3. Oligomer restriction.
4. Oligomer hybridization.
5. Reverse dot-blot.

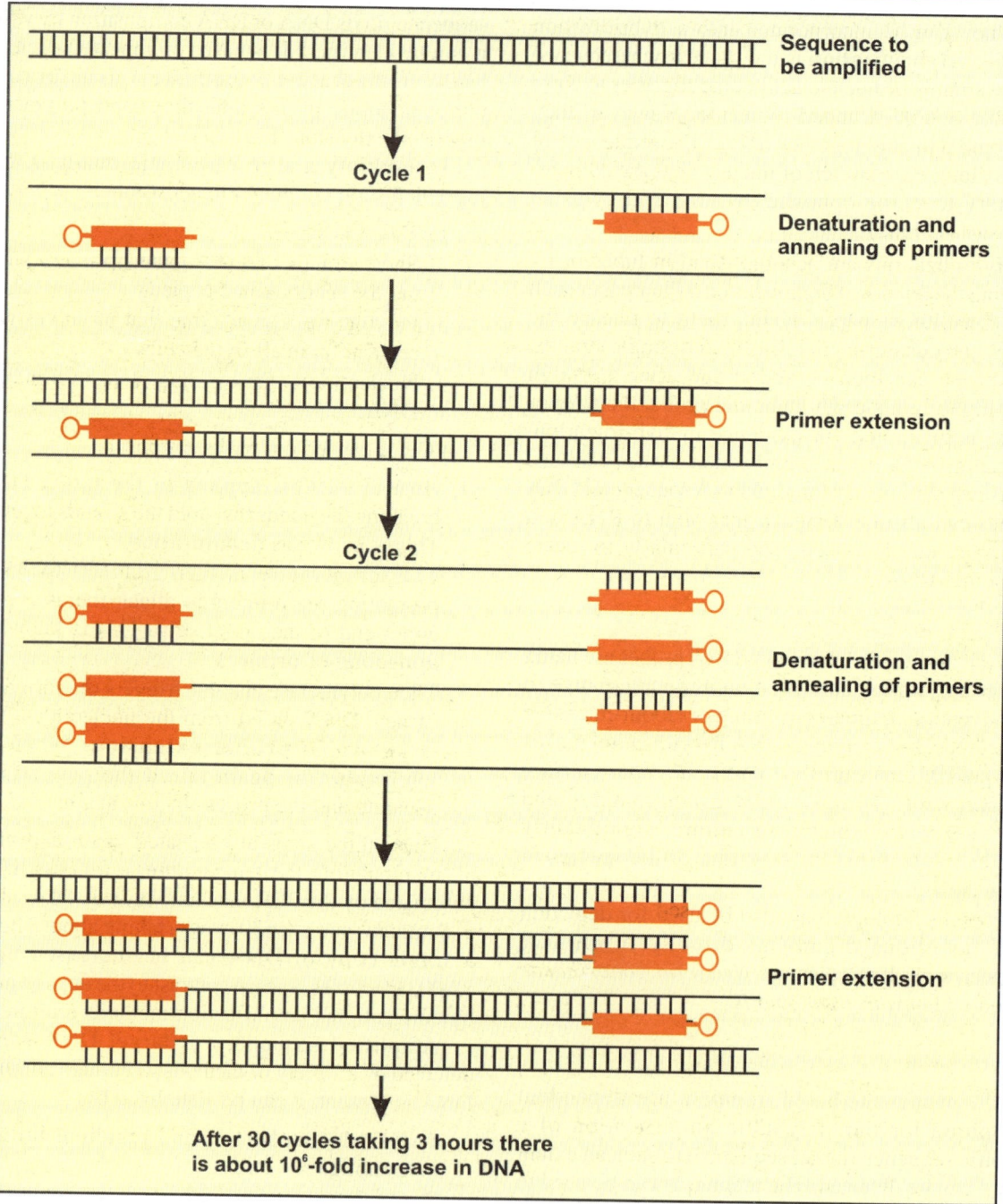

Fig. 7.7. Polymerase chain reaction.

Applications of PCR

The development of PCR or gene amplification method in 1983 is a major methodological break-through in molecular biology. Within a short span, this method has found its way into nearly every type of laboratory from forensic to ecology and from diagnosis to pure research. Applications of PCR in clinical laboratory are given in Table 7.2.

Table 7.2. Applications of PCR in clinical laboratory

Diagnosis of infections due to:

Viruses	HIV-1, HIV-2, HTLV-1, cytomegalovirus, human papillomavirus, herpes simplex viruses, hepatitis B virus, HCV, HDV, HEV, rubella virus, Epstein-Barr virus, varicella-zoster virus, human herpes viruses 6 and 7, parvovirus B19, enteroviruses, coxsackieviruses, echoviruses, rhinoviruses, measles virus, rotavirus, adenovirus, respiratory syncytial virus.
Bacteria	*Mycobacterium tuberculosis, Mycobacterium avium* complex, *Legionella pneumophila, Chlamydia trachomatis, Mycoplasma pneumoniae, Helicobacter pylori, Burkholderia pseudomallei, Campylobacter* spp., *Corynebacterium diphtheriae, Leptospira interrogans, Streptococcus pyogenes, Streptococcus pneumoniae, Yersinia enterocolitica.*
Fungi	*Candida* spp., *Cryptococcus neoformans, Aspergillus* spp., *Pneumocystis jiroveci.*
Protozoa	*Toxoplasma gondii, Trypanosoma cruzi, Enterocytozoon bieneusi, Encephalitozoon hellem, Plasmodium* spp.

KEY FACTS

- *DNA* molecule is composed of two chains of nucleotides wound together in the form of ***double helix***
- *DNA replication* is the synthesis of new strands of DNA using original DNA strands as templates; DNA-dependent DNA polymerase is the main enzyme that mediates DNA replication

- *Genetic variation* in bacteria can occur either by ***mutation*** or ***gene transfer***
- ***Mutation*** is a random, undirected, heritable variation caused by an alteration in the nucleotide sequence at some point of the DNA of the cell, which may be due to ***addition, deletion*** or ***substitution of one or more bases***
- ***Gene transfer*** in bacteria may occur by ***conjugation, transduction, transformation*** or ***transposition***
- ***Plasmids*** are ***extrachromosomal, double-stranded circular DNA molecules*** capable of ***independent replication*** within the bacterial host
- The ***clinical relevance*** of plasmids lies in the fact that they code for antibiotic resistance, resistance to heavy metals, exotoxin production and sex pilus formation
- ***Transposons*** are '***jumping genes***' that move from one site to another either within or between the DNA molecules
- DNA probes used in ***diagnostic microbiology*** are labelled (with chemicals or radioactive phosphate groups) pieces of DNA that can be used to detect specific sequences of DNA of the pathogen (in the clinical sample) by pairing with the complementary bases
- The ***polymerase chain reaction*** is a widely used technique that ***enables multiple copies of a DNA molecule to be generated by enzymatic amplification of target DNA sequence***

IMPORTANT QUESTION

Write short notes on:
(a) Lac operon
(b) Mutation
(c) Transformation
(d) Transduction
(e) Conjugation
(f) Fertility factor
(g) Resistance plasmid
(h) Transposable genetic elements
(i) Polymerase chain reaction
(j) DNA probes

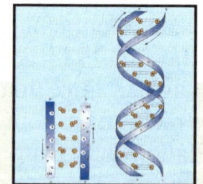

Chapter 8

Infection

Skin, alimentary tract and other mucous membranes are continually contaminated by microorganisms from the environment. Based on their relationship they can be divided into saprophytes and parasites.

Saprophytes (*sapros*, decayed; and *phyton*, plant) are free-living microbes that live on dead or decaying organic matter. They are found in soil and water. They are generally incapable of multiplying on living tissues. However, sometimes when host resistance is lowered some saprophytes like *Bacillus subtilis* may cause infection.

Parasites are the microorganisms that can enter and multiply in hosts. They are of two types – **micro-parasites** which include viruses, bacteria, fungi and protozoa, and **macroparasites** which include helminths.

Pathogens (*pathos*, suffering; and *gen*, produce; i.e., disease-producing) are the microorganisms which are capable of producing disease in man and animals. They are of two types – opportunists and primary pathogens.

Opportunistic pathogens rarely cause disease in individuals with intact immunological and anatomical defences. In immunocompromised hosts these bacteria are able to cause disease. Coagulase-negative staphylococci are normally carried on the human skin where they cause no harm. However, introduction of these organisms into anatomical sites in which they are not normally found may lead to infection.

Primary pathogens are the organisms which are capable of causing disease in previously healthy individuals with intact immunity.

Commensals (organisms of normal flora) are the microorganisms which live in complete harmony with the host without causing any damage to it. For the first nine months of life, the human foetus is in a sterile environment protected from microbes. This state of sterility comes to an abrupt end at the time of birth when the newborn is confronted with the mother's vaginal microbes and environmental organisms. The infant skin is colonized first, followed by the oropharynx, gastrointestinal tract and other mucosal surfaces. The organisms differ at different parts of the body (Table 8.1). This is due to local environmental factors which tend to select certain species. These organisms obtain their nutrition from the secretions and waste products of the body.

INFECTION

The lodgement and multiplication of a parasite in or on the tissue of a host is known as infection.

Table 8.1. Normal flora at various sites of the body

Site	Organisms
Skin	*Staphylococcus epidermidis, S. aureus, Candida* spp. *Clostridium* spp., diphtheroids, α-haemolytic and nonhaemolytic streptococci, *Acinetobacter* spp., *Bacteroides* spp.
Nares and nasopharynx	*S. aureus, S. epidermidis, Corynebacterium* spp., *Peptostreptococcus* spp., *Fusobacterium* spp., *Streptococcus* spp., *Neisseria* spp. including *N. meningitidis, S. pneumoniae, Prevotella* spp., yeasts
Mouth	*S. epidermidis, S. aureus, S. mitis, S. sanguis, S. salivarius, S. mutans, Peptostreptococcus* spp., *Veillonella* spp., *Actinomyces israelii, Bacteroides* spp., *Treponema denticola, T. refringens, Neisseria* spp., lactobacilli, *Candida* spp., *Entamoeba gingivalis, Trichomonas tenax*
Oropharynx	*S. aureus, S. epidermidis, S. pneumoniae, S. mitis, S. mutans, S. milleri, S. sanguis, S. salivarius, Moraxella catarrhalis, H. parainfluenzae, H. influenzae,* anaerobic streptococci, *Bacteroides* spp., *Prevotella* spp., *Porphyromonas* spp., *Fusobacterium necrophorum, S. pyogenes, N. meningitidis*
Gastrointestinal tract	*Bacteroides* spp., *Clostridium* spp., Enterobacteriaceae, *Fusobacterium* spp., *Peptostreptococcus* spp., *Peptococcus* spp., *S. aureus, Lactobacillus* spp., yeasts
Genitourinary tract	*Lactobacillus* spp., *Bacteroides* spp., *Clostridium* spp., *Peptostreptococcus* spp., *S. aureus, S. epidermidis,* diphtheroids, group B streptococci, *Candida albicans*
Conjunctiva	*Corynebacterium* spp., *S. epidermidis,* nonhaemolytic streptococci, neisseriae

Types of infection

1. *Primary infection:* Initial infection with a parasite is known as primary infection.
2. *Reinfection:* Subsequent infection with the same parasite in the same host is known as reinfection.
3. *Secondary infection:* When the primary infection lowers the resistance of the host and the latter gets infection with another organism it is known as secondary infection.
4. *Cross infection:* When a patient already suffering from a disease acquires a new infection it is known as cross infection.
5. *Nosocomial infection:* When cross infection is acquired by the patient during his stay in the hospital it is known as hospital-acquired or hospital-associated or nosocomial infection.
6. *Iatrogenic infection:* When the infection is acquired during therapeutic or investigative procedures, it is known as iatrogenic or physician-induced infection.
7. *Subclinical infection:* When the clinical symptoms of an infection are not apparent it is known as subclinical infection.
8. *Latent infection:* When a parasite, after infection, remains in a latent or hidden form for some time and it proliferates and produces clinical disease when the host resistance is lowered, it is known as latent infection.

SOURCES OF INFECTION

Infections may be endogenous, due to the organisms of the normal flora, and exogenous, due to the organisms derived from a source outside the body.

Endogenous infections

These are also referred to as autoinfections. Organisms of normal flora are usually non-pathogenic but occasionally they may lead to infection. For example, the most viridans streptococci are the normal flora of the mouth but when there is abnormality of the heart like rheumatic heart disease and injury to the oral cavity like tooth extraction or fractured mandible, these organisms enter into the blood stream and settle down on the heart leading to infective endocarditis. In both the above examples, two conditions are fulfilled: the organism initiating infection does so in an area of the body remote from its normal habitat and infection develops only where there is some tissue abnormality lowering local tissue resistance.

Exogenous infections

Most of the infections are exogenous in origin. The sources of exogenous infections are as under:

1. Human cases and carriers.

2. Animal cases and carriers.
3. Insects.
4. Environment.

1. Human cases and carriers

The commonest source of human infection is man himself who may be a patient or a carrier. Infections due to some organisms are acquired mainly or exclusively from ill persons, e.g., AIDS, syphilis, gonorrhoea, pulmonary tuberculosis, leprosy, hepatitis B, measles, mumps, influenza, polio-myelitis, etc.

A **carrier** is a person who harbours the pathogenic microorganisms without suffering from it. There are several types of carriers:

- *Healthy carrier:* One who harbours the pathogen but has never suffered from the disease caused by it.
- *Convalescent carrier:* One who has recovered from the disease but continues to harbour the pathogen on his body.
- *Temporary carrier:* When carrier state lasts for less than six months.
- *Chronic carrier:* When carrier state lasts for years or may be for the life of the patient.
- *Paradoxical carrier:* Who acquires the organisms from another carrier.
- *Contact carrier:* Who acquires the organisms from a patient.

Carriers are very important source of infection. For example, a person acquires organisms from a patient of meningococcal meningitis and becomes a contact carrier. He is then a source of infection for other persons (patient → carrier → patient).

2. Animal cases and carriers

Certain pathogens are capable of causing infection in both man and animals. Therefore, animals may act as a source of infection of such organisms. The infection may be acquired by contact with the animal, animal bite and ingestion of milk or meat. Infection in animals may be asymptomatic and these animals may serve as reservoir for human infections. These are known as **reservoir hosts**. Infectious diseases transmitted from animals to man, either directly or indirectly via a vector, are known as **zoonoses**.

In these infections man is generally an end host and there is rarely any secondary spread from the patient to other persons or back to animals.

3. Insects

Blood-sucking insects such as mosquitoes, ticks, mites, flies, and lice act as a source of a number of human and animal infections. Insects transmitting pathogens are known as **vectors**.

4. Environment

This includes soil, water and food. A few infective diseases of man are caused by saprophytic microbes derived from soil and vegetation. Some pathogens can survive in the soil for very long periods. For example, spores of tetanus and gas gangrene bacilli remain viable in the soil for several decades and serve as a source of infection. The normal habitat of these organisms is the human and animal intestines and they enter the soil through their faeces. Eggs of the parasites like roundworms and hookworms survive and develop in the soil and cause human infection. Water contaminated with polio virus, and hepatitis A and E viruses acts as a source of these infections.

MODES OF SPREAD OF INFECTION

Pathogenic organisms can spread from one host to another by a variety of mechanisms. These include:

1. Inhalation

Respiratory infections such as common cold, influenza, measles, mumps, tuberculosis and whooping cough are acquired by inhalation. These organisms are shed into the environment by patients in secretions of nose or throat during sneezing, coughing, talking and other forceful expiratory activities. These activities expel a spray of droplets. **Large droplets** more than 0.1 mm in diameter fly forwards and downwards from the mouth to the distance of a few feet and they reach the floor within a few seconds or they may fall on the eyes, face, mouth and clothes of the person standing in front of the producer of the spray. Small droplets, less than 0.1 mm in diameter, evaporate immediately to become minute residue or **droplet nuclei** and remain airborne and may be inhaled into the nose, throat or lungs.

2. Ingestion

Intestinal infections like hepatitis A and E and most of the parasitic infections are acquired by ingestion. The source of these infections is the faeces of the patients or carriers. The faeces containing pathogens may contaminate the water supply or it may contaminate the eatables through the houseflies.

3. Contact

Infection may be acquired by direct or indirect contact with the patient. Sexually transmitted diseases (STD) such as syphilis, gonorrhoea, trichomoniasis, herpes simplex type 2, hepatitis B and C, and AIDS are acquired by direct contact. The term **contagious disease** may be used for the disease acquired by direct contact, and disease acquired by other modes, through inanimate objects, as **infectious disease**.

4. Contamination of wounds

The infections may be caused by:

- Organisms present in the nose or throat of the patient himself or of nurses or doctors. Pathogenic staphylococci and streptococci derived from respiratory tract are important causes of wound and burn infection.
- Airborne spread of organisms from the infected wounds of other patients.
- Contact with infected hands, clothing or other articles.
- Spores of *Clostridium tetani* and *C. perfringens* are present in the soil. These get inoculated into the host tissue following severe wounds leading to tetanus and gas gangrene respectively.

5. Blood-sucking arthropods

In some diseases, blood-sucking insects play an important role in the spread of infection, e.g., malaria from one individual to another.

Insects normally become infected by biting a human or animal host in whose blood the causative organism is present. After this there is an interval, known as **extrinsic incubation period**, during which the insect is incapable of transmitting the infection. During this period the organisms multiply in the body of the insect.

Arthropods transmit infection in four ways:

- The infective agent gains access to the salivary glands of the insect and the organisms enter into the wound caused by the insect bite along with the saliva, e.g., transmission of malaria by female anopheles mosquito.
- The infective agent multiplies in the intestinal tract of the insect and during feeding it is regurgitated into the wound, e.g., transmission of bubonic plague by rat flea.
- The agent multiplies in the intestinal tract and is excreted in the faeces. These are deposited by the insect besides the wound when it bites and due to irritation caused by insect bite, are scratched by the victim into the wound, e.g., transmission of rickettsial diseases.
- The infective agent multiplies in the coelomic cavity of the insect and infection is due to contamination of the wound of bite with the coelomic fluid of an insect that has been crushed in its vicinity by the victim, e.g., transmission of louse-borne relapsing fever.

6. Iatrogenic and laboratory infections

If meticulous care in asepsis is not taken, infections like AIDS, and hepatitis B, C and D may sometimes be transmitted during therapeutic and investigative procedures such as injections, lumbar puncture, blood transfusion, dialysis, and heart and kidney transplant surgery. These are known as iatrogenic or physician-induced infections. Laboratory personnel handling infectious material and doing mouth-pipetting are particularly at risk.

7. Congenital

Some microorganisms like *Toxoplasma*, rubella virus, cytomegalovirus, herpes simplex virus, *Treponema pallidum*, human immunodeficiency virus, malaria parasites, etc. can cross the placental barrier and infect the foetus in utero. This is known as **vertical transmission**. This may result in abortion, miscarriage or still birth. Live infants may be born with manifestations of the disease.

FACTORS PREDISPOSING TO MICROBIAL PATHOGENICITY

Pathogenicity denotes the ability of a microbial species to cause disease, while the term **virulence** refers to the same property in a strain of the species. Bacterial virulence factors can be defined as the components and products of the bacterial cell which confer on the bacterium the potential to harm the host. Virulence may undergo spontaneous or induced variation.

Enhancement of virulence of a strain is termed as **exaltation**. This can be induced by serial passage of a strain in an experimental animal. Reduction of virulence of a strain is termed **attenuation**. This can be induced by repeated passage through unfavourable hosts and repeated culture in artificial media.

DETERMINANTS OF VIRULENCE

1. Adhesion

Many bacteria possess on their surface colonization factors or adhesins. These usually occur on fimbriae. Through adhesins bacteria attach specifically on the receptors present on the host cells. They are, therefore, responsible for tissue tropism. Adhesion is necessary to avoid innate host defence mechanisms such as peristalsis in the gut and the flushing action of mucus, saliva and urine which remove nonadherent bacteria. Loss of adhesins may render a strain avirulent.

2. Invasion of tissues

Invasiveness signifies the ability of an organism to penetrate a tissue after it adheres to a cell surface. Some bacteria can invade tissues in the absence of physical injury, e.g., *Neisseria meningitidis* in nasal epithelium and salmonellae in intestinal epithelium. These organisms are endocytosed by epithelial cells, transported across these cells within vacuoles and released into the submucosal space, from which they invade the underlying tissues.

3. Capsules

Cell wall in many bacteria is enclosed by a protective gelatinous covering layer known as capsule. It contributes to the virulence of the bacteria by inhibiting phagocytosis.

4. Streptococcal M protein

The M protein present on the surface of *S. pyogenes* binds both fibrinogen and fibrin to the bacterial cell wall thus masking the bacterial receptors from complement.

5. Bacterial toxins

These are substances produced by or present in bacteria, which have a direct toxic action on tissue cells. Two major types of toxin have been described – endotoxins and exotoxins (Table 8.2).

Endotoxins

They are components of the outer membrane of Gram-negative bacteria. They are lipopolysaccharide (LPS) in nature and are released from the bacterial surface by natural lysis of the bacteria or by disintegration of the organisms *in vitro*. The endotoxic activity of LPS resides in its lipid A moiety. The latter is not destroyed by autoclaving, hence infusion of a sterile solution containing endotoxin can cause serious illness. They are poor antigens and the toxicity is not completely neutralized by the homologous antibodies. They cannot be toxoided. Endotoxins exert a wide spectrum of effects on the host, the most dramatic of which are fever and the shock syndrome associated with Gram-negative bacterial sepsis. Man is particularly sensitive to minute amounts of endotoxins and often a mild Gram-negative bacterial infection will cause fever. Larger amounts of endotoxin may cause irreversible shock seen in association with a fulminating Gram-negative bacteraemia.

Exotoxins

They are produced extracellularly by both Gram-positive and Gram-negative bacteria. They are highly potent even in small amounts and constitute some of the most poisonous substances known. **Botulinum toxin is the most poisonous followed by tetanus toxin.** Minimum lethal dose of botulinum toxin for a mouse is 0.03 ng and for humans may be 1 μg. It has been estimated that 3 kg of this toxin can kill all the inhabitants of the world. Exotoxins are heat-labile, protein in nature and have enzymatic activity. Some exotoxins can be partially denatured by

Table 8.2. Differences between exotoxins and endotoxins

Exotoxins	Endotoxins
1. Proteins with high molecular weight ranging from 10,000–900,000.	Lipopolysaccharide in nature. Lipid A portion is probably responsible for the toxicity.
2. Heat-labile. The toxicity is destroyed by heating above 60°C.	Heat-stable; can withstand heat over 60°C without losing toxicity.
3. Highly antigenic; stimulate formation of antitoxin which neutralizes toxin.	Weakly antigenic; do not stimulate the formation of anti-toxin. Antibodies against only polysaccharide component are raised.
4. Actively secreted by the cells; diffuse into the surrounding medium.	Form integral part of the cell wall; do not diffuse into surrounding medium. These can be obtained only by cell lysis.
5. Converted into toxoid by formaldehyde.	Cannot be toxoided.
6. Action often enzymic.	No enzymic action.
7. Specific pharmacological effect for each exotoxin.	Non-specific action of all endotoxins.
8. Highly specific for particular tissue, e.g., tetanus toxin for CNS.	Non-specific in action.
9. Very high potency (one mg of botulinum or tetanus toxin can kill more than one million guinea-pigs).	Low potency (one mg of extracted somatic antigen can kill one mouse).
10. Do not produce fever in the host.	Usually produce fever in the host.
11. Produced by both Gram-positive bacteria and Gram-negative bacteria.	Produced by Gram-negative bacteria only.
12. Frequently controlled by extrachromosomal genes (e.g., plasmids).	Synthesis directed by chromosomal genes.

treatment with formaldehyde to generate toxoids which lack toxicity but retain antigenicity inducing protective immunity when used as vaccines. Some exotoxins like diphtheria toxin consist of two fragments A and B. The toxin binds to the specific receptors, on the host cell surface, through fragment B (binding) and then toxic or enzymatic A fragment causes cell damage.

6. Resistance to killing by phagocytic cells

Some pathogens like tubercle bacilli can be readily ingested (phagocytosed) by macrophages and other phagocytes but they resist intracellular killing by preventing fusion of phagosome with lysosome. These organisms rather multiply inside these cells. Other bacteria such as *Staphylococcus aureus* and *N. gonorrhoeae* are able to resist the action of lysosomal components following fusion.

KEY FACTS

- *Pathogens* are microorganisms which are capable of producing disease in man

- *Commensals* (organisms of normal flora) are the microorganisms which live in complete harmony with the host without causing any damage to it
- **Lodgement and multiplication** of a parasite in or on the tissue of a host is known as *infection*
- Infection may be *endogenous*, due to the organisms of the normal flora, and *exogenous*, due to the organisms derived from a source outside the body
- *Sources* of exogenous infections are human cases and carriers, animal cases and carriers, insects and environment
- **Endotoxins are the lipopolysaccharide** components of cell walls of Gram-negative bacteria and hence, by definition, Gram-positive bacteria do not have endotoxins
- **Exotoxins** are **produced by both Gram-positive and Gram-negative bacteria**
- **Biological effects of endotoxins** of bacteria include fever, hypotension, activation of complement cascade, disseminated intravascular coagulation and increased phagocytic activity of macrophages

- **Attenuated exotoxins** of bacteria are called toxoids; they are not toxic but antigenic and hence used in protective vaccines
- Pathogenic organisms can spread from one host to another by inhalation, ingestion, contact, contamination of wounds, blood sucking arthropods, and by vertical transmission
- Infectious diseases are responsible for 30% of the world's disease burden
- Toxins of bacteria are classified as **endotoxins** and **exotoxins.**

IMPORTANT QUESTIONS

1. Discuss:
   (a) Sources of infection
   (b) Spread of infection
2. Tabulate differences between exotoxins and endotoxins.
3. Enumerate and discuss determinants of virulence of bacteria.

SECTION B
Immunogy

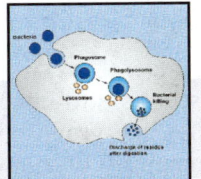

Chapter 9

Immunity

Immunity refers to resistance of a host to pathogens and their toxic products. It is of two types:

1. Innate immunity
   (a) Non-specific ⎤ Species, Racial, Individual
   (b) Specific ⎦
2. Acquired immunity
   (a) Active
      • Natural
      • Artificial
   (b) Passive
      • Natural
      • Artificial

1. INNATE IMMUNITY

It is due to genetic and constitutional make-up of an individual. Prior contact with microorganisms or their products is not essential. It may be specific against a particular organism or non-specific. Innate immunity may be further divided into species, racial or individual immunity.

Species immunity

It is total or relative resistance to a pathogen shown by all the members of a species. For example, all human beings are resistant to plant pathogens and many animal pathogens. Rat is strikingly resistant to diphtheria whilst guinea-pig and man are highly susceptible. This is due to physical and biochemical differences between the tissues of different host species which determine if a pathogen can multiply in them.

Racial immunity

Within a species, there may be marked racial differences in resistance to infection, e.g., in the USA, Negroes are more susceptible to tuberculosis than whites. Racial differences in immunity are known to be genetic in origin. A hereditary (genetic) abnormality of red blood cells (sickling) confers immunity to infection by *Plasmodium falciparum* because such RBCs cannot be parasitized by these parasites. This may provide survival advantage to such individuals in malaria-infested areas.

Individual immunity

Different individuals in a race differ in their resistance to microbial infections. The genetic basis of individual immunity is apparent from the observation that if one homozygous twin develops tuberculosis, there is a 75% chance that the other twin will develop overt tuberculosis. In contrast, for heterozygous twins, there is only 33% chance that the second twin will contract overt disease.

Factors influencing innate immunity

1. Age

In general, very young and very old are more susceptible to infectious diseases than persons in other age groups. This appears to be due to the immaturity of immune system in very young and gradual waning of immune response in very old. Foetus in utero is protected from maternal infection by placental barrier. But some pathogens such as HIV cross this barrier leading to foetal infection, while others like *Toxoplasma gondii*, rubella and cytomegalovirus lead to congenital malformations.

Newborn animals are more susceptible to experimental infection than adult animals, e.g., coxsackievirus causes fatal infection in suckling mice but not in adult mice. On the other hand, in many diseases such as measles, mumps, poliomyelitis and chickenpox, the clinical illness is more severe in adults than in children. This may be due to more active immune response which leads to greater tissue damage.

2. Hormonal influences and sex

There is an increased susceptibility to infection in endocrine disorders such as diabetes mellitus, hypothyroidism and adrenal dysfunction. The reason for this increased susceptibility is not known but it may be related to hormone activity. For example, glucocorticoids are antiinflammatory agents. They inhibit the ability of phagocytes to ingest foreign particles. Staphylococcal, streptococcal and certain fungal infections such as candidiasis, occur more frequently in diabetics. Pregnant women are more susceptible to microbial infections due to increased steroid levels during pregnancy. In general, incidence and death rate from infectious diseases is greater in males than in females. However, in case of hepatitis A and whooping cough, morbidity and mortality is higher in females than in males.

3. Nutritional factors

Both antibody-mediated and cell-mediated immunity are lowered in malnutrition. Protein calorie malnutrition:

- lowers factor B and C3 of the complement system,
- decreases the interferon response, and
- inhibits neutrophil activity.

Similarly, deficiency of vitamin A, vitamin C, folic acid and zinc predisposes to certain infections.

Mechanism of innate immunity

1. Mechanical barriers and surface secretions

The intact skin and the mucous membranes provide a high degree of protection against pathogens. If skin is damaged, as in case of injury or burns, infections may be a serious problem. Skin is a very effective barrier because of unusual structure of outermost epithelial layer which is composed mainly of keratin which is indigestible by most microorganisms, and thus protects the living cells of the epidermis from microorganisms and their toxins. Even more important than this are the fatty acids secreted by the sebaceous glands, propionic acid produced by the normal flora of the skin and high salt concentration in drying sweat. Secretions from sebaceous glands contain both saturated and unsaturated fatty acids that kill many bacteria and fungi.

We have a specialized epithelial lining in our respiratory and gastrointestinal tract to minimize infection. Mucous membrane is composed of specialized epithelial cells which secrete a sticky substance called mucus. This traps dust. In respiratory tract there are also ciliated cells, which move the dust-laden mucus up and out of respiratory tract (**mucociliary escalator**) enabling it to be swallowed or coughed out. When swallowed they are destroyed in the stomach's highly acidic environment and digestive juices. Should a pathogen survive in stomach, it usually cannot penetrate mucous membrane lining the entire gastrointestinal tract and if it escapes the respiratory mucociliary escalator, it would be met by phagocytes lining the alveoli.

The mouth is constantly bathed in saliva which has an inhibitory effect on many microorganisms. Tubercle bacilli are resistant to phagocytosis and thus might escape attack by macrophages in the alveoli. Nicotine from cigarettes can paralyse the mucociliary escalator. This exposes cigarette smokers to bacterial infection leading to chronic bronchitis.

Gastrointestinal tract

Four factors protect gastrointestinal tract from infection:

1. Physical barrier produced by mucus secreting epithelial cells.
2. Secretory IgA antibodies produced here.
3. Highly acidic environment of stomach may hydrolyze microbial invaders.
4. Already established normal flora such as *Escherichia coli* serves to inhibit invasion and repopulation by pathogenic microparasites. However, normal flora is a double-edged weapon. If body resistance is lowered it may lead to opportunistic infections.

Urogenital tract

Kidneys produce sterile urine which travels down the ureter to the bladder and passes out through the urethral opening. Although urethra has normal flora, invading microorganisms usually do not gain access to the bladder. It is mainly due to frequent flushing of urethra by sterile urine. However, if organisms have mechanism to attach to epithelial cells lining the tract even frequent flushing might not evacuate them. Because of short urethra, bladder infection is more common in females than in males.

Conjunctiva

Conjunctiva is continually being assaulted by microbe-laden dust. Whenever the dust hits the conjunctiva we blink and tears are produced. Tears mechanically wash away the particles and a hydrolytic enzyme, lysozyme, destroys most viruses and bacteria.

2. Humoral defence mechanisms

Many microbicidal substances are present in the tissues and body fluids. These are non-specific. There is no specific recognition of the microorganism and the response is not enhanced by re-exposure to the same antigen. They are responsible for innate immunity. Following are the bactericidal substances present in the tissues and body fluids:

Lysozyme

This is a basic protein of low molecular weight (approximately 20,000 daltons) found in high concentrations in polymorphonuclear leucocytes as well as in most tissue fluids except CSF, sweat and urine. It functions as a mucolytic enzyme, splitting sugars of the structural mucopeptide of the cell wall of many Gram-positive bacteria leading to their lysis. It may also play a role in the intracellular destruction of some Gram-negative bacteria.

Basic polypeptides

Several basic proteins, derived from tissues and blood cells, possess antibacterial activity. These include spermine and spermidine which can kill tubercle bacilli and some staphylococci. Other antibacterial substances include arginine and lysine-containing proteins, protamine and histone. Basic polypeptides such as leukins extracted from leucocytes and plakins from platelets have antibacterial effect.

Complement

(See Chapter 11)

Interferons

These are a family of antiviral agents produced by cells stimulated by live or killed viruses and certain other inducers. A number of molecules have been described. α and β interferons are part of innate immunity, and γ interferon is produced by T cells as part of acquired immunity.

3. Cellular defence mechanisms

Microparasites that penetrate the physical barriers are confronted, in addition to humoral defence mechanism, by non-specific cellular defences. Cellular defence against microparasites is provided by **phagocytes** and a subpopulation of lymphocytes known as **natural killer (NK) cells**. Phagocytes are classified into microphages and macrophages. **Microphages** are polymorphonuclear leucocytes and **macrophages** consist of histiocytes which are the wandering amoeboid cells seen in tissues, fixed reticuloendothelial cells and monocytes of blood. In connective tissue they are known as histiocytes, in kidneys as mesangial cells, in bones as osteoclast, in brain as microglial cells, in lungs as alveolar macrophages, in liver as Kupffer cells, and in spleen, lymph nodes and thymus as sinus lining macrophages.

Phagocytic cells reach the site of inflammation in large numbers. They engulf, kill and digest bacteria. On the other hand, viral invasion is countered by NK cells. Residing in the peripheral lymphoid organs, NK cells recognize virus-infected cells, bind to them and subsequently lyse them. NK cells have also been implicated in host defence against cancers. They are thought to recognize the changes in the cell membranes of transformed cells in a mechanism similar to that used to combat virus infection. Fungi are confronted by polymorphonuclear leucocytes, macrophages and NK cells.

Phagocytic cell engulfs microparasite by extending pseudopodia around it. These fuse and microorganism is internalized into a vacuole (**phagosome**) which fuses with lysosomes found in the cell to form **phagolysosome** (Fig. 9.1). Microparasites are subjected to the lytic enzymes in the phagolysosome and are destroyed.

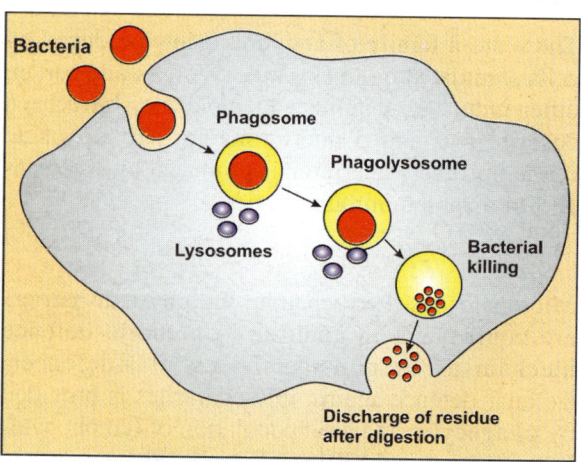

Fig. 9.1. Events of phagocytosis.

Eosinophils are polymorphonuclear leucocytes with cytoplasmic granules and bilobed nucleus. Their number in the blood of normal individuals is 3–5%. But in patients with parasitic infections and allergies their number increases. They are not efficient phagocytic cells. However, their granules possess molecules that are toxic to parasites. Large parasites such as helminths cannot be internalized. Therefore, they must be killed extracellularly.

4. Fever

A rise in temperature following infection is a natural defence mechanism. It inhibits or kills the infecting organisms. Before penicillin era, therapeutic induction of fever was employed for destruction of *Treponema pallidum* in patients suffering from syphilis. Fever also stimulates production of interferon and helps in recovery from virus infection.

5. Inflammation

It is the cellular and vascular response to injury such as invasion by an infectious agent, exposure to a noxious chemical or physical trauma. The signs of inflammation are redness, swelling, heat, pain and disturbed or altered functions. Inflammation leads to vasodilation, increased vascular permeability and cellular infiltration. **Polymorphonuclear leucocytes** escape into the tissues by diapedesis and accumulate in large numbers attracted by the chemotactic substances released at the site of injury. They then phagocytose microorganisms and their products. Because of increased vascular permeability, there is an **outpouring of plasma** which helps to dilute the toxic products present. In addition, plasma contains a number of non-specific (complement, properdin, beta lysin, leukins and plakins) and specific (antibodies) inhibitors.

2. ACQUIRED IMMUNITY

Most potential pathogens are checked by innate immunity before they establish an overt infection. If these defences are breached the acquired immune system is called into play. The resistance that an individual acquires during his lifetime is known as acquired immunity. It is antigen-specific and may be antibody-mediated or cell-mediated. It is of two types – active immunity and passive immunity (Table 9.1 and Fig. 9.2).

Both active and passive immunity may be further divided into natural and artificial.

Active immunity

This involves the active involvement of the person's own immune apparatus leading to the synthesis of antibodies and/or the production of immunocompetent cells (ICCs). It appears only after a **lag (latent) period**, i.e., the time

Table 9.1. Differences between active and passive immunity

Active immunity	Passive immunity
1. Produced actively by host's immune system as a result of antigenic stimulation.	Received passively by the host. No participation of host's immune system.
2. Induced by infection or by contact with antigens.	Conferred by administration of antibodies.
3. Long-lasting.	Transient.
4. Immunity effective only after a lag period, i.e., time required for generation of antibodies and immuno-competent cells.	Immunity effective immediately.
5. During development of active immunity there is often a negative phase during which the level of measurable immunity may actually be lower than before antigenic stimulus. This is due to antigen combining with the pre-existing antibodies and lowering its level.	No negative phase.
6. Immunological memory present, therefore, subsequent challenge (secondary response) is more effective.	No immunological memory. Subsequent administration of antibodies is less effective due to immune elimination.
7. More effective and confers better protection.	Less effective and provides inferior immunity.
8. Not applicable in immunodeficient individuals.	Applicable in immunodeficient individuals

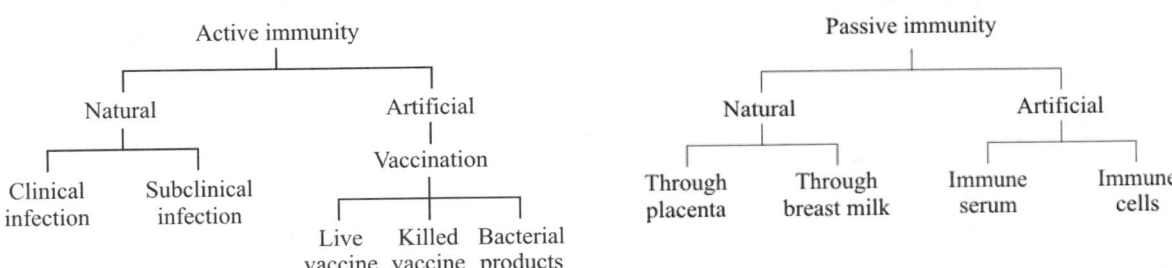

Fig. 9.2. Types of immunity.

required for generation of antibodies and ICCs. During development of active immunity there is often a negative phase during which the level of measurable immunity may actually be lower than before antigenic stimulus. This is due to antigen combining with preexisting antibodies and lowering its level.

If an individual who has been actively immunized against an antigen, experiences the same antigen subsequently, the immune response occurs more quickly and more abundantly than during the first encounter. This is known as **secondary response**.

Immune system is able to retain the memory of a prior antigenic exposure for long periods and produces a secondary type response when encountered with the same antigen. This is known as **immunological memory**.

Natural active immunity

Natural active immunity results either from a subclinical or clinical infection. A large majority of adults in the developing countries possess natural active immunity to poliomyelitis due to repeated subclinical infections with poliovirus during childhood. Some infections like diphtheria, whooping cough, measles and mumps induce long-lasting immunity. Others such as common cold and influenza confer immunity which lasts for a short time.

- In case of influenza, short-lived immunity is due to the ability of influenza virus to undergo antigenic variation, so that immunity following first infection is not effective against second infection due to an antigenically different virus.

- In common cold the apparent lack of immunity is because the same clinical picture can be produced by infection with a large number of different viruses. In general, immunity following bacterial infections is generally less permanent than that following viral infections.
- In some infections like syphilis and malaria, immunity lasts only till original infection remains active. This is known as **concomitant immunity** (previously called **premunition** or **infection-immunity**). Once the disease is cured the patient becomes susceptible again.

Artificial active immunity

This is the resistance induced by vaccines which are preparations of live or killed microorganisms or their products:

1. **Bacterial vaccines**
   (a) *Live:*
      - B.C.G. for tuberculosis
      - Ty 21a for typhoid
   (b) *Killed:*
      - TAB for enteric fever
      - Cholera
      - Pertussis
   (c) Bacterial products
      - Tetanus toxoid
      - Diphtheria toxoid
      - Capsular polysaccharide of meningococci
      - Capsular polysaccharide of *Haemophilus influenzae* type b
2. **Viral vaccines**
   (a) *Live:*
      - Sabin vaccine for poliomyelitis or oral polio vaccine (OPV)
      - 17D vaccine for yellow fever
      - MMR vaccine for measles, mumps, rubella
      - Varicella-zoster
   (b) *Killed:*
      - Salk vaccine for poliomyelitis
      - Neural and non-neural vaccines for rabies
      - Influenza
      - Hepatitis A
      - Hepatitis B
      - Japanese encephalitis

Live vaccines initiate a sort of mini infection without causing disease. The immunity following vaccination, therefore, parallels that following natural infection. However, it is of lower order than that induced by infection. Since live vaccines undergo limited multiplication in the body, therefore, number of organisms required in a dose is less; single doses may be sufficient and they are relatively cheaper. Live vaccines may be administered orally (e.g., oral polio-vaccine). They provide more effective and more lasting immunity than killed vaccines. Some of them can be given as combined vaccines, e.g., measles, mumps, rubella (MMR) vaccine.

Killed vaccines are generally less immunogenic than live vaccines and protection lasts only for a short period. Therefore, they have to be administered repeatedly. At least two doses are required. First dose is known as **primary** and subsequent doses as **booster doses**. In killed vaccines since the organisms are killed, therefore, larger number of these are required in each dose. Oral route for killed vaccines is generally not effective. Antibody response to killed vaccines is improved by addition of adjuvants, for example, aluminium phosphate adjuvant vaccine for cholera.

Passive immunity

The immunity that is transferred to a recipient in a ready-made form is known as passive immunity. Here the recipient's immune system plays no active role. There is no lag or latent period, the immunity is effective immediately after passive immunization. There is no negative phase. It confers only transient immunity lasting usually for days or weeks till the antibodies are metabolized and eliminated. There is no secondary type response. Rather subsequent administration of antibodies is less effective due to **immune elimination**.

Following first injection of antibody, its elimination is only by metabolic breakdown but during subsequent injections its elimination is much quicker because metabolic breakdown is combined with immune elimination as it combines with antibodies to horse serum that would have been produced following first injection. This happens when horse (foreign) serum is used. Immune elimination is not a problem when human serum is used. Because of its immediate action it is employed where instant immunity is required as in case of protection against tetanus, gas gangrene and diphtheria following exposure.

Natural passive immunity

This is the resistance transferred from mother to foetus through placenta. IgG antibodies can cross placental barrier to reach the foetus. After birth, immunoglobulins are passed to the newborn through the breast milk. Human colostrum is rich in IgA antibodies which are resistant to digestion in stomach and small intestine, hence confers immunity in the neonate up to three months of age. Human foetus acquires some ability to synthesize IgM antibodies from twentieth week of gestation, but its immunological capacity is still inadequate at birth. It is only by the age of three months that the infant acquires a satisfactory level of immunological independence. Until then, maternal antibodies give passive protection against infectious diseases of the infant.

Transport of antibodies across placenta is an active process, therefore, the concentration of antibodies in foetal blood may sometimes be higher than that seen in the mother. These antibodies are generally against all common infectious diseases in the locality. Therefore, most paediatric infections are commoner after the age of three months when maternal immunoglobulins disappear. By active immunization of mother during pregnancy the immune status of the neonate can be improved. Therefore, immunization of pregnant women with tetanus toxoid is recommended in countries where neonatal tetanus is common.

Artificial passive immunity

This is the immunity transferred passively to the recipient by administration of antibodies. This is done by administration of hyperimmune sera of man or animals. For example, tetanus antitoxin is prepared in horses by active immunization of horses with tetanus toxoid, bleeding them and separating the serum. Similarly, diphtheria antitoxin and gas gangrene antitoxin are also prepared. However, since these antitoxins are foreign proteins and are liable to

cause serious or even fatal hypersensitivity reactions, these should be administered only after testing for hypersensitivity. After first administration, it is removed by metabolism and following subsequent injections by metabolism and immune elimination. Therefore, immunity conferred is short-lived.

Sera collected from patients convalescing from infectious diseases contain high levels of specific antibodies. Convalescent sera have, therefore, been employed for passive immunization against viral infections such as measles and rubella. Sera of healthy adults contain antibodies against infectious agents prevalent in a community. Therefore, sera from a large number of individuals can be collected and used for passive immunization. Placenta provides a convenient source of human immunoglobulins. Human immune serum does not lead to any hypersensitivity reaction, therefore, there is no immune elimination and its half-life is more than that of animal sera. However, with human serum there is a grave risk of transmission of human immunodeficiency virus and hepatitis B, C and D viruses.

Indications of passive immunization

- To provide immediate protection to a non-immune individual exposed to an infection, when there is insufficient time for active immunization, e.g., administration of tetanus antitoxin and gas gangrene antitoxin to a non-immune individual with crushing roadside injury, and administration of diphtheria antitoxin to a non-immune child exposed to diphtheria.

- Administration of anti-Rh (D) IgG to Rh-negative mother, bearing Rh-positive baby at the time of delivery to prevent Rh isoimmunization.

- For suppression of active immunity, when it is injurious, for example, administration of anti-lymphocytic serum for suppression of lymphocytes in transplantation surgery to suppress the immune response towards the transplant.

Combination of active and passive immunization may also be employed. For example, a person exposed to tetanus may be injected tetanus antitoxin on one arm and tetanus toxoid on the other with separate syringes followed by full course of tetanus toxoid. Diphtheria antitoxin and diphtheria toxoid can also be practised similarly.

ADOPTIVE IMMUNITY

Injection of immunologically competent lymphocytes is known as adoptive immunity. Instead of whole lymphocytes, an extract of immunologically competent lymphocytes known as **transfer factor** can be used. This has been attempted in the treatment of lepromatous leprosy.

LOCAL IMMUNITY

This means immunity at a particular site, generally the site of invasion and multiplication of pathogen. For example, in case of poliomyelitis, parenteral vaccine provides systemic immunity. The antibodies neutralize virus only after blood invasion. It does not prevent multiplication of the virus at the site of entry, the gut mucosa, and its faecal excretion. However, when live oral vaccine is given it leads to local immunity. Similarly, live influenza vaccine administered intranasally provides local immunity while killed influenza vaccine evokes humoral antibody response. Local immunity is conferred by **secretory IgA antibodies** produced locally by plasma cells present on mucosal surfaces or in secretory glands.

HERD IMMUNITY

Overall level of immunity in a community is known as herd immunity. When a large number of individuals in a community (herd) are immune to a pathogen the herd immunity to a pathogen is said to be satisfactory. When herd immunity is low, epidemics are likely to occur on the introduction of the pathogen. This is due to the fact that a larger number of individuals are susceptible.

KEY FACTS

- The *innate system* of immune defence consists of a formidable *barrier to entry* and *second-line phagocytes and circulatory soluble factors*

- *The cells which mediate immunity include lymphocytes and phagocytes*. Lymphocytes recognize antigens on pathogens. Phagocytes internalize pathogens and degrade them
- The main phagocytic cells are *polymorphonuclear neutrophils* and *macrophages*
- *Specificity and memory* are two essential features of acquired immunity. The immune system mounts a more effective immune response on second and subsequent encounters with a particular antigen
- *Phagocytic cells* reach the site of inflammation in large numbers. They engulf, kill and digest bacteria. On the other hand viral invasion is countered by NK cells
- The *influx of polymorphs* and *increase in vascular permeability* constitute the potent antimicrobial acute inflammatory response
- Natural infection may produce **lifelong protection** against reinfection with the same pathogen, with induction of memory T and B lymphocytes
- Some infectious diseases can be prevented by vaccination in childhood with live attenuated or inactivated pathogens or their products
- Injection of immunologically competent lymphocytes is known as *adoptive immunity*
- Immunity at the site of invasion and multiplication of a pathogen is known as *local immunity*
- Overall level of immunity in a community is known as *herd immunity*
- Immune system exists to protect the body against threats from outside (pathogens) and inside (cancer)
- Components of innate immune system include *phagocytes, natural killer cells*, the *alternative complement pathway* and *inflammation*

IMPORTANT QUESTIONS

1. Discuss mechanism of innate immunity.
2. Tabulate differences between active and passive immunity.
3. Write short notes on:
   (a) Innate immunity
   (b) Acquired immunity

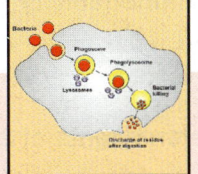

Chapter 10

Antigen and Antibody

ANTIGEN

Antigens (*anti*body *gen*erators) are substances that can stimulate an immune response and, given the opportunity, react specifically by binding with the effector molecules (antibodies) and effector cells (lymphocytes) produced. Most antigens are proteins, but some are carbohydrates, lipids or nucleic acids. Some antigens are more immunogenic or capable of eliciting an immune response, than others. Some antigens such as proteins may possess a number of small chemical groups that are called antigenic determinants or **epitopes** which can bind specifically to antigen binding site (**paratope**) of the antibody molecule (Fig. 10.1) and T cell receptors. Each determinant can stimulate the formation of a particular kind of antibody or effector cell. Thus a pure protein antigen may give rise to many distinct antibodies and effector cells.

Incomplete antigen or hapten

This is a chemical substance of low molecular weight that cannot induce an immune response by itself. Nevertheless, haptens can induce a response if combined with larger molecules (normally proteins) which serve as carriers. This response requires assistance from T helper (Th) lymphocytes. In

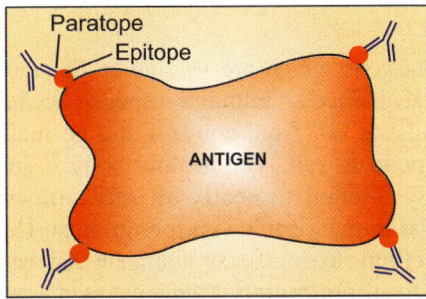

Fig. 10.1. Epitopes of antigen and paratopes of antibody.

contrast to complete antigens, haptens contain a single epitope. In response to hapten carried on carrier particle, antibodies are produced not only against the hapten but also against the carrier particle. Haptens are of two types:

1. **Complex haptens:** These can combine with specific antibodies to form precipitate, e.g., capsular polysaccharide of pneumococci.
2. **Simple haptens:** These combine with specific antibodies but no precipitate is produced (non-precipitating). This is due to the univalent character of simple haptens, whereas complex haptens are polyvalent, since it is assumed that precipitation requires the antigen to have two or more antibody combining sites.

Immunogenicity

This refers to the ability of an antigen to stimulate an immune response.

Determinants of antigenicity

1. Size

Antigenicity depends upon the molecular weight. Very large molecules such as haemocyanins are highly antigenic and particles with low molecular weight (less than 5,000) are non-antigenic or feebly so. Low molecular weight substances may be rendered antigenic by absorbing them on large inert particles such as bentonite or kaolin. Some low molecular weight substances such as picryl chloride and penicillin may be antigenic when applied on the skin, probably by combining with tissue proteins.

2. Foreignness

Only antigens which are foreign to the individual (non-self) induce an immune response because host distinguishes self from non-self and normally does not respond to self. The healthy body is immunologically tolerant to nearly all self antigens, that would be immunogenic in a foreign host. However, under certain circumstances tolerance may be broken leading to **autoimmunity**. Antigenicity of a substance is related to the degree of its foreignness. Antigens from other individuals of the same species are less antigenic than those from other species.

3. Chemical nature

Proteins and polysaccharides are most antigenic. Lipids and nucleic acids are less antigenic. Their antigenicity is enhanced by combination with proteins. However, all proteins are not antigenic. A well-known exception is gelatin. The presence of an aromatic radical appears to be essential for antigenicity and the absence of aromatic amino acids such as tyrosine in gelatin is responsible for its non-antigenicity.

4. Susceptibility to tissue enzymes

Only those substances which can be metabolized and are susceptible to the action of tissue enzymes behave as antigens. Antigens introduced into the body are degraded by the host into the fragments of appropriate size containing antigenic determinants. Phagocytosis and intracellular enzymes appear to play an essential role in breaking down antigens into immunogenic fragments. Substances insusceptible to tissue enzymes such as polystyrene latex and synthetic polypeptides which are not metabolized in the body, are not antigenic.

Antigenic specificity

It is determined by chemical grouping and acid radicals. Antigenic specificity varies with the position of antigenic determinant, i.e., whether it is in *ortho*, *meta* or *para* positions. However, antigenic specificity is not absolute. Cross reactions can occur between antigens which bear stereochemical similarities.

Species specificity

Tissues of all individuals in a species contain species-specific antigens. However, some degree of cross-reactivity is seen between antigens from related species. **Species-specific antigens possess forensic applications in the identification of species of blood and seminal stains.**

Isospecificity

Isoantigens are antigens found in some but not all members of a species. On the basis of isoantigens a species may be divided into different groups. The best example of isoantigens is human blood group antigens on the basis of which all humans can be divided into different groups: A, B, AB and O. Each of these groups may be further divided into Rh-positive or Rh-negative. **This carries clinical importance in blood transfusion, isoimmunization during pregnancy and disputed paternity.**

Histocompatibility antigens

These are the antigens present on the cells of each individual of a species. Histocompatibility typing is essential in organ/tissue transplantation from one individual to another within a species. These antigens are associated with plasma membrane of tissue cells and are responsible for evoking immunological response against graft unless it is antigenically identical to that of the recipient. These antigens are encoded by genes known as histocompatibility genes which collectively constitute **major histo-compatibility complex** (MHC). These are located on short arm of chromosome 6. MHC products present on the surface of leucocytes are known as **human leucocyte-associated (HLA) antigens**. These have been studied extensively in organ transplantation. Major histocompatibility antigens in man and mouse are known as HLA and H2 respectively (see Chapter 17).

Autospecificity

Autologous or self antigens are ordinarily non-antigenic. However, hidden or sequestrated antigens that are not normally found free in circulation or tissue fluids are not recognized as self antigens. For example, **lens protein** which is normally confined within the capsule of the lens, and antigens that are absent during the embryonic life and develop later, such as **spermatozoa**, are also not recognized as self antigens. But if these antigens are released into the tissues, as for instance following injury to lens or damage to the testis, antibodies are produced against them. This is one of the mechanisms of pathogenesis of autoimmune diseases. Cells or tissues may undergo **antigenic alteration** as a result of infection or irradiation and may thus become immunogenic leading to **autoimmunity**.

Organ specificity

Some organs such as brain, kidney and lens protein of different species share the same antigens. These are known as organ-specific antigens. The neuroparalytic complications following antirabic vaccination, with neural vaccines, are a consequence of brain-specific antigens shared by sheep and man.

Heterogenetic (heterophile) specificity

Same or closely related antigens occurring in different biological species, classes and kingdoms are known as heterogenetic or heterophile antigens. The best example of such heterophile antigens is the **Forssman antigen** which is a lipid carbohydrate complex widely distributed in man, animals, birds, plants and bacteria. It is absent in rabbits, therefore, anti-forssman antibody can be prepared in these animals. Examples of tests based on the principle of heterophile antigens used in diagnostic serology are as under:

1. Weil-Felix reaction

It is an agglutination test in which patient sera are tested for agglutinins to O antigens of nonmotile strains of *Proteus* OX2, OX19 and OXK. Cross reaction between O antigen of these strains of *Proteus* and certain rickettsial antigens is the basis of this test.

2. Paul-Bunnell test

In patients with infectious mononucleosis heterophile antibodies appear in the serum of the patient. These antibodies agglutinate sheep erythrocytes. This test is known as Paul-Bunnell test.

3. Cold agglutinin test

Agglutination of human O group erythrocytes at 4°C by the sera of patients suffering from primary atypical pneumonia.

4. Agglutination of Streptococcus MG

Agglutination of *Streptococcus* MG by the sera of the patients of primary atypical pneumonia.

ANTIBODY

Antibodies or immunoglobulins (Igs) are γ globulins which are produced in response to antigenic stimulation. These react specifically with the antigens which stimulated their production. Igs are produced by plasma cells and to some extent by lymphocytes also. All antibodies are Igs, but all Igs (e.g., myeloma proteins) are not antibodies. On the basis of physicochemical and antigenic structure Igs can be divided into five distinct classes or isotypes namely IgG, IgA, IgM, IgD and IgE. They differ from each other in size, charge, carbohydrate content and amino acid composition. Within certain classes there are subclasses that show slight differences in structure and function from other members of the class. If injected into animals they induce the formation of antibodies that can be used to differentiate between the different isotypes serologically.

Antibody Structure

IgG has been studied extensively and serves as a model of basic structural unit of all Igs. It is a Y-shaped four polypeptide chain molecule. Of the four chains, two each are light (L) and heavy (H). These are held together by disulphide bonds (Fig. 10.2). L chain has a molecular weight of 25,000 daltons and H chain 50,000 daltons. H chains are structurally and antigenically distinct for each class and are designated with Greek letters α (alpha), δ (delta), ε (epsilon), γ (gamma) and μ (mu) in IgA, IgD, IgE, IgG and IgM respectively. L chains are of two types – κ (kappa) and λ (lambda). A molecule of Ig may have either κ or λ chains but never both together. κ and λ chains occur in a ratio of about 2 : 1 in human serum.

IgG when treated with proteolytic enzyme papain in the presence of cysteine cleaves it into three fragments. Two identical fragments (45,000 daltons each) still possess the antigen-binding sites and are thus named **fragment antigen binding** or **Fab**. These two fragments represent bivalency of IgG molecule. The third fragment (50,000 daltons) which lacks the ability to bind to antigen can be crystallized. It is, therefore, known as **fragment crystallizable (Fc)**.

Functions of Fc

- Binds complement leading to complement fixation.
- Binds to cell receptors (FcRs).
- Determines passage of IgG across the placental barrier.
- Determines skin fixation and catabolic rate.
- Antigenic determinants that distinguish one class of antibody from another are also located on Fc fragment.

Treatment of the IgG antibody molecule with proteolytic enzyme pepsin cleaves H chains on the carboxyterminal side of the interchain disulphide bonds of the hinge region. Therefore, 2 Fab fragments remain united. This fragment is designated as **F(ab´)₂** with two antigen-binding sites. Pepsin also degrades part of the Fc portion to small peptides and leaves a dimer of the carboxyterminal quarter of the chain, termed **pFc´**.

When IgG is treated with reducing agent, such as mercaptoethanol in the presence of urea, the disulphide bonds are reduced releasing four peptide chains – two heavy and two light.

Immunoglobulin domains

Two H chains are always identical in a given molecule and the same is true of L chains. Each H chain of IgG contains 440 amino acids while each L chain contains 220 amino acids. H chain has four domains of 110 amino acids each, while L chain has two domains of 110 amino acids each (Fig. 10.3). The antigen combining sites of the molecule are at its aminoterminal end. These are composed of both H and L chains. Of the 220 amino acids, those that constitute carboxyterminal half of L chain occur in a constant sequence. This part of the chain is called **constant region** (C_L). Only two sequence patterns are seen in constant region of κ and λ chains. On the other hand, amino acid sequence in aminoterminal half of the L chain is highly variable; the variability determines the immunological specificity of the antibody molecule. It is, therefore, called **variable region** (V_L).

A similar pattern is seen in H chains. The variable region of H chain, however, is only 25% as long as constant region. The variable region of H chain like that of L chain has highly variable sequence of amino acids and is known as V_H. The constant region of H chain is divided into three portions C_H1, C_H2 and C_H3. The infinite range of specificity of Igs depends upon the variability of amino acid sequences at the variable regions of H and L chains which form antigen combining sites.

Fd piece

It is the portion of H chains present in Fab fragment. H chains carry a carbohydrate moiety which is distinct for each class of immunoglobulins.

Each Ig peptide chain has internal disulphide links in addition to interchain disulphide bonds which bridge H and L chains. These intrachain disulphide bonds form loops in the peptide chain and each of the loops is completely folded to form a globular domain and each domain has its separate function. Variable region domains V_L and V_H are responsible

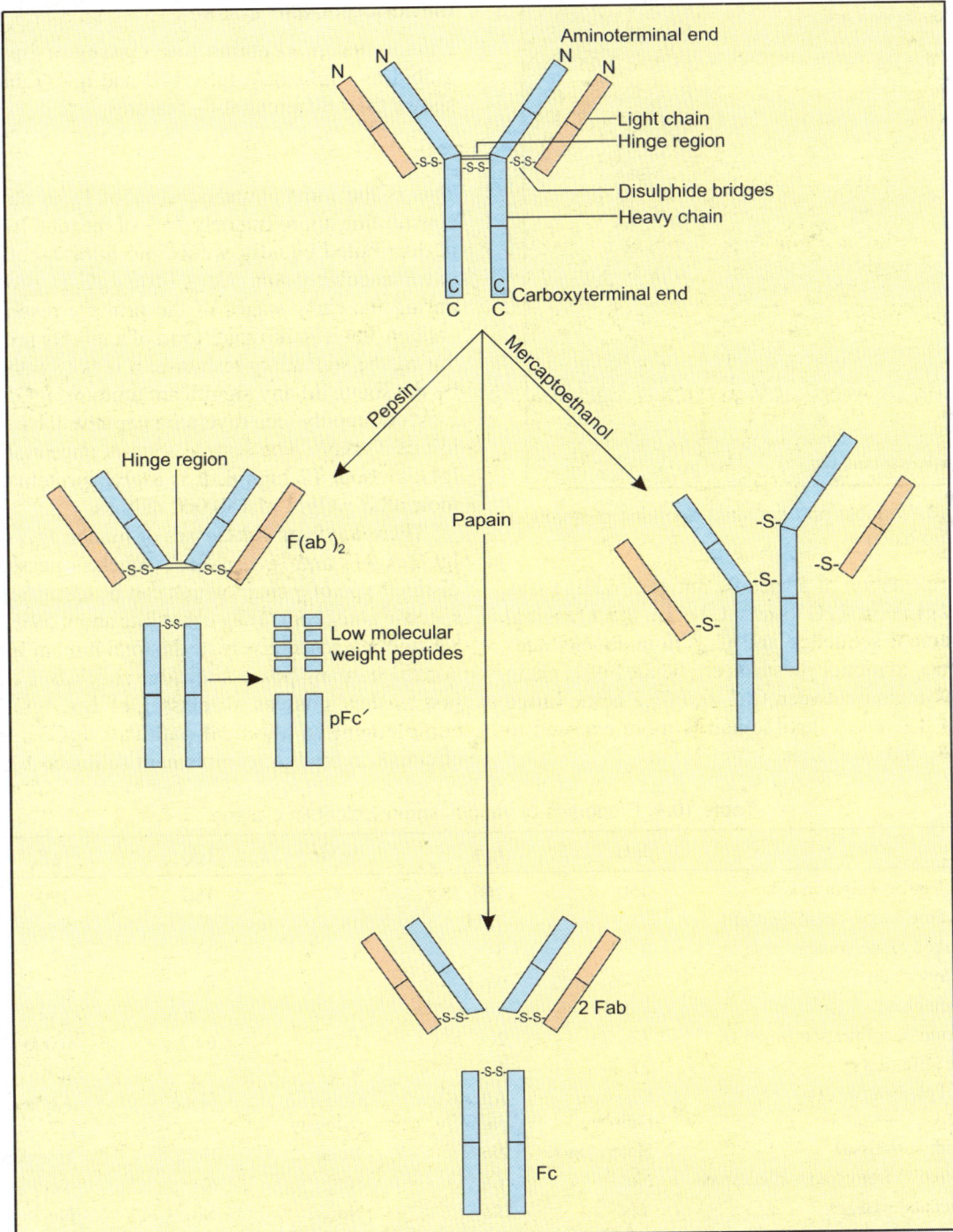

Fig. 10.2. Basic immunoglobulin structure.

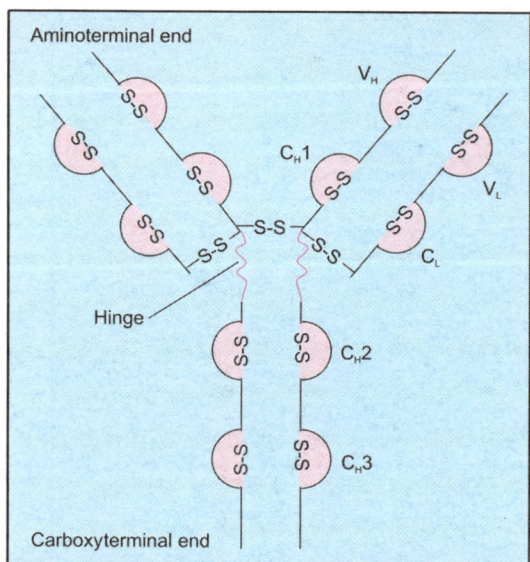

Fig. 10.3. Variable and constant domains of immuno-globulin molecule.

for the formation of a specific antigen-binding site. C_H2 region in IgG binds C1q in the classical complement sequence and C_H3 domain mediates adherence to monocyte surface. The area of H chain in the C region between C_H1 and C_H2 is the **hinge region**. It is more flexible and is more exposed to enzymes and chemicals.

Immunoglobulin classes

Human serum contains five classes of immuno-globulins – IgG, IgA, IgM, IgD and IgE. Table 10.1 shows their differentiating features.

Immunoglobulin G

This is the most abundant class of Ig in the body constituting approximately 75% of the total Igs. This is distributed equally within the intravascular and extravascular pools. Very little IgG is produced during the early stages of the primary response to antigen, but it is the major form of antibody produced during the secondary response. It is not synthesized by the foetus in any significant amount. IgG is also most commonly seen **myeloma protein**. It has a half-life of 21 days. The normal serum concentration of IgG is about 12 mg/ml. It is a glycoprotein with a molecular weight of 150,000 daltons.

There are **four subclasses** of human IgG (IgG1, IgG2, IgG3 and IgG4). Each subclass possesses a distinct type of γ chain which can be identified with specific antiserum. They constitute about 59%, 30%, 8% and 3% respectively of the total human IgG. All normal humans possess all four subclasses of IgG, just as they possess all classes of Igs. IgG binds complement in classical pathway. IgG3 is most effective in binding complement followed by IgG1

	IgG	IgA	IgM	IgD	IgE
1. Molecular weight in kDa	150	160, 385	900	180	190
2. Sedimentation coefficient(s)	7	7, 11	19	7	8
3. Carbohydrate content (%)	3	8	12	13	12
4. Heavy chain	$\gamma_1, \gamma_2, \gamma_3, \gamma_4$	α_1, α_2	μ	δ	ϵ
5. Light chain	κ or λ	κ or λ	κ or λ	κ or λ	κ or λ
6. Serum concentration (mg/ml)	12	2	1.2	0.03	0.00004
7. Half-life (days)	21	6	5	3	2
8. Complement binding	Classical pathway	Alternative pathway	Classical pathway	None	None
9. Binding to tissue	Heterologous	None	None	None	Homologous
10. Secretion from serous membranes	No	Yes*	No	No	Yes
11. Placental passage	Yes	No	No	No	No
12. Heat stability (56°C)	Yes	Yes	Yes	Yes	No

Table 10.1. Properties of various immunoglobulin classes

* Secretory IgA.

and IgG2. It can bind to protein A (from *Staphylococcus aureus*) and protein G (from group G streptococci). *IgG is the only class of Igs that can cross the placenta and is responsible for the protection of the infant during first few months of life. However, subclass IgG2 does not cross the placenta.* IgG is also found, along with IgA, in milk during the first few weeks after birth, providing additional protection if the infant is breast-fed.

Macrophages and monocytes bear Fc receptors (FcRs) which bind to the Fc portion of IgG1 and IgG3 in C_H3 domain. Such binding permits these cells to exhibit antibody-dependent cellular toxicity. IgG usually exhibits high affinity for antigens leading to efficient neutralization of toxins. Among null cells, a distinct subpopulation of cytotoxic cells has been recognized which also possesses FcRs for Fc part of IgG. They are capable of lysing or killing target cells sensitized with IgG. They are known as **killer cells**. They are responsible for **antibody-dependent cell-mediated cytotoxicity (ADCC)**. Platelets also possess FcRs for Fc portion of IgG leading to aggregation, degranulation and release of histamine. IgG is the only Ig which has the property of fixing to guinea-pig skin.

Catabolism of IgG is unique in that it varies with its serum concentration. When its level is raised, as in chronic malaria, kala-azar or myeloma, the IgG synthesized against a particular antigen will be catabolised rapidly and may result in the particular antibody deficiency. Conversely, in hypogamma-globulinaemia, the IgG given for treatment will be catabolised slowly.

IgG participates in most immunological reactions such as complement fixation, precipitation and neutralization of toxins and viruses. Passively administered IgG suppresses the homologous anti-body synthesis by a feedback process. This property is utilized for prevention of isoimmunization of Rh-negative mother bearing Rh-positive baby by administration of anti-Rh (D) IgG at the time of delivery.

Immunoglobulin M

It is so named because it is a macroglobulin at least five times larger than IgG. It is a glycoprotein with molecular weight of 900,000–1,000,000 daltons (millionaire molecule). It is present on the surface of virtually all uncommitted B cells. About 10% of normal serum Igs consist of this class. The normal serum level of IgM is 1.2 mg/ml. It has a half-life of about 5 days. IgM normally exists as a pentamer, consisting of 5 Ig subunits (Fig. 10.4).

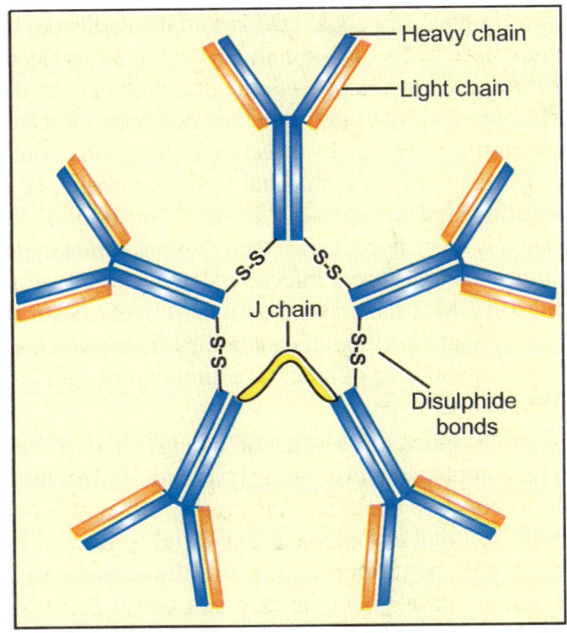

Fig. 10.4. IgM immunoglobulin.

In contrast to IgG, IgM remains almost exclusively in the serum and is not usually found extravascularly in body cavities or secretions. Therefore, IgM is believed to be responsible for protection against blood invasion by microorganisms. Penta-meric IgM is apparently too large to cross the placenta. The H μ chain has four C_H domains rather than three as seen in H chains of IgG. H chains are held together by disulphide bonds. There is an additional peptide chain called the **joining (J) chain**. The J chain may be largely responsible for the polymerization process, which occurs shortly before the molecule is secreted by plasma cell.

IgM contains 10 Fab fragments, and thus 10 antigen-binding sites. Therefore, theoretically it can bind to 10 antigen molecules. However, it appears that many antigens are so large that when bound to one site, they physically prevent the binding of another antigen molecule to an adjacent binding site. Thus, generally, IgM is capable of binding as few as five molecules of antigen.

Phylogenetically IgM is the oldest Ig class. It is usually the first antibody to appear following stimulation by an antigen. However, IgM synthesis is usually not prolonged, and IgG antibodies soon become the most prevalent class. IgM is also the earliest to be synthesized by foetus beginning by about **20 weeks of gestation**. As it cannot cross the placental barrier, the presence of IgM in the foetus or newborn indicates intrauterine infection. Its detection is, therefore, useful for the diagnosis of congenital syphilis, rubella, HIV infection and toxoplasmosis. IgM antibodies are relatively short-lived, hence their demonstration in the serum indicates recent infection. Treatment of serum with 0.12 M 2-mercaptoethanol selectively destroys IgM without affecting IgG antibodies. This provides a simple method for differential estimation of IgG and IgM antibodies.

IgM is much more efficient than IgG in its ability to fix complement, promoting lysis and death of most Gram-negative bacteria. This greater efficacy is due to the fact that complement may bind to several Fc regions of pentameric IgM simultaneously thus initiating complement cascade and target cell lysis with a single molecule.

Isohaemagglutinins (anti-A and anti-B), and antibodies to *Salmonella* Typhi O antigen and Wassermann reaction antibodies in syphilis are usually IgM. In certain disease states such as lupus erythematosus and rheumatoid arthritis, IgM may occur in monomeric form in high concentration. Monomeric IgM has lower avidity for antigen than does the pentameric form. A single molecule of IgM can bring about haemolysis, whereas 1,000 IgG molecules are required for the same effect. IgM is also more effective than IgG in opsonization, bactericidal action and in bacterial agglutination. However, in neutralization of toxins and viruses, it is less active than IgG.

Immunoglobulin A

The basic structure of IgA is similar to that of IgG. It contains two identical light chains (either κ or λ) and two heavy α chains. It is the second most abundant class, constituting about 15% of human serum Igs where it exists as a monomeric Ig. More important form is the dimeric form, known as **secretory IgA (sIgA)**. It is the predominant class of Igs in secretions such as milk, tears, nasal secretions, saliva, perspiration, genitourinary secretions and seromucous secretions.

On mucus surfaces sIgA antibodies form an antibody paste and is believed to play an important role in local immunity against respiratory and intestinal pathogens. sIgA is relatively resistant to digestive enzymes and reducing agents. Many infectious organisms cause disease by attaching to glycoproteins on the surface of epithelial cells of secretory gland. If this adhesion is sufficiently strong, the organism will divide, establish a colony and cause disease by any of a number of mechanisms, e.g., secretion of toxins that cause local and systemic injury. Secretory IgA when present in the secretions prevents attachment of organisms to epithelial cells thus preventing adhesion, colonization and infection.

Serum IgA is principally a monomeric 7S molecule with a molecular weight of 160,000 daltons. Secretory IgA is synthesized by plasma cells in the subepithelial tissue and secreted as a dimer containing four heavy chains, four light chains and one **J chain** which is similar to J chain found in pentameric IgM (Fig. 10.5). sIgA also possesses an additional structural unit called secretory component (SC). It is synthesized not in lymphoid cells but in epithelial cells of glands of intestine, and the respiratory tract and is attached to IgA molecules at their Fc portions producing 11S dimer with a molecular weight of 385,000 daltons. sIgA is relatively resistant to digestive enzymes, which may be due to the secretory component. IgA does not fix complement in classical

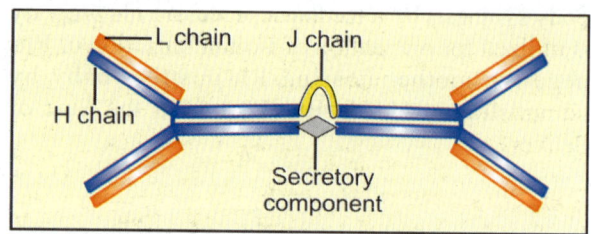

Fig. 10.5. Secretory IgA.

pathway but can activate the alternative complement pathway. It promotes phagocytosis and intracellular killing of microorganisms.

There are two subclasses of IgA in humans – IgA1 and IgA2. In serum, IgA1 constitutes 80%–90% of IgA while sIgA consists of about equal amounts of the two subclasses.

Certain streptococci and pathogenic *Neisseria* produce proteases that specifically cleave the heavy chain of IgA1. IgA2 is resistant to such cleavage because it has a shorter hinge region and lacks the proline-rich site cleaved by the proteases.

Immunoglobulin D

Like other monomeric antibodies IgD is composed of two light and two heavy chains. The latter are designated as δ chains. It contains about 13% carbohydrate. Its molecular weight is 180,000 daltons. It does not bind complement. It does not cross placenta and does not bind to cells via Fc region. IgD is present on the surface of B lymphocytes which are destined to differentiate into antibody-producing plasma cells and its serum concentration is very low (0.03 mg/ml). Reaction of antigen with surface immunoglobulin may lead to cell differentiation and antibody synthesis.

Immunoglobulin E

It resembles IgG structurally. Its molecular weight is 190,000 daltons. Its half-life is about two days. It does not fix complement or cross placental barrier. In contrast to other Igs it is heat-labile and gets inactivated by heating it at 56°C for 30 minutes. It is susceptible to 2-mercaptoethanol. It is chiefly produced in the linings of the respiratory and intestinal tracts. It is present in extremely low concentrations (0.00004 mg/ml) in the serum. But raised serum levels are seen in atopic (type I hypersensitivity) conditions like asthma and hay fever.

Most of a person's IgE is fixed to the surface of mast cells and basophils and when a specific antigen binds with IgE bound to mast cell or basophil membrane, the reaction results in the release of pharmacologically active substances such as histamine and serotonin which dilate capillaries, increase vascular permeability and cause bronchial constriction. Fc portion of IgE binds to the Fc receptors present on the surface of mast cells and basophils leaving antigen-binding sites free to react with specific antigen.

So far, no beneficial effect of IgE has been identified. It has been observed that IgE levels may rise following infections with parasites especially helminths. It has been suggested that mast cell-bound IgE reacts with antigens on the parasite followed by release of histamine. This results in increased vascular permeability followed by influx of plasma and cells (particularly eosinophils) and destruction of parasite. IgE mediates **Prausnitz-Kustner reaction**.

From available information it appears that:

- IgG   Protects the body fluids
- IgA   Protects the body surfaces
- IgM   Protects the blood stream
- IgE   Mediates type I hypersensitivity
- IgD   Role not known

KEY FACTS

- *Antigens* are substances that can stimulate an immune response and, given the opportunity, react specifically by binding with the effector molecules (antibodies) and effector cells (lymphocytes)
- Same or closely related antigens occurring in different biological species, classes and kingdoms are known as *heterogenetic* or *heterophile antigens*
- *Antibodies* or immunoglobulins are γ globulins which are produced in response to antigenic stimulation. These react specifically with the antigens which stimulated their production
- *The immunoglobulins have a basic unit of two light chains and two heavy chains in a light-heavy-heavy-light arrangement*
- *There are five classes of antibody – IgG, IgA, IgM, IgD and IgE*
- *Circulating antibodies* recognize antigen in serum and tissue fluids
- *The infinite range of specificity of immunoglobulins* depends upon the *variability of amino acid sequences* at the variable regions of heavy and light chains which form *antigen combining sites*

- Antibodies neutralize antigens, induce killing of target cells by complement and natural killer cells and opsonize particles for phagocytosis
- IgG is the ***most abundant*** class of immunoglobulin in the body constituting approximately 75% of total immunoglobulins
- ***Joining (J) chain*** is present in **IgM** and **secretory IgA**
- **Secretory IgA** is relatively ***resistant to digestive enzymes***, which may be due to the ***secretory component*** of this immunoglobulin
- In contrast to other immunoglobulins, **IgE** is **heat-labile** and gets inactivated by heating at 56°C for 30 minutes

IMPORTANT QUESTIONS

1. Write short notes on:
   (a) Heterophile antigens
   (b) Immunoglobulin G
   (c) Immunoglobulin A
   (d) Immunoglobulin M
2. Define antigen and discuss determinants of antigenicity.
3. Draw labelled diagram of immunoglobulin G and tabulate differences between IgG, IgA and IgM.

Chapter 11

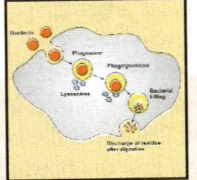

The Complement System

The term **complement** (C) is applied to a system of components present in the serum of man and animals. It consists of nine different proteins denoted C1–C9. The fraction C1 occurs in serum as calcium ion dependent complex, which on chelation with EDTA yields three protein subunits called C1q, C1r and C1s. Thus C is made up of 11 different proteins. Complement proteins differ in their electrophoretic mobility and molecular weight having sedimentation coefficient ranging from 4S–11S. These differences permit their separation by physical methods. Though some of its components are stable, C as a whole is heat-labile undergoing spontaneous denaturation slowly at room temperature and in 30 minutes at 56°C. Serum deprived of C activity by heating it at 56°C for 30 minutes is said to be inactivated.

The amount of C present in the serum cannot be increased by immunization. It is, biologically, of considerable importance as an amplifier of immune reactions involving humoral antibodies and is believed to play an important role in the defence of the body against microbial infections. C does not bind to free antigen or antibody but only to antibody which has combined with its antigen. C binding site is located on the C_H2 domain of the Fc portion of IgM and IgG molecules only. These sites are not exposed when antibodies are in the uncombined state.

However, after antibody combines with antigen the C binding site is exposed.

C is normally present in the body in an inactive form but can be activated to form an enzyme cascade. The cascade is a series of reactions in which the preceding components act as enzymes on the succeeding components cleaving them into dissimilar fragments. The larger fragments join the cascade and the smaller fragments are released which often possess biological effects which contribute to defence mechanism by:

- Initiating an inflammatory response.
- Causing the destruction of parasites, bacteria, virus-infected cells or red blood cells.
- Clearing dead cells and immune complexes.
- Detoxifying endotoxins.
- Effecting release of histamine from mast cells.

There are **two activation mechanisms** through which complement system executes its role. These are known as classical pathway and alternative or properdin pathway. The former requires the presence of antibody for activation. In contrast, the alternative pathway does not need antibody and can be triggered by the mere presence of bacterial or viral components. For example, the lipopolysaccharide layer of Gram-negative bacterial cell wall is enough to activate alternative pathway. However, both these pathways lead to the same physiological consequences, i.e., opsonization, cellular activation and lysis. But the initiation process is different. Component C3 forms the connection between the two pathways and the binding of the molecule to the surface is the key process in complement activation.

Classical pathway of complement activation

Activation of classical pathway of complement requires the presence of antibody, either IgM or IgG, bound to cell surface antigen or as an antigen-antibody immune complex. All the 11 proteins of the complement comprise the classical complement pathway. All are designated by C followed by the number of the component (complement's protein). Inactive components are described as C1, C2, C3 and so on. Activated forms are designated by placing a bar over the number, for example, $\overline{C2}$ represents activated C2 which is actually C2b.

The classical pathway (Fig. 11.1) is initiated when C1 interacts with the Fc portion of either cell-bound Ig (IgG or IgM) or immune complex. This interaction results in the sequential activation of C4, C2 and C3 and leads to the formation of complex cleaving enzymes. Activation of C5, C6, C7, C8 and C9 then completes the cascade and results in the formation of the **C5 to C9 membrane attack complex (MAC)**, which can lyse the cell. C1 is composed of one molecule of C1q, and two molecules each of C1r and C1s. C1q binds to Fc portion of the antibody molecule. Binding of this component of C1 causes a conformational change in the C1 complex that leads to the autoactivation of C1r.

This then converts C1s into an active esterase that acts on C4 to produce C4a and a reactive C4b. C4a is released and less than 1% of the C4b becomes attached to the cell membrane. Unbound molecules of C4b are rapidly inactivated. $\overline{C1s}$ also cleaves C2 into two components – C2a, larger component, and C2b, smaller component. C2a attaches itself to membrane-bound C4b to form a new active protease, $\overline{C4b2a}$, which is called C3 convertase since it can bind and cleave the next inactive complement component in the sequence, C3.

The newly formed C3 convertase, $\overline{C4b2a}$ cleaves C3 into two fragments, C3a and C3b. The larger C3b fragment attaches to both the cell membrane and $\overline{C4b2a}$ complex, while the smaller fragment, C3a, is released to the body fluids. C3a has chemo-

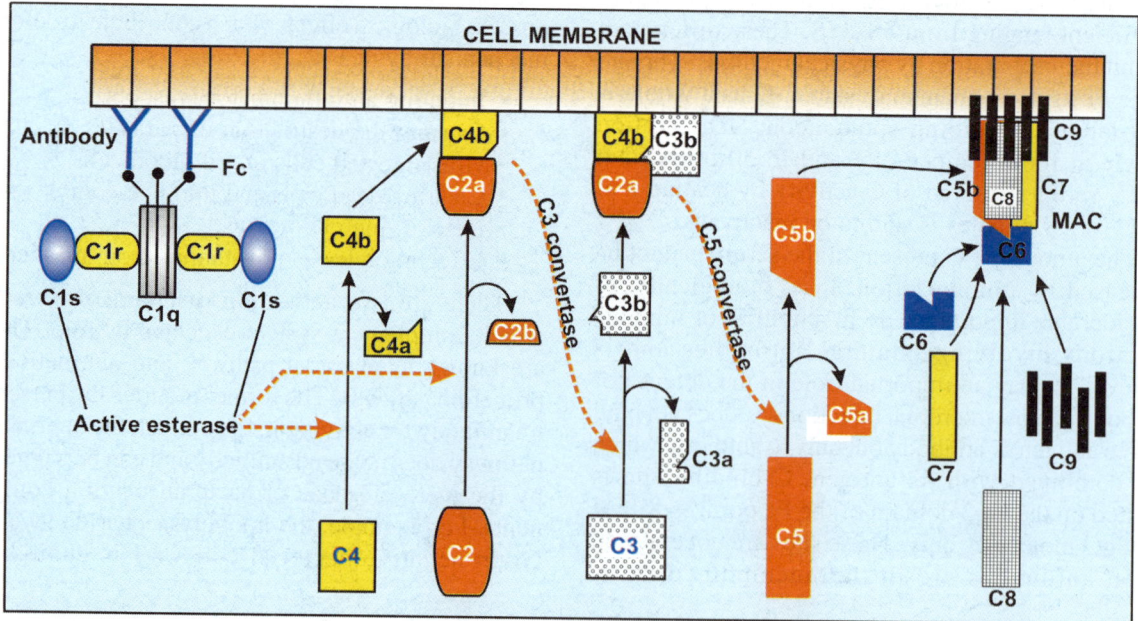

Fig. 11.1. Classical pathway of complement activation.

tactic and anaphylatoxic properties. $\overline{C4b2a3b}$ is termed C5 convertase. It cleaves C5 into two products, C5a and C5b. C5a which is a powerful chemotactant of neutrophils and monocytes and has anaphylatoxic activity is released when formed and C5b attaches to the cell membrane. The binding of $\overline{C5b}$ leads to the uncovering of a binding site for C6 and C7 on the molecule, producing a stable complex $\overline{C5b67}$.

This trimolecular complex attaches to the membrane surface and enables C8 to join. C8 then binds several C9 molecules. About 10–18 protein units of C9 attach to $\overline{C5b678}$ base to form a long hollow tube. This is a stable complex and is referred to as **membrane attack complex (MAC)**. This creates a **membrane pore** or lesion, that is 100 Å in diameter leading to cell death. Pores in the cell membrane created by MAC may also permit degradative enzymes in the area to enter and destroy cellular organelles contributing to target cell death.

Alternative or properdin pathway of complement activation

This pathway does not require the presence of specific antibodies. C3 is the major component of C. In the classical pathway, activation of C3 is achieved by the C3 convertase ($\overline{C4b2a}$). *The activation of C3, without the prior participation of C142, is known as the alternative or properdin pathway of complement activation*. The overall result of this pathway is the same as that of classical pathway but the C3 and C5 convertases for alternative pathway are different from those of classical pathway. A wide range of chemically unrelated substances are known to activate alternative pathway. These (other than antigen-antibody complexes) include:

- Yeast cell walls.
- Bacterial endotoxins.
- Rabbit (not sheep) RBCs.
- Snake venom proteins.
- A protein termed 'nephritic factor' found in the serum of patients with diseases such as glomerulonephritis.

The fact that these products can activate the alternative pathway directly, without the need of antibody is of considerable importance because it allows for defence against infection prior to initiation of an immune response.

There are at least three normal serum proteins that, when activated together with C3, form a functional C3 convertase and a C5 convertase. These are factor B, factor D and properdin. These are normal serum proteins, and the alternative pathway is routinely being activated in the absence of any stimulus. In the absence of initiators, the initial complexes of the alternative pathway are rapidly destroyed. In the presence of the initiators, such complexes are stabilized and complement is activated to form the MAC as in case of classical pathway.

Intrinsically, C3 undergoes a low level of hydrolysis of an internal thioester bond to generate C3b. Nonimmune activators, such as repeating polysaccharide units or the lipopolysaccharide found on the cell walls of some microbes split up C3 into C3a and C3b. There are a wide variety of pathogens that can be recognized within minutes after they come in contact with plasma. Organisms sensitive to attack by the alternative pathway include bacteria, fungi, certain viruses, virus-infected cells, parasites and certain tumour cells. C3b, in the presence of Mg^{++}, binds to these foreign surfaces and interacts with plasma protein factor B forming C3bB (Fig. 11.2).

The factor B portion of C3bB complex is split by factor D into two fragments, Ba and Bb. Ba is released during reaction and Bb remains bound to C3b forming C3bBb. The newly formed $\overline{C3bBb}$ is a C3 convertase of alternative pathway. $\overline{C3bBb}$ splits more C3 to C3a and C3b. The newly formed C3b binds more factor B. This continues until the membrane surface is saturated with $\overline{C3bBb}$. The result is opsonization of the cell or particle by neutrophils. The soluble C3a, that is released upon cleavage of C3, has chemotactic and anaphylatoxic activity, which can initiate an inflammatory response. C3 convertase $\overline{C3bBb}$ can bind additional C3b to produce C5 convertase ($\overline{C3bBb3b}$). This activates terminal lytic complement sequence, C5 to C9.

Thus activation of either classical or alternative pathway leads to the formation of C3 convertases ($\overline{C4b2a}$ or $\overline{C3bBb}$). These cleave C3 into C3a and C3b. The latter combines with C3 convertases forming C5 convertases ($\overline{C4b2a3b}$ or $\overline{C3bBb3b}$).

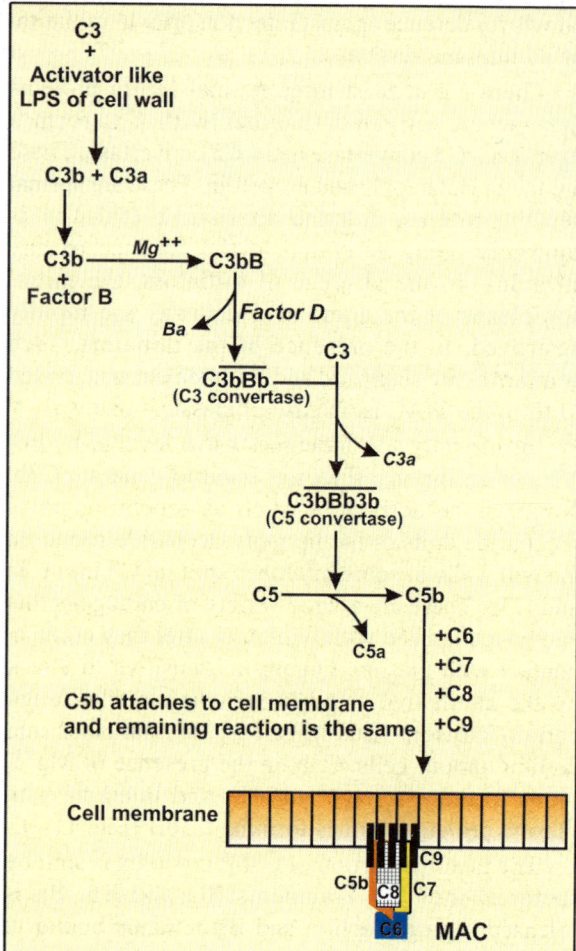

Fig. 11.2. Alternative pathway of complement activation.

These split C5 into C5a and C5b. C5b then binds C6, C7, C8 and several molecules of C9 to form MAC which initiates lysis of target cells in both pathways.

Biological effects of complement

1. Complement mediates **immunological membrane damage.** This results in bacteriolysis and cytolysis. Different cells vary in their susceptibility to complement-mediated lysis. Gram-negative bacteria are generally sensitive to lysis, while Gram-positive are killed without lysis. Neutralization of certain viruses requires the participation of C, e.g., neutralization of herpes virus by IgM antibody requires the binding of C1, C4 and possibly C3 too.

2. C fragments released during cascade reaction help in **amplifying the inflammatory response.** Proteolytic cleavage of C3 and C5, in either the classical or alternative pathway, generates two potent mediators of inflammation, C3a and C5a. Mast cells and basophils possess receptors for C3a and C5a. Binding of C3a or C5a to these receptors causes these cells to release histamine. This may lead to contraction of the uterus, trachea, arteries, atrium of the heart and intestines, and increased vascular permeability leading to oedema. C5a, in addition exerts a series of unique effects on white blood cells. These include:

   • Degranulation and lysosomal enzyme release.
   • Promotes adherence of granulocytes to the endothelium.
   • Induces chemotactic migration of granulocytes. $\overline{C5b67}$ is also chemotactic. C4a has weak anaphylatoxic activity. It is weakly spasmogenic and increases vascular permeability. Therefore, redness, pain, swelling and heat of inflammation is due to the action of C4a, C3a, C5a and histamine.

3. Phagocytes such as macrophages, monocytes and neutrophils possess surface receptors for C3b. If immune complexes have activated the complement system, the C3b bound to them facilitates their recognition and ingestion by these phagocytes. This facilitated phagocytosis is referred to as **opsonization**.

4. Complement participates in **type II (cytotoxic)** and **type III (immune complex) hypersensitivity** reactions. The destruction of erythrocytes, following incompatible blood transfusion is an example of type II hypersensitivity. Participation of C is required for the production of immune complex diseases such as serum sickness and Arthus reaction (type III hypersensitivity).

5. Several serum C components are lowered in many autoimmune diseases such as systemic lupus erythematosus and rheumatoid arthritis. These may, therefore, be involved in the pathogenesis of **autoimmune diseases.** C plays a major role in the pathogenesis of autoimmune haemolytic

anaemia, paroxysmal nocturnal haemoglobinuria and hereditary angioneurotic oedema.

6. C3 and C6 participate in coagulation process.

7. C bound to antigen-antibody complexes adheres to erythrocytes. This is known as **immune adherence.** It contributes to defence against pathogenic microorganisms as such adherent particles are rapidly phagocytosed. C3 and C4 are necessary for immune adherence.

KEY FACTS

- *The complement system*, a multicomponent triggered enzyme cascade, attracts phagocytic cells to the microbes which engulf them
- Complement can be activated by classical and alternative pathways
- The amount of complement present in the serum cannot be increased by immunization
- Complement participates in type II and type III hypersensitivity

- Several serum complement components are lowered in many autoimmune diseases such as systemic lupus erythematosus and rheumatoid arthritis. They may, therefore, be involved in the pathogenesis of autoimmune diseases
- Complement mediates immunological membrane damage
- C fragments released during cascade reaction help in amplifying the inflammatory response
- C3 and C4 mediate immune adherence
- C3 and C6 participate in coagulation process

IMPORTANT QUESTIONS

1. What is the sequence of events when the classical pathway of the complement system is activated?
2. How does complement contribute to defence against infection?
3. Write short notes on:
   (a) Alternative pathway of complement activation
   (b) Biological effects of complement.

Chapter 12

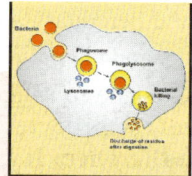

Antigen–Antibody Reactions

When an antigen is mixed with its specific antibody, in the presence of electrolytes at a suitable temperature and pH, they combine with each other in an observable manner.

In the body they form the basis of:
- Antibody-mediated immunity in infectious diseases.
- Tissue injury in some types of hypersensitivity and autoimmune diseases.

In the laboratory, they help in the diagnosis of:
- Infectious diseases.
- Noninfectious agents such as enzymes.

These reactions can be used for the detection and quantitation of either antigen or antibody. Antigen-antibody reactions *in vitro* are known as serological infections.

CHARACTERISTICS OF ANTIGEN-ANTIBODY REACTIONS

- Antigen-antibody reaction is specific but cross-reactions may occur. This is due to antigenic similarity or relatedness.
- Antigen-antibody combination is firm but reversible.
- There is no denaturation of antigen or antibody during the reaction.
- Binding takes place on the surface. Therefore, surface antigens are more relevant.
- Entire molecules react. Therefore, when an antigenic determinant present on a large molecule or a carrier particle reacts with antibody, whole molecules or particles are agglutinated.

For better understanding of antigen-antibody reactions a few terms are defined below:

Affinity: Intensity of the attraction between an antibody-combining site and an antigenic determinant.

Avidity: Strength of the bond after the formation of antigen-antibody complexes.

Sensitivity: Ability of a test to identify correctly all those who have the disease, i.e., true positives. A 90% sensitivity means that 90% of the diseased persons screened by the test will give a true positive and 10% a false negative result.

Specificity: Ability of a test to identify correctly all those who do not have the disease, i.e., true negatives. A 90% specificity means that 90% of non-diseased persons screened by the test will give a true negative and 10% a false positive result. In other words, 10% of non-diseased persons will be wrongly classified as diseased when they are not.

METHODS USED TO DETECT AND QUANTITATE ANTIGEN AND ANTIBODY

A number of methods can be used to determine the presence or amount of antigens and antibodies. Measurement may be in terms of mass (e.g., mg nitrogen) or more commonly as units or titre. **Antibody titre** is the highest dilution of serum which gives an observable reaction with the antigen in a particular test.

1. *Agglutination:* If the antigen is on the surface of particulate material, such as a bacterium or a red blood cell, the end result is a clumping of the cells or agglutination.
2. *Precipitation:* A soluble antigen may form an antigen-antibody complex that becomes too large to stay in solution and the result is a precipitation.
3. *Antitoxin:* An antibody may neutralize a bacterial toxin. Antibody neutralizing the toxin is known as antitoxin.
4. *Neutralizing antibodies:* An antibody may neutralize viruses so that they cannot infect susceptible cells. These are known as neutralizing antibodies.
5. *Opsonins:* Antibodies which react with bacterial cells to make them more easily phagocytosed by leucocytes are known as opsonins.

However, multiplicity of antibody names does not mean that different types of antibodies exist for each reaction. Thus, if a soluble antigen is mixed with specific antibody it leads to precipitation and when the same antigen is coated on particles such as polystyrene beads, the same specific antibody will agglutinate the beads or enhance their phagocytosis. With this in mind, a number of antigen-antibody reactions used to detect the presence of antigen or antibody in clinical specimens are described below.

Precipitation reactions

Precipitation

When a soluble antigen is mixed with its specific antibody in the presence of electrolytes at a suitable temperature and pH, the antigen-antibody complex forms an insoluble precipitate. This precipitate usually settles down at the bottom of the tube. Precipitation can take place in liquid media and in gels such as agar, agarose and polyacrylamide. The process of precipitation can be hastened by electrically driving the antigen and antibody.

Flocculation

When instead of sedimenting the precipitate remains suspended as floccules, the reaction is called flocculation.

Zone phenomenon

If a series (10–12) of tubes is set up (Fig. 12.1), each

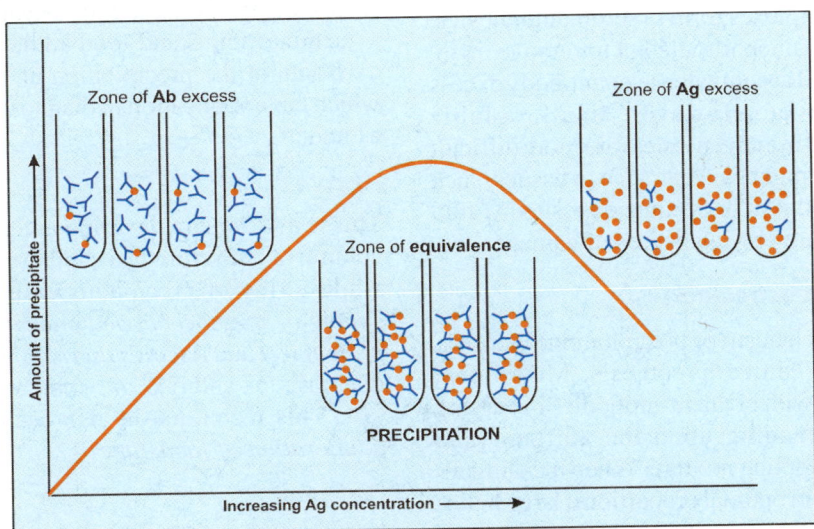

Fig. 12.1. Zone phenomenon.

containing a constant amount of antiserum, and increasing amounts of antigen are added to the tubes in the row, precipitation will be found to occur most rapidly and abundantly in one of the middle tubes, in which antigen and antibody are in optimal or equivalent proportion. In the preceding tubes, in which the antibody is in excess, and in the later tubes, in which the antigen is in excess, the precipitation will be weak or absent. Therefore, the amount of precipitation will be seen to increase along the row, reaching a maximum and then falling off with higher antigen concentration.

If the amounts of precipitate in different tubes are plotted on a graph, the resulting curve will have **three phases** – an ascending part (**prozone** or zone of antibody excess), a peak (**zone** of equivalence), and a descending part (**postzone** or zone of antigen excess). This is called **zone phenomenon**. Assay of supernatant solution will show that those tubes containing too little antigen still contain free antibody and in the tubes with antigen excess, little precipitate forms, although soluble immune complexes and free antigens are present in the supernatant fluid. Only in tubes of maximum precipitation is all antibody removed from solution. *The prozone is of importance in clinical serology, as sera rich in antibody may sometimes give false negative result, unless several dilutions are tested.*

If immune complexes form in serum, monocytes, neutrophils and eosinophils attempt to remove them. Complexes formed at equivalence or antibody excess are easily removed. However, small, soluble complexes formed in antigen excess are more difficult to remove. These might gain entrance to tissues, such as glomeruli of kidneys or become deposited within vessel walls causing varying degree of damage.

Mechanism of precipitation

To explain the mechanism of precipitation, Marrack, 1934 proposed a lattice hypothesis. Multivalent antigens combine with bivalent antibodies in varying proportions, depending upon the antigens and antibodies in the reacting mixture. When the antigens and antibodies are in optimal proportion a large lattice is formed consisting of alternating antigen and antibody molecules. Therefore, most abundant preci-

pitation occurs when both antigens and antibodies are in optimal proportion. In antibody excess each antigen or two combine with an independent molecule of antibody. Therefore, the lattice does not enlarge. Similarly, in antigen excess the lattice does not enlarge (Fig. 12.2).

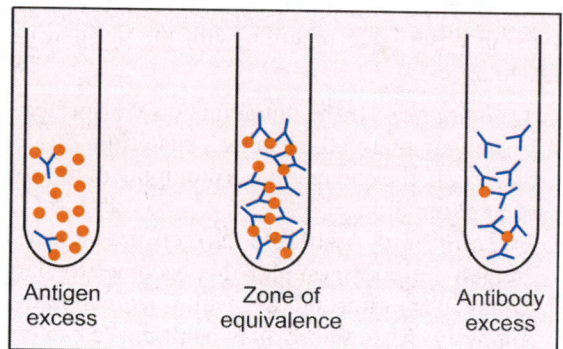

| Antigen excess | Zone of equivalence | Antibody excess |

Fig. 12.2. Lattice formation.

Applications of precipitation reactions

1. The precipitation test may be carried out for both qualitative and quantitative determination of both antigen and antibody. It is a very sensitive test for detecting antigens and is relatively less sensitive for detection of antibodies. The precipitation test is capable of detecting as little antigen proteins as 1 µg.
2. It can be used for identification of blood and seminal stains and food adulterants.

Some of the precipitation and flocculation tests which have application in diagnostic bacteriology are as under:

Ring test

This test is done by layering antigen solution over a column of antiserum in a capillary tube. After a short while a ring of precipitate forms at the interface. *Typing of streptococci and pneumococci, C-reactive protein test and Ascoli's thermoprecipitin test* for the diagnosis of anthrax, are some of the uses of ring test. This technique is also used for *detection of adulteration of foodstuffs.*

Slide test

This is an example of flocculation test. When a drop each of antigen and antiserum are placed on a slide and mixed by shaking, floccules appear. *VDRL, a most widely used test* for the diagnosis of syphilis, is an example of slide flocculation test.

Tube test

Flocculation test can be carried out in the tubes also. *Kahn test* for syphilis and *standardization of toxins and toxoids* are examples of tube flocculation.

Immunodiffusion (precipitation in gel)

When an antibody and its antigen are placed in an agar gel they diffuse towards each other and form an opaque band of precipitation at the junction of their diffusion front. Precipitation in gel has several advantages over precipitation in liquid medium:

- The reaction appears as a distinct band of precipitation which can be stained for better visibility and preservation.

- Since each antigen-antibody reaction gives rise to one line of precipitation, therefore, different number of antigens in a mixture can be detected.
- This technique also indicates *identity, cross-reaction* and *nonidentity* between different antigens.

Types of immunodiffusion tests

1. Single diffusion in one dimension (Oudin procedure)

Antibody is incorporated in agar gel in a test tube. Antigen solution is then layered over it. The antigen diffuses downwards and wherever it reaches in optimum concentration with antibody a line of precipitation is formed (Fig. 12.3A). As more antigen diffuses, the line of precipitation moves downwards. Number of lines of precipitation indicates the number of antigens and antibodies present.

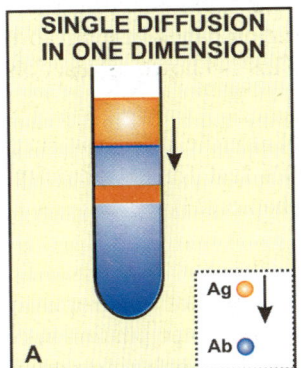
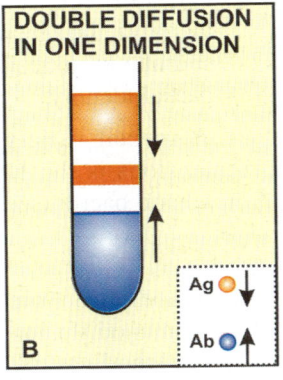
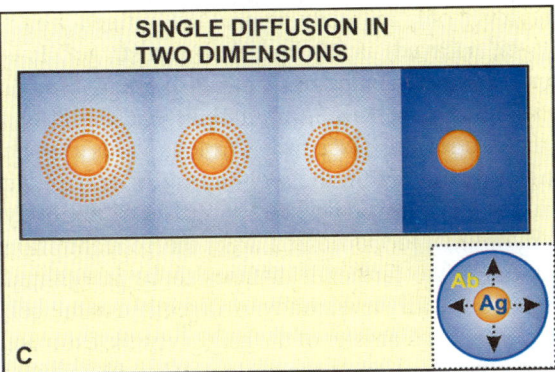

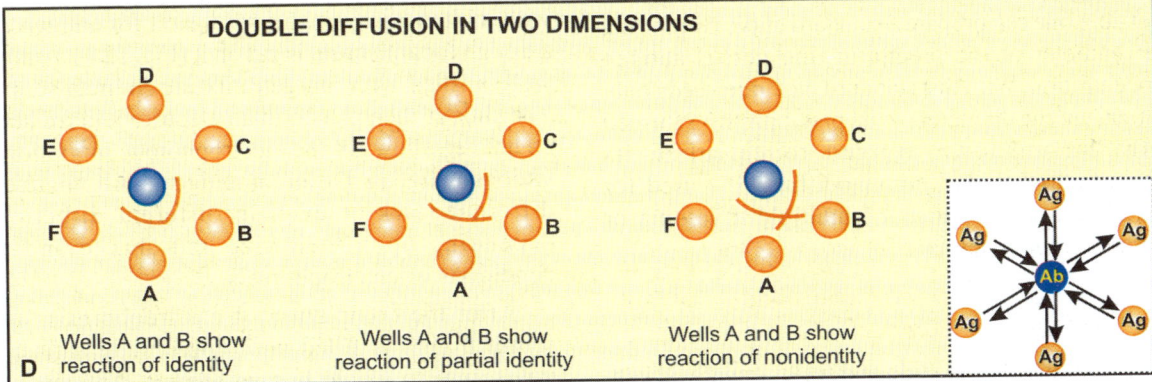

Fig. 12.3. Immunodiffusion.

2. Double diffusion in one dimension (Oakley-Fulthorpe)

Antibody is incorporated in agar gel in a test tube. Above this is placed a column of plain agar which in turn is overlaid with antigen, either as liquid or incorporated into agar (Fig. 12.3B). Antigen and antibody diffuse (double diffusion) towards each other (in one dimension) through the intervening column of plain agar and form a band of precipitation where they meet in optimum concentration.

3. Single diffusion in two dimensions (radial immunodiffusion)

This method is used to quantitate the amount of a specific antigen present in a sample and can be used for many antigens. The most widely used diagnostic application of this procedure is to measure the amount of various Ig classes (IgG, IgA, IgM, IgD and IgE) in patient serum.

Here monospecific antiserum (antiserum containing only antibody against the antigen which is to be assayed) is incorporated in agar gel. It is poured on a glass slide or a petri dish and a number of wells are punched into it, and different dilutions of the antigen are placed into various wells. As the antigen diffuses from the well, a ring of precipitate forms at that position where antigen and antibody are in optimal proportions. Larger the concentration of antigen, the farther it diffuses to be in optimal proportions with the antibody incorporated in the gel. Therefore, the diameter of the ring gives the estimate of the concentration of the antigen (Fig. 12.3C).

Using known concentrations of the antigen in question, one can prepare a standard curve by plotting the diameter of the precipitin ring versus antigen concentration. With this standard plot, one needs only to measure the diameter of the precipitin ring formed with the unknown antigen to calculate its concentration. Radial immunodiffusion is used for the laboratory diagnosis of multiple myeloma or agammaglobulinaemia.

4. Double diffusion in two dimensions (Ouchterlony procedure)

Agar is poured on the slide and wells, usually seven, are punched in it using a template. The known antiserum is placed in the central well and different antigens in surrounding wells. One of these contains known positive antigen. It acts as a positive control. This technique is also useful for comparing different antigens for the presence of identical or cross-reacting components. The samples are placed in adjacent wells, and the corresponding antibody is placed in the central well.

1. *Reaction of identity:* If two precipitin bands fuse completely (Fig. 12.3D), the pattern is termed reaction of identity. It indicates that the antigens in the adjoining wells are identical.

2. *Reaction of nonidentity:* If unrelated antigens are placed in adjacent wells, they diffuse towards central well containing antibodies for both, the two precipitin bands form independently and cross each other. This is known as reaction of nonidentity.

3. *Reaction of partial identity:* If the antigens in the two adjacent wells are cross-reacting (partial identity), the precipitation bands fuse but form a spurlike projection. This is known as reaction of partial identity.

A special variety of double diffusion in two dimensions is the **Elek's test** for toxigenicity of diphtheria bacilli (see Chapter 23).

5. Immunoelectrophoresis

Immunoelectrophoresis combines electrophoresis and immunodiffusion (immune precipitation in gel). This method can be used for analyzing complex antigens in biological fluids. A glass slide is covered with molten agar or agarose. A well for antigen and a trough for antiserum is cut on it (Fig. 12.4). Antigen well is filled with antigen mixture (human serum). The slide is then placed in an electric field for about an hour to allow for the electrophoretic migration of various antigens. Different antigens will migrate at different rates or even in different directions, depending upon their size and charge and the conditions of electrophoresis.

After the completion of electrophoresis, antiserum trough is filled with appropriate antiserum (antiserum to whole human serum). Antigens and antibodies diffuse towards each other, resulting in

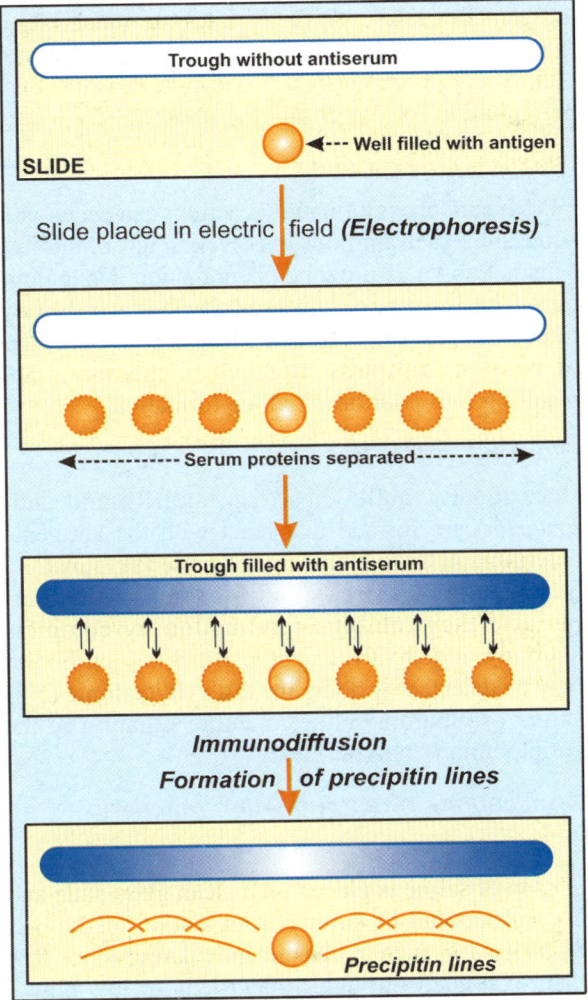

Fig. 12.4. Immunoelectrophoresis.

the formation of precipitin bands, for individual antigens and antibodies, whenever they are both in zones of optimal proportions, in 18–24 hours. Because immunoelectrophoresis uses electric charge in addition to diffusion, it is more likely to separate antigen than is simple diffusion alone. By this method, over 30 different antigens can be identified in human serum. This technique is useful for detection of normal and abnormal serum proteins.

6. Electroimmunodiffusion

Immunodiffusion is a slow process. The development of precipitin lines can be speeded up by electrically driving antigens and antibodies in a gel, rather than simply allowing them to come in contact by diffusion. Of these, one dimensional double electroimmuno-diffusion and one dimensional single electroimmuno-diffusion are used frequently in the clinical laboratory.

1. *One-dimensional double electroimmuno-diffusion (counterimmunoelectrophoresis or CIE):* This method can be used for those antigens and antibodies that migrate in opposite directions in electric field. The wells are punched about 1 cm apart in an agar slab on a glass plate. Antigen and antibody solutions are placed in wells towards cathode and anode sides respectively. Electric field is then applied electrophoresing both antigens and antibodies from separate wells. The antigen migrates towards antibody and antibody migrates towards antigen. A precipitin band is formed, in between the two wells, where they meet in optimum proportions (Fig. 12.5). This method has several advantages over simple diffusion in agar:

• The electrophoresis forces the reactants into a small area allowing the detection of small quantities of antigens and antibodies. Therefore, **it is 10 times more sensitive than simple diffusion in agar**.

• It is a rapid assay. Precipitin bands may form in just 30 minutes.

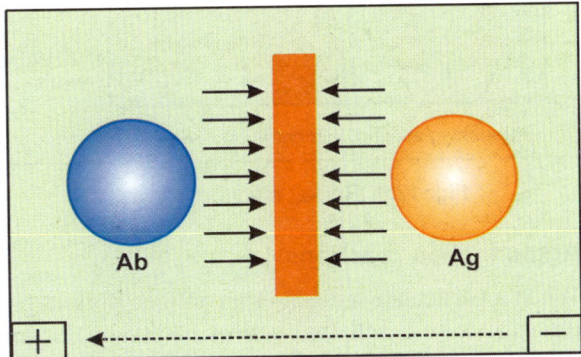

Fig. 12.5. Counterimmunoelectrophoresis.

This method is used for detection of various antigens such as:

• hepatitis B surface antigen (HBsAg) and alpha-fetoprotein in serum;

- meningococcal and cryptococcal antigens in CSF; and
- anti-DNA antibody in the serum of patients with several autoimmune disorders.

2. *One-dimensional single electroimmuno-diffusion (rocket electrophoresis):* As in case of radial immunodiffusion, wells are cut in an agarose gel slab on a glass plate. Agarose contains the antiserum to the antigen of interest. The antigen, in increasing concentrations, is placed in wells. The antigen is then electrophoresed into the agarose containing antibody that does not migrate. The pattern of immunoprecipitation resembles a rocket (hence the name), since precipitation occurs along the moving boundary of antigen, as it migrates into the agarose (Fig. 12.6). The height (distance from the antigen well to the top of the precipitin band) is proportional to the antigen concentration. The main application of this technique, therefore, is for quantitative estimation of antigen.

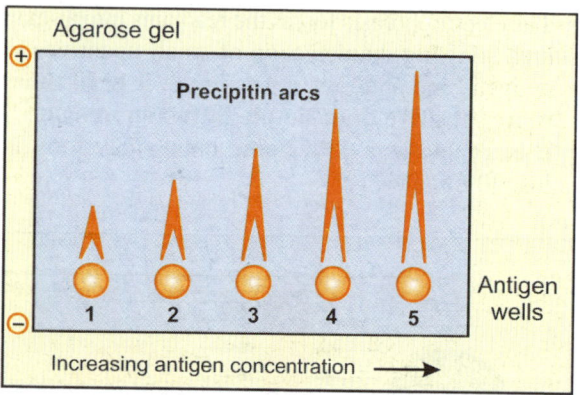

Fig. 12.6. Rocket electrophoresis.

Agglutination reactions

When a particulate antigen or an antigen present on the surface of a cell (red cell or bacterium) or an inorganic particle (e.g., polystyrene latex coated with antigen) is mixed with its antibody in the presence of electrolytes at a suitable temperature and pH, the particles are clumped or agglutinated. This reaction is analogous to precipitation reaction, in that antibody merely acts as a bridge to form a lattice network of antibody and cells or inorganic particles coated with antigen. Because cells or particles are much larger than soluble antigen, therefore, they aggregate into clumps. Agglutination reaction is more sensitive than precipitation for detection of antibodies.

Prozone phenomenon

False negative agglutination reactions can occur with some antisera in antibody excess (first few dilutions). This is known as prozone phenomenon. Unagglutinated cells in prozone actually have antibody molecules adsorbed on their surface, with both sites of bivalent antibody attached to the same cell resulting into poor or no lattice formation.

Blocking antibodies

Occasionally, antibodies (e.g., anti-Rh and anti-*Brucella*) are formed that react with the antigenic determinants on a cell but do not cause agglutination. Such antibodies are called blocking antibodies, because they inhibit agglutination by complete antibody added subsequently. Blocking antibodies may be detected by doing the test in hypertonic (5%) saline or albumin saline, or more reliably by the antiglobulin (Coombs') test.

Applications of agglutination reactions

Slide agglutination

A drop of saline is placed on a clean glass slide and a small amount of culture from a solid medium is emulsified in it by means of inoculating loop. It is then examined through a hand lens or low-power microscope that the suspension is even and bacteria are not autoagglutinable. Then with a platinum loop a drop of specific antiserum is placed on the slide near the bacterial suspension. The serum and the bacterial suspension are then mixed and examined with naked eye or with hand lens or under low-power microscope for the evidence of agglutination within a minute. Slide agglutination test is rapid and convenient, but in order to obtain rapid agglutination serum is used undiluted or in low dilutions.

Uses:
- Identification of bacterial isolates (e.g., *Salmonella* spp., *Shigella* spp. and *Vibrio cholerae*) from clinical specimens. This method is practicable only when clumping of organisms occurs instan-

taneously or within a minute because clumping occurring after a minute may be due to drying of the fluid.

- Blood grouping and cross matching.

Tube agglutination

This is done in round-bottomed test tubes or perspex plates with round-bottomed wells. A fixed volume of a particulate antigen suspension is added to an equal volume of serial dilutions of the patient serum in test tubes or perspex plates. Following several hours of incubation at 37°C, agglutination is seen at the bottom of the tubes. **The titre of the serum is given as the reciprocal of the highest dilution that causes clumping.** Thus, the serum that agglutinates at a dilution of 1 : 256 is reported to have a titre of 256 and if the test has been carried out in 1 ml volumes, the titre of the serum is 256 units/ml of serum.

Uses:
Serological diagnosis of:
- Enteric fever (Widal test)
- Brucellosis
- Typhus fever (Weil–Felix reaction)
- *Streptococcus* MG agglutination
- Cold agglutination
- Paul–Bunnel test

In the **Widal test** used for the diagnosis of enteric fever, two types of antigens are used – the flagellar (H) antigen and somatic (O) antigen. H antigen is a formolised suspension of the organisms which on combination with antibody, forms large, loose and fluffy clumps resembling wisps of cotton-wool. For H agglutination conical (Dreyer's) tubes are used. O antigen is prepared by treating the bacterial suspension with alcohol. On combination with antibody it forms fine granular deposit resembling chalk powder at the base of round-bottomed (Felix) tubes, whereas, negative reaction shows a compact button-like deposit (Fig. 12.7).

Tube agglutination test for brucellosis may be complicated by prozone phenomenon and the presence of blocking antibodies. To avoid false negative results due to prozone, several dilutions of the serum should be tested. *Blocking antibodies may*

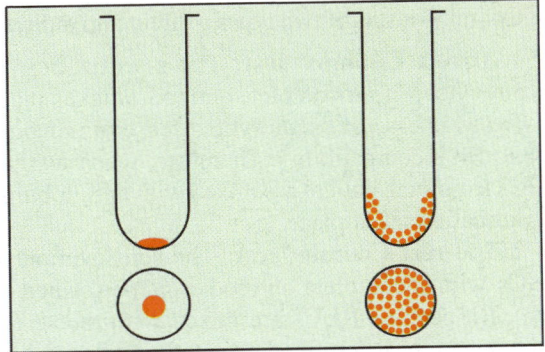

Fig. 12.7. Tube agglutination test.

be detected by doing the test in hypertonic (5%) saline, albumin saline or more reliably by the antiglobulin (Coombs') test. Rh antibodies are also blocking antibodies.

Weil-Felix reaction for serodiagnosis of typhus fever and *Streptococcus* **MG agglutination** for the diagnosis of primary atypical pneumonia are the examples of **heterophile agglutination test** (see Chapter 10). Red blood cells are used as antigens in **cold agglutination** and **Paul-Bunnell test.** IgM antibodies capable of agglutinating human red cells at 0–4°C (cold agglutinins) are sometimes found in certain human diseases including primary atypical pneumonia, malaria, trypanosomiasis and acquired haemolytic anaemia. Sera of the patients suffering from infectious mononucleosis agglutinate sheep RBCs.

Antiglobulin (Coombs') test

Anti-Rh antibodies are of IgG type, but they normally do not agglutinate Rh-positive RBCs (blocking antibodies). The inability of these antibodies to agglutinate is perhaps due to the presence of insufficient antigenic determinants on the RBCs to permit the antibody to overcome the normal electrostatic repulsion that exists among RBCs. When sera containing blocking anti-Rh antibodies are mixed with Rh-positive red cells, the antibody coats the surface of erythrocytes but they are not agglutinated. When such antibody-coated erythrocytes are washed to free all unattached protein and are treated with anti-human gammaglobulin (**antiglobulin or Coombs' serum**), the cells are agglutinated.

Coombs' test is of two types – direct and indirect.

1. **Direct Coombs' test:** The sensitization of erythrocytes with incomplete antibodies takes place *in vivo* as in case of haemolytic disease of newborn due to Rh incompatibility. Therefore, when washed RBCs from such patient are mixed with antiglobulin, agglutination takes place.

2. **Indirect Coombs' test:** The sensitization of RBCs with incomplete antibodies is performed *in vitro*. Rh-positive RBCs are mixed with the serum to be tested for Rh-antibodies and then after a short incubation and washing, antiglobulin is added. If the test serum contained anti-Rh antibodies, agglutination will take place.

Coombs' test is also useful for demonstrating nonagglutinating (blocking) antibodies in brucellosis.

Passive (indirect) agglutination

A precipitation reaction can be converted into agglutination reaction by coating soluble antigen onto the surface of carrier particles such as RBCs, latex, bentonite and gelatin particles. Such test is more convenient and more sensitive for detection of antibodies. Most polysaccharide and lipopolysaccharide antigens may be adsorbed by simple mixing with the cells. For adsorption of protein antigens, tanned red cells are used. Some of the examples of passive agglutination are given below:

- In rheumatoid arthritis, **RA factor** (an anti-gammaglobulin autoantibody) appears in the serum of the patient. It acts as an antibody to human IgG. Latex polystyrene beads coated with denatured human IgG when mixed with patient serum leads to agglutination of latex polystyrene beads.
- Latex particles coated with antibodies to meningococci, *Haemophilus influenzae* type b and pneumococci can be used to detect corresponding antigens in cases of **pyogenic meningitis.**
- Latex agglutination tests are also widely used for detection of hepatitis B, antistreptolysin O, C-reactive protein, human chorionic gonadotropin hormone and many other antigens.
- One of the most widely used passive agglutination test employing erythrocytes is *Treponema pallidum* **haemagglutination (TPHA)** for serological diagnosis of treponemal infection.

- For the detection of **anti-HIV antibodies**, gelatin particles can be sensitized (coated) with inactivated HIV antigen. When these sensitized particles are mixed with the patient serum or plasma these particles are agglutinated if the anti-HIV antibodies are present in the sample. The test procedure is extremely simple using a microtitre technique and is particularly suitable for mass screening of specimens. The test is time-saving and results are readable by the naked eye after about two hours.

When, instead of antigen, antibody is adsorbed on the carrier particles in tests for estimation of antigens, the technique is known as **reversed passive agglutination**.

Coagglutination

This is based upon the principle that most strains of *Staphylococcus aureus* (especially Cowan strain I) possess protein A on their surface. Protein A binds IgG molecules, non-specifically, through Fc region leaving specific Fab sites free to combine with specific antigen. When suspension of such sensitized staphylococcal cells is treated with homologous (test) antigen, the antigen combines with free Fab sites of IgG attached to staphylococcal cells leading to visible clumping of staphylococci within two minutes. This is known as coagglutination (COA).

COA test can be used for detecting the presence of bacterial antigens in serum, urine and CSF. For example, typhoid bacillus antigen is consistently present in the blood in the early phase of disease, and also in the urine of the patients. This antigen can be detected by COA test. Similarly, meningococcal, pneumococcal and *Haemophilus* antigens can be detected by COA test in the CSF. Identification of *Neisseria gonorrhoeae* and serogrouping of β-haemolytic streptococci A, B, C, D and G can also be carried out by COA test.

Complement fixation test (CFT)

The ability of antigen-antibody complexes to fix complement is made use of in complement fixation test (CFT). This is a very versatile and sensitive test. This can detect as little as 0.04 µg of antibody nitrogen and 0.1 µg of antigen. CFTs include **Wassermann reaction** and **Reiter protein complement** fixation test (RPCFT) for the serodiagnosis of syphilis. Similarly, CFTs for the identification of various viral antigens are also available.

In most of the cases fixation of complement with antigen-antibody complex causes in itself no visible effect. Therefore, it is necessary to use an **indicator system** consisting of sheep red cells coated with anti-sheep red cell antibody. Complement lyses antibody coated red cells. CFT, therefore, is performed in two stages.

Stage 1: Test serum (for the detection of antibody) and the antigen are mixed in the presence of carefully measured amount of complement and then incubated at 37°C for 1 hour. If the test serum contains antibody then antigen-antibody complexes are formed and complement gets fixed on it.

Stage 2: Indicator system, antibody-coated sheep red cells, is added to determine whether the complement has been fixed in stage 1 reaction or not. If the complement has been taken up during stage 1 reaction then it will not be available to lyse the red cells. Therefore, a positive CFT is indicated by absence of lysis of red cells whilst a negative test, with unused complement, is shown by lysis of the red cells (Fig. 12.8).

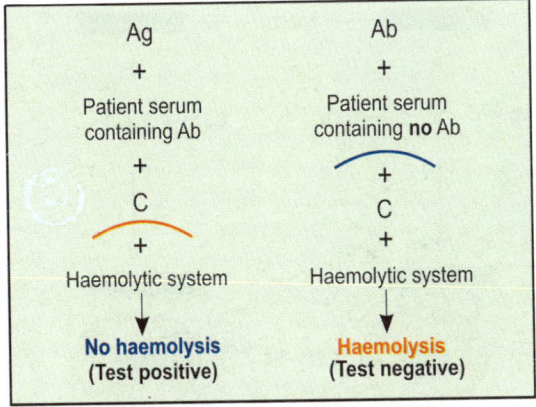

Fig. 12.8. Complement fixation test.

The antigen in this test may be soluble or particulate. Prior to commencement of test the serum should be inactivated by heating it at 56°C for 30 minutes to destroy any complement activity serum may have and also to remove some non-specific

inhibitors of complement. The source of complement for laboratory use is guinea-pig serum. Guinea-pig serum is first titrated for complement activity. One unit or **minimum haemolytic dose (MHD)** of **complement** is the highest dilution of guinea-pig serum that lyses one unit volume of washed sheep RBCs in the presence of excess of haemolysin (amboceptor) within a fixed time (usually 30–60 minutes) at 37°C. Similarly, amboceptor should also be titrated. **One MHD of haemolysin** may be defined as highest dilution of the serum that lyses one unit volume of washed sheep RBCs in the presence of excess complement within a fixed time (usually 30–60 minutes) at 37°C.

Anti-complementary effect

Non-specific adsorption of complement may give false positive results. Some sera may develop anti-complementary properties on ageing, and after bacterial contamination. Haemolysed blood serum also has anti-complementary effect.

Other tests employing complement

Immune adherence

Some bacteria, like *Vibrio cholerae* and *Treponema pallidum*, react with specific antibody in the presence of complement and particulate material such as erythrocytes or platelets; the bacteria are aggregated and adhere to the cells. This is known as immune adherence. **Adherence occurs through the activated C3b component of complement.**

Treponema pallidum immobilization test

The test serum is incubated anaerobically with a suspension of live treponemes and complement. If antibodies are present, the treponemes will be found to be immobilized.

Cytolytic or cytocidal tests

When *V. cholerae* is mixed with its antibody in the presence of complement, the bacterium is killed and lysed.

Neutralization tests

These are of two types – virus neutralization tests and toxin neutralization tests.

Virus neutralization tests

Neutralization of viruses by their antibodies in a patient serum may be quantitated by their ability to reduce the infectivity of a stock virus preparation. The test serum is diluted serially, incubated with a known amount of virus and the mixture is then added to indicator systems – animals, embryonated hen's egg and tissue culture. The highest dilution of serum ablating infectivity in 50% of virus-serum mixtures tested is taken as the titre. **Neutralization of bacteriophages can be demonstrated by plaque inhibition test.** When bacteriophages are seeded in appropriate dilution on lawn cultures, plaques of lysis are produced. Specific antiphage serum inhibits plaque formation.

Toxin neutralization

Bacterial exotoxins are highly antigenic and their activity may be completely neutralized by appropriate concentrations of specific antibody. Antibody to bacterial exotoxin is usually referred to as antitoxin. Bacterial endotoxins are poorly antigenic and their toxicity is not neutralized by antisera.

The neutralizing capacity of an antitoxin can be assayed by neutralization test in which mixture of toxin and antitoxin is injected into a susceptible animal and the least amount of antitoxin that prevents death or disease in the animal is estimated. In case of diphtheria toxin, which in small doses causes cutaneous reaction, neutralization test can be carried out on the human skin. The **Schick test** is based on the ability of circulating antitoxin to neutralize the diphtheria toxin given intradermally. Neutralization (no reaction) indicates immunity, and erythema and induration indicates susceptibility to diphtheria.

If a toxin has a demonstrable *in vitro* effect, this effect can be neutralized by specific antitoxin. For example, antistreptolysin O, present in the serum of the patient suffering from *Streptococcus pyogenes* infection, neutralizes the haemolytic activity of the streptococcal O haemolysin. Another example of *in vitro* toxin-antitoxin neutralization is **Nagler's reaction.** *Clostridium perfringens* produces α-toxin which is a phospholipase (lecithinase-C). This produces opalescence in serum or egg yolk media. This reaction is specifically neutralized by the antitoxin.

Opsonization

A substance, such as complement or antibody, that can bind to the surface of a cell or a particle, making it more readily phagocytosed is known as opsonin. Enhanced complement-mediated phagocytosis can occur either in the presence or absence of antibody. Phagocytes such as macrophages, monocytes and neutrophils possess surface receptors (CR1) for C3b and Fc receptors for antibody. If immune complexes have activated the complement system then Fc and CR1 receptors, present on the phagocyte, bind Fc region of antibody and C3b bound on immune complexes respectively thus facilitating their phagocytosis. This facilitated phagocytosis by antibody and complement is known as **immune opsonization.**

In contrast, **nonimmune opsonization** requires only C3b (opsonin) for opsonization. Bacteria in the blood stream can activate the alternative pathway and generate C3b, which coats the bacteria. C3b binds to CR1 receptors present on the phagocytes thus facilitating their phagocytosis. Viruses, soluble immune complexes and tumour cells are also opsonized and removed by the same mechanism (Fig. 12.9).

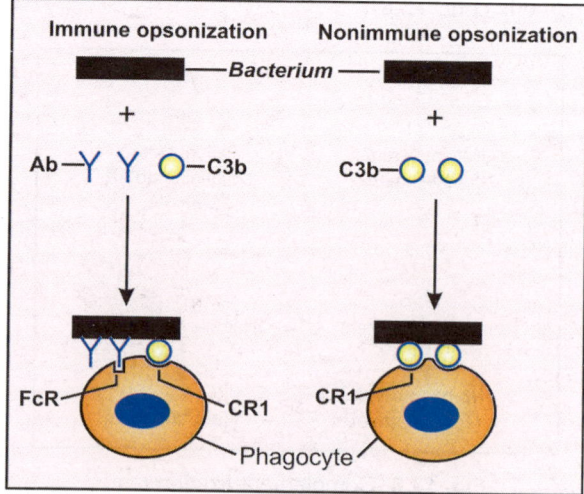

Fig. 12.9. Opsonization.

Immunofluorescence

Fluorescent dyes absorb invisible UV light between 290–495 nm and emit visible longer wavelength (525 nm) green light. Therefore, if microorganisms or tissue cells are stained with a fluorescent dye and examined under the microscope with UV light instead of visible light they are seen as bright objects against a dark background. This principle is used in fluorescence microscopy. Coons and his colleagues (1942) showed that fluorescent dyes, such as fluorescein isothiocyanate (FITC), can be conjugated to antibodies (without affecting their specificity) permitting their ready detection, when attached to an antigen associated with a cell. Immunofluorescence (IF) is now used extensively to detect:

- Tissue antigens.
- Antibodies to tissues including autoantibodies.
- The antigens of infecting organisms in the body.
- Antigen-antibody complexes.

It is more sensitive than precipitation and complement fixation test. Fluorescence can be observed under a fluorescence microscope (FM), which contains a high intensity UV light source (mercury lamp) instead of visible light. Two types of filters are fitted in the FM:

1. *Primary filter:* It is fitted close to the lamp. This ensures the maximum emission of radiation (UV light) of the required wavelengths.

2. *Secondary filter:* It is placed in the eyepiece to cut out UV rays which might damage the observer's eye.

Fluorescence-staining techniques are of two types – direct and indirect (Fig. 12.10).

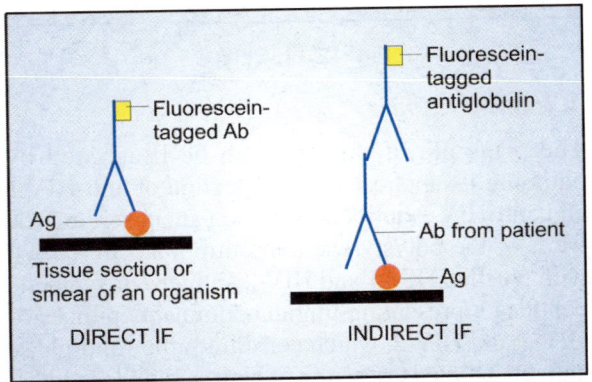

Fig. 12.10. Immunofluorescence.

Direct IF

This consists of bringing fluorescein-tagged antibodies in contact with antigens (bacteria, viruses and other antigens) fixed on a slide (e.g., in the form of a tissue section or a smear of an organism), allowing them to react, washing off excess antibody and examining under FM. The site of union of the labelled antibody with its antigen can be seen by the apple-green fluorescent areas on the slide. **Direct IF is routinely used as a sensitive method of diagnosing rabies, by detection of rabies virus antigens in brain smears.** A disadvantage of this method is that separate fluorescent conjugates have to be prepared against each antigen to be tested.

Indirect IF

This method can be used for detection of specific antibodies in sera or other body fluids and also for identifying antigens. The disadvantage of direct IF, mentioned above, is overcome by this method. An example of this method is the **fluorescent treponemal antibody test for the diagnosis of syphilis.** Here a drop of the patient serum is placed on a smear of *T. pallidum* on a slide and after incubation, the slide is washed well to remove all free serum, leaving behind only antibody, if present, coated on the surface of the treponemes. Whether or not the patient serum contains antibodies to *T. pallidum* is shown by means of a fluorescein-tagged antihuman gammaglobulin (antiglobulin).

If patient serum contains anti-treponemal antibodies fluorescein-tagged antiglobulin will react with it. After washing away all the unbound fluorescent conjugate, when the slide is examined under FM the treponemes will be seen as bright objects against a dark background. If the patient serum is negative for anti-treponemal antibodies, there will be no antibody coating on the treponemes and, therefore, they will not take up the fluorescent conjugate. Therefore, they will not fluoresce. The advantage of this technique is that a single antihuman gammaglobulin fluorescent conjugate can be employed for detecting human antibody to any antigen. Indirect IF is also a convenient method for detecting autoantibodies that have bound to membrane antigens, *in vivo*.

The direct method is simple and rapid to perform with fewer nonspecific reactions, however, it is less sensitive. The indirect method is more sensitive and gives brighter fluorescence, however, due to increased cross-reactivity it is less specific.

Radioimmunoassay (RIA)

RIA is a very sensitive and specific method. It involves the use of either antiserum or more usually antigen labelled with ^{125}I. The amount of radioactive label bound to antigen-antibody complex can be measured, and hence the concentration of antigen or antibody in a specimen can be determined. RIA permits measurement of analytes up to picogram (10^{-12} gram) quantities. It has been used to measure a variety of serum proteins including Igs, hormones, drugs, tumour markers and viral antigens. RIA is based on the competition of radiolabelled, known antigen and unlabelled, unknown antigen for limited binding sites on known specific antibody in solution or attached to a plate or tube (solid phase).

To establish an assay, antibody must be produced against the known antigen and the antigen radiolabelled, e.g., with ^{125}I. A standard curve is established by adding fixed amounts of radiolabelled antigen, specific antibody and increasing concentrations of known unlabelled antigen to a series of tubes or wells in a plastic microtitre plate. Following incubation, the amount of labelled antigen bound to antibody is determined after separation from free labelled antigen in a gamma spectrometer. If a test serum contains antigen for the antibody, then there is competition with labelled antigen. This appears as reduction in the amount of labelled antigen bound in the complex. The concentration of the antigen in the sample can be determined from the standard curve.

Enzyme immunoassay (EIA)

Enzyme immunoassay is an important immunological method for detecting and measuring antigens or antibodies. It is based on the same principle as that of radioimmunoassay. The key difference is that for enzyme immunoassays the antigen or antibody is conjugated to an enzyme rather than a radioactive isotope. The enzyme is then detected by its ability to convert a colourless substance to a coloured one.

Obviously the method requires that, in the enzyme immunoglobulin conjugate, the enzyme retains its enzymatic activity and the antigen or antibody its immunological activity.

Enzyme immunoassays have become very popular in view of their high sensitivity, safety, economy and the simple instrumentation requirements. Solid-phase immunoassays are more widely used. Such systems are called enzyme-linked immunosorbent assays (ELISAs). The ELISA can be used to detect and determine concentrations of antigen or antibody. The test may be done in polystyrene well (microtitre plate) or tube. Different types of ELISA have been developed (Fig. 12.11).

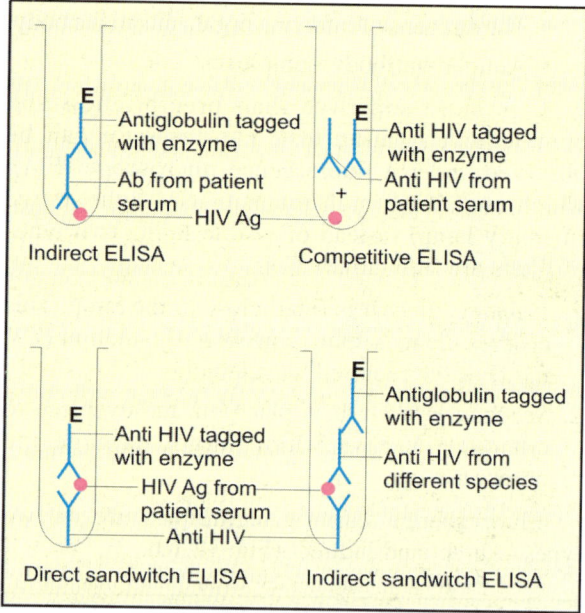

Fig. 12.11. ELISA.

1. Indirect ELISA

The principle of this test can be illustrated by outlining its application for detection of anti-HIV-1 and anti-HIV-2 antibodies in the patient serum. The wells of the polystyrene microtitre plate are coated with purified HIV-1 and HIV-2 antigens or synthetic peptides representing immunodominant epitopes of HIV-1 and HIV-2, which constitutes the solid-phase antigen. Diluted test serum or plasma sample is added to such a well and incubated. If antibodies specific for HIV-1 and/or HIV-2 are present in the test sample they will form stable complexes with antigens coated on the well. Well is then washed and a conjugate of goat antihuman immunoglobulin, which has been labelled with the enzyme horseradish peroxidase, is added. If the antigen-antibody complex is present, the peroxidase conjugate will bind to the complex and remains in the well. The conjugate fraction remaining free in the well is removed by washing and the presence of enzyme immobilized on the complexes is shown by incubation in the presence of a colourless enzyme substrate (orthophenylene-diamine dihydrochloride solution). Incubation with enzyme substrate produces a yellow-orange colour in the test well. If the sample contains no anti-HIV-1 and/or anti-HIV-2, then the labelled antibody cannot be found and no colour develops. The absorbance value of each well is read by an ELISA plate reader at wavelength of 492 ± 2 nm.

2. Competitive ELISA

The principle of this test too can be illustrated by outlining its application for detection of anti-HIV antibodies in the patient serum. The wells of the polystyrene microtitre plate are coated with HIV antigens which constitutes the solid-phase antigen. The test sample and human anti-HIV, which has been labelled with the enzyme horseradish peroxidase, are incubated in such a well. When the sample contains no anti-HIV, solid-phase antigen/labelled antibody complex will be formed. The incubation with enzyme substrate produces a yellow-orange colour in the test well. If anti-HIV is present in the test sample, it competes with the labelled antibody for the available solid-phase antigen and no colour or reduced colour develops.

3. Sandwich ELISA

The most frequently used ELISA for detecting microbial antigen is the sandwich solid-phase ELISA. It is of two types:

(i) Single-antibody or direct sandwich ELISA

Antibody is attached to the solid-phase. The test sample is then exposed to the solid-phase antibody, to which the antigen, if present, will bind. The solid-phase antibody-antigen complex is then rinsed free

of unbound test sample and exposed again to antibodies reactive against the test antigen and conjugated with the enzyme. The conjugated antibody will react with the antigen held to the solid-phase by the first antibody, forming an **antibody-antigen-antibody sandwich on the solid-phase**. The solid-phase sandwich is again separated from unreacted test sample by rinsing. The second antibody (conjugated to an enzyme) can be detected with an appropriate substrate. This is a single antibody or direct sandwich ELISA.

(ii) Double-antibody or indirect sandwich ELISA

In the double-antibody ELISA the second antibody as above is not conjugated with the enzyme. The second antibody can be detected by treating it with an antiimmunoglobulin-enzyme conjugate. In the double-antibody ELISA, the second antibody of the sandwich must be from a different species than the solid-phase antibody, otherwise, the antiimmuno-globulin conjugate reacts with the solid-phase antibody, producing high background activity.

ELISA is a simple and versatile technique. It needs only microlitre quantities of reactants. ELISA kits are commercially available for the detection of anti-HIV, hepatitis B surface antigen and rotavirus. ELISA kits have also been developed for detecting:

- *Entamoeba histolytica* antigens in faeces.
- *Toxoplasma* antigens in the patient serum.
- *Haemophilus influenzae* antigens in spinal fluid.
- β-haemolytic streptococcal antigens in spinal fluid.
- Hepatitis A virus in stools.
- Respiratory syncytial virus in pharyngeal secretions.
- Adenovirus antigens in nasopharyngeal specimens.
- Labile enterotoxin of *Escherichia coli* in stools.

Chemiluminescence immunoassay (CLIA)

Chemiluminescence refers to a chemical reaction emitting energy in the form of light. As radioactive conjugates are employed in RIA, fluorescent conjugates in fluorescence microscopy and enzymes in ELISA, chemiluminescent compounds such as luminol or acridinium esters are used in CLIA as the label to provide the signal during the antigen-antibody reaction. The signal (light) can be amplified, measured and the concentration of analyte calculated. The method has been fully automated.

Western blotting

Western blotting is analogous to Southern blotting, for isolated DNA, and Northern blotting, for isolated RNA. In Western blotting, protein antigens are separated according to their electrophoretic mobility and molecular weight by polyacrylamide gel electrophoresis, then blotted onto nitrocellulose paper by standard blotting procedure. The patient serum is allowed to react with the blot. Antibodies attached to separated viral antigens on the nitrocellulose paper are detected by enzyme tagged-antihuman gamma-globulin. Enzyme substrate is subsequently added which indicates positive test. The substrate changes colour in the presence of enzyme and permanently stains the nitrocellulose paper. The position of the band on the paper indicates the antigen with which the antibody has reacted.

Immunoelectron microscopy

When the virus particles, for example, rotavirus and hepatitis A virus in stool, are scanty in the specimen they can be treated with specific antisera. It leads to clumping of virus particles which can be seen under electron microscope. This is known as immuno-electron microscopy and it finds application in detection of some viruses causing diarrhoea.

Capsule swelling or Quellung reaction

Mixing capsulated bacteria, such as *S. pneumoniae* and *Klebsiella pneumoniae*, with homologous antibody makes possible the direct microscopic visualization of capsules. Binding of the homologous type specific antibody increases the refractility and apparent thickness of the capsule thus making direct microscopic visualization of the capsule possible.

Immunoenzyme test

Some stable enzymes, such as peroxidases, can be conjugated with antibodies. Antigens in tissue sections can be detected by treating them with peroxidase conjugated specific antibody. If the tissue section possesses specific antigen then antigen-enzyme conjugated antibody complexes will be formed which can be detected by treatment with enzyme substrate.

KEY FACTS

- *Antigen-antibody reactions are specific* but cross-reactions may occur
- When a *soluble antigen* is mixed with its *specific antibody* in the presence of *electrolytes* at a *suitable temperature* and *pH*, the antigen-antibody complex forms an *insoluble precipitate*
- When a *particulate antigen* or an *antigen* present on a cell or an inorganic particle is mixed with its *antibody* in the presence of *electrolytes* at a suitable *temperature and pH*, the particles are *clumped or agglutinated*
- The ability of *antigen-antibody complexes* to *fix complement* is made use of in *complement fixation test*
- A substance, such as complement or antibody, that can bind to the surface of a cell or a particle, making it more readily phagocytosed is known as *opsonin*
- Radioactive conjugates are employed in radio-immunoassay, fluorescent conjugates in fluorescence microscopy, enzymes in enzyme-linked immunosorbent assay and chemiluminescent compounds are used in chemiluminescence immunoassay.

IMPORTANT QUESTION

Discuss principle and clinical applications of:
(a) ELISA
(b) Agglutination reactions
(c) Precipitation reactions
(d) Coagglutination test
(e) Antiglobulin (Coombs') test
(f) Immunofluorescence

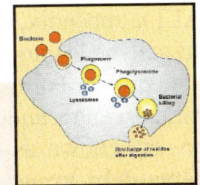

Chapter 13

Structure and Functions of Immune System

Immune responses are mediated by a variety of cells, and by the soluble molecules they secrete. Lymphocytes (B cells and T cells), phagocytes (mononuclear phagocytes, neutrophils and eosinophils), and auxiliary cells (basophils, mast cells and platelets) are the cellular components of immune system. *Antibodies produced by B cells; cytokines produced by T cells and mononuclear phagocytes; complement produced by mononuclear cells; inflammatory mediators produced by basophils, mast cells and platelets; and interferon produced by infected tissue cells are the soluble mediators of immune system.*

Immune response to an antigen is of two types:

1. **Humoral or antibody-mediated immunity** (AMI) which is mediated by antibodies produced by plasma cells.
2. **Cell-mediated immunity** (CMI) which is mediated directly by sensitized lymphocytes.

Lymphoid organs can be classified into primary (central) lymphoid organs and secondary (peripheral) lymphoid organs. Thymus and bursa of Fabricius are primary lymphoid organs. They are responsible for cellular and humoral immune response respectively. The equivalent of the avian bursa of Fabricius, in mammals, is bone marrow.

Lymphocytes, like other circulating blood cells, arise from the differentiation of a single pleuripotent stem cell. In early embryonic development, blood cell precursors are found in foetal liver and other tissues; in postnatal life, the stem cells reside in bone marrow. They can differentiate in several ways. In liver and bone marrow, stem cells may differentiate into cells of red cell series or into cells of lymphoid series. Lymphoid stem cells evolve into two main lymphocyte population, B cells and T cells. If a stem cell is to become a T cell, it leaves the bone marrow and emigrates to the thymus where it differentiates further under the influence of the thymic micro-environment and soluble factors produced by the thymic epithelium. The resulting T cells are responsible for specific cell-mediated immunity.

However, if the lymphoid stem cell is destined to become a B cell it remains in the bone marrow (in case of birds it emigrates to bursa of Fabricius, a gut appendage) where it undergoes several more differentiative steps before it gains the ability to produce and secrete antibody in response to the presence of infectious organisms. After acquiring immunocompetence, both T and B cells leave their primary site of differentiation and emigrate to the peripheral lymphoid organs (Fig. 13.1). These include lymph nodes, spleen, gut-associated lymphoid tissue (GALT), appendix, tonsils and adenoids.

B cells seed into outer cortex in germinal follicles and medullary cords of peripheral lymph nodes and germinal centre and mantle layer of spleen. These areas are known as **bursa-dependent** or **thymus-independent areas**. T cells seed into paracortical areas of lymph nodes and white pulp of spleen around the central arterioles. These areas are known as **thymus-dependent areas**. Here, in the peripheral lymphoid organs, they encounter with infectious organisms that have escaped the innate defence system.

CELLS OF THE IMMUNE SYSTEM

Lymphocytes

Of the many cells involved in specific response to antigen, lymphocytes are the most important effector cells. They are small, round, 5–15 μm in diameter and are found in peripheral blood, lymph, lymphoid organs and in many other tissues. In peripheral blood, they constitute 20–40% of the leucocyte population, while in lymph and lymphoid organs they form the predominant cell type. They may be small (5–8 μm), medium (8–12 μm) and large (12–15 μm). The small lymphocytes are most numerous. They may be short-lived (life-span about two weeks) or long-lived (life-span three years or more or even for life). Short-lived

cells are effector cells in immune response, while long-lived cells act as memory cells. Long-lived cells are mainly thymus-derived. Lymphopoiesis takes place in the bone marrow, central lymphoid organs and peripheral lymphoid organs.

Lymphocytes possess antigen recognition mechanism on their surface, enabling each cell to recognize only one or a small number of antigens. Two major classes of lymphocytes are recognized which are designated **T cells** and **B cells**. T and B cells are indistinguishable by conventional light microscopy.

Classification of lymphocytes on the basis of surface markers makes use of two important characteristics:

1. Cluster of differentiation or cluster determinant (CD).
2. Antigen recognition receptors.

1. Cluster of differentiation or cluster determinant

CDs represent families of surface glycoprotein antigens that can be recognized by specific antibodies produced against them. Thus a cell displaying CD1 is identified by the binding of antibodies against CD1. Each class of leucocyte displays a diagnostic pattern of CDs, for example:

- CD3 is expressed only by T cells.
- CD19 is expressed only by B cells.

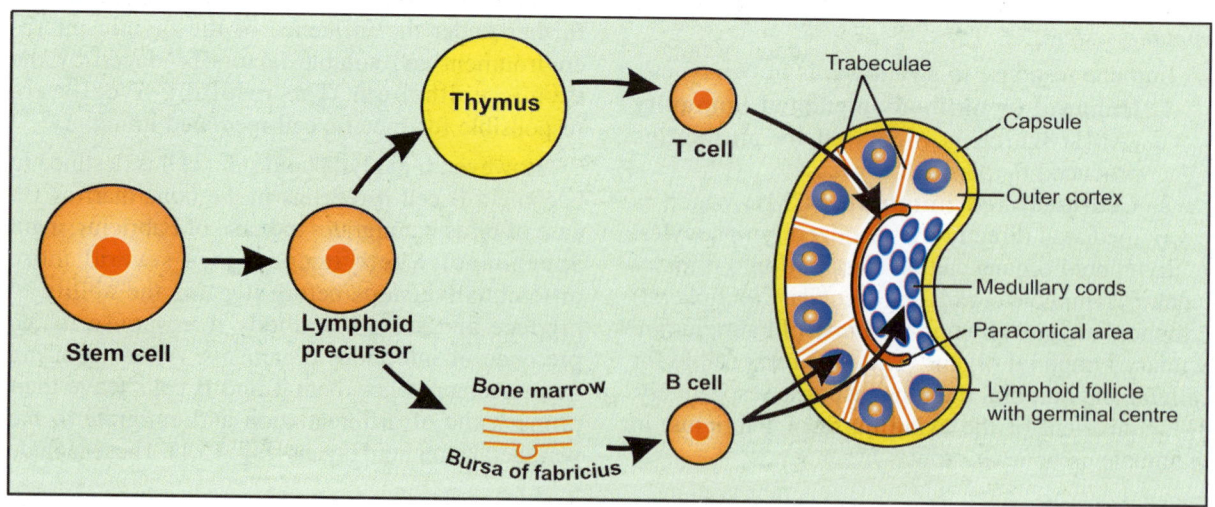

Fig. 13.1. Development of T and B cells.

- CD64 is expressed only by monocytes.
- CD66 is expressed only by granulocytes.
- CD68 is expressed only by macrophages.
- On the other hand, CD18 and CD45 are expressed by a variety of leucocyte types.
- A total of more than 150 CDs are known.

2. Antigen recognition receptors

These include membrane-bound (surface) immuno-globulins (mIgs or sIgs) in B cells, and T cell receptors (TCRs) in T cells. In contrast to CDs, which can serve as diagnostic feature for all leucocytes, antigen recognition receptors are limited to B and T lymphocytes only. These receptors are required for B and T cells to be antigen reactive. Both mIgs and TCRs serve as specific surface receptors, recognizing and interacting with only single antigenic determinant on the antigen. Reaction of antigens with mIgs and TCRs activates B cells and T cells respectively, leading to proliferation and differentiation.

Thus the antigen specificity of the mIgs in B cells and TCRs in T cells is predetermined, and the sole effect of antigen is to select out a cell with appropriate surface receptor and induce it to clonally expand and differentiate into a cell that will produce the antibody it has been predetermined to make or produce specific clones of effector T cells respectively.

B lymphocytes

Lymphocytes possessing mIgs are termed B cells. They arise from pleuripotent stem cells in bone marrow, they mature in bone marrow itself and then emigrate to the peripheral lymphoid organs where, upon contact with antigen, they can differentiate into antibody-producing **plasma cells.** Each B cell possesses about 10^5 mIg molecules, primarily of IgM and IgD classes. Following activation, immuno-globulins of other classes might also reside on B lymphocyte membranes. Immature B cells do not possess mIg receptors.

A single B cell or a clone of B cells possess mIg receptors specific for only one (monospecific) antigenic determinant. Thus billions of B cells display a diversity of receptors capable of reacting with any antigenic determinant that might be encountered. Receptor immunoglobulin and secreted immuno-globulin of a single cell or clone of cells are identical in the variable regions of the antibody molecule.

Most B cells and macrophages, and certain activated T cells express class II major histocompatibility gene products or immune associated (Ia) antigens in the mouse, and HLA-DR antigens in humans. Receptors for the Fc portion of IgG (FcR) are found on all B cells, macrophages and certain subsets of T cells. Some cells express receptors for other classes of immunoglobulin as well. These receptors bind antigen-antibody complexes. Receptors for C3 component of complement are found on most B cells. These are known as complement receptors (CRs). These receptors are thought to play a role in the regulation of the B cell response to antigen. Because of the presence of CRs on the surface of B cells they bind to sheep RBCs which have been coated with antibody and complement forming EAC rosettes. They undergo blast transformation on treatment with bacterial endotoxins.

T lymphocytes

Pleuripotent stem cells in the bone marrow give rise to precursor T cells, which migrate to the thymus (Fig. 13.2). Once they enter the cortex of the thymus they are known as **thymocytes**. As T cells mature, their surface antigens including CDs and TCRs change. Monoclonal antibodies are used to identify the antigenic subsets of T cells. Approximately 65% of mature T cells that leave the thymus display CD2+CD3+CD4+CD8–TCR+ phenotype (CD4+ cells), while approximately 35% display CD2+CD3+CD4–CD8+TCR+ phenotype (CD8+ cells). A very small number express neither CD4 nor CD8 and consequently have a phenotype of CD2+CD3+ CD4–CD8–TCR+ (CD4–CD8– cells).

T cell subsets

Four distinct subsets of T cells are known. Two each of these are regulator and effector cells.

Regulator cells:

1. *Helper T cells (Th cells):* They possess CD2, CD3 and CD4 surface antigens. They help in the antigen-specific activation of B cells and effector T cells.
2. *Suppressor T cells (Ts cells):* They possess CD2, CD3 and CD8 surface antigens. They suppress expression of immune response by other lymphocytes.

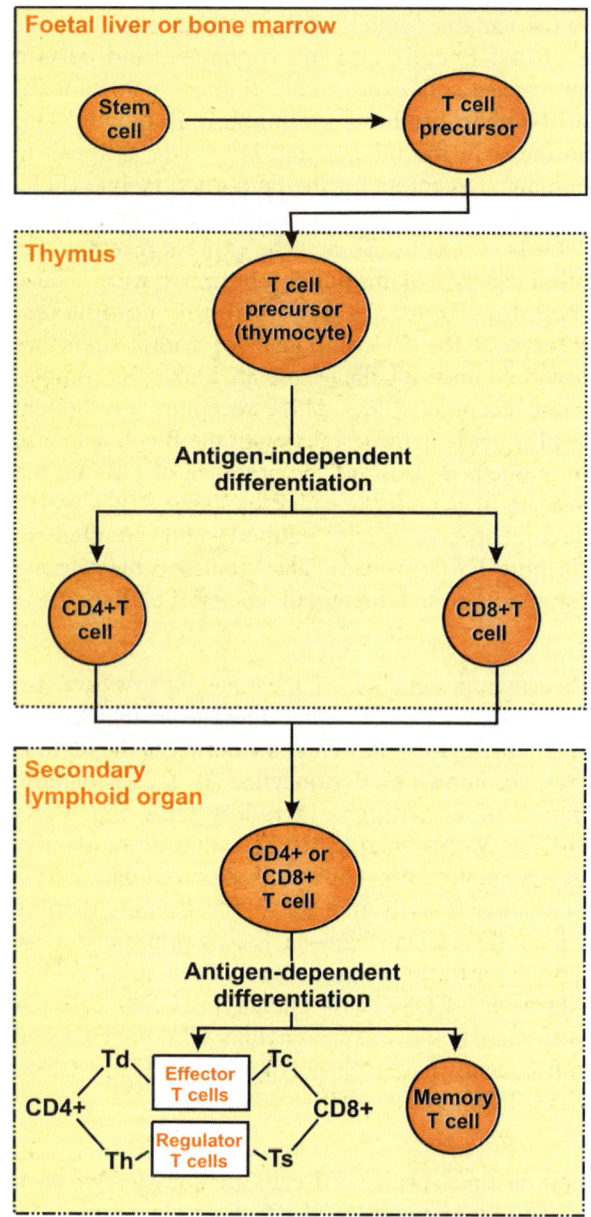

Fig. 13.2. T cell differentiation.

Effector cells:

1. *Delayed-type-hypersensitivity T cells (Td cells):* They possess CD2, CD3 and CD4 surface antigens. They are involved in delayed hypersensitivity and cell-mediated immune responses.

2. *Cytotoxic T cells (Tc cells):* They possess CD2, CD3 and CD8 surface antigens. They are also involved in cell-mediated immune responses and lyse target cells by direct cell-cell contact.

Immune response is regulated by mutually opposing influence of Th and Ts cells. Overactivity of Th or decreased activity of Ts causes abnormal immune responses as seen in autoimmunity. Diminished Th function or increased activity of Ts leads to immunodeficiency.

During maturation and differentiation in thymus, T cells also learn to recognize self-major histocompatibility (MHC) antigens. CD4+ cells recognize class II MHC antigens and CD8+ cells recognize class I MHC antigens.

T cells bind to sheep RBCs at 37°C forming SRBC or E rosettes while B cells do not. They undergo blast transformation, evidenced by enhanced DNA synthesis, on treatment with mitogens such as phytohaemagglutinin (PHA) and concanavalin A (Con A).

Table 13.1 summarises differences between T cells and B cells.

Table 13.1. Differences between T and B lymphocytes		
Property	**T cell**	**B cell**
1. Antigen recognition receptors	TCRs	mIgs
2. Surface glycoprotein antigens	CD3	CD19
3. Receptors for Fc piece of immunoglobulins (FcR)	–*	+
4. Receptors for C3 component of complement (CRs)	–	+
5. EAC rosette	–	+
6. E rosette	+	–
7. Thymus specific antigens	+	–
8. Blast transformation on treatment with	PHA and Con A	Bacterial endotoxins

* Certain subsets of T cells possess FcR

Null cells

A small proportion (5%) of lymphocytes that lack distinguishing phenotypic markers characteristic of T or B lymphocytes are known as null cells or non-T and non-B lymphocytes. They do not possess TCRs or mIgs. A few null cells in the circulation might be immature T or B cells.

Killer cells or K cells

A subpopulation of null cells possess surface receptors for Fc part of IgG. They are capable of lysing or killing target cells sensitized by IgG antibody. They are known as killer or K cells. They are responsible for antibody-dependent cell-mediated cytotoxicity (ADCC) in contrast to the action of cytotoxic T lymphocytes which are independent of antibody.

Natural killer or NK cells

Another subpopulation of null cells is natural killer or NK cells. These are large lymphocytes containing azurophilic granules in the cytoplasm. They are, therefore, known as large granular lymphocytes (LGL). NK cells are capable of non-specific killing of virus-transformed target cells and are involved in allograft and tumour rejection.

Plasma cells

Plasma cells are fully differentiated antibody-synthesizing cells. Antigenically stimulated B cells undergo blast transformation, becoming successively plasmablasts, intermediate transitional cells and plasma cells. It is an oval cell, about twice the size of a small lymphocyte. It has an eccentric nucleus, abundant rough endoplasmic reticulum, numerous mitochondria and prominent Golgi apparatus. Plasma cells are end cells and have a short life-span of two or three days. A plasma cell secretes an antibody of a single specificity of a single antibody class and of a single light chain type. However, in primary antibody response plasma cell produces IgM initially and later it may switch onto IgG production. Lymphocytes, lymphoblasts and transitional cells may also synthesize immunoglobulins to some extent.

Antigen-presenting cells (APCs)

A number of different cell types have been described as APCs. In addition to presenting antigen to effector lymphocytes, many of these cells perform non-specific immunological functions such as phagocytosis and cytotoxicity. Induction of humoral or cell-mediated immunity cannot occur efficiently in the absence of APCs, i.e., with lymphocytes alone. APCs include dendritic cells that are found in skin (Langerhans' cells), thymus, lymph node, spleen and other secondary lymphoid organs and macrophages which include monocytes as blood macrophages and histiocytes as tissue macrophages.

The processing and presentation of antigen by macrophages to T cells require that both the cells possess surface determinants coded by the same MHC genes. T cells can accept the processed antigen only if it is presented by macrophages carrying on its surface the self-MHC determinant known as immune-associated or Ia antigen. When the macrophage bears a different Ia antigen, it cannot cooperate with T cell. This is known as **MHC restriction**.

Functional activity of macrophages may be enhanced by lymphokines, complement components and interferon. Activated macrophages are not antigen specific. They secrete a number of biologically active substances like interleukin-1. They can bind immune complexes by means of FcRs or CRs, which are present on their surface, and then engulf and digest them. Macrophages can also exhibit ADCC reactions. Role of macrophages in innate immune response is discussed in Chapter 9.

OTHER CELLS INVOLVED IN IMMUNOLOGICAL RESPONSES

Neutrophils

Approximately 60% of the circulating leucocytes in humans are neutrophils. Their primary function is phagocytosis of foreign or dead cells and pinocytosis of pathological immune complexes. They can also exhibit ADCC. They are capable of rapid activation and mobilization in response to chemotactic stimuli such as bacterial products or activated components of complement (C5a). A variety of receptors, e.g., FcRs, CR1 and CR2 are increasingly displayed following activation. They constitute predominant cell type in inflammation.

Eosinophils

These are granulocytes containing prominent acidophilic granules. They account for 3–5% of the white blood cells. During allergic conditions and during certain parasitic infections the number of eosinophils may increase dramatically. They can engulf and remove immune complexes by phago-cytosis/pinocytosis. They possess FcRs and can mediate ADCC. They can bind to worm larvae such as schistosomulae coated with IgG, degranulate and release toxic proteins which damage the parasites.

Basophils and mast cells

Basophils comprise less than 1% of white blood cells. Basophils and their tissue counterparts, mast cells, possess basophilic granules. These granules contain pharmacological mediators of type I hypersensitivity. IgE antibodies get attached to FcRs present on the surface of mast cells and basophils. When stimulated with allergen, granules release their contents. Basophils also possess FcRs for IgG and CRs for C3a, C3b and C5a.

KEY FACTS

- *The immune system is able to recognize and respond to many antigens* by generating great diversity in the antibodies produced by B cells

- Each lymphocyte expresses either antibody or a TCR with a single specificity for antigen
- A lymphocyte bearing a complementary antibody or TCR on its surface will bind antigen, be *activated*, *proliferate* to form *a clone*, and also form a large pool of *memory cells*
- Many antigens require *T cell help* before they can activate B cells, and the interactions are mediated by a variety of *soluble cytokines*
- *Immune response* to antigen is of two types – humoral or *antibody mediated immunity* and *cell-mediated immunity*
- *T cell subsets* include *regulator cells* (Th cells and Ts cells) and *effector cells* (Td cells and Tc cells)

IMPORTANT QUESTIONS

1. Write short notes on:
   (a) Subsets of T lymphocytes
   (b) B lymphocytes
2. Tabulate differences between T cells and B cells.

Chapter 14

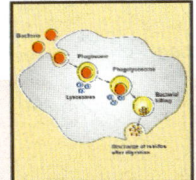

Immune Response

Specific reactivity following an antigenic stimulus is known as the immune response. It is of two types:

- Humoral or antibody-mediated immunity (AMI).
- Cell-mediated immunity (CMI).

AMI provides defence against most extracellular bacterial pathogens and viruses that infect through the respiratory and intestinal tract. It also participates in immediate (types I, II, III and V) hypersensitivity reactions and certain autoimmune diseases.

CMI protects against fungi, most of the viruses and intracellular bacterial pathogens like *Mycobacterium leprae*, *M. tuberculosis*, *Brucella* and *Salmonella*, and parasites like *Leishmania* and trypanosomes. It also participates in allograft rejection, graft versus host reaction, delayed hypersensitivity and certain autoimmune diseases. It provides immunological surveillance and immunity against cancer.

HUMORAL OR ANTIBODY-MEDIATED IMMUNE RESPONSE

The antibody response to stimulation by antigen can be described as primary humoral response and secondary humoral response.

Primary humoral response

Phases (Fig. 14.1)

1. **Lag phase:** After first injection of the antigen there is a long lag phase of several days before antibody appears. During this period the antigen binds specifically to cells displaying complementary antigen receptors. These cells are stimulated to divide forming a **clone of effector cells and memory cells**. The lag phase depends upon the kind and amount of antigen given, the route of administration, species of animal and its health. Usually antibodies, produced by effector B cells, appear in 5–10 days.

2. **Log phase:** As the lag period ends, the titre of antibody gradually increases over a period of a few days to a few weeks.

3. **Plateau or steady phase:** There is equilibrium between antibody production and catabolism.

4. **Phase of decline:** Catabolism exceeds the production of antibody and the titre falls.

Secondary humoral response

If the same animal is subsequently exposed to the same antigen there occurs a temporary fall in the level of antibodies due to the combination of the antigen

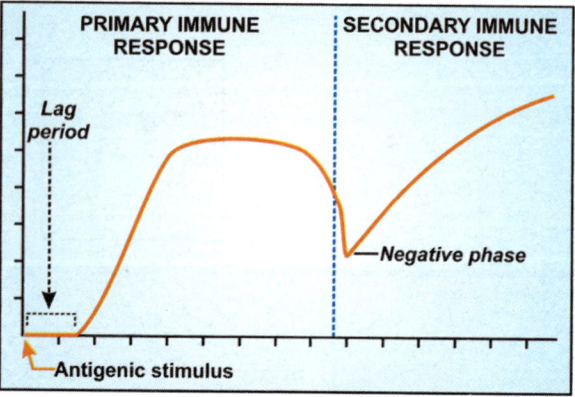

Fig. 14.1. Immune response.

with preexisting antibody. This is known as **negative phase.** After two to three days a marked increase in antibody level becomes evident. This goes on increasing for several days thus exceeding the initial level. This is also known as **booster response**. The booster response is attributed to the persistence of antigen sensitive 'memory cells' following the primary response.

The antibody formed in primary response is predominantly IgM and in secondary response IgG. The first dose is known as **priming dose** and subsequent injection as **booster dose**. Both these doses are particularly essential in case of killed vaccines. With live vaccines a single dose is usually sufficient as multiplication of organisms in the body provides a continuing antigenic stimulus that acts both as priming and booster doses.

Fate of antigen in tissue

Antigens introduced subcutaneously are mainly localized in the draining lymph nodes, only a small amount being found in the spleen. On the other hand, antigens introduced intravenously are rapidly localized in the spleen, liver, bone marrow, kidneys and lungs. 70–80% of these are broken down by reticulo-endothelial (R.E.) cells and excreted in the urine.

Production of antibodies

Antigen processing and presentation

Antigens are presented to immunocompetent cells (ICC) by antigen-presenting cells (APC) – macro-

phages and dendritic cells. With many antigens (T cell-dependent antigens such as proteins and erythro-cytes), processing by macrophages is pre-requisite for antibody formation. But for T cell-independent antigens, such as polysaccharides, antibody production does not require T cell participation. APC can ingest antigen, degrade it and present it to T cell. T cell is able to recognize only when the processed antigen is presented on the surface of APC, in association with MHC molecules to the T cell carrying the T cell receptor (TCR) for the epitope.

The antigen has to be presented complexed with MHC class II in case of CD4 (helper T/Th) cells and for CD8 (cytotoxic T/Tc) cells with MHC class I molecules.

T and B cell activation

The activation of Th cell requires two signals for activation. The first signal is a combination of the TCR with the MHC class II-complexed antigen. The second signal is interleukin-1 (IL-1) which is produced by APC. The activated Th cell produces IL-2 and other cytokines required for B cell stimulation. These include IL-4, IL-5 and IL-6 which act as B cell growth factor (BCGF) and B cell differentiation factor (BCDF). They activate B cells which have combined with their respective antigens to clonally proliferate and differentiate into antibody-secreting plasma cells. A small proportion of B cells, instead of being transformed into plasma cells, become long-lived memory cells producing a secondary type of response to subsequent contact with the antigen. B cells carry surface receptors which consist of IgM or other immunoglobulin classes. A plasma cell secretes an antibody of a single specificity of a single antibody class (IgM, IgG or any other single class). However, in primary humoral response, plasma cells secrete IgM and later switch over to form IgG.

CD8 (cytotoxic T/Tc) cells are activated when they come into contact with antigens presented along with MHC class I molecules. They also need a second signal IL-2, which is secreted by activated Th cells. On contact with a target cell carrying the antigen on its surface, the activated Tc cells release cytokines that destroy the target, which may be virus-infected or tumour cells. Some Tc cells also become memory cells.

Theories of antibody production

These fall into two groups:

1. Instructive theories.
2. Selective theories.

Instructive theories postulate that an ICC is capable of synthesizing antibodies of all specificities. An antigen encounters an ICC and instructs it to produce the complementary antibody. On the other hand, selective theories postulate that ICCs have only restricted immunological range. The antigen selects its ICC and stimulates it to synthesize its antibody. The most accepted theory is the clonal selection theory.

Clonal selection theory

This theory was proposed by Burnet (1957). This theory states that during immunological development a large number of lymphocytes capable of reacting with different antigens are formed. Cells with immunological reactivity with self-antigens are eliminated during embryonic life. Such clones are known as **forbidden clones**. *Their persistence or development in the later life leads to autoimmunity.* Each ICC is capable of reacting with one antigen. Contact with specific antigen leads to cellular proliferation to form clones which synthesize antibodies.

Monoclonal antibodies

Principle

If an antigen is injected into an animal, the latter produces different types of antibodies against various epitopes of the antigen. The antibodies thus generated are polyclonal in nature. This means different clones of antibody secreting cells are simultaneously synthesizing the antibody. Different molecules will have different specificities and affinities. In all microbial infections, body reacts with polyclonal antibody production. When these polyclonal antisera are used in bacterial test systems, **cross-reactivity** often occurs.

A single antibody-forming cell or clone produces antibodies directed against specific epitope of the antigen. Such antibodies produced by a single clone and directed against a single antigenic determinant are called monoclonal antibodies (MCA). In nature, MCA are produced in multiple myeloma where only one clone secretes a particular type of antibody. MCA can be generated in the laboratory. The theory of MCA production is based on clonal selection hypothesis of Burnet (1959) and the method for production of MCA was described by Kohler and Milstein in 1975, for which they were awarded Nobel Prize for Medicine in 1984.

The main breakthrough was not that a single line of monoclonal antibody producing cells could be isolated, but rather that the mouse splenic lymphocytes could be fused with mouse myeloma cells to produce **hybrid cells (hybridoma)**. Among the two cell types chosen for fusion, one provides the hybrid cell immortality (**myeloma cell**) while the other (**splenic plasma cell**) provides the antibody producing capacity. Such hybridomas can be maintained indefinitely in culture and continue to form MCA.

Technique

- Lymphocytes from the spleen of mice immunized with desired antigen are fused with mouse myeloma cells grown in culture and deficient in the enzyme hypoxanthine phosphoribosyl transferase (HPRT) (Fig. 14.2).

- The fused cells are placed in a basal culture medium containing hypoxanthine, aminopterin and thymidine (HAT medium).

- Only hybrid cells possessing properties of both the splenic lymphocytes (HPRT+) and myeloma cells (HPRT–) can grow in culture. Normal lymphocytes cannot replicate indefinitely and unfused myeloma cells are killed by the aminopterin in HAT medium.

- The peritoneal cavity of mice, preferably of the same strain that was used for initial immunization step, can be used to grow the selected hybrid cell clone. First the peritoneal cavity is injected with an organic irritant such as pristane to produce chemical peritonitis. Next the selected hybrid cell line is injected into the peritoneal cavity. Within days, a tumour known as hybridoma develops. This tumour produces large quantities of MCA that can be harvested by aspirating ascitic fluid from mouse's peritoneal cavity.

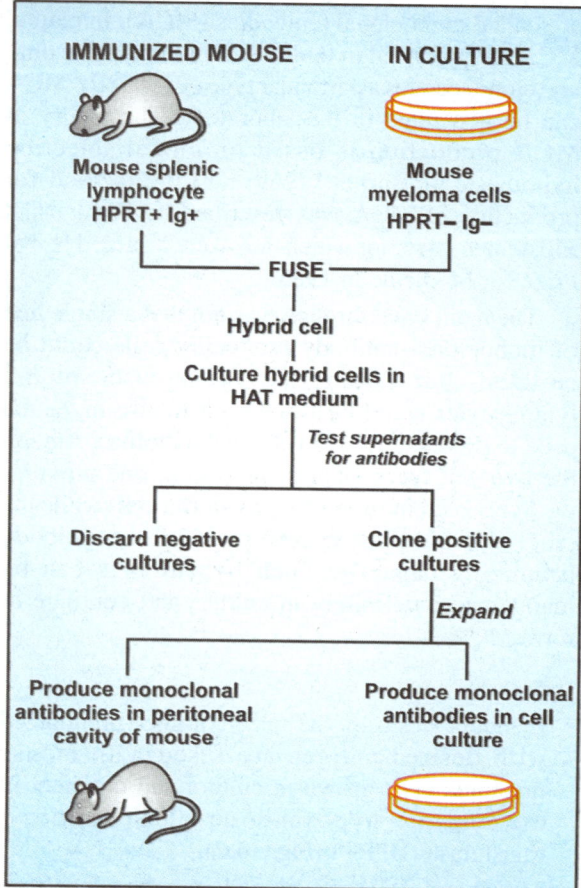

Fig. 14.2. Production of monoclonal antibodies.

- A tumour-bearing mouse will survive for 4–6 weeks, during which time large quantities of antibody can be recovered.
- Hybridomas can also be grown in tissue cultures where highly purified antibodies are produced without contamination from serum, ascites proteins or the cross-reactivity of histocompatibility antibodies derived from mouse tissues.

Applications of monoclonal antibodies

Monoclonal antibodies have been produced for specific epitopes of a wide variety of viruses, bacteria (including mycobacteria), parasites and fungi. Many of the commercial systems using direct fluorescence and enzyme-linked assays utilize monoclonal antibody conjugates.

Adjuvants

Adjuvants are compounds that potentiate the immune response when mixed and administered with antigens. They contribute to greater and more prolonged antibody production and increased effector cell counts. They act in several ways:

1. Sustained release of antigen from the depot
2. Stimulate lymphocytes nonspecifically.
3. Activate macrophages.

Types of adjuvants

A number of substances such as aluminium hydroxide or phosphate and an aqueous solution of an antigen may be emulsified in light mineral oil so that tiny water droplets containing antigen are dispersed throughout the oil (water-in-oil emulsion). The emulsion forms a depot of antigen in the tissues from which small quantities of antigen are released slowly sometimes for a year or more. This is known as **Freund's incomplete adjuvant**.

Complete Freund's adjuvant: It possesses killed mycobacteria in addition to incomplete adjuvant. Besides increasing humoral immune response, it induces high degree of cellular immunity (delayed hypersensitivity) as well. However, this adjuvant cannot be used in humans, because it produces local granuloma, and must be replaced by other adjuvants such as alum or killed *Bordetella pertussis*.

Immunosuppressive agents

Immunosuppressive agents are those which inhibit the immune response of macrophages, and B and T lymphocytes leading to lowered capacity to phagocytosis or to produce immunoglobulins and lymphokines. Organ and bone marrow transplantation became practicable on a large-scale only after powerful immunosuppressive drugs became available. They may also be used to control autoimmune responses or to prevent allergic reactions.

A wide range of physical, chemical and biological agents have been tried (Table 14.1). Some of these were soon dropped because the margin of safety was too small and toxic effects too pronounced.

- X-irradiation is more cytotoxic to replicating cells and has been used to prolong transplant survival and to control certain autoimmune conditions.

Table 14.1. Immunosuppressive agents

PHYSICAL AGENTS
- X-irradiation
- Surgery

CHEMICAL AGENTS
- *Alkylating agents*
  - Cyclophosphamide
  - Nitrogen mustard
- *Corticosteroids*
- *Antimetabolites*
  - Folic acid antagonists (methotrexate)
  - Analogues of purine (6-mercaptopurine and azathioprine)
  - Cytosine
  - Uracil (5-fluorouracil)
- *Miscellaneous*
  - Cyclosporine

BIOLOGICAL AGENTS
- Antilymphocytic serum

- Corticosteroids and cyclosporine impair maturation of activated cells by suppressing production of interleukins (ILs). Corticosteroids are antiinflammatory drugs that diminish the responsiveness of both B and T cell pools. They can inhibit production of IL-1 and IL-2. Prolonged use of corticosteroids may lead to hypertension, bone necrosis, cataract and mental disturbances.

- Cyclosporine has been widely used as an immuno-suppressant in organ transplantation. It causes immune suppression by inhibiting the production of IL-2. It may have adverse side-effects affecting the liver and kidney.

- Cytotoxic drugs, such as azathioprine or cyclophosphamide, act on various stages of nucleic acid synthesis preventing replication of active lymphocytes. Azathioprine, used in renal transplant, inhibits T cells, but not B cell responses. Cyclophosphamide, used in bone marrow recipients, selectively prevents B cell replication.

T cell population can be depleted by use of antilymphocytic serum produced in horses. This destroys body's T cell pool but leaves antibody production intact. Unfortunately, it also reduces the ability of the body to fight viral infection.

CELL-MEDIATED IMMUNE RESPONSES

Cell-mediated immunity (CMI) normally refers to specific acquired immunity, which is accomplished by effector T cells and macrophages rather than B cells and antibodies. This includes allograft rejection, delayed hypersensitivity (DH) and cytotoxic reactions against intracellular parasites. As in case of antibody-mediated immune response, cell-mediated immune response can also be divided into primary and secondary cell-mediated immune responses.

Primary cell-mediated immune response

This is produced by initial contact with a foreign antigen. Foreign antigen is presented by antigen-presenting cells (APCs) to T cells leading to their activation. T cells possess antigen recognition receptors known as T cell receptors (TCRs) that recognize foreign antigen and a self-MHC molecule on the surface of the APC (Fig. 14.3). Because of the specificity of the TCRs only particular cells become activated. These cells proliferate and produce specific clones of effector T cells (Th, Tc, Td and Ts). Cell-mediated immune response develops after several days of antigenic challenge.

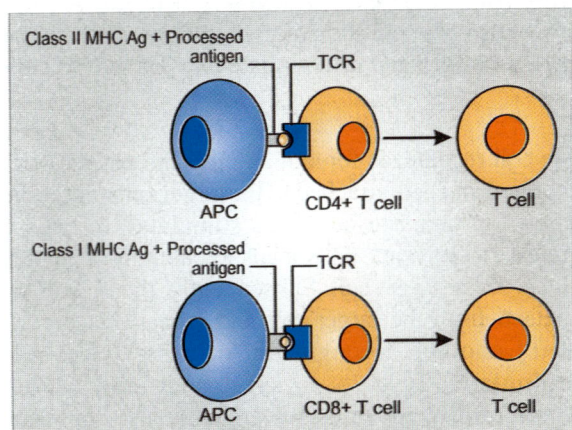

Fig. 14.3. Cell-mediated immune response.

Secondary cell-mediated immune response

If the same host is subsequently exposed to the same antigen, then the secondary cell-mediated immune response is usually more pronounced and occurs more rapidly. Because of the availability of specific memory cells, an increased number of effector cells are produced.

T cell differentiation

APCs, such as macrophages, phagocytose the antigen and degrade it. Subsequently, portions of antigen become associated with MHC antigens and are expressed on APC's surface. Two modes of processing are known (Fig. 14.3):

- One mode is seen in case of processing of phago-cytosed material such as bacteria. The antigenic material dissociated from the bacteria is associated with class II MHC molecules probably within the phagosome. MHC-antigen complex then expresses on the surface of the APC.
- Second mode is seen in processing antigens derived within the cell, for example, viral antigens synthe-sized in infected cell. However, this antigenic determinant associates with class I MHC molecule probably in the endoplasmic reticulum. MHC-antigen complex then expresses on the surface of the APC.

CD8+ cells recognize the combination of foreign antigen and class I MHC antigen and differentiate into Tc and Ts lymphocytes while CD4+ cells recognize the combination of antigen and class II MHC antigen and differentiate into Th and Td cells.

Lysis of target cell

Tc cell recognizes foreign antigen and class I MHC antigen and gets attached to the target cell expressing these on their surface. This stimulates Tc cells to release **cytolysins**. This leads to calcium-dependent lysis of the target cell. Subsequently, the Tc cell can detach from the target cell and repeat this process with another. Recognition of target cells also stimulates Tc cells to synthesize and secrete **interferon-γ**, and thus they probably also contribute to some extent to macrophage activation.

Delayed hypersensitivity

Delayed hypersensitivity (DH) or **type IV hyper-sensitivity** is the clinically observable outcome of cell-mediated immune reaction in the tissues of a sensitized individual. The immune response to

proteins of the tubercle bacillus, observed by Robert Koch in 1880, has served a general model for DH. When a small dose of purified antigen (tuberculin) is injected intradermally in an individual sensitized to tuberculoprotein by prior infection or immuni-zation, an indurated inflammatory reaction develops at the site of inoculation within 48–72 hours. It is characterized by erythema due to increased blood flow to the damaged area and induration due to infiltration with a large number of mononuclear cells, mainly T lymphocytes and about 10–20% macro-phages.

Mechanism

On initial exposure the antigen is engulfed by the macrophage. It then presents the antigen to specific T lymphocytes that can recognize the foreign antigen on its surface. These T cells clone, and two subsets (Td and Tc) are created. On subsequent exposure to the antigen, Td cells secrete lymphokines. These are glycoproteins which exert a regulatory effect chiefly on macrophages. These include **chemotactic factor (CF)** which attracts macrophages, **migration inhibiting factor** (MIF) which impedes their move-ment from the site of infection, **macrophage stimulating factor** (MSF) which stimulates macro-phage migration to the site of antigen and **macro-phage activating factor** (MAF) which keeps them at the site of infection and causes them to actively phagocytose and destroy foreign cells at the site of infection. Activated macrophages release their degra-dative lysosomal enzyme into the tissues where the antigen is located thus leading to localized inflamma-tory response. This can lead to necrosis and fibrosis of the host tissue and destruction of infecting agents.

A second subset of T cells, Tc lymphocytes, is also generated. They also play a role, as described above, under lysis of target cells.

Cytokines

These are biologically active substances produced by cells that influence other cells. They are referred to as **lymphokines** if they are derived from lympho-cytes and **monokines** if they are derived from mono-cytes and macrophages. Interleukins are a family of cytokines that function primarily as growth and differentiation factors. Cytokines have been named

Table 14.2. Source and activity of cytokines

Cytokine	Source	Activity
Macrophage stimulating factor (MSF)	Td cells	Stimulates macrophage migration to the site of action
Macrophage activating factor (MAF)	Td cells	Restricts macrophage movement and increases phagocytic activity
Migration inhibiting factor (MIF)	Td cells	Inhibits migration of macrophages
Chemotactic factor (CF)	Td cells	Stimulates chemotaxis of macrophages
Interferon-gamma (IFN-γ)	Th, Td and NK cells	Increases cytotoxicity of NK cells and macrophages
Interleukin-1 (IL-1)	NK cells, APCs, B cells and T cells	Promotes growth and expression of fibroblasts, NK cells, B cells and T cells
Interleukin-2 (IL-2)	Th cells	Promotes B cell differentiation and T cell growth
Interleukin-3 (IL-3)	Th cells	Acts as a growth factor for bone marrow stem cell
Interleukin-4 (IL-4)	Th cells	Acts as a growth factor for macrophages, mast cells, B cells and T cells
Interleukin-5 (IL-5)	Th cells	Promotes B cell growth, antibody production and maturation of eosinophils
Interleukin-6 (IL-6)	Macrophages	Promotes B cell growth
Interleukin-7 (IL-7)	Bone marrow stromal cells	Stimulates B cell and T cell proliferation
Interleukin-8 (IL-8)	Mononuclear cells, endothelial cells and skin fibroblasts	Stimulates chemotaxis of neutrophils and T cells
Interleukin-9 (IL-9)	Activated T cells	Stimulates proliferation of IL-3 dependent myeloid cells and mast cells
Interleukin-10 (IL-10)	Th cells	Inhibits production of IFN-γ and other cytokines
Interleukin-11 (IL-11)	Bone marrow stromal cells	Induces acute phase proteins
Interleukin-12 (IL-12)	T cells	Activates natural killer (NK) cells
Interleukin-13 (IL-13)	T cells	Inhibits mononuclear cell functions
Interleukin-14 (IL-14)	T cells	Stimulates proliferation of activated B cells, inhibits immunoglobulin production
Interleukin-15 (IL-15)	Monocytes	Proliferation of T cells and activated B cells
Interleukin-16 (IL-16)	Eosinophils, CD8+ T cells	Chemoattraction of CD4+ T cells
Interleukin-17 (IL-17)	CD4+ T cells	Release of IL-6, IL-8
Interleukin-18 (IL-18)	Hepatocytes	Induces production of interferon-γ, induces NK cell activity

based on the biological effects they produce. Various cytokines are given in Table 14.2.

Detection of CMI

Development of CMI can be detected by following methods:

1. Skin test for DH.

2. Transformation of cultured sensitized T lymphocytes on contact with antigen.
3. Target cell destruction: killing of cultured cells by T lymphocytes sensitized against them.
4. Migration inhibiting factor (MIF) test (Fig. 14.4).

MIF test is most commonly employed. If a piece of capillary tube containing peritoneal exudate cells

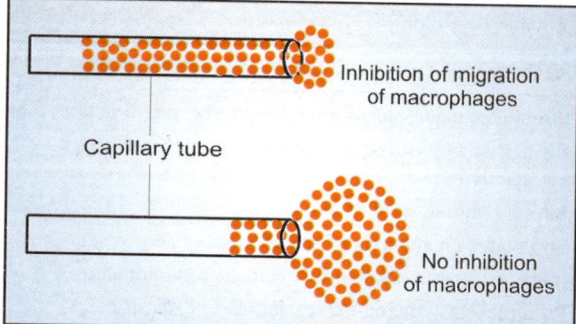

Fig. 14.4. Inhibition of migration of macrophages.

(macrophages and a few lymphocytes) is placed in a tissue culture chamber containing tissue culture fluid and no antigen, the macrophages migrate out of the open end of the tube into culture fluid to form a fan-like pattern. However, if the macrophages are obtained from a guinea-pig sensitized to tuberculo-protein, addition of tuberculin to the culture chamber will inhibit migration.

Transfer factor

Lawrence (1954) reported transfer of CMI in man by injection of extract from the leucocytes from immunized individual. The extract from the leuco-cytes contains a soluble factor called transfer factor (TF). The transferred immunity is specific in that CMI can be transferred only to those antigens to which the donor is sensitive.

TF is a nucleopeptide with a molecular weight of 2,000–4,000 daltons. It is non-antigenic. It is resistant to trypsin but gets inactivated by heating at 56°C in 30 minutes. The mode of action of TF is not known. It appears to stimulate the release of lymphokines from sensitized T lymphocytes. It does not promote antibody synthesis. TF has been used in patients with:

- T cell deficiency (Wiskott-Aldrich syndrome).
- Disseminated infections associated with deficient CMI (lepromatous leprosy, tuber-culosis and mucocutaneous candidiasis).
- Malignant melanoma and other types of cancer.

IMMUNOLOGICAL TOLERANCE

Immunological tolerance may be defined as a state of unresponsiveness to specific antigens. This

unresponsiveness is specific to antigens to which the individual is tolerant. Response to other antigens is unaffected. Two forms of tolerance can be identified – natural tolerance and acquired tolerance.

Natural tolerance

It is nonresponsiveness to self-antigens. This arises during foetal development, when the immune system is being formed and maturing. If this tolerance breaks down and body responds to self molecules then an autoimmune disease will develop. Dizygotic cattle twins, which are genetically dissimilar, share the same placental circulation in utero. As adults, each twin fails to mount immune response to histo-compatibility antigens on the cells of the other twin. Thus they accept transplants from each other. This could be accounted for by induction of specific immunological tolerance during foetal life. Based on this observation of Owen (1945), Burnet and Fenner (1949) suggested that the unresponsiveness of individuals to self-antigens was due to the contact of the immature immunological system with self-antigens during embryonic life.

Any antigen that comes into contact with the immunological system during its embryonic life would be recognised as a self-antigen and would not induce any immune response. They postulated that tolerance could be induced against foreign antigens if they were administered during embryonic life. Medawar and his colleagues (1953) proved it experimentally. When skin graft from one inbred strain of mice (CBA) is applied on a mouse of another strain (A), it is rejected. But if CBA cells are injected into foetal or newborn A strain mice, the latter when grow up will freely accept skin grafts from CBA mice.

Certain strains of mice that are genetically deficient in the C5 complement component make vigorous antibody response when immunized with pure C5 taken from normal animals. Normal animals (which are not deficient in C5) do not respond to similar immunization.

Acquired tolerance

It arises when a potential immunogen induces a state of unresponsiveness to itself. This has consequences for host defences since the presence of a tolerogenic epitope on a pathogen may compromise the ability of the body to resist infection. For acquired tolerance to be maintained the tolerogen must persist or be repeatedly administered. This is probably necessary because of the continuous production of new B and T cells that must be rendered tolerant.

A number of factors influence the induction of tolerance. These include species and immuno-competence of the host, physical nature, dose and route of administration of antigen. Rabbits and mice can be rendered tolerant more rapidly than guinea-pigs and chickens. Higher the degree of immuno-competence of the host, the more difficult it is to induce tolerance. Therefore, embryos and newborns are particularly susceptible for induction of tolerance.

It is easier to induce tolerance to a soluble macro-molecule than to an aggregated antigen. For example, when human gammaglobulin is heat aggregated, it is highly immunogenic in mice, but when de-aggregated it is tolerogenic. This is probably due to the fact that aggregated antigens are readily phago-cytosed by macrophages, where they can be presented to antibody-forming cells thus inducing antibody synthesis. On the other hand, soluble antigens are not so easily processed and may be more effective in inducing the Ts suppressor circuit.

The induction of tolerance is dose-dependent. Generally high doses of antigen tolerize B cells, while minute doses given repeatedly tolerize T cells. A moderate dose of the same antigen might be immunogenic. The route of administration is also important. Intravenously administered antigens have faster contact with more cells at the highest concentration of tolerogen. Moreover, an intravenous injection rapidly reaches the spleen to which Ts cells migrate leading to tolerance.

Tolerance can be overcome spontaneously or by injection of cross-reacting immunogens. For example, tolerance to bovine serum albumin in rabbits can be abolished by immunization with cross-reacting human serum albumin.

Mechanism of tolerance

Tolerance can arise through three possible mechanisms:

1. *Clonal deletion:* In embryonic life clones of B and T cells possessing receptors that recognize self-antigens are selectively deleted or eliminated and, therefore, no longer available to respond upon subsequent exposure to that antigen. This is known as clonal deletion.

2. *Clonal anergy:* Clones of B and T cells expressing receptors that recognize self-antigen might remain but they cannot be activated. This is known as clonal anergy.

3. *Suppression:* Clones of B and T cells expressing receptors that recognize self-antigens are preserved. Antigen recognition might be capable of causing activation, however, expression of immune response might be inhibited or blocked through active suppression.

KEY FACTS

- After *first injection of the antigen* there is a long *lag phase* of several days before *antibodies appear*
- *Second contact* with antigen *stimulates* the pool of *memory cells* to produce a *larger and faster response* than primary reaction
- Unlimited expansion of clones is restricted by antigen concentration and antibody feedback T cell suppression
- *Cell-mediated immunity* refers to specific acquired immunity, which is accomplished by *effector T cells* and *macrophages*
- **Cytokines** are biologically active substances produced by cells that influence other cells
- Reactivity to self is prevented by a variety of *tolerance mechanisms*

IMPORTANT QUESTION

Write short notes on:
(a) Primary and secondary humoral response
(b) Monoclonal antibodies
(c) Cytokines
(d) Burnet's clonal selection theory

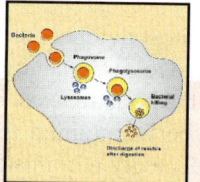

Chapter **15**

Hypersensitivity & Autoimmunity

HYPERSENSITIVITY

Hypersensitivity is an abnormal immune response which produces physiological or histopathological damage in the host. It may be divided into five types:

Type I	Anaphylactic
Type II	Cytotoxic
Type III	Immune complex
Type IV	Cell-mediated or delayed
Type V	Stimulatory or antireceptor

Type I, II, III and V hypersensitivity depend on the interaction of antigen with humoral antibodies and are known as immediate type reactions, although some are more immediate than others. Immediate hypersensitivity reactions develop in less than 24 hours after reexposure to an antigen. Type IV hypersensitivity or delayed hypersensitivity is mediated by T lymphocytes. Delayed hyper-sensitivity reactions develop in 24–48 hours.

Type I hypersensitivity: Anaphylactic

It is **mediated by IgE antibody** and is due to the powerful effects of histamine and other vasoactive amines. Hypersensitivity may be local or generalized, depending upon the amount of histamine released, the site of its release and route of stimulating antigen. Generally, small amount of antigen administered to mucous membrane or skin will induce local anaphylaxis, whereas larger amounts may induce a generalized reaction and antigen administered systemically may cause generalized anaphylaxis. Local anaphylaxis is exemplified by such conditions as hay fever and asthma. Systemic anaphylaxis is a shock-like condition that can occur in individuals who are intensely allergic to such things as bee venom, penicillin and horse serum.

An antigenic substance that can trigger the allergic state is known as **allergen**. It may be a protein or chemically complex low molecular weight substance. Most allergens are considered weakly immunogenic and most people do not respond to them adversely. However, an allergic person is often sensitive to several different allergens.

Mechanism of type I hypersensitivity

In order to produce type I hypersensitivity an individual must first come in contact with an antigen and produce IgE antibodies. These antibodies bind to mast cells and basophils (Fig. 15.1). Basophils are found in the circulation while mast cells (or fixed basophils) are located in lymphoid regions of respiratory tract, gastrointestinal tract, reproductive tract, skin and lining of blood vessels including capillaries. They have large number of vesicles containing pharmacologically potent compounds like histamine and serotonin.

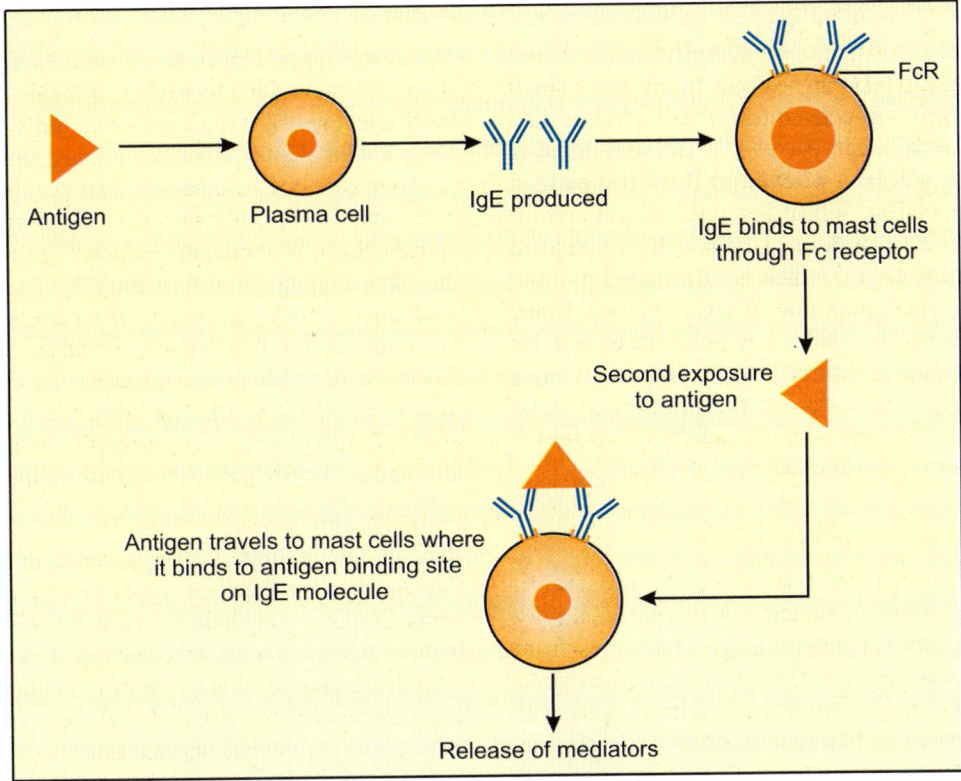

Fig. 15.1. Antigen-induced mediator release from mast cell.

Thus **after first exposure** allergen-specific IgE is fixed to the mast cells and basophils, thereby sensitizing them. The part of the IgE molecule that binds to the surface of mast cells and basophils is the Fc portion. These cells possess high affinity receptors specific for Fc portion of IgE antibodies. Thus Fab portion of IgE remains exposed. IgE antibodies can remain attached on these cells for up to six weeks. Such an individual is said to be **sensitized**.

After a second exposure the allergen travels to the mast cells and basophils, where it binds to antigen-binding site on IgE molecule. Antigen-antibody binding triggers the process of degranulation through which the mast cell explosively discharges its pharmacologically active agents. These include histamine, serotonin, bradykinin, slow-reacting substance of anaphylaxis (SRS-A), platelet-activating factors, eosinophil chemotactic factor of anaphylaxis and prostaglandins.

Of these, histamine is the most abundant and fastest acting. It induces smooth muscle contraction, release of mucus, vasodilation and increased capillary permeability. All these reactions can have profound effects. For example, excessive smooth muscle contraction and release of mucus in respiratory tract can close the air passages of trachea and bronchi, causing asphyxiation and death by suffocation.

Another target area is the uterus. Pregnant women who are severely allergic may abort the foetus during an attack of histamine release and subsequent smooth muscle contractions in the uterus. Histamine also induces increased capillary permeability leading to oedema. Thus there is extensive loss of blood fluids into the tissues. This may lead to circulatory shock and death.

Cutaneous anaphylaxis

If a person is suspected to be allergic to a particular substance, a **skin test** can be done. In this test a small dose of allergen is injected intradermally. In less than 30 minutes results can be read. If the individual is allergic there will be a **wheal and flare response** at the site of injection. Wheal is a pale central area of puffiness due to oedema (caused by increased capillary permeability) which is surrounded by flare (caused by hyperaemia due to vasodilation). Since the injection site is small, it is possible to test for hypersensitivity to hundreds of substances on a person's back. The wheal and flare response can be used to determine the specific substance to which the atopic person is sensitive.

Prausnitz-Kustner (PK) reaction

Prausnitz and Kustner in 1921 demonstrated transmission of IgE-mediated type I hypersensitivity by injecting serum containing IgE antibodies from allergic person into the skin of a normal or non-allergic person. Serum from Kustner, who was hypersensitive to certain species of cooked fish, was injected intracutaneously in Prausnitz (normal) followed 24 hours later by an intracutaneous injection of cooked fish, to which Kustner was sensitive, into the same site in Prausnitz. This led to wheal and flare reaction within 20 minutes. As IgE antibody is homocytotropic, the test has to be carried out on human skin, therefore, there is risk of transmission of hepatitis B and C viruses, and human immunodeficiency virus.

Anaphylaxis in vitro (Schultz-Dale phenomenon)

In 1910, Schultz and Dale demonstrated that sensitized strips of smooth muscle contract, *in vitro*, following exposure to antigen. Thus intestinal and uterine muscle strips from a sensitized animal (guinea-pig) held in Ringer's solution bath contract vigorously on addition of specific antigen. Smooth muscle strips can be passively sensitized by bathing them in serum from a hypersensitive animal. The actual test is done by adding the antigen and observing subsequent contractions.

Atopy

The term atopy refers to chronic human allergic states. These include **hay fever**, **allergic asthma** and **food allergies**. The antigens commonly involved in atopy are inhalants (pollen, house dust, animal dander or other types of fine particles suspended in air) or ingestants (milk, milk products, eggs, meat, fish or cereal). Some of them are contact allergens, to which the skin and conjunctiva may be exposed. The mechanism of development of atopy is essentially the same as that of systemic anaphylaxis. Atopy is likely to develop when allergen is localized or absorbed slowly, on the other hand systemic anaphylaxis is likely to develop if large quantities of allergen are quickly distributed throughout the body.

Hay fever (allergic rhinitis)

It is an IgE-mediated allergic reaction that affects the mucosal surfaces of upper respiratory tract. It leads to nasal congestion, headache, running nose, watery eyes, itching and sneezing. The specific stimuli that cause allergic rhinitis include antigenic components of grass, weed and tree pollens, dust, mites, animal dander, organic dusts, components of tobacco smoke, and noninfectious components of fungal and bacterial allergens. If the allergen cannot be removed, then antihistaminics are the pharmacological agents of choice for the treatment of allergic rhinitis since histamine seems to be the major mediator of this allergy.

Allergic asthma

It is a severe form of respiratory allergy. It leads to contraction of the trachea and bronchi. The specific stimuli that cause allergic asthma include airborne allergens. In addition, asthma-producing foods such as milk, milk products, eggs, meat, fish or cereal may also precipitate allergic asthma. Some patients may even be sensitive to normal microbial flora leading to endogenous asthma. The main mediators of this allergy are serotonin and SRS-A. Therefore, anti-histaminics are not able to reverse the smooth muscle contraction. The drug of choice for the treatment of this allergy is adrenaline (epinephrine). It is dispensed as atomizers for quick delivery. In addition, cortico-steroids and cromolyn sodium have proved beneficial in treating attacks of allergic asthma.

Food allergies

Food allergy occurs in infants and children, but is uncommon in adults. Certain foods such as eggs, milk, peanuts, seafoods, citrus fruits and chocolate are frequent causes of food allergy. Consumption of the food in a patient with food allergy leads to nausea, vomiting, diarrhoea and cramps with typical urticaria and wheezing or upper airways congestion. Best cure for food allergy is to avoid that food unless it is a common ingredient of prepared foods such as flour.

Desensitization

This is accomplished by actually injecting the person with offending allergen. The patient is injected with very small doses of allergen repeatedly over a long period of time (months). The dose is progressively increased until the person no longer reacts to the allergen. However, some persons may get relapse after years.

Following small earlier injections, the allergens react with IgE antibodies attached to mast cells and basophils leading to degranulation. This process goes on till all the IgE antibodies are consumed. Subsequently, in response to higher doses IgG antibodies are produced in place of IgE antibodies. IgG antibodies are known as **blocking antibodies** because they are able to bind to the allergen in the blood stream before they reach IgE attached to the mast cells thus blocking degranulation. Most subclasses of IgG (with the exception of IgG4) cannot bind to mast cells. Another theory states that this type of immunotherapy stimulates the expression of suppressor T cells which block IgE antibody production by B cells. Therefore, the level of IgE antibodies falls and symptoms disappear.

Type II hypersensitivity: Cytotoxic reaction

This involves the combination of IgG and IgM serum antibodies with foreign antigenic components on a cell surface. Alternatively, a free foreign antigen or hapten such as a drug or microbial product may be adsorbed onto a cell membrane, which subsequently combines with antibody.

Clinically, antibody-mediated reactions occur in following situations:

1. Drug-induced immune haemolytic anaemia

A type II hypersensitivity reaction involving haemolytic anaemia may be induced by administration of certain drugs. Drugs such as antibiotic penicillin, and alpha-methyldopa for the treatment of hypertension can bind to the surface of red blood cell and form an antigenic complex with the surface of these cells. This can bring about the production of complement-fixing antibody to the drug. Reaction of this antibody with the RBC-bound drug activates the complement system, resulting in RBC lysis and anaemia.

2. Transfusion reactions

When a person receives incompatible blood transfusion, the antibodies normally present in recipient's serum agglutinate and lyse donor RBCs with the liberation of free haemoglobin into the plasma. This leads to jaundice, fever and failure of kidney function. Serum of the donor may also agglutinate and lyse recipient's RBCs. For example, transfusion of group O whole blood or plasma to group A or group B or group AB recipients may lead to haemolysis. But this reaction is mild since the donor's serum gets considerably diluted in the circulation of the recipient.

3. Rh incompatibility

Rh antibodies are major cause of **haemolytic disease of newborn (HDN)**, and lead to destruction of transfused red cells. When an Rh-negative woman carries an Rh-positive foetus, she may be immunized against Rh antigen by passage of foetal red cells into maternal circulation. Minor transplacental leaks may occur any time during pregnancy, but it is during delivery that foetal cells enter the maternal circulation in large numbers. Therefore, the mother is usually immunized only at first delivery, and consequently, the first child escapes damage (except where the woman has been sensitized already by prior Rh incompatible blood transfusion). During subsequent pregnancy, Rh antibodies of IgG class pass from the mother to the foetus and damage its erythrocytes. The clinical features of HDN may vary from a mere accentuation of the physiological jaundice in the newborn to erythroblastosis foetalis or intrauterine death due to hydrops foetalis.

4. Autoimmune haemolytic anaemia, agranulocytosis and thrombocytopenia

Some persons develop antibodies against their blood elements, resulting in autoimmune haemolytic anaemia, agranulocytosis or thrombocytopenia.

5. Anaemia due to infectious diseases

A variety of infectious diseases due to *Salmonella* and mycobacteria are associated with haemolytic anaemia. Studies in *Salmonella* infections have revealed that the haemolysis is due to an immune reaction against a lipopolysaccharide bacterial endotoxin that becomes coated onto the erythrocytes of the patient.

Type III hypersensitivity: Immune complex

If an antigen is not cell-bound but is rather small and soluble, the body can encounter severe difficulties if it is repeatedly exposed to that antigen. Antigen-antibody complexes formed under these conditions may lead to type III or immune complex-mediated hypersensitivity. Monocytes and macrophages are very efficient at binding and removing large precipitating antigen-antibody complexes. They can also eliminate the smaller complexes made in antibody excess but are relatively inefficient at removing those formed in antigen excess. The formation of antigen-antibody complexes in serum, with subsequent deposition of the complexes in tissues, is the key event in type III hypersensitivity. Antigen-antibody complexes can then activate serum complement, platelets and phagocytes, all of which lead to tissue damage.

Arthus reaction (local immune complex disease)

Arthus (1903) observed that when rabbits were repeatedly injected subcutaneously with normal horse serum, the initial injections were without any local effect, but with later injections, there occurred intense local reaction consisting of oedema, induration and haemorrhagic necrosis. This is known as Arthus reaction. The tissue damage is due to formation of local precipitating immune complexes which are deposited on the endothelial lining of the blood vessels. Antigen-antibody complexes can then trigger and activate complement leading to inflammation and tissue damage.

Serum sickness (systemic immune complex disease)

This is a systemic form of type III hypersensitivity. This develops in persons who receive a single injection of a high concentration of horse antitoxin against tetanus, gas gangrene, diphtheria, etc. for prophylactic and therapeutic purposes. Seven to 12 days after the injection, patient may develop fever, lymphadenopathy, splenomegaly, arthritis, glomerulonephritis, endocarditis, vasculitis, urticarial rash, abdominal pain, nausea and vomiting. It is due to the immune response to horse antigens and it has also been encountered in allergic reactions to certain drugs. After 7–12 days, antibodies to horse antigens appear while horse antigens are still persisting because a large dose was administered. Initially they form antigen-antibody complexes in antigen excess. These soluble complexes can circulate and get deposited in various sites throughout the body particularly in skin, joints, kidneys and heart.

Antigen-antibody aggregates can fix complement leading to inflammation and tissue damage as discussed above. The plasma level of complement falls due to massive complement activation and fixation by antigen-antibody complexes. Initially, the circulating immune complexes are in antigen excess and produce inflammatory lesions, but as antibody production rises, the immune complexes increase in size as zone of equivalence is reached. These larger immune complexes are more easily phagocytosed and cleared by the cells of reticuloendothelial system of liver and spleen. Once all immune complexes are removed from the circulation, symptoms are usually resolved within a week.

Type IV hypersensitivity: Cell-mediated or delayed

Type IV hypersensitivity or delayed hypersensitivity (DH) is the clinically observable outcome of cell-mediated immune reaction in the tissues of a sensitized individual. The reaction is not brought about by circulating antibodies and B lymphocytes but by sensitized T lymphocytes and macrophages. It is named delayed hypersensitivity because it appears in 24–48 hours after the presensitized host encounters the antigen, while immediate hypersensitivity reactions develop in ½–12 hours (Table 15.1). The mechanism of delayed hypersensitivity is given in Chapter 14. Two types of DH are recognized – tuberculin (infection) type and contact dermatitis type.

1. Tuberculin (infection) type

The immune response to the tubercle bacillus, observed by Robert Koch in 1880, has served a general model for DH. When a small dose (1–3 units) of tuberculin or purified protein derivative (PPD) is injected intradermally in an individual sensitized to tuberculoprotein by prior infection or immunization, an indurated inflammatory reaction, 10 mm or more in diameter, develops at the site of injection within 48–72 hours. It is characterized by erythema due to increased blood flow to the damaged area and induration due to infiltration with a large number of mononuclear cells, mainly T lymphocytes and about 10–20% macrophages. In unsensitized individuals, the tuberculin injection provokes no response. Cell-mediated hypersensitivity reactions are seen in a number of chronic infectious diseases due to mycobacteria, protozoa and fungi.

2. Contact dermatitis type

Contact dermatitis is cell-mediated allergic reaction that occurs when certain substances like metals (nickel and chromium), dyes (picryl chloride and dinitrochlorobenzene), drugs such as penicillin, and toiletries come in contact with skin. Sensitization is particularly liable to occur when contact is with an inflamed area and when chemical is applied in an oily base. Application of antibiotic ointments frequently provokes sensitization. The substances involved are not antigenic by themselves but may acquire antigenicity on combination with skin proteins. Subsequent contact with allergen in a sensitized individual leads to contact dermatitis. The lesions vary from macules and papules to vesicles which break down leaving behind raw weeping areas typical of acute eczematous dermatitis.

This hypersensitivity can be detected by **patch test**. The allergen is applied to the skin under an adherent dressing. Sensitivity is indicated by itching, appearing in 4–5 hours and local reaction which may vary from erythema to vesicle or blister formation in 24 hours.

Type V hypersensitivity: Stimulatory or antireceptor

This is an antibody-mediated hypersensitivity. Here antibody reacts with a key surface component such as a hormone receptor and switches on or stimulates the cell. An example of this type of hypersensitivity is the thyroid hyperactivity in Graves' disease due to **thyroid stimulating autoantibody**.

Normally thyroid stimulating hormone (TSH) from pituitary gland binds to thyroid cell receptors. This activates adenyl cyclase in the membrane which

Characteristic	**Type I**	**Type II**	**Type III**	**Type IV**
Approximate time to develop clinical signs	1/2–8 hours	5–12 hours	3–8 hours	24–48 hours
Reaction mediators	IgE, histamine, serotonin, SRS-A, etc.	IgG, IgM and complement	IgG, IgM, complement, neutrophils, eosinophils and lysosomal enzymes	T cells, macrophages and lymphokines
Response to intradermal injection of antigen	Wheal and flare	—	Erythema and oedema	Erythema and induration
Passive transfer with	Serum	Serum	Serum	T cells
Examples	Anaphylaxis, asthma, hay fever and, food and insect allergies	Transfusion reaction, HDN and drug-induced allergy	Arthus reaction and serum sickness	Tuberculin test, contact dermatitis, graft rejection and tumour immunity.

Table 15.1. Comparison of hypersensitivity reactions

converts ATP to AMP. The latter stimulates activity of thyroid cells thus secreting thyroxine. **The thyroid stimulating antibody present in the sera of thyrotoxic patients is an autoantibody directed against receptors for TSH.** This antibody, therefore, binds to these receptors and brings about the same effect as that of TSH.

AUTOIMMUNITY

Normally we do not form potentially destructive antibodies and T cells against our own cells because our body has developed tolerance to self-antigens. However, sometimes we can produce antibodies and T cells against our own cell or tissue components leading to autoimmune diseases. **Autoimmunity may, therefore, be defined as immune response to self-antigens, which can generate autoantibodies and autocytotoxic T cells.**

Mechanism of autoimmunity

There are several possible mechanisms involved in the development of autoimmunity:

1. Forbidden clones

According to clonal selection theory, antibody-forming lymphocytes capable of reacting with different antigens are formed. Clones of cells that have immunological reactivity with self-antigens are eliminated during embryonic life. Such clones are called forbidden clones. Their persistence or development in later life by somatic mutations can lead to autoimmunity.

2. Hidden or sequestrated antigen

Certain self-antigens are present in closed systems and are not accessible to immune system. An example is the **lens antigen of the eye**. The lens protein is enclosed in its capsule and does not circulate in the blood. Therefore, immunological tolerance against this antigen does not develop during foetal life. When the lens protein antigen leaks out, following cataract surgery or injury to the eye, it leads to immune response and damage to the other eye.

Another example of hidden antigen is seen in case of **sperm antigens**. Since sperms develop only at puberty, therefore, the sperm antigens cannot induce tolerance during foetal life. Sperms may enter into blood stream following injury of the testes and mumps orchitis. Virus probably damages the basement membrane of seminiferous tubules leading to the leakage of sperms and initiation of an immune response resulting in orchitis.

3. Neoantigens or altered antigens

Cells or tissues may undergo antigenic alteration by physical agents such as irradiation. Photosensitivity or cold allergy may be due to altered antigens by light and cold respectively. Several chemical agents including drugs can combine with cells and tissues and alter their antigenic structure. Skin contact with a variety of chemicals may lead to contact dermatitis. Drug-induced anaemia, leucopenia and thrombocytopenia often have autoimmune basis. Viruses and other intracellular pathogens may induce alterations of cell antigens leading to autoimmunity.

4. Cross-reacting antigens

Immunological damage may result from immune response induced by cross-reacting foreign antigens. For example, **Semple rabies vaccine** consists of infected sheep brain tissue inactivated with phenol. Its injection elicits an immune response against sheep brain antigens. This may lead to damage to patient's nervous tissue due to cross-reaction between human and sheep brain leading to encephalitis.

Immunological injury may be due to cross-reacting antigens present on microorganisms causing infection. An important example of this is the non-suppurative sequelae of *Streptococcus pyogenes* infection which include **acute rheumatic fever and acute glomerulonephritis**. M protein of *S. pyogenes* and heart of man share antigenic characteristics. The immune response induced by repeated streptococcal infections can, therefore, damage the heart. Nephritogenic strains of *S. pyogenes* share antigens with renal glomeruli. Therefore, immune response following infection with such strains may lead to acute glomerulonephritis. It has been suggested that antibodies raised against *Treponema pallidum* antigens cross-react with certain blood group antigens bringing about the anaemia.

5. Mutation

Immunocompetent cells may acquire an unnatural responsiveness to self-antigens by mutation.

6. Activity of helper and suppressor T cells

Helper T (Th) cells facilitate B cell response to many antigens. Suppressor T (Ts) cells inhibit antibody production by B cells. Optimal antibody response depends on the balanced activity of Th and Ts cells. *Overactivity of Th cells or decreased activity of Ts cells may lead to autoimmunity.*

Autoimmune diseases

These include systemic lupus erythematosus, rheumatoid arthritis, systemic sclerosis (scleroderma), dermatomyositis, and polyarteritis nodosa. Rheumatic fever is also sometimes classified as autoimmune disorder.

Systemic lupus erythematosus

Systemic lupus erythematosus (SLE) is a chronic multisystem disease of autoimmune origin. Patients have a variety of antibodies directed against cell nuclei, intracytoplasmic cell constituents, immunoglobulins, thyroid and other organ specific antigens. This indicates that the fundamental defect in SLE is a failure of the regulatory mechanisms that sustain self-tolerance. SLE is predominantly a disease of women with a female to male ratio of 9 : 1.

Antinuclear antibodies (ANAs) are directed against several nuclear antigens. Several techniques are used to detect ANAs. The most commonly used method is indirect immunofluorescence, which detects a variety of nuclear antigens, including DNA, RNA, and proteins. Four basic patterns are recognized:

1. *Homogenous or diffuse nuclear staining* usually reflects the presence of antibodies to chromatin, histones, and occasionally double-stranded DNA.
2. *Peripheral or rim staining* indicates the presence of antibodies to double-stranded DNA.
3. *Speckled pattern* indicates the presence of antibodies to non-DNA nuclear constituents.
4. *Nucleolar pattern* refers to the presence of a few discrete spots of fluorescence within the nucleus. This indicates the presence of antibodies to nucleolar RNA.

The immunofluorescence test for ANAs is positive in virtually every patient with SLE. Therefore, this test is very sensitive, but it is not specific because patients with other autoimmune diseases are frequently positive. Furthermore, 5–15% of normal individuals have low titres of these antibodies. Anti-DNA antibodies can also be detected by RIA or ELISA.

In tissues, nuclei of damaged cells react with ANAs, lose their chromatin pattern, and become homogenous, to produce so called **LE bodies**. Related to this phenomenon is the **LE cell**, which is readily seen *in vitro*. Basically the LE cell is any phagocytic leucocyte (neutrophil or macrophage) that has engulfed the denatured nucleus of an injured cell. For the demonstration of LE cells, the withdrawn blood is agitated with the beads in the tube for 30 minutes either manually or on a rotator. It is then incubated at 37°C for 30 minutes to 1 hour, shaking intermittently thus exposing their nuclei to ANAs. The binding of ANAs to nuclei denatures them, and subsequent fixation of complement renders antibody-coated nuclei strongly chemotactic for phagocytic cells. The blood is centrifuged, the cells from the buffy coat are withdrawn, thin-smear is prepared and stained with Leishman stain. It is examined under oil-immersion objective for LE cells which are indicated by bluish purple mass in the cytoplasm of a neutrophil. The LE cell test is positive in up to 70% of the patients with SLE.

Antinuclear antibodies can also be detected by agglutination of latex particles coated with deoxyribonucleoprotein. It is more specific and sensitive than LE cell test.

Oral manifestations

Patients with SLE are affected by a variety of orofacial disorders, including characteristic oral lesions, nonspecific ulcerations, salivary gland disease, and temporomandibular disorders. The oral lesions of SLE are caused by vasculitis and appear as frank ulceration or mucosal inflammation. Some individuals with SLE or discoid lupus have discoid-appearing oral lesions.

The lip lesions often have a central atrophic and occasionally ulcerated area with small white dots, surrounded by a keratinized border composed of small radiating white striae. The intraoral lesions are somewhat different because of the thinner epithelium;

they are composed of a central depressed red atrophic area surrounded by a 2–4 mm elevated keratotic zone that dissolves into small white lines.

Another oral sign of SLE is **xerostomia** secondary to Sjögren's syndrome. Xerostomia can significantly increase the occurrence of dental caries and candidiasis, especially when patients are being treated with steroids or immunosuppressive agents.

Systemic sclerosis (Scleroderma)

Systemic sclerosis is a chronic disease of unknown etiology characterized by abnormal accumulation of fibrous tissue in the skin and multiple organs. The skin is most commonly affected, but the gastrointestinal tract, kidneys, heart, and lungs also are frequently involved. In some patients, the disease appears to remain confined to the skin for many years, but in the majority, it progresses to visceral involvement with death from renal failure, cardiac failure, pulmonary insufficiency, or intestinal malabsorption.

Systemic sclerosis can be classified into two groups on the basis of its clinical course:

1. **Diffuse scleroderma**, characterized by initial widespread skin involvement, with rapid progression and early visceral involvement.
2. **Limited scleroderma**, with relatively minimal skin involvement, often confined to the fingers and face. Involvement of the viscera occurs late, and hence the disease in these patients generally has a fairly benign course.

Oral manifestations

The clinical signs of scleroderma of the mouth and jaws are consistent with findings elsewhere in the body. The lips become rigid and the oral aperture narrows considerably. Skin folds are lost around the mouth, giving a masklike appearance to the face. Tongue may become hard and rigid, leading to difficulty in speaking and swallowing. Involvement of oesophagus causes dysphagia. When the soft tissues around the temporomandibular joint are affected, they restrict movement of the mandible causing pseudoankylosis.

The linear form of localized scleroderma may involve the face as well as underlying bone and teeth.

Radiographic findings include calcinosis of the soft tissues around the jaws and uniform thickening of the periodontal membrane, especially around the posterior teeth in less than 10% of patients.

When the facial tissues and muscles of mastication are extensively involved, the pressure exerted will cause resorption of the mandible. This resorption is particularly apparent at the angle of the mandible at the attachment of the masseter muscle. The coronoid process, condyle, or area of attachment of the digastric muscles may also be damaged by the continual pressure.

Dermatomyositis

Dermatomyositis is an inflammatory disorder of the skin as well as skeletal muscles. It is characterized by a distinctive skin rash that may accompany or precede the onset of muscle disease. The disease occurs most frequently during childhood and between the fourth and sixth decade of life. Most studies have found a preponderance of female patients over male patients.

It usually begins with a symmetric and painless weakness of the proximal muscles of the arms, legs, and trunk. The weakness is progressive and characteristically spreads to the face, neck, larynx, pharynx, and heart. Muscle involvement may become severe enough to confine the patient to bed or cause death due to failure of the respiratory muscles.

Oral manifestations

These include weakness of the pharyngeal and palatal muscles, which causes difficulty in swallowing (dysphagia) and nasal speech (dystonia). The muscles of mastication and the facial muscles may also be involved, causing difficulty in chewing. Oral mucosa may show shallow ulcers, erythematous patches, and telangiectasis. More characteristic are the facial skin lesions which may present as a "butterfly" rash (similar to the lesions of SLE) or as a swelling of the eyelids, face or lips. Lilac-coloured eyelids secondary to stasis of blood in multiple telangiectasias is also a common finding. Calcinosis of the soft tissues is seen especially in children. These calcified nodules may appear in the face and may show up on dental radiographs. The tongue may also become rigid due to severe calcinosis.

Rheumatoid arthritis

Rheumatoid arthritis (RA) is a chronic systemic inflammatory disorder that may affect many tissues and organs – skin, blood vessels, heart, lungs, and muscles, but principally attacks the joints producing a non-suppurative proliferative synovitis that often progresses to destruction of articular cartilage and ankylosis of joints. It is generally considered to be an autoimmune disease. Both humoral and cell-mediated immune reactions are believed to be important in the pathogenesis of RA.

The synovial membrane is usually infiltrated by large number of lymphocytes and plasma cells. There is an increased amount of immunoglobulins (IgG, IgM and IgA) in the serum and synovial fluid and there is deposition of immune complexes in the synovium. **About 80% of individuals with RA have autoantibodies to the Fc portion of autologous IgG called rheumatoid factors.** These are mostly IgM antibodies but they may be of other classes (IgG and IgA). RF may be absent in some (seronegative) and may be found in some non-RA patients such as systemic lupus erythematosus, dermatomyositis and even in otherwise healthy people. RF is detected by agglutination of latex particles coated with IgG.

Oral manifestations

Patients with long-standing active RA have an increased incidence of periodontal disease, including loss of alveolar bone and teeth. The treatment of RA can cause oral manifestations. The long-term use of methotrexate and other antirheumatic agents such as D-penicillamine and NSAIDs can cause stomatitis. Cyclosporine may cause gingival overgrowth.

KEY FACTS

- *Type I hypersensitivity* is mediated by *IgE antibodies*
- *IgE antibodies bind to specific receptors on mast cells and basophils*
- *Type I hypersensitivity leads to anaphylaxis, hay fever, atopic dermatitis and allergic asthma*
- Severity of symptoms depends on IgE antibodies and the quantity of allergen
- *Type II hypersensitivity* is mediated by IgG or IgM antibodies against cell surface or extracellular matrix antigens
- *Transfusion reactions to erythrocytes* are produced by antibodies to blood group antigens which may occur naturally or may have been induced by previous blood transfusion or during pregnancy
- Antibodies damage cells and tissues by activating complement
- *Haemolytic disease of newborn* occurs when maternal antibodies to foetal blood group antigen cross the placenta and destroy the foetal erythrocytes
- *Persistence of antigen* from continued infection or in autoimmune disease can lead to **immune complex disease**
- *Immune complexes* can form both in the circulation, leading to systemic disease, and at local sites such as the lungs
- *Two types of type IV hypersensitivity* are recognized – tuberculin (infection) type and contact dermatitis type
- Overactivity of Th cells or decreased activity of Ts cells may lead to *autoimmunity*

IMPORTANT QUESTION

Write short notes on:
(a) Type I hypersensitivity
(b) Type II hypersensitivity
(c) Type III hypersensitivity
(d) Type IV hypersensitivity
(e) Mechanism of autoimmunity
(f) Systemic lupus erythamatosus
(g) Systemic sclerosis
(h) Dermatomyositis
(i) Rheumatoid arthritis

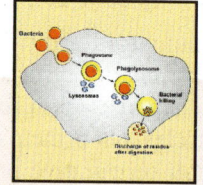

Chapter 16

Immunodeficiency Diseases

Immunodeficiency diseases are the conditions where the defence mechanism of the body is impaired leading to repeated microbial infections and sometimes enhanced susceptibility to malignancies. These include defects in all components of immune system, including B, T and NK lymphocytes, phagocytic cells and complement proteins. Patients with defects in immunoglobulins, complement proteins or phagocytosis are very susceptible to recurrent infections with encapsulated bacteria such as *Haemophilus influenzae*, *Streptococcus pneumoniae* and *Staphylococcus aureus*. These are called **pyogenic infections**, because the bacteria give rise to pus formation. On the other hand, patients with defects in cell-mediated immunity, i.e., in T cells, are susceptible to overwhelming, even lethal, infections with microorganisms that are ubiquitous in the environment and to which normal people rapidly develop resistance. For this reason these are called **opportunistic infections**.

Immunodeficiencies may be classified as primary or secondary. **Primary immunodeficiencies** are due to the abnormalities in the development of the immune mechanisms. **Secondary immunodeficiencies** are secondary to some other disease process affecting the normal functioning of some part of the lymphoid tissues, drugs, malnutrition and

ionizing radiations used to treat cancer. Since 1981, the most common immunodeficiency disease is acquired immunodeficiency syndrome (AIDS).

PRIMARY IMMUNODEFICIENCY SYNDROMES

Attempts have been made to classify primary immunodeficiency disorders. Table 16.1 lists well-known primary immunodeficiency syndromes.

A. Humoral immunodeficiencies (B cell defects)

X-linked (congenital) agammaglobulinaemia or Bruton's disease

This is the first immunodeficiency disease to have been recognised. It was described by Bruton in 1952. As an X-linked disease, it is seen almost entirely in males, but sporadic cases have also been described in females. It is characterized by recurrent infections with pyogenic bacteria, such as pneumococci, streptococci, staphylococci and *Haemophilus*. The most common type of infections include sinusitis, pneumonia, otitis, furunculosis, meningitis and septicaemia. Most patients afflicted with this disease remain well during the first six to nine months of life, presumably by virtue of maternally transmitted immunoglobulins.

Table 16.1. Primary immunodeficiency syndromes

**HUMORAL IMMUNODEFICIENCIES
(B CELL DEFECTS)**
- X-linked (congenital) agammaglobulinaemia (Bruton's disease)
- Transient hypogammaglobulinaemia of infancy
- Common variable immunodeficiency
- Selective IgA deficiency
- Selective IgM deficiency
- Immunodeficiency with elevated IgM

CELLULAR IMMUNODEFICIENCIES
- Thymic hypoplasia (DiGeorge's syndrome)
- Purine nucleoside phosphorylase (PNP) deficiency

**COMBINED IMMUNODEFICIENCIES
(B AND T CELL DEFECTS)**
- Cellular immunodeficiency with abnormal immunoglobulin synthesis (Nezelof's syndrome)
- Ataxia telangiectasia
- Immunodeficiency with thrombocytopenia and eczema (Wiskott-Aldrich syndrome)
- Immunodeficiency with thymoma
- Severe combined immunodeficiency diseases
  - Swiss-type agammaglobulinaemia
  - Adenosine deaminase deficiency
  - Reticular dysgenesis

COMPLEMENT IMMUNE DEFICIENCY DISORDERS

DISORDERS OF PHAGOCYTOSIS
- Chronic granulomatous disease
- Myeloperoxidase (MPO) deficiency
- Leucocyte G6PD deficiency
- Chediak-Higashi syndrome

Because their T cell-mediated responses are normal, individuals with Bruton's agammaglobulinaemia can normally handle viral, fungal, protozoal and some bacterial diseases. But there are some important exceptions to this generalization. These patients seem to be very susceptible to echovirus and enterovirus infections. They are also at increased risk for development of *Pneumocystis jiroveci* pneumonia. Persistent generalized infections with *Giardia lamblia* may give rise to malabsorption. These observations indicate a role of antibodies in resistance against these agents. Allograft rejection, in patients with Bruton's disease, is normal and delayed hypersensitivity to tuberculin can be demonstrated. Autoimmune diseases like rheumatoid

arthritis, lupus erythematosus, dermatomyositis and others occur with increased frequency in patients with Bruton's disease.

The basic defect in this disorder is a failure of pre-B cells to differentiate into mature B cells. Tonsils and adenoids are atrophic. Lymph node biopsy reveals a depletion of cells of bursa-dependent areas. Plasma cells and germinal centres are absent even after antigenic stimulation. B cells are absent or remarkably decreased in the circulation and there is an absence or deficiency of all the five classes of serum immunoglobulins. Pre-B cells are found in normal numbers in bone marrow. These diseases can be treated by routine injections of normal immunoglobulins.

Transient hypogammaglobulinaemia of infancy

This is due to an abnormal delay in the initiation of IgG synthesis in some infants. It involves infants of both sexes and is not a common entity. Normally infants start producing their own antibodies by 3–7 months, but in infants with this condition antibody production starts by 6–11 months of age. Lymphocytes show no abnormality in the percentage of cells in different subpopulations. Gammaglobulin therapy is not indicated in this condition, as it may contribute to prolongation of immunodeficiency by a negative feedback inhibition of IgG synthesis.

Common variable immunodeficiency

Common variable immunodeficiency is also known as late onset hypogammaglobulinaemia because it usually manifests only by 15–35 years of age. The patient may have normal-sized or enlarged tonsils, lymph nodes and spleen. The serum immunoglobulin and antibody deficiency are usually as profound as in X-linked disorder and the kinds of infections experienced and bacterial etiologic agents involved are generally the same for the two defects. This may also be associated with an increased incidence of autoimmune disease. B cells may be present in circulation in normal numbers, but they appear defective in being unable to differentiate into plasma cells and secrete immunoglobulins. Thus this defect appears to be caused by abnormal terminal differentiation of the B cell line. The total immunoglobulin level is usually less than 300 mg per 100 ml, with IgG less than 250 mg per 100 ml. Increased suppressor T cell and decreased helper T cell activity has been proposed as a cause of this disorder. Treatment of this condition is by administration of gamma-globulin preparations intramuscularly or intra-dermally.

Selective IgA deficiency

Absence or near absence of serum and secretory IgA is thought to be the most common well-defined immunodeficiency disorder. Because of the deficiency of secretory IgA, infections occur predominantly in the respiratory, gastrointestinal and urogenital tracts. Serum concentration of other immunoglobulins are usually normal in patients with selective IgA deficiency. Anti-IgA antibodies are present in the sera of nearly half of the patients with selective IgA deficiency and administration of IgA-containing solutions to these patients may lead to severe or fatal anaphylactic reactions.

Selective IgM deficiency

Selective IgM deficiency may occur occasionally. These patients develop septicaemia due to meningococci and other Gram-negative bacteria, pneumococcal meningitis, tuberculosis, recurrent staphylococcal pyoderma, periorbital cellulitis, bronchiectasis, otitis and other respiratory infections.

Immunodeficiency with elevated IgM

This disorder is characterized by low IgA and IgG levels with either a normal or more frequently with elevated IgM. Patients with this defect may develop recurrent pyogenic infections, including otitis media, sinusitis, pneumonia and tonsillitis during first or second year of life. In addition, patient may develop autoimmune disorders such as thrombocytopenia, neutropenia and haemolytic anaemia. Some patients develop malignant infiltration with IgM producing cells. T cell functions, in these patients, are usually normal.

B. Cellular immunodeficiencies (T cell defects)

Thymic hypoplasia (DiGeorge's syndrome)

Thymic hypoplasia results from a congenital malformation affecting the third and fourth pharyngeal pouches. These structures give rise to the thymus, parathyroid glands, and portions of lips, ears and the aortic arch. Therefore, in addition to thymic hypoplasia the parathyroid glands are also either hypoplastic or totally absent. The functions of both these organs are essential for survival, the thymus for the formation of competent T cells to carry out cellular immune functions and parathyroid for the production of the hormone, parathormone, which regulates calcium levels in the blood. Most of these infants have additional developmental defects affecting the face, ears, heart and great vessels.

In these patients thymus is usually rudimentary and T cells are deficient or absent in the circulation. They are similarly depleted in thymus-dependent areas of the lymph nodes and spleen. Thus infants with this defect are extremely vulnerable to viral, fungal and protozoal infections. Susceptibility to intracellular bacteria is also increased, because phagocytic cells that eliminate them require T cell-derived signals for activation. The B cell system and serum immunoglobulins are entirely unaffected.

Purine nucleoside phosphorylase (PNP) deficiency

The lack of enzyme PNP because of a gene defect in chromosome 14 results in impaired metabolism of cytosine and inosine to purine. These patients show decreased T cell proliferation leading to decreased T cell-mediated immunity and recurrent or chronic infections.

C. Combined immunodeficiencies (B and T cell defects)

Cellular immunodeficiency with abnormal immunoglobulin synthesis (Nezelof's syndrome)

In this condition there is depressed cell-mediated immunity associated with decreased, normal or increased levels of most of the five immunoglobulin classes. Patients present during infancy with recurrent or chronic pulmonary infections, failure to thrive, oral or cutaneous candidiasis, chronic diarrhoea, recurrent skin infections, Gram-negative sepsis, urinary tract infections and severe varicella. Other findings include lymphopenia, neutropenia and eosinophilia. The thymus is small and peripheral lymphoid tissues are hypoplastic and demonstrate paracortical lymphocyte depletion. Bone marrow transplantation, thymus transplantation and transfer factor have been used for treatment with success in some cases. For the treatment of microbial infections adequate antimicrobial therapy is essential.

Ataxia telangiectasia

Ataxia telangiectasia is a multisystem defect involving vascular, endocrine, nervous and immune systems. Clinically, patient develops cerebral ataxia, oculocutaneous telangiectasia, chronic sino-pulmonary disease, ovarian dysgenesis, a high incidence of malignancy and variable humoral and cellular immunodeficiency. Mental capacity, immune status and other physiological conditions deteriorate with time. The majority of patients lack IgA and IgE antibodies. Some patients possess antibodies to IgA. Cell-mediated immunity is also defective leading to impairment of delayed hypersensitivity and graft rejection. Severe infections begin to occur during the first year of life. Death occurs due to sinopulmonary infections early in life, or malignancy in the second or third decade.

Immunodeficiency with thrombocytopenia and eczema (Wiskott-Aldrich syndrome)

Wiskott-Aldrich syndrome is an X-linked recessive disease characterized by bleeding, eczema and recurrent infections. The bleeding is due to thrombo-cytopenia, eczema from elevated IgE levels and recurrent bacterial, viral and fungal infections from abnormalities in cell-mediated (thymic hypoplasia) and antibody-mediated (lymphoid hyperplasia) immunity. B and T cell numbers are normal initially, but by six years of age there is a profound loss of cell-mediated immunity. Transfer factor and foetal thymus transplants have been tried with some benefit.

Immunodeficiency with thymoma

This syndrome consists of thymoma with impaired cell-mediated immunity and agammaglobulinaemia. This usually occurs in adults. They may also have eosinophilia or eosinopenia, haemolytic anaemia, agranulocytosis, thrombocytopenia and pancyto-penia. Antibody formation is poor and progressive lymphopenia develops. Several patients with this disorder have been shown to have excessive suppressor T cell activity.

Severe combined immunodeficiency diseases

Severe combined immunodeficiency diseases (SCID) include syndromes in which patients lack both B and T cells. Many distinct patterns of severe combined immunodeficiency have been described:

(a) Swiss-type agammaglobulinaemia

This is inherited either through a sex-linked pattern or as an autosomal-recessive trait. Such persons are born with stem-cell defects and lack both antibody and cell-mediated immunity. They have agamma-globulinaemia with lymphocytopenia.

(b) Adenosine deaminase deficiency

Certain types of immune deficiency disorders arise as a consequence of reduced enzymatic activity. One such example of a SCID has a genetically inherited enzyme deficiency disorder. The enzyme that is deficient in this disorder is adenosine deaminase (ADA), an enzyme involved in purine metabolism. In these patients, T cell deficiency is more profound than B cell deficiency. ADA levels are low in all the tissues, including red blood cells. The mechanism by which this deficiency causes SCID is not clear. It is, however, believed that deficiency of this enzyme leads to accumulation of adenosine and deoxy-adenosine triphosphate, which are toxic to lympho-cytes, particularly of T cell lineage.

Infants with these severe immune disorders are vulnerable to all forms of viral, fungal and bacterial infections, and most die during the first year of life. A number of such cases have been successfully treated by transplantation of normal histocompatible bone marrow. This suggests that these patients have normal thymus, and bursa-equivalent tissues and the basis of their B and T cell deficiency is defective lymphoid stem cells.

(c) Reticular dysgenesis

This is the most serious form of SCID. Here the defect is in the development of the multipotent bone marrow stem cell. The individual is born without any white blood cells, neither phagocytes nor lymphocytes. This is known as reticular dysgenesis. As a result of this disorder there is the absence of immunologically competent cells. A baby with this disorder usually dies within the first year of life from recurrent, intractable infections.

D. Complement immune deficiency disorders

Various components of complement are involved in phagocytosis, antibody killing of bacteria, lysis of viruses, virus-infected cells, tumour cells, histamine release by mast cells and basophils, and chemotaxis of phagocytic neutrophils and monocytes. Some animals and humans have been found to possess genetic defects that result in complete absence of one or another complement component.

Deficiency of C1 and C4 is associated with systemic lupus erythematosus. In C2 deficiency, there appear to be few problems probably because the alternative pathway of complement can still be used. The absence of C3 component is associated with increased susceptibility to bacterial infections, such as pneumonia, meningitis and septicaemia.

Persons deficient in C5 to C8 can be asymptomatic for years and then develop infections caused by *Neisseria meningitidis* and *N. gonorrhoeae* and immune complex syndromes with rheumatoid-like symptoms. So far, there is no known disease with deficiency of C9.

E. Disorders of phagocytosis

Phagocytosis may be impaired either by intrinsic defects within the phagocytic cells such as enzyme deficiency or extrinsic defects due to deficiency of opsonic antibody, complement or due to drugs or antineutrophil antibodies. Phagocytic dysfunction leads to increased susceptibility to infections.

Chronic granulomatous disease

Chronic granulomatous disease (CGD) is a frequently fatal genetic disorder in which there is a deficiency of NADPH oxidase. Individuals with CGD possess polymorphonuclear leucocytes that phagocytose invading bacteria normally but are unable to kill many of the ingested microorganisms because engulfment of bacteria is not followed by activation of oxygen-dependent killing mechanisms. Many bacteria produce hydrogen peroxide, which can be utilized by neutrophils to form bactericidal compounds. However, bacteria like *Staphylococcus aureus* and those belonging to the family Enterobacteriaceae possess catalase, which inactivates hydrogen peroxide and thus prevents its utilization by the neutrophils. Against such bacteria the CGD neutrophils are defenceless. Therefore, CGD is characterized by repeated bacterial infections most commonly caused by these organisms.

Myeloperoxidase (MPO) deficiency

In this rare disease, leucocytes are deficient in MPO. Phagocytes from MPO-deficient patients produce H_2O_2 and possess other cidal mechanisms that involve superoxide. They generally remain well and free from recurrent infections, however, they are liable to develop recurrent *Candida albicans* infection.

Leucocyte G6PD deficiency

In this rare disease leucocytes are deficient in glucose 6 phosphate dehydrogenase. These patients show diminished bactericidal activity after phagocytosis leading to repeated bacterial infections.

Chediak-Higashi syndrome

Chediak-Higashi syndrome (CHS) is an autosomal recessive disorder. The individuals with this syndrome suffer from recurrent infections similar to those seen in persons with CGD. Polymorphonuclear leucocytes in patients with CHS possess large (giant) lysosomes. These abnormal lysosomes do not fuse readily with a cytoplasmic phagosome.

Oral manifestations of primary immunodeficiency disorders

Patients with T lymphocyte abnormalities have a higher incidence of oral disease than patients with B lymphocyte disorders have. T lymphocyte abnormalities lead to chronic fungal and viral infections, which are more likely to occur in oral mucosa than are the bacterial infections seen in B lymphocyte deficiencies. A consistent oral sign noted in patients with T cell diseases such as thymic hypoplasia or ataxia telangiectasia is chronic oral candidiasis. Herpes simplex virus infections are also common in patients with T cell disease.

The infections may be localized to the mouth but frequently become disseminated and are potentially lethal if not treated with antiviral medications. Other oral signs seen with T cell deficiencies include the dermal and mucosal telangiectases of ataxia telangiectasia. Congenital defects of the mouth and jaws (including cleft palate, micrognathia, bifid uvula, and short philtrum of the upper lip) have also been seen in patients with thymic hypoplasia. In patients with ataxia telangiectasia, hypotonia of facial muscles and atrophy of the skin gives rise to characteristic dull expression; drooling can also be problem.

The major sign in patients with B-cell abnormalities is recurrent bacterial infections that frequently involve the respiratory tract. The most common of these infections that comes to the attention of dentists is chronic maxillary sinusitis.

Neutropenia and neutrophil dysfunction syndromes commonly cause oral ulcers, but immunoglobulin deficiencies do not.

SECONDARY IMMUNODEFICIENCY

Acquired deficiencies of immunological mechanisms can occur secondarily to a number of disease states such as metabolic disorders, malnutrition, malignancy and infections or after exposure to drugs and chemicals. Secondary immunodeficiency is far more common than primary immunodeficiency.

Deficiency of immunoglobulins can be brought about by excessive loss of protein through diseased kidneys or via the intestine in protein-losing enteropathy. Malnutrition and iron deficiency can lead to depressed immune responsiveness, particularly in cell-mediated immunity. Irradiations, cytotoxic drugs and steroids often have undesirable effects on the immune system. Infections with human immunodeficiency, measles and other viruses are often immunosuppressive.

Raised immunoglobulin levels are seen in certain disorders of plasma cells due to malignant proliferation of a particular clone or group of plasma cells. In these conditions, such as chronic lympho-

cytic leukaemia and multiple myeloma each malignant clone will produce one particular type of antibody. This leads to decreased synthesis of normal immunoglobulins and increased susceptibility to bacterial infections. Cell-mediated immunity is depressed in lymphoreticular malignancies like Hodgkin's lymphoma, obstruction to lymph circulation and infiltration of the thymus-dependent areas of lymph nodes with nonlymphoid cells as in lepromatous leprosy.

Acquired immunodeficiency syndrome (AIDS), which has assumed pandemic proportion, is the most important of secondary immunodeficiency diseases (see chapter 30).

KEY FACTS

- In **immunodeficiency disease** the defence mechanism of the body is impaired leading to *repeated microbial infections*
- **Primary immunodeficiencies** are due to the abnormalities in the development of the immune mechanisms
- **Secondary immunodeficiencies** are secondary to some other disease process affecting the normal functioning of some parts of lymphoid tissues, drugs, malnutrition and ionizing radiations used to treat cancer
- Since 1981, the most common immunodeficiency disease is *acquired immunodeficiency syndrome* (AIDS)
- Patients with T lymphocyte abnormalities have a higher incidence of oral disease than patients with B lymphocyte disorders have

IMPORTANT QUESTIONS

1. What are immunodeficiency diseases? Differentiate between primary and secondary immunodeficiencies.
2. List well-known primary immunodeficiency syndromes. Describe Bruton's disease.
3. Write short notes on:
   (a) DiGeorge's syndrome
   (b) Wiskott-Aldrich syndrome
   (c) Chediak-Higashi syndrome
   (d) Oral manifestations of immunodeficiency disorders

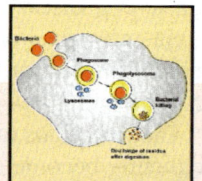

Chapter 17

Immunology of Transplantation & Malignancy

Transplantation of normal tissues and organs from one animal to another has been extensively studied. Most of the experimental work on transplantation has been done on mice, an animal species easy to breed and handle in the laboratory. The aim of tissue and organ transplantation from one person to another is to replace diseased tissues and organs. The tissue or organ transplanted is known as the **transplant** or **graft**. The individual from whom the transplant is obtained is known as **donor** and the individual on whom it is applied, the **recipient**.

Types of grafts

1. **Autografts:** Grafts from one part of the body to another in the same individual are known as autografts. Autografts survive and function for the life time of the individual.
2. **Isografts:** Grafts between genetically identical individuals (identical twins).
3. **Allografts:** Grafts between members of the same species (allogeneic individuals) but of different genetic constitution.
4. **Xenografts:** Grafts between members of different species.

A xenograft and an allograft do not survive. Except in case of uniovular twins, the transplantation of a tissue from one human to another amounts to an allograft. Grafts between ordinary brothers and sisters or between parents and offsprings, or even between dissimilar twins are examples of allografts. Allografts survive longer than xenografts but are ultimately rejected.

ALLOGRAFT REACTION

When a skin graft from an animal is applied on a genetically unrelated animal of the same species (allograft), for the first few days it behaves as an autograft. It is quickly vascularized and looks healthy. By about fourth day, it slowly becomes dark because of diminished circulation due to stasis followed by thrombosis and haemorrhage. The graft is invaded by lymphocytes and macrophages and in about two weeks, the graft sloughs off due to ischaemic necrosis. In addition, antibodies are believed to play a significant role in this process. The sequence of events resulting in the rejection of an allograft is known as **first-set reaction**.

If in an animal, which has rejected a graft by first-set reaction, another graft from the same donor is applied, it will lead to a hyperacute or immediate rejection response. This is accomplished by cytolytic leucocytes and complement-mediated antibody lysis of transplanted cells. The initial vascularisation may not occur, if it does, it is poor and is halted abruptly.

Thrombosis of vessels is a feature. The graft is rejected much sooner in three to five days. This is known as **second-set reaction**.

The cells of an individual express a unique set of membrane antigens called **histocompatibility antigens**, which immunologically define a person's cell type as specifically as do fingerprints. The information about the synthesis of these antigens is stored on **histocompatibility genes**. Everyone on earth, with the possible exception of identical twins, has a personal set of histocompatibility genes and gene products (histocompatibility antigens). These genetically defined histocompatibility antigens, some of which are found on the surface of all body cells, serve to discriminate self from non-self.

Only those grafts in which there is a complete identity between the genetic constitution of the donor and the recipient (their histocompatibility genes and antigens are identical) survive and function. The rejection of an allograft has an immunological basis. This is evident from the specificity of the second-set reaction. Accelerated rejection is seen only if the second graft is from the same donor as the first. Application of a skin graft from another donor will evoke only the first-set reaction.

Mechanism of allograft rejection

Presentation of foreign cell MHC antigens is one of the initial events of first-set reaction. Once blood vessels communicate with the graft, graft antigens can travel to the lymph nodes where they activate lymphatic T cells. The activated lymphocytes give rise to expanded clones of specific Tc, Th and Td cells. Tc cells can enter the circulation directly, while Td cells remain in the lymph nodes and mobilize phagocytic leucocytes via the release of soluble lymphokines. Tc cells eventually reach the transplantation site, enter the blood vessels of the graft, and proceed to destroy the grafted tissue by repeated cell to cell toxicity.

In second-set reactions, the memory of foreign antigenic cells is so vivid that the blood vessels of the second graft are destroyed almost as soon as they are established. This rapid response is brought about primarily by Tc cells which are rapidly activated. The additional participation of circulating complement fixing antibodies and NK cells might contribute to graft rejection. The infiltration of neutrophils, macrophages and Tc cells, which are already present in the circulation, follows soon leading to rapid and irreversible rejection of foreign tissue transplanted to the host a second time.

MAJOR HISTOCOMPATIBILITY COMPLEX

Genes mediating graft rejection in mice are called the histocompatibility genes or H genes or H loci. A large number of H loci exist widely spread throughout the mouse genome. The products of the different H genes differ greatly in their ability to induce graft rejection. The strongest locus is known as major histocompatibility complex (MHC) in contrast to weaker loci (minor histocompatibility loci) which are more than 30. The MHC in mouse is referred to as **H-2 complex**.

The MHC in humans is known as the **human leucocyte antigen (HLA) complex.** The genes that code for the HLA antigens are found on the short arm of sixth pair of chromosome (one paternal and one maternal). The MHC genes are contained within four HLA loci known as A, B, C and D (Fig. 17.1). There are many different alleles at each of HLA-A, HLA-B and HLA-C loci, although any individual will possess a maximum of two at each locus (one on each chromosome). The A locus is associated with segregant series of 24 alleles, the B locus with 52 alleles and the C locus with 11 alleles. The various

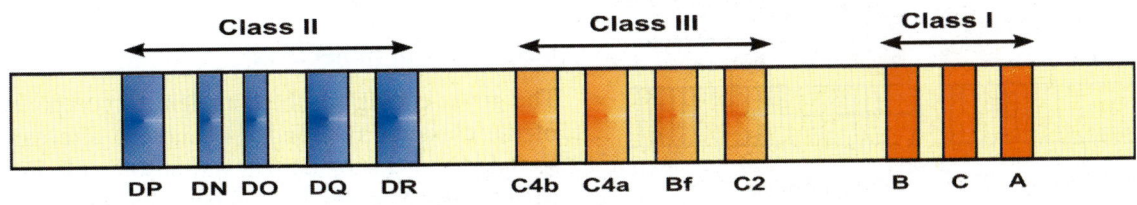

Fig. 17.1. HLA complex.

alleles are assigned the letters signifying the locus followed by a number signifying the allele. For example, HLA-A10 implies an HLA allele number 10 belonging to the locus A.

There are three classes of genes in these HLA loci: class I, class II and class III genes which code for the corresponding molecules (antigens).

MHC class I molecules

In humans the genes encoding the major transplantation antigens are HLA-A, HLA-B and HLA-C loci. The products of these loci are known as class I antigens. Class I antigens are membrane-bound glycoprotein in nature. They are composed of two polypeptide chains (Fig. 17.2). The smaller of the two polypeptide chains is known as β_2-microglobulin (β_2-M). It is not encoded by genes within the MHC, but by the gene located on chromosome 2. It has a molecular weight of 12,000 daltons. The larger polypeptide chain of class I antigen is encoded by a gene present on HLA-A, HLA-B and HLA-C regions. It is known as a chain and has a molecular weight of 44,000 daltons. It has five structural domains. Three external globular domains (α_1, α_2 and α_3) held in place by disulphide bonds and non-covalent interactions, a transmembrane portion and a short cytoplasmic tail. β_2-M is non-covalently associated with the α_3 domain. The globular protein formed by these two peptides is present on the surface of virtually all nucleated cells, with probable exception of ova, sperms and amniotic cells, in man. They are involved in recognition of target cells by cytotoxic T cells. The cytotoxic T cells recognize antigen only if presented simultaneously with class I antigens.

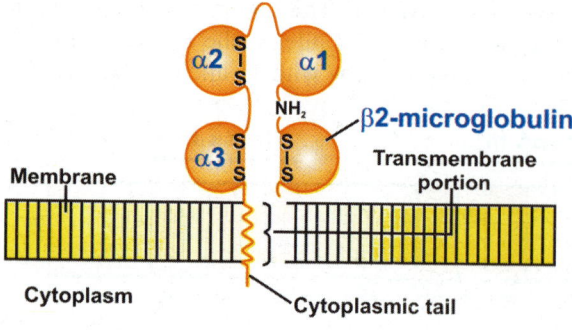

Fig. 17.2. Class I MHC antigens.

MHC class II molecules

Class II antigens are encoded by the HLA-DP, HLA-DQ and HLA-DR loci (all of which reside within the HLA-D region of HLA complex), for which there are multiple alleles in the population. They are glycoproteins consisting of two polypeptide chains (α and β) held together by non-covalent interactions (Fig. 17.3). Both these chains are inserted into the cell membrane and have molecular weights of 33,000 and 25,000 daltons respectively. Each chain is composed of two extracellular domains (α_1, α_2 and β_1, β_2), a transmembrane portion and a cytoplasmic tail. The tissue distribution of class II MHC antigens is relatively limited. In man, they are normally found on immunologically reactive cells such as B lymphocytes, macrophages, monocytes and activated T lymphocytes.

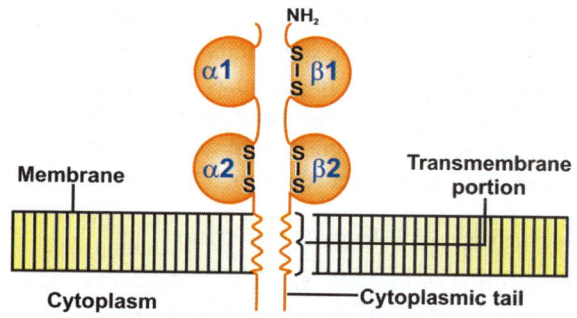

Fig. 17.3. Class II MHC antigens.

Class I and class II MHC antigens are members of the immunoglobulin superfamily. Both the class I and class II MHC-encoded proteins are structurally related to immunoglobulin and are involved in cell-cell interaction in the generation and regulation of immune responses. As such, they are members of the larger group of proteins called the immunoglobulin superfamily.

MHC class III molecules

The genes coding for the complement components of the classical (C2 and C4) and the alternative (properdin or factor B) pathway also reside in the MHC genes complex located between MHC class I and class II regions (Fig. 17.1).

HISTOCOMPATIBILITY TESTING

For matching of donor and recipient for transplantation following procedures are undertaken:

ABO grouping

When tissue transplantation is anticipated, grouping and crossmatching of blood from donor and recipient are performed as a first step. If there exists any discrepancy in the ABO blood group, then the use of the prospective donor's tissue is absolutely contraindicated because blood group antigens are strong histocompatibility antigens.

Tissue typing (detection of MHC antigens)

Class I antigens are identified by means of antisera, therefore, the term serologically defined antigens is applied to them. Antisera used to detect class I antigens are obtained from:

- multiparous women, individuals who have received multiple blood transfusions,
- individuals who have received and rejected grafts, and
- volunteers who have been immunized with cells from another individual with a different HLA haplotype.

   Following methods are used:

(a) **Lymphoagglutination test:** When donor and recipient lymphocytes are mixed with a panel of specific antisera, agglutination of lymphocytes is seen with specific antiserum.

(b) **Lymphocytotoxicity test:** Donor and recipient lymphocytes are incubated with a panel of antisera directed against specific class I MHC antigens followed by addition of complement. Lysis of cells is seen with specific antiserum.

   MHC class II antigens are identified by the method known as mixed lymphocyte culture (MLC) assay. This can determine a possible match between donor and recipient class II antigens. In this test, donor and recipient lymphocytes are mixed together in a tube containing a radioactive DNA precursor. Donor or stimulator cells are irradiated to prevent DNA synthesis and proliferation. If the class II antigens are foreign, the responder cells will be stimulated to divide. As the stimulated cells replicate

their DNA, they incorporate the radioactive precursor. The amount of radioactivity incorporated into cells can then be easily measured and quantitated.

Uses of HLA typing

HLA typing is used primarily for the following:

- Determination of HLA compatibility prior to transplantation.
- Paternity testing.
- Anthropologic studies.
- Establishing HLA disease associations.

   HLA typing was first done to identify HLA compatible donors and recipients for organ transplantation. The collaborative transplant study has demonstrated that the graft survival rate of HLA-identical (two haplotypes) transplants is superior to that of grafts matched for one haplotype. HLA matching has a statistically significant and clinically important impact on the short and long-term graft survival for most of the organ transplants (kidney, liver, bone marrow, etc.).

   Matching at HLA-D locus has a strong effect on kidney graft survival but in long term (5 years or more) the desirability of reasonable HLA-B, and to a lesser extent HLA-A, matching also becomes apparent. It has now been firmly established that multiple blood transfusions prior to grafting have a significant beneficial effect on survival but its mechanism is still not clear.

   In heart transplants, graft survival is significantly influenced by the extent of HLA compatibility. Full HLA matching is of course not practical but single DR mismatch gives 90% survival for three years.

   Successful corneal transplants have been performed without recourse to tissue typing or immunosuppression. Cornea is an immunologically privileged site. It lacks lymphatic drainage and the small amount of antigen released into the blood stream from graft is not sufficient to trigger a cellular response. But HLA typing may be very important in corneal transplantation in those cases where the recipient's eye is chronically inflamed.

   HLA typing demonstrating that the putative father and child do not share any haplotype is usually accepted by the courts as excluding the possibility that a given male is the father.

GRAFT VERSUS HOST REACTION

Under certain circumstances the immunologically competent cells of the graft react against antigens of the host (recipient), the reverse of the normal transplantation reaction. Such a reaction is known as graft versus host reaction (GVH). Following conditions are necessary for the development of GVH:

1. The host's immunological responsiveness must be either destroyed or so impaired (following whole-body irradiation) that he cannot reject a graft (allograft or xenograft).
2. There is HLA incompatibility between the donor and the host (recipient).
3. The graft (bone marrow, lymphoid tissue, splenic tissue, etc.) contains immunocompetent cells. MHC antigens of recipient activate transplanted immunocompetent cells which lead to the production of antibodies, lymphokines, activated phagocytes, Tc cells, etc. They attack the recipient cells leading to the death of the recipient.

FOETUS AS A GRAFT

Foetus is always a mixture of maternal and paternal genes, therefore, foetal MHC antigens are always different from those of the mother. In spite of this foetus is not treated as foreign transplanted tissue and rejected. On the other hand, it grows and develops inside the uterus of the mother for more than nine months because of immunosuppressant factors made by foetus, placenta and mother.

1. Cells of the placenta produce mucoproteins which coat foetal cells, thus masking histocompatibility antigens and prevent recognition.
2. Placental giant cells can produce soluble inhibitory factor which suppresses T cell proliferation and antibody production, and induces a population of Ts cells. Immunosuppression is also due to hormones (human chorionic gonadotropin, produced by placenta, and the high levels of maternal progesterone produced during pregnancy).
3. The mother produces specific blocking antibodies to foetal antigens of the foetal cells thus blocking immune recognition and immune attack by maternal Tc cells.

4. Major foetal serum protein, α-fetoprotein, can stimulate the formation of Ts cells, and the amniotic fluid contains immunosuppressive phospholipids. These factors contribute to immunosuppression in the mother.
5. β_1-glycoprotein, of foetal origin, can be found in maternal plasma. It has been shown to inhibit maternal cellular immunity.

These factors depress immune system of the mother, however, it is usually not life-threatening because most of the response is localized in the uterus.

Why the foetus does not reject the mother? It may be due to the fact that the developing immune system of the foetus cannot respond.

MHC RESTRICTION

Limitation imposed upon activation of an immune response, unless antigen presentation occurs in association with either a class I or a class II MHC antigen is known as MHC restriction. Tc and Ts cells recognise the combination of foreign antigen and class I MHC antigens, whereas Td and Th cells recognize foreign antigen in association with class II antigens. Therefore, in addition to transplantation reactions, MHC antigens are involved in immune surveillance, for example in viral infection. Both class I and class II antigens operate in this phenomenon.

Antigen presenting cells (APCs) or virus-infected cells, present viral antigen in association with class I molecules which is recognized by T cell receptors of Tc cell, and in association with class II molecules which is recognized by T cell receptors of Th cells. Binding of class I molecule/viral antigen complex to Tc cell receptors stimulates expansion of cytotoxic cells. Binding of class II molecule/viral complex to Th cell receptors stimulates expansion of Th cells. Release of interleukin-1 (IL-1) from APCs promotes both proliferation and differentiation responses to Tc and Th cells and IL-2, produced by activated Th cells, stimulates clonal expansion of Tc cells. Tc cells then recognize and destroy target cells expressing both self class I molecules and viral antigens.

MINOR HISTOCOMPATIBILITY ANTIGENS IN MAN

Very little is known about minor histocompatibility (mH) in man. However, evidence suggests that mH antigens also play a role in graft rejection because graft rejections have been observed in cases with complete HLA match.

TUMOUR IMMUNOLOGY

When a cell undergoes malignant transformation, it acquires new surface antigens and may lose some normal antigens. A tumour can, therefore, be considered as an allograft and be expected to induce an immune response.

Tumour antigens

Tumour antigens that elicit an immune response have been demonstrated in many experimentally induced tumours and in some human cancers. They can be broadly classified into two categories:

1. Tumour-specific antigens (TSAs)

They are present only on the membranes of malignant cells and not on normal cells. They induce immune response when tumour is transplanted to syngeneic animals. Different tumours possess different TSAs, even though induced by the same carcinogen. In contrast, TSA of virus induced tumours is virus-specific in that all tumours produced by one virus possess the same antigen, even if the tumours are in different animal strains or species.

2. Tumour-associated antigens (TAAs)

These are present on tumour cells and also on some normal cells. Since they are also present on some normal cells, therefore, they do not evoke an immune response and are of little significance in tumour rejection. Detection of these antigens is nevertheless of value in the diagnosis of certain tumours and antibodies raised against them can be useful for immunotherapy. TAAs fall into three categories:

(i) Tumour-associated carbohydrate antigens (TACAs)

They represent abnormal forms of widely expressed glycoproteins and glycolipids such as mucin-associated antigen detected in pancreatic and breast cancers.

(ii) Oncofoetal antigens

These are foetal antigens which are found in embryonic and malignant cells, but not in normal adult cells. The best known examples are α-feto-protein in hepatomas and carcinoembryonic antigen in carcinoma of the colon, pancreas, lung, stomach and breast.

(iii) Differentiation antigens

They are peculiar to the differentiation state at which cancer cells are arrested. For example, CD10, an antigen expressed in early B lymphocytes, is expressed in B cell leukaemias and lymphomas. Similarly, prostate-specific antigen is expressed on normal as well as cancerous prostatic epithelium. Both serve as useful differentiation markers in the diagnosis of lymphoid and prostatic cancer.

Immune response in malignancy

Both cell-mediated and antibody-mediated immunity have antitumour activity. As with virus-infected cells and foreign grafts, the T lymphocytes play a major role in the destruction of tumour cells in mammals. T cell activation generates helper T (Th), delayed-type hypersensitivity T (Td) and cytotoxic T (Tc) cells. Of special interest is the role played by Td cells. These cells affect tumour killing by means of the lymphokines that they release.

NK cells are lymphocytes that are capable of destroying tumour cells without prior sensitization. After activation with IL-2, NK cells can lyse a wide range of human tumours, including many that appear to be nonimmunogenic for T cells. So NK cells may provide the first line of defence against many tumours. In addition to direct lysis of tumour cells, NK cells can also participate in antibody-dependent cellular cytotoxicity (ADCC).

Activated macrophages also exhibit some selective cytotoxicity against tumour cells *in vitro*. T cell derived cytokine (interferon-gamma) activates macrophages which acquire antitumour activity.

Humoral mechanisms may also participate in tumour cell destruction by activation of complement and induction of ADCC by NK cells.

Immunosurveillance

It has been postulated that the primary function of cell-mediated immunity is to destroy malignant cells that arise by somatic mutation. Such malignant mutations are believed to occur frequently and would develop into tumour but for the constant vigilance of the immune system. The strongest argument for the existence of immunosurveillance is the increased frequency of cancers in immunodeficient hosts. About 5% of persons with congenital immuno-deficiencies develop cancers about 200 times the expected prevalence. Immunosuppressed transplant recipients and patients with AIDS have more malignancies. Therefore, inefficiency of immuno-surveillance, either as a result of ageing or in congenital or acquired immunodeficiencies, leads to an increased incidence of cancer.

Tumour escape mechanism

Most cancers occur in persons who do not suffer from any overt immunodeficiency. It is, therefore, evident that tumour cells must develop mechanisms to escape or evade the immune system in immunocompetent hosts. Several such mechanisms may be operative:

- *Weak immunogenicity:* Some tumours are weakly immunogenic, so in small numbers they do not elicit an immune response. But when their numbers increase enough to provoke immune response the tumour load may be too great for the host's immune system to mount an effective response.
- *Modulation of surface antigens:* Certain tumour cells can transfer antigens from their surface to the cytoplasm or they may shed or stop expressing the surface antigens thus making the tumour cells immunologically invisible.
- *Masking tumour antigens:* Certain cancers produce copious amounts of a mucoprotein called sialomucin. It binds to the surface of the tumour cells. Since sialomucin is a normal component, the immune system does not recognize these tumour cells as foreign.
- *Induction of immune tolerance:* Some tumour cells can synthesize various immunosuppressants. They may also activate specific Ts cells. Both these suppress the effector T and B cell clones.

- *Production of blocking antibodies:* Some tumour cells invoke immune system to produce blocking antibodies that cannot fix and activate complement, so lysis of tumour cell is not possible. Blocking antibodies also cover the surface of cancer cells, preventing Tc cells from binding to hidden receptors.
- *Reduced levels of HLA class I molecules:* In some instances, tumour cells express reduced levels of HLA class I molecules. This impairs presentation of antigenic peptides to cytotoxic T cells.

Immunotherapy of cancer

Immunotherapy of cancer is of two types:

1. Antigen-nonspecific treatment

This activates the cells of the immune system in a generalized manner which destroy the tumour cells. BCG vaccine when injected directly into certain solid tumours may lead to tumour regression. This may also be administered by scarification in which deep scratches are made in the thigh and BCG vaccine applied on the scratches. Antitumour effect of BCG is believed to be due to activation of macrophages and NK cells. Treatment with BCG has been reported to be useful in malignant melanomas, stage I lung cancer, bladder cancer and certain leukaemias.

Corynebacterium parvum has also been shown to possess antitumour activity. It appears to activate macrophages and B cell function. When used in conjunction with cyclophosphamide (chemo-therapeutic agent) a synergistic antitumour effect is achieved. This therapy has been reported to be beneficial in various types of lung cancers and metastatic breast cancer.

Instead of using live bacteria, synthetic immuno-stimulants structurally derived from the bacterial cell walls of *Mycobacterium bovis* (muramyl dipeptides) and *C. parvum* (trehalose diesters) may be used. When used in combination, they act synergistically to give enhanced antitumour activity by activating macrophages against cancer cell.

Other nonspecific immune modulators include thymic hormones (thymosine, thymopoietin, thymic humoral factor and thymic serum factor) to restore T cell function, interferon to stimulate NK cell function, tuftsin (tetrapeptide located in the H chains of γ globulin) to stimulate phagocytic cells and IL-2 to stimulate killing of cancer cells by Tc cells, NK cells and macrophages. Bone marrow transplantation is another approach to the treatment of some neoplastic diseases such as leukaemia.

2. Antigen-specific treatment

This includes:

- *Vaccination with tumour antigens:* This provides immunity against specific tumour type.
- *Treatment with immune RNA:* This stimulates humoral and cell-mediated immune responses.
- *Treatment with transfer factor:* This stimulates cell-mediated immune response and release of lymphokines.
- *Modification of tumour antigenicity:* The immunogenicity of the tumour cell can be increased by treatment with neuraminidase, which removes sialomucin covering tumour antigens.
- *Monoclonal antibodies:* These can be raised against TAAs. These, when administered, either alone or tagged with a cytotoxic drug, will bind to and specifically destroy only cancer cells.

KEY FACTS

- Cells of an individual express a unique set of membrane antigens called *histocompatibility antigens*
- Major histocompatibility complex in humans is known as *human leucocyte antigen (HLA) complex*
- **Genes** that code for HLA antigens are found on *the short arm of sixth pair of chromosome*
- There are three **classes of genes** in HLA loci – *class I, class II and class III genes* which code for the corresponding molecules (antigens)
- **Immunologically competent cells** of the graft may react against *antigens of the host* (graft versus host reaction)
- When a cell undergoes malignant transformation, it acquires new surface antigens and may lose some normal antigens

IMPORTANT QUESTIONS

1. Define various types of grafts? Describe allograft reaction.
2. What is the mechanism of graft rejection?
3. What is major histocompatibility complex? Describe various classes of MHC molecules.
4. What are histocompatibility antigens? Describe various procedures for histocompatibility testing.
5. Name and describe various tumour antigens.
6. Discuss immunotherapy of cancer.
7. Write short notes on:
   (a) Tumour escape mechanism
   (b) Graft versus host reaction
   (c) Foetus as a graft
   (d) MHC restriction

Chapter 18

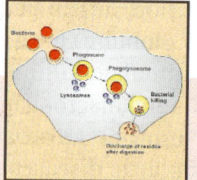

Immunohaematology

Life-saving property of transfused blood became clear during the Second World War, and thereafter blood transfusion quickly became a routine hospital function. Without blood transfusion treatment of severe haemorrhage is difficult or impossible and many surgical procedures cannot be safely attempted. Haematological conditions such as thalassaemia, haemophilia, leukaemia and aplastic anaemia cannot be treated effectively without the support from blood transfusion service.

The ABO system is the most important of all the blood group systems and its discovery by Landsteiner (1900) made blood transfusion possible. Subsequently, other blood groups (MN, P, Rh, Lutheran, Lewis, Kell, Duffy, Kidd, Diego, Yt, Kg, Dombroc and Colton) were reported. ABO and Rh are the major blood group antigens.

ABO BLOOD GROUP SYSTEM

The ABO system contains four blood groups. The blood group is determined by the presence or absence of two distinct antigens A and B on the surface of the erythrocytes. Distribution of ABO antigens on red blood cells and antibodies in the serum is shown in Table 18.1. An individual with blood group A possesses antigen A on its RBCs and its serum possesses anti-B antibodies. Similarly B, AB and O

Table 18.1. Distribution of ABO antigens on the red blood cells and antibodies in the serum

Blood group	Antigens on red blood cells	Antibodies in serum	Occurrence (%) in India
A	A	Anti-B	22
B	B	Anti-A	33
AB	A and B	None	5
O	None	Anti-A and Anti-B	40

groups possess B, A and B, and no antigen on their RBCs and anti-A, none, and anti-A and anti-B antibodies in their sera respectively. Forty per cent individuals in India have O group followed by B (33%), A (22%) and AB (5%).

Anti-A and anti-B isoantibodies appear in the serum of infants by about the age of six months and persist thereafter. These are called natural antibodies, because they are seen to arise without any apparent antigenic stimulation. However, it is believed that they develop as a result of cross-immunization with bacteria of family Enterobacteriaceae that colonize the infant's gut. These bacteria have outer membrane oligosaccharides strikingly similar to those A and B antigens in the human body. Therefore, a newborn with group A will not have anti-B in his or her serum,

152

since there has been no opportunity to undergo cross-immunization. When the intestine is eventually colonized by the normal microbial flora, the infant will start to develop anti-B, but will not produce anti-A because of tolerance to his or her own blood group antigens.

Immune isoantibodies may develop following ABO incompatible pregnancy or transfusion. More commonly, they result from injection of substances containing blood group-like antigens such as horse serum or bacterial vaccines made from media containing horse serum. **Natural antibodies are saline agglutinating while immune isoantibodies are albumin agglutinating.** The latter generally cause more severe transfusion reactions.

Ideally, the donor and recipient should belong to the same ABO group. It used to be held that O group cells could be transfused to recipients of any group as they possessed neither A nor B antigen. Hence O group was designated as the 'universal donor'. The anti-A and anti-B antibodies in the transfused O blood do not ordinarily cause any damage to red cells of A, B and AB group recipients because they will be rendered ineffective by dilution in the recipient's plasma. But some O group plasma may contain isoantibodies in high titres (1 : 200 or above) so that the damage to the recipient's cells may result. This is known as **dangerous O group**. Transfusion of large quantities of O group blood to persons of another group may also cause reactions. **Anti-A antibody in O group blood is generally more potent than anti-B.** Hence O group is more likely to cause reaction when given to group A recipient, than to those of B group. *While O group blood may be transfused to a patient of any other group in dire emergency, this practice should never be employed as a routine.*

Due to the absence of isoantibodies in plasma, AB group persons were designated 'universal recipients'. AB group donors may not always be available due to their rarity and it may, on occasion, be necessary to use donors of other groups. In such cases **group A blood is safer than B, because anti-A antibody is usually more potent than anti-B**.

Blood groups are inherited by simple Mendelian laws. Their synthesis is determined by allelomorphic genes A, B and O. Genes A and B give rise to corresponding antigens but O does not produce any antigen.

H antigen

Red cells of all ABO groups possess a common antigen, the H antigen, which is the precursor for the formation of A and B antigens. Due to its universal distribution, H antigen is not ordinarily important in grouping or blood transfusion. However, Bhende et al. (1952) from Bombay (now Mumbai) reported a very rare instance in which A and B antigens as well as H antigens were absent from the red cells. This is known as **Bombay or Oh blood group**. Sera of these individuals have anti-A, anti-B and anti-H antibodies, therefore, they can accept the blood only from the same rare blood group.

A, B and H antigens are glycoproteins. In addition to erythrocytes, they are also present in almost all the tissues and fluids of the body. A and B antigens have also been extracted and purified commercially from stomach of hogs and horses. Anti-A antibodies can be obtained from the albumin gland of the snails. Because anti-A harvested from snails has a very high titre, as much as 2.5 litres of potent reagent can be prepared from one snail.

RH BLOOD GROUP SYSTEM

Rh antibodies are clinically most significant after anti-A and anti-B antibodies. Almost all Rh antibodies result from immunization by pregnancy or blood transfusion. Rh antibodies are major cause of haemolytic disease of new born (HDN) and lead to destruction of transfused cells. When an Rh-negative woman carries an Rh-positive foetus, she may be immunized against Rh antigen by the passage of foetal red cells into maternal circulation. Minor transplacental leaks may occur any time during pregnancy, but it is during delivery that foetal cells enter the maternal circulation in large numbers. Therefore, the mother is usually immunized only at first delivery and consequently the first child escapes damage (except when the woman has already been sensitized by prior Rh incompatible blood transfusion). During subsequent pregnancy, Rh antibodies of the IgG class pass from the mother to the foetus and damage its erythrocytes. The clinical features of HDN may vary from **a mere accentuation of the physiological jaundice in the newborn to erythroblastosis foetalis or intrauterine death due to hydrops foetalis**.

Most Rh antibodies belong to IgG class. Being incomplete antibodies, they do not agglutinate Rh-positive cells in saline. A minority are complete (saline agglutinating) antibodies of IgM class. These are not relevant in the pathogenesis of haemolytic disease as they do not cross the placenta.

HDN does not affect all issues of Rh-incompatible marriages. Its incidence is much less than the expected figures. This is due to:

1. **Immunological unresponsiveness to Rh antigens:** Not all Rh-negative individuals form Rh antibodies following antigenic stimulation. Some fail to do even after repeated injections of Rh-positive cells. They are called '**non-responders**'. The reason for this immunological unresponsiveness is not known.

2. **Foetomaternal ABO incompatibility:** Rh immunization is more likely to result when mother and foetus possess the same ABO group. When Rh and ABO incompatibility co-exists, Rh sensitization from the mother is rare. In this situation the foetal cells entering the maternal circulation are destroyed rapidly by the ABO antibodies before they can induce Rh antibodies.

3. **Number of pregnancies:** As explained above the first child usually escapes disease. The risk increases with each successive pregnancy.

Rh isoimmunization can be prevented by administration of 100–300 mg of anti-Rh IgG prepared from human volunteers, at the time when the antigenic stimulation is expected to take place, i.e., immediately after delivery. To be effective, this should be employed from first delivery onwards.

ABO haemolytic disease

Maternofoetal ABO incompatibility is very common but only in a proportion of these, haemolytic disease occurs in the newborns, because in persons of blood group A or B, natural antibodies are IgM in nature, therefore, they cannot cross the placenta to harm the foetus. But in persons with blood group O, the isoantibodies are predominantly IgG in nature. Therefore, ABO haemolytic disease is seen largely in O group mothers having A or B foetus. As ABO haemolytic disease is due to naturally occurring maternal isoantibodies, it may occur even in first birth, without prior immunization. ABO haemolytic disease is much milder than Rh disease.

It has been shown that some diseases may influence blood group antigens. Some blood group antigens have been reported to become weak in leukaemia and other malignancies. The reason for this is not known. Group A persons have been shown to acquire B antigen following septicaemia, intestinal obstruction and carcinoma of colon or rectum. The antigen is believed to come from infecting microorganisms.

COMPLICATIONS OF BLOOD TRANSFUSION

The complications of blood transfusion may be divided into immunological and non-immunological.

Immunological complications

Immunological complications may be caused by red cell, leucocyte or platelet incompatibility or allergic reaction to plasma components. **Red cell incompatibility** leads to acute intravascular haemolysis or the red cells may be coated by antibodies and engulfed by phagocytes, removed from the circulation and subjected to extravascular lysis. Haemolysis may also be due to transfusion of group O whole blood or plasma to group A or group B or group AB recipients.

Leucocyte incompatibility may cause fever, pulmonary infiltrates, dyspnoea, non-productive cough and chest pain. The risk of these reactions can be reduced by using leucocyte-poor red cells. Fever is sometimes a complication of blood transfusion. Leucoagglutinins are probably the commonest cause of fever. Platelet incompatibility, allergy and infection may also lead to fever.

Allergic reactions may be caused by interaction of patient's preformed reagins with transfused allergens. When allergic reactions develop administer antihistaminics during transfusion.

Non-immunological complications

Non-immunological complications of blood transfusion include transmission of infectious agents and circulatory overload. Infectious agents which may be transmitted during blood transfusion may be viruses, bacteria and protozoa (Table 18.2). Circulatory overload may be due to massive transfusion.

Table 18.2. Non-immunological complications of blood transfusion

TRANSMISSION OF INFECTIOUS AGENTS

Viruses
- Hepatitis B virus*
- Hepatitis C virus*
- Human immunodeficiency virus 1* and 2*
- Human T cell lymphotrophic virus 1 and 2
- Cytomegalovirus

Bacteria
- *Treponema pallidum**
- *Leptospira interrogans*
- *Borrelia burgdorferi*

Parasites
- *Plasmodium* spp.*
- *Babesia* spp.
- *Trypanosoma cruzi*
- *Leishmania donovani*
- *Toxoplasma gondii*

CIRCULATORY OVERLOAD

* Mandatory tests in India

KEY FACTS

- **ABO blood group** is determined by the presence or absence of *two distinct antigens A and B* on the surface of erythrocytes
- Forty percent individuals in India have O group followed by B (33%), A (22%) and AB (5%)
- Red cells of all ABO groups posses a common antigen, **the H antigen** which is precursor for the formation of A and B antigens
- Rarely, H antigen is absent from red cells; this is known as **Oh or Bombay blood group**
- **Rh antibodies** are major cause of *haemolytic disease of new born* and lead to *destruction of transfused cells*
- Most Rh antibodies belong to IgG class
- **Maternofoetal ABO incompatibility** is very common but *only in a proportion of these haemolytic disease occurs* because in persons of blood group *A or B, natural antibodies are IgM in nature,* therefore, they cannot cross the placenta to harm the foetus

IMPORTANT QUESTIONS

1. Discuss ABO blood group system.
2. Name various blood group systems and discuss Rh blood group system.
3. What is haemolytic disease of new born? Why is its incidence much less than the expected figures?
4. What are the complications of blood transfusion?

SECTION C
Systemic Bacteriology

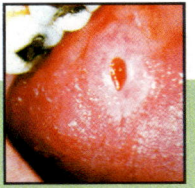

Chapter 19

Staphylococcus

Genus *Staphylococcus* contains 40 defined species, 20 of which are known to be associated with colonization and/or infection of man. Of the 20 species found in man, one (*S. aureus*) is coagulase-positive and 19 coagulase-negative. Not all coagulase-negative staphylococci (CoNS) have been isolated from human infections.

Staphylococci were first seen in pus by Koch in 1878, were first cultivated in liquid medium by Pasteur in 1880 and named so by Sir Alexander Ogston in 1881. The name *Staphylococcus* was derived from Greek words *staphyle* (bunch of grapes) and *kokkos* (grain or berry).

STAPHYLOCOCCUS AUREUS

Morphology

They are spherical cocci about 0.8–1.0 μm in diameter. They are arranged characteristically in grape-like clusters. Cluster formation is due to cell division occurring in more than one plane with daughter cells remaining close together. In smear from pus, the cocci appear singly or in pairs, clusters or short chains of three or four cells (Figs. 19.1 and 19.2). They are non-motile (non-flagellated), non-sporing and, with the exception of rare strains, non-capsulated. They are Gram-positive but old and phagocytosed organisms may be Gram-negative.

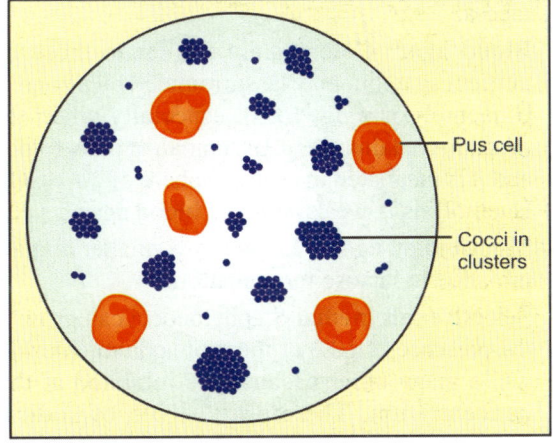

Fig. 19.1. Staphylococci and pus cells.

Cultural characteristics

They are aerobes and facultative anaerobes. Optimum temperature for growth is 37°C, range being 12–44°C. Optimum pH is 7.5. They can grow well on ordinary media.

1. **Nutrient agar:** After overnight incubation at 37°C, colonies are 1–2 mm in diameter with a smooth glistening surface. They are opaque and easily emulsifiable. Most strains produce golden-yellow (*aureus*) pigment, though some strains may

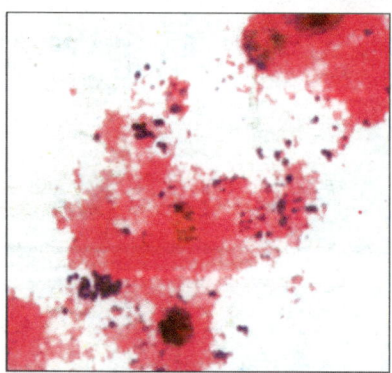

Fig. 19.2. Staphylococci in Gram-stained smear of pus.

form white (non-pigmented) colonies. Pigment production occurs optimally at 22°C and only in aerobic cultures. Pigment is not formed in liquid media.

2. **Blood agar:** Colonies are similar to those on nutrient agar, but may be surrounded by a zone of β-haemolysis (Fig. 19.3), especially when the medium contains sheep, ox, human or rabbit blood and it is incubated in an atmosphere of 20% CO_2. Haemolysis is weak on horse blood agar.

3. **MacConkey agar:** Colonies are smaller and are pink due to lactose fermentation.

4. **Selective salt media:** Staphylococci can grow in the presence of 10% or more of sodium chloride, while many other bacteria are inhibited at this concentration. Therefore, 7–10% of sodium

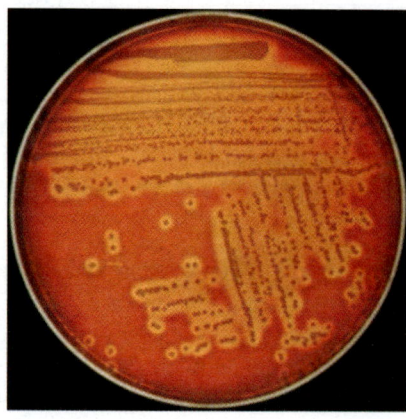

Fig. 19.3. Growth of *Staphylococcus aureus* on blood agar showing β-haemolysis.

chloride may be added to nutrient agar. Salt agar is useful for isolation of staphylococci from food, dust, faeces and pus where mixed bacterial flora are expected. The appearance of colonies on these media is similar to those on nutrient agar.

5. **Enrichment salt medium:** 10% sodium chloride may be added to cooked meat broth. This may be used for primary enrichment.

6. **Mannitol salt agar:** 1% mannitol, 7.5% sodium chloride and 0.0025% phenol red is added to nutrient agar. This is both selective and indicator medium. Most strains of *S. aureus* ferment mannitol, therefore, due to the production of acid their colonies are surrounded by yellow zones. Otherwise the colonies resemble those seen on nutrient agar.

Susceptibility to physical and chemical agents

Staphylococci are usually killed by a temperature of 60°C in 30 minutes but some strains are killed by heating at 62°C in 30 minutes. Disinfectants such as chlorhexidine, hexachlorophane and phenol kill staphylococci rapidly. But mercuric chloride is a poor disinfectant for them. They are very sensitive to aniline dyes; thus they are inhibited on blood agar medium containing 1 in 500,000 crystal violet, which permits the growth of streptococci.

Before the introduction of penicillin, most of the strains of *S. aureus* were sensitive to this antibiotic but from 1945 onwards penicillinase-producing (penicillin-resistant) strains were encountered. Similarly, they have also developed resistance against sulphonamides and other antibiotics. The drug-resistance in staphylococci is due to:

- Penicillinase (β-lactamase) production, which is usually controlled by genes located on a plasmid although chromosomally mediated control has also been shown. Penicillinase plasmid may also carry markers for resistance to heavy metals such as mercury, arsenic, cadmium, lead and bismuth and other antibiotics such as erythromycin, and fusidic acid. Penicillinase plasmids are transmitted to the sensitive staphylococci by transduction and also possibly by conjugation.

- Resistance to penicillins and cephalosporins may be produced by a reduction in affinity of the penicillin-binding proteins of the staphylococcal cell wall for β-lactam antibiotics.

Biochemical reactions

S. aureus is catalase-positive and oxidase-negative. Catalase production by staphylococci may function to inactivate toxic hydrogen peroxide and free radicals formed by myeloperoxidase system within phagocytic cells after ingestion of microorganisms. It ferments glucose, maltose, lactose, sucrose and mannitol with the production of acid but no gas. Of these fermentation reactions, fermentation of mannitol carries diagnostic significance because most strains of *S. aureus* ferment mannitol while most strains of *S. epidermidis* and *S. saprophyticus* are mannitol-negative. In addition, *S. aureus* is indole-negative, MR-positive, VP-positive, urease-positive, hydrolyzes gelatin and reduces nitrates to nitrites. Most strains are lipolytic, therefore, when grown on media containing egg-yolk, produce a dense opacity. They also produce phosphatase.

Bacteriophage typing

Phages of *S. aureus* have a narrow host range and lyse only some other strains of the same species. Therefore, for epidemiological studies and tracing the source of infection, strains of *S. aureus* can be distinguished from one another by their patterns of susceptibility to lysis by an internationally recognized set of 23 standard typing phages (Table 19.1). Lysis of a culture by one phage is often associated with lysis by one or more other phages. Staphylococci can seldom be characterized by lysis by a single phage,

Table 19.1. Typing set of staphylococcal phages

Lytic group	Designation of phages in lytic group
I	29, 52, 52A, 79, 80
II	3A, 3C, 55, 71,
III	6, 42E, 47, 53, 54, 75, 77, 83A, 84, 85
IV	–
V	94, 96
Unclassified	81, 95

but many different patterns of lysis are obtained with a set of phages. Differences between these patterns are used to make fine distinction between staphylococcal strains.

The strain to be typed is inoculated on a plate of nutrient agar to produce a lawn culture. Drops of various phages at their routine test dilution (RTD) are applied over marked squares. After overnight incubation at 30°C the culture will be observed to be lysed by some phages but not by others. The phage type of a strain is expressed by designation of the phages that lyse it. Thus, if a strain is lysed only by phages 3C, 55 and 71, it is called phage type 3C/55/71.

Determinants of pathogenicity or virulence factors of Staphylococcus aureus

S. aureus possesses a large number of cell-wall associated factors and extracellular toxins and enzymes (Table 19.2 and Fig. 19.4), which contribute to the ability of the organism to overcome the body's defence and to invade, propagate, survive and produce disease in the host.

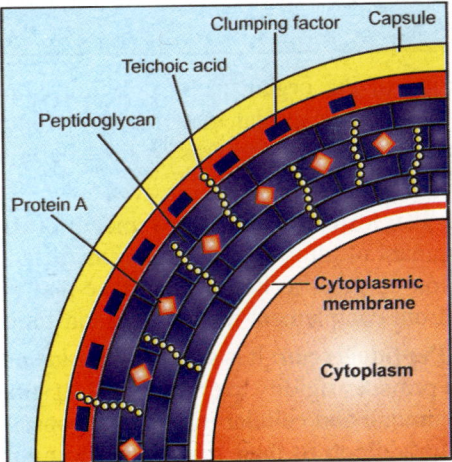

Fig. 19.4. Cell wall associated factors of *Staphylococcus aureus*.

Cell wall associated

1. **Capsular polysaccharide:** A few strains of *S. aureus* are encapsulated and these tend to be more virulent than the non-capsulated strains. The capsule is composed of antigenic polysaccharide. It prevents

Table 19.2. Determinants of pathogenicity or virulence factors of *Staphylococcus aureus*

CELL WALL ASSOCIATED
- Capsular polysaccharide
- Teichoic acid
- Peptidoglycan
- Protein A
- Clumping factor

EXTRA CELLULAR FACTORS
- Haemolytic toxins (Haemolysins)
  - α lysin
  - β lysin
  - γ lysin
  - δ lysin
- Leucocidin
- Epidermolytic toxins
- Enterotoxins
- Toxic shock syndrome toxin-1

EXTRA CELLULAR ENZYMES
- Coagulase
- Staphylokinase
- Hyaluronidase
- Deoxyribonuclease
- Lipase
- Phospholipases
- Proteases

ingestion of the organism by polymorphonuclear leucocytes. The capsular material may promote the adherence of the organisms to host cells and to prosthetic devices.

2. **Teichoic acid:** It is a major antigenic determinant of all strains of *S. aureus*. It facilitates adhesion of cocci to host cell surface and protects them from complement mediated opsonization.

3. **Peptidoglycan:** It is a polysaccharide polymer which provides rigidity to the cell wall. It stimulates both humoral and cellular immune responses in the host. In addition to their role in providing rigidity and resilience to the staphylococcal cell wall, peptidoglycan and teichoic acid also have several biologic activities that are thought to contribute to virulence.

4. **Protein A:** Protein A is a group-specific antigen found in the cell wall of about 90% strains of *S. aureus* (especially Cowan I strain). It has a molecular weight of 13,000 daltons. It is chemotactic, anti-

complementary, antiphagocytic, mitogenic, potentiates natural killer cells, and elicits platelet injury and hypersensitivity reaction.

Protein A binds IgG molecules, non-specifically, through Fc region leaving specific Fab sites free to combine with specific antigen. When suspension of such sensitized cells is treated with homologous (test) antigen, the antigen combines with free Fab sites of IgG attached to staphylococcal cells leading to visible clumping of staphylococci within two minutes. This is known as **coagglutination** (see chapter 12).

5. **Clumping factor (bound coagulase):** It is a surface component that causes the organisms to clump when mixed with plasma. This factor reacts directly with fibrinogen in plasma, causing rapid cell agglutination. It can be detected by emulsifying a few colonies of the bacteria in a drop of normal saline on a clean glass slide and mixing it with a drop of rabbit plasma. Prompt clumping of the organisms indicates the presence of clumping factor (bound coagulase). Since this factor is detected by performing the test on a slide, therefore, the test is known as **slide coagulase test**. Almost all the clumping factor producing strains of *S. aureus* produce coagulase, whereas 12% of coagulase producing strains may not produce clumping factor. This factor is also not detectable in capsulated strains of *S. aureus*.

Extracellular toxins

S. aureus produces a variety of extracellular toxins, including haemolysins, leucocidin, epidermolytic toxins, enterotoxins and toxic shock syndrome toxin-1.

1. **Haemolysins:** Almost every strain of *S. aureus* produces one or more of four haemolytic, membrane-damaging exotoxins known as α, β, γ and δ lysins. They are antigenically distinct and differ from one another in their activity against the red blood cells of different animal species, lethal activity, dermo-necrosis and leucocidal activity (Table 19.3).

α lysin (α toxin): Of the four haemolysins produced by *S. aureus*, α lysin is the most important in pathogenicity. In cultures, it is produced only under aerobic conditions and its production is enhanced by a high concentration of carbon dioxide. It is a protein

Table 19.3. Properties of α, β, γ and δ haemolysins produced by *Staphylococcus aureus*

Property	Haemolysin			
	α	**β**	**γ**	**δ**
Lysis of red blood cells of				
• Sheep	++++	++++	++++	++++
• Rabbit	++++	+	++++	++++
• Horse	–	–	–	++++
• Man	–	+	++++	++++
Lethal activity	++++	±	±	+
Dermonecrosis	+	–	–	+
Leucocidal activity	+	–	+	+

consisting of a single polypeptide chain, with a molecular weight of 28,000–30,000 daltons. It is inactivated at 60°C, however, its activity is regained paradoxically, if it is further heated to between 80–100°C. This is due to the fact that the toxin combines with a heat-labile inhibitor at 60°C but at higher temperature (80–100°C) the inhibitor is inactivated thus toxin regains its activity. Above 100°C toxin itself gets inactivated.

The α toxin lyses rabbit and sheep erythrocytes. It is leucocidal and when injected intradermally into mice and rabbits it is dermonecrotic and when injected intravenously in these animals it is lethal. It is known to damage smooth muscles, is toxic for human macrophages and platelets, and causes degranulation of polymorphonuclear leucocytes through disruption of their lysosomes.

β lysin (β toxin): β lysin is strongly active on sheep and weakly active on rabbit and human red blood cells. It does not lyse horse red blood cells. This is a phospholipase C. It acts specifically on sphingomyelin and lysolecithin. Therefore, the susceptibility of red cells from different species depends upon their sphingomyelin content. β lysin gives rise to **'hot-cold' haemolysis,** the cells that have been exposed to the lysin at 37°C lyse only when cooled to 4°C.

γ lysin (γ toxin): γ lysin acts on sheep, rabbit and human red blood cells but not on those of horse.

δ lysin (δ toxin): δ lysin is a polypeptide with a molecular weight of 1600 daltons. It lyses red blood cells of sheep, rabbit, horse and man. It also possesses lethal, dermonecrotic and leucocidal activity.

2. Leucocidin: Leucocidin consists of two protein components. On the basis of their migration in carboxymethylcellulose columns they are designated F (fast) and S (slow) components. These components act synergistically to damage polymorphonuclear leucocytes and macrophages, and to produce dermonecrosis.

3. Epidermolytic toxins (exfoliative toxins): Many strains of *S. aureus*, mainly belonging to phage group II, produce two types of epidermolytic toxin (types A and B). They are proteins with a molecular weight of 30,000 and 29,500 daltons respectively. Epidermolytic toxin A is heat-stable and its production is determined by a chromosomal gene. On the other hand, epidermolytic toxin B is heat-labile and plasmid-controlled.

4. Enterotoxins: About 40% of all clinical isolates of *S. aureus* produce enterotoxins which are exotoxins that cause food-poisoning in man. These have also been implicated in some cases of **pseudo-membranous enterocolitis** seen in patients after antibiotic therapy. Enterotoxins are proteins with molecular weights of 26,000–30,000 daltons. These are heat-stable, resisting boiling for 30 minutes. Therefore, once formed enterotoxins might not be destroyed even if food is heated sufficiently to kill all viable staphylococci. These are also not destroyed by gut enzymes. Nine antigenic types (A, B, C_1, C_2, C_3, D, E, H and I) of enterotoxins have been identified. Enterotoxin F is now known as toxic shock syndrome toxin-1. Type A toxin is responsible for most cases.

5. Toxic shock syndrome toxin-1 (TSST-1): TSST-1 is produced by certain strains of *S. aureus*. Most of the strains producing TSST-1 belong to phage group I. TSST-1 is a protein with a molecular weight of 22,000 daltons. It is antigenic and most persons over 30 years of age have circulating anti-bodies.

TSST-1 and the enterotoxins are now recognized as **superantigens,** i.e., they are potent activators of T lymphocytes resulting in the liberation of cytokines such as tumour necrosis factor, and they bind with high affinity to mononuclear cells. These characteristics partly explain the florid and multisystem nature of the clinical conditions associated with these toxins.

Extracellular enzymes

1. **Coagulase:** *S. aureus* produces an extracellular enzyme called coagulase. It activates a coagulase-reacting factor (CRF) normally present in plasma, causing the plasma to clot by the conversion of fibrinogen to fibrin. Clotting does not occur with plasma of certain species like guinea-pig which lack CRF. CRF is similar to prothrombin but is probably not identical with it. Coagulase is produced during the logarithmic phase of growth in a variety of media. Eight antigenic types (A–H) have been described. Most human strains produce coagulase A.

All coagulase-producing staphylococci are, by definition, *S. aureus* and as a result, coagulase production is considered the best laboratory evidence for the potential pathogenicity of *Staphylococcus*. However, there is no conclusive proof of the role of coagulase as a virulence factor because coagulase-negative mutants of *S. aureus* are no less virulent than the parent strain. Coagulase may act to coat the bacterial cells with fibrin, rendering them resistant to opsonization and phagocytosis.

Coagulase (tube coagulase) test: 0.1 ml of an overnight broth culture or broth suspension from an agar plate culture made up to the same density is mixed with 0.5 ml of a 1 in 10 dilution of human or rabbit plasma. The mixture is incubated in a water bath at 37°C for three to six hours. If positive, the plasma clots and does not flow when the tube is inverted. If clot does not appear it is left overnight at room temperature and re-examined. On continued incubation, the clot may be lysed by fibrinolysin produced by some strains. Controls with plasma alone, and known coagulase-positive and coagulase-negative cultures must be set up with each batch of tests. Human, rabbit or pig plasma which are rich in CRF can be used. Oxalate, EDTA or heparin are suitable anticoagulants. **Citrated plasma should not be used because contaminating Gram-negative bacilli may utilize the citrate and produce false positive reaction.**

For slide coagulase see clumping factor.

2. **Staphylokinase (fibrinolysin):** Many strains of *S. aureus* that do not produce β lysin may produce staphylokinase. It is a protein with a molecular weight of 13,000–15,000 daltons. It has fibrinolytic activity. It is antigenically and enzymatically distinct from streptokinase produced by *Streptococcus pyogenes*. Fibrinolysin may break down fibrin clots and allow spread of infection to contiguous tissues.

3. **Hyaluronidase:** More than 90% strains of *S. aureus* produce hyaluronidase, but the amount varies widely. It hydrolyzes hyaluronic acid present in the intercellular ground substance of connective tissue, thus facilitating the spread of the organisms to adjacent areas.

Other extracellular enzymes produced by *S. aureus* and their activities are as under:

Extracellular enzyme	Activity
1. Deoxyribonuclease	Degrades DNA
2. Lipase	Degrades lipid
3. Phospholipases	Degrade phospholipids
4. Proteases	Cause proteolysis

Pathogenicity

About 35–50% of normal adults carry *S. aureus* in the anterior nares. Other sites of colonization include intertriginous skin folds, perineum, axillae, and vagina. Skin carriage rates of 10–20% are found in most areas of the body except the hands, where up to 40% of swabs may yield *S. aureus*. These organisms are acquired from the nose by contact (transients) and their elimination from the nose by antibiotic treatment results in cessation of skin carriage. These can also be removed from the skin by washing.

Staphylococci shed by patients and carriers contaminate fomites such as handkerchiefs, bed linen and blankets, and may persist on them for days or weeks. **Staphylococcal disease may follow endogenous or exogenous infection.** The mode of transmission may be by contact, direct or through fomites or by airborne droplets.

S. aureus is an **opportunistic pathogen** in that it causes infection most commonly at sites of lowered host resistance, e.g., damaged skin or mucous membranes or haematomas in the cancellous tissue of a long bone. Those with respiratory tract viral infections, such as influenza and measles, and diabetic patients are also more susceptible to staphylococcal infections.

Staphylococcal diseases may be classified as cutaneous and deep infections, exfoliative diseases, food poisoning and the toxic shock syndrome.

Cutaneous infections: These include wound and burn infection, pustules (small cutaneous abscesses), furuncles or boils (large cutaneous abscesses), carbuncles, styes, impetigo and pemphigus neonatorum.

Deep infections: These include osteomyelitis, periostitis, tonsillitis, pharyngitis, sinusitis, broncho-pneumonia, empyema, septicaemia, meningitis, endocarditis, breast abscess, renal abscess and abscesses in other organs.

Exfoliative diseases: These lesions are produced by the strains of *S. aureus* which produce epidermo-lytic toxins. These toxins separate the outer layer of epidermis from the underlying tissues leading to **blistering disease**. The most dramatic manifestation of these toxins is **scalded skin syndrome** or **Ritter's disease** in which toxin spreads systemically in individuals that lack neutralizing antitoxin. Extensive areas of the skin are involved. Patient develops painful rash which sloughs off and skin surface resembles scalding.

Staphylococcal scalded skin syndrome (SSSS) occurs primarily in newborns and previously healthy young children. In adults, it occurs most commonly among patients with chronic renal failure and those with compromised immune systems. Although the mortality rate is low (0–7%) in cases seen among children, the rate in adults is as high as 50%.

Food-poisoning: It is caused by staphylococcal enterotoxin. Enterotoxin is a preformed toxin already present in contaminated food before consumption. Food is often contaminated by a food handler, who is either a carrier of *S. aureus* or is suffering from staphylococcal skin infection. Milk and milk products, and animal products like fish and meat kept at room temperature after cooking are mainly incriminated. When kept at room temperature, the contaminating staphylococci multiply and produce enterotoxin. It may also be produced in uncooked food contaminated with *S. aureus* and kept at room temperature. The enterotoxin is heat stable, resisting heat at 100°C for 10–40 minutes, therefore, it is not inactivated by brief cooking.

Patient develops nausea, vomiting and diarrhoea 2–6 hours after consumption of food containing preformed enterotoxin of *S. aureus*. It is a self-limiting condition.

Toxic shock syndrome (TSS): It is a multisystem illness characterized by high fever, headache, confusion, conjunctival reddening, subcutaneous oedema, vomiting, diarrhoea, scarlatiniform rash and fine desquamation of the hands and feet. Severe cases progress to acute renal failure, disseminated intravascular coagulation, peripheral gangrene, profound hypotensive shock and death.

Initially, the disease was noted most frequently in women, with onset mainly occurring during menstruation. Investigations of initial cases noted an association between the onset of disease and the use of hyperabsorbable tampons. Subsequently, TSS has been reported in both males and females as a complication of staphylococcal abscesses, osteo-myelitis and postsurgical wound infections.

Laboratory diagnosis (Flowchart 19.1)

Specimens

Specimens to be collected include pus from suppu-rative lesions, blood from a patient with pyrexia of unknown origin, midstream urine from a patient with urinary tract infection, sputum from a patient with bronchopneumonia, and faeces, food remains and vomit from cases of food poisoning. Nasal and perineal swabs may be collected from suspected carriers.

Microscopy

Examine a Gram-stained smear of pus or wound exudate which may show pus cells and Gram-positive cocci in clusters (Fig. 19.2).

Culture

The specimens are cultured on a blood agar plate. Specimens, where staphylococci are expected to be outnumbered by other bacteria (e.g., wound swab and faeces), are inoculated on selective media like salt agar. The inoculated media are incubated at 37°C for 24 hours. Next day, the plates are inspected for golden-yellow or white colonies and are confirmed by slide coagulase test. On blood agar plate, look for haemolysis around the colonies (Fig. 19.3). Other tests which may be carried out include tube coagulase, mannitol fermentation, DNAse and

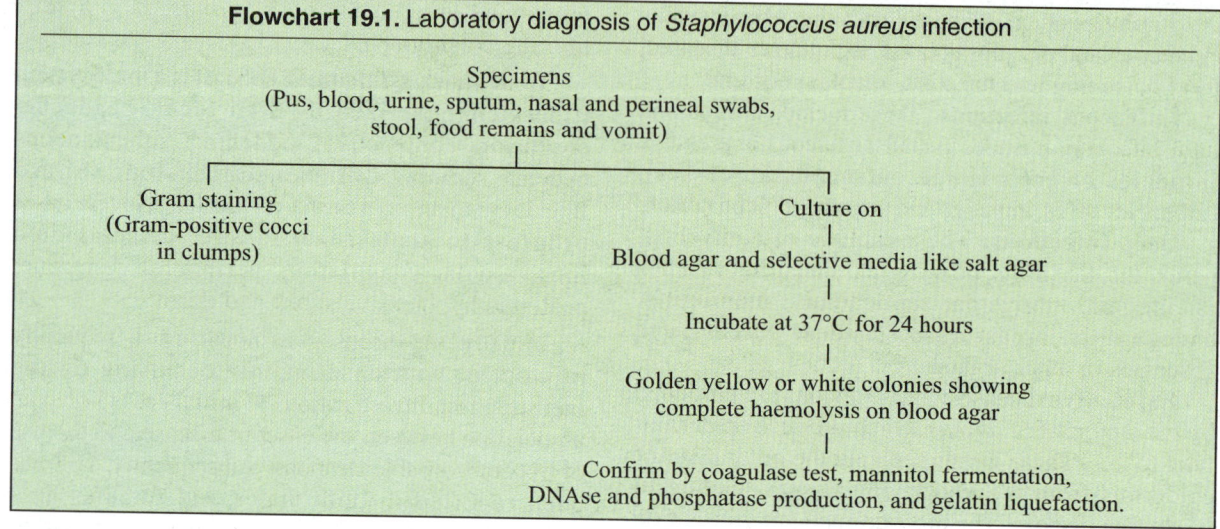

Flowchart 19.1. Laboratory diagnosis of *Staphylococcus aureus* infection

Specimens
(Pus, blood, urine, sputum, nasal and perineal swabs,
stool, food remains and vomit)

Gram staining
(Gram-positive cocci
in clumps)

Culture on

Blood agar and selective media like salt agar

Incubate at 37°C for 24 hours

Golden yellow or white colonies showing
complete haemolysis on blood agar

Confirm by coagulase test, mannitol fermentation,
DNAse and phosphatase production, and gelatin liquefaction.

phosphatase production, and gelatin liquefaction. As a guide to treatment, antibiotic sensitivity tests should be done and for epidemiological purposes bacteriophage typing may be done.

Treatment

Since drug resistance is common among staphylococci, therefore, appropriate antibiotic should be chosen by antibiotic sensitivity test. Benzyl penicillin is the most effective antibiotic, if the strain is sensitive. Cloxacillin, oxacillin, flucloxacillin and methicillin are penicillinase-resistant penicillins. In serious infections they may be combined with an aminoglycoside or fusidic acid. First and second-generation cephalosporins are also effective but third-generation cephalosporins should be avoided. Clindamycin is useful in cases of osteomyelitis. Patients allergic to penicillins may be given erythromycin, vancomycin or first-generation cephalosporins. Methicillin-resistant strains are also resistant to other penicillins and cephalosporins. However, they may be sensitive to vancomycin, rifampin, fusidic acid and ciprofloxacin.

COAGULASE-NEGATIVE STAPHYLOCOCCI

Coagulase-negative staphylococci (CoNS) form part of the normal flora of the skin. Some species of CoNS, e.g., *S. epidermidis* and *S. saprophyticus*, can produce human infections. They are morphologically similar to *S. aureus* and the methods for isolation are the same. Their colonies are white (non-pigmented) and they can be distinguished from *S. aureus* by their failure to coagulate plasma and by their lack of clumping factor and DNAse.

Staphylococcus epidermidis

The role of *S. epidermidis* as an aetiologic agent of disease has become increasingly evident. Infections caused by *S. epidermidis* are predominantly hospital acquired. Some of the predisposing factors are instrumentation procedures such as catheterization, prosthetic heart valve implantation, and immuno-suppressive therapy. Infections caused by this organism include endocarditis of native and prosthetic valves, intravenous catheter infections, CSF shunt infections, peritoneal dialysis, catheter-associated peritonitis, bacteraemia, osteomyelitis, wound infections, vascular graft infections, prosthetic joint infections and mediastinitis. *S. epidermidis* is probably the most common cause of hospital-acquired urinary tract infections.

Many strains of *S. epidermidis* can adhere to plastic catheters and prosthetic devices. Adherence of CoNS to plastic prosthetics is, most likely, facilitated by nonspecific binding related to electrical charge and/or hydrophobic interactions between the bacterial surface and the surface of plastic devices. Many strains of *S. epidermidis* are capable of

Table 19.4. Differences between three species of *Staphylococcus*

Character	S. aureus	S. epidermidis	S. saprophyticus
Production of			
• Coagulase	+	–	–
• DNase	+	–	–
• Phosphatase	+	– / weak +	–
• Toxin	+	–	–
Anaerobic fermentation of mannitol	+	–	–
Protein A in the cell wall	+	–	–
Novobiocin resistance	–	–	+

producing large amounts of polysaccharide glycocalyx known as slime. It is produced readily when the bacteria are growing on a solid surface such as a plastic catheter allowing the formation of microcolonies. Slime has been thought to play a role in the adherence of staphylococci to surfaces. Slime-producing strains also utilize this adherence factor to inhibit the action of lymphocytes and neutrophils.

Staphylococcus saprophyticus

S. saprophyticus is a well documented pathogen causing primarily acute urinary tract infections in young healthy sexually active women. In this population *S. saprophyticus* is the most common cause of cystitis after *Escherichia coli*. When present in urine cultures, it may be found in low numbers and yet considered significant. It is found to adhere more effectively to the epithelial cells lining the urogenital tract.

S. saprophyticus can be differentiated from *S. epidermidis* from its novobiocin resistance (Table 19.4).

KEY FACTS

- **Staphylococci with streptococci** constitute the main group of **medically important Gram-positive cocci**. The former occur in clumps and are catalase-positive and the latter occur in chains and are catalase-negative

- Staphylococcal infections range from the trivial to the rapidly fatal. They can be very difficult to treat, especially those contracted in hospitals, because of remarkable ability of staphylococci to acquire antibiotic resistance determinants

- *Staphylococcus aureus* is one of the most common causes of **bacterial infections**, and is also an important cause of intoxications such as **food-poisoning** and **toxic shock syndrome**

- *Staphylococcus epidermidis* is an important cause of **prosthetic implant infections**

- *Staphylococcus saprophyticus* causes urinary tract infections, especially **cystitis in women**

IMPORTANT QUESTIONS

1. Discuss pathogenicity and laboratory diagnosis of *Staphylococcus aureus* infection.
2. Write short notes on:
   (a) Coagulase
   (b) Coagulase-negative staphylococci
   (c) Toxic shock syndrome
   (d) Toxins and enzymes produced by *Staphylococcus aureus*.

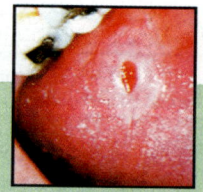

Chapter 20

Streptococcus

The genus *Streptococcus* includes three of the most important pathogens:

1. *S. pyogenes*, the causative agent of sore throat, which can lead to rheumatic fever, and acute glomerulonephritis.
2. *S. agalactiae*, the most frequent cause of sepsis in newborns.
3. *S. pneumoniae*, a leading cause of pneumonia and meningitis in persons of all ages.

Streptococci are catalase-negative, Gram-positive, non-sporing, spherical or ovoid cells. Most group A, B, and C strains produce capsules composed of hyaluronic acid. Cell division occurs in one plane, therefore, they are arranged in pairs or chains. With the exception of some species, they are non-motile. Majority of them are aerobes and facultative anaerobes but some are obligate anaerobes. Most of the former grow in air but some require the addition of CO_2 for growth.

They grow poorly in simple media but their growth is greatly enhanced by the addition of fermentable carbohydrates (e.g., glucose) and blood or serum. Their G + C content is 30–46 mol %. Streptococci form part of the normal flora of man and animals. They inhabit various sites, notably the upper respiratory tract, and usually live harmlessly as commensals. However, some species, of which *S. pyogenes* is the most important, are highly pathogenic. Streptococci were discovered in 1874 by Billroth but their important characteristics were described for the first time by Rosenbach in 1884.

Classification

Streptococci are divided into facultative anaerobes and obligate anaerobes. Genus *Peptostreptococcus* is obligate anaerobe (see Chapter 26). Based upon their haemolytic properties, facultative anaerobic streptococci can be classified into three groups (Table 20.1):

1. **α-haemolytic streptococci:** The colonies are surrounded by a narrower zone (1–2 mm in diameter) of haemolysis, with unhaemolysed RBCs persistent in an inner zone and complete haemolysis in an outer zone. The reason why some RBCs are spared is not known. Green discoloration of haemolysed zone takes place due to the formation of an unidentified reduced product of haemoglobin. The streptococci producing α-haemolysis are also known as **viridans streptococci**. They are not part of Lancefield's classification because they do not have C carbohydrate. They are widely found as normal flora in upper respiratory tract of humans. They are often seen as opportunistic pathogens.

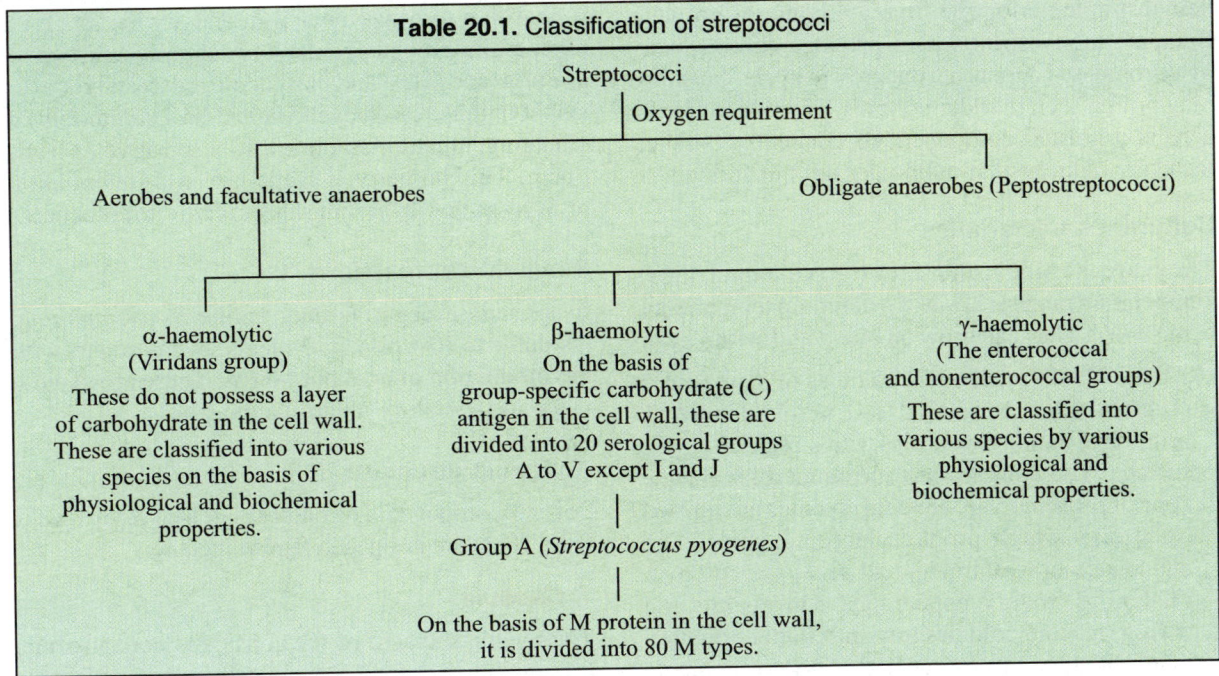

Table 20.1. Classification of streptococci

Streptococci

Oxygen requirement

Aerobes and facultative anaerobes | **Obligate anaerobes (Peptostreptococci)**

α-haemolytic (Viridans group)

These do not possess a layer of carbohydrate in the cell wall. These are classified into various species on the basis of physiological and biochemical properties.

β-haemolytic

On the basis of group-specific carbohydrate (C) antigen in the cell wall, these are divided into 20 serological groups A to V except I and J

Group A (*Streptococcus pyogenes*)

On the basis of M protein in the cell wall, it is divided into 80 M types.

γ-haemolytic (The enterococcal and nonenterococcal groups)

These are classified into various species by various physiological and biochemical properties.

2. **β-haemolytic streptococci:** These organisms produce a wide (2–4 mm in diameter) clear zone of complete haemolysis in which no red blood cell is visible on microscopic examination.

3. **γ-haemolytic streptococci:** These organisms do not produce any haemolysis or discoloration on blood agar. *Enterococcus faecalis* is an important organism of this group.

On the basis of group-specific carbohydrate (C) antigens in the cell wall, β-haemolytic streptococci are divided into 20 serological groups from A to V except I and J. These are known as Lancefield groups. Group A β-haemolytic strains, which are responsible for many important human infections, are given the species name *S. pyogenes*.

STREPTOCOCCUS PYOGENES

Morphology

They are Gram-positive, spherical cocci about 0.6–1.0 μm in diameter. They occur in chains of varying lengths. Chain formation is due to the cocci dividing in one plane only and the daughter cells failing to separate completely (Fig. 20.1). In actively spreading

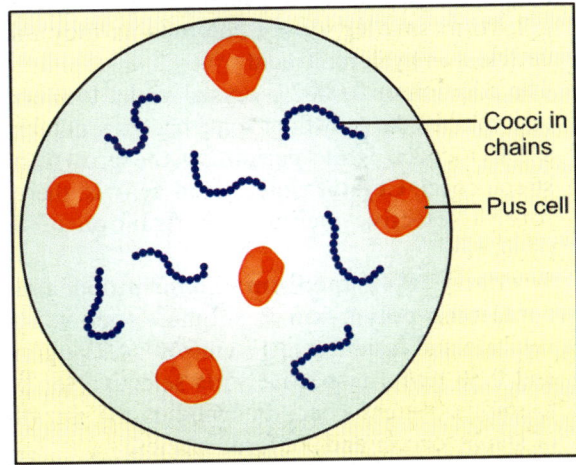

Cocci in chains

Pus cell

Fig. 20.1. Streptococci in Gram-stained smear of pus.

lesions within the tissues, diplococcal and individual coccal forms are common, whereas in purulent exudates from walled-off lesions and in artificial culture media, chain formation is a rule. Chains are longer in liquid than in solid media. They are non-motile, non-sporing and some strains produce a capsule of hyaluronic acid, which may be demonstrable during the first 2–4 hours of growth. Because many strains also produce the enzyme hyaluronidase later during the growth cycle, capsules may not be seen in older cultures. Since hyaluronic acid is a normal component of connective tissue, therefore, anticapsular antibodies are not formed.

Cultural characteristics

They are aerobes and facultative anaerobes. Temperature range is 22–40°C, optimum temperature being 37°C. They can grow on blood and serum agar.

- After 24 hours incubation, colonies of *S. pyogenes* on **blood agar** are small (0.5–1 mm in diameter), semitransparent, grey-white with a matt or glossy surface. The colonies are surrounded by a wide zone of β-haemolysis. Mucoid colonies are formed by strains which produce large capsules. The abundance of hyaluronic acid gives the colony a glistening, watery appearance. On ageing and drying, mucoid colonies turn into flatter, rougher, matt colonies. Streptococci that do not generate hyaluronic acid or do not retain it as a capsular gel, form smaller glossy colonies as they are deficient in hyaluronic acid.
- The addition of 0.0002% crystal violet to blood agar inhibits the growth of some bacteria, notably staphylococci, while permitting the growth of streptococci. **Crystal violet blood agar** is, therefore, a selective medium for isolation of *S. pyogenes*.
- Similarly, **PNF medium** (horse blood agar containing polymyxin B sulphate, neomycin sulphate and fusidic acid 17 units/ml, 4.25 µg/ml and 0.50 µg/ml respectively) is selective for β-haemolytic streptococci, but inhibits the growth of staphylococci and coliform species.

Susceptibility to physical and chemical agents

S. pyogenes is a delicate organism. It can be killed by heating at 54°C for 30 minutes. However, if protected from sunlight, it can survive in dust for months. It is also killed by usual strengths of disinfectants, but is more resistant to crystal violet than many other bacteria including *Staphylococcus aureus* hence it is used for preparation of selective media. It

is sensitive to benzylpenicillin and a wide range of other antimicrobial agents. It is naturally resistant to aminoglycosides and has acquired resistance to sulphonamides, tetracyclines and less commonly to clindamycin and macrolides. It is sensitive to bacitracin. This property is made use in differentiation of *S. pyogenes* from other haemolytic streptococci.

Biochemical reactions

It is catalase-negative and, unlike *S. pneumoniae*, insoluble in 10% bile. It ferments several sugars with the production of acid but no gas. These are of little value in laboratory identification.

Antigenic structure

Several components of bacterial cell of *S. pyogenes* (Fig. 20.2) are antigenic. These include:

1. Capsule

The hyaluronic acid of the capsule is nonantigenic, presumably because it is chemically indistinguishable from the hyaluronic acid of ground substance of animal connective tissue. Capsule has only a weak antiphagocytic effect.

2. Cell wall

Cell wall is composed of an outer layer of protein, a middle layer of group-specific carbohydrate and an inner layer of peptidoglycan.

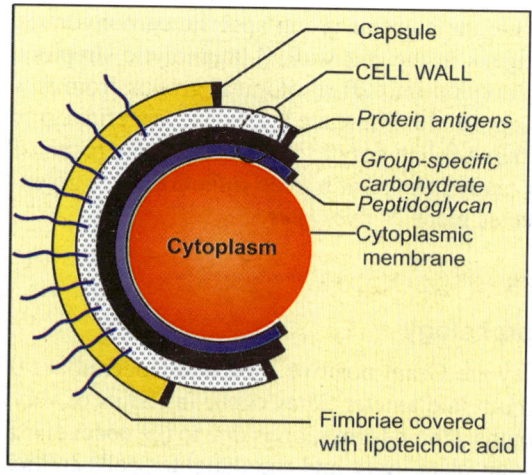

Fig. 20.2. Components of *Streptococcus pyogenes*.

(a) **Peptidoglycan:** Peptidoglycan is responsible for cell wall rigidity. It also has biologic properties such as pyrogenic and thrombolytic activity.

(b) **Group-specific carbohydrate:** Carbohydrate antigen of haemolytic streptococci can be extracted by a number of methods like Lancefield acid extraction, enzyme (produced by *Streptomyces albus*) extraction and formamide extraction. It gives specific precipitate with sera prepared by injecting killed whole cells into rabbits. On the basis of group-specific carbohydrate antigens contained in the cell wall, haemolytic streptococci have been divided into 20 groups (A to V except I and J). These are known as Lancefield groups. *S. pyogenes* belongs to Lancefield group A. **All streptococci except the viridans group have a layer of carbohydrate.**

(c) **Proteins:** *S. pyogenes* produces three surface protein antigens (M, T and R) that are useful in serologic typing:

- **M protein:** It is the most important. It acts as a virulence factor by inhibiting phagocytosis. Specific anti-M antibody develops after infection which enhances phagocytosis. **M protein extends through the capsule as fine fimbriae.** They are covered with lipoteichoic acid. They enable the organism to attach to epithelial cells. M protein is acid- and heat-stable and trypsin-sensitive. It is antigenic and antisera can be raised against it. On the basis of antigenic differences in the M protein, *S. pyogenes* is divided into more than 80 M types. M protein can be extracted by Lancefield acid extraction method and M typing is performed by capillary tube precipitation tests using type-specific antisera and acid extract.

- **T protein:** It is resistant to pepsin and trypsin but is heat- and acid-stable. It is present in many serotypes of *S. pyogenes*. T typing is done by slide agglutination test using trypsin-treated whole streptococci.

- **R protein:** It is destroyed by pepsin and not by trypsin. Typing systems employing the R surface antigens are not commonly used.

Various structural components of *S. pyogenes* exhibit antigenic **cross-reaction with different tissues** of the human body, e.g., capsular hyaluronic acid, cell wall protein, cell wall carbohydrate, cytoplasmic membrane and peptidoglycan cross-react with human synovial fluid, myocardium,

Table 20.2. Structural components of *Streptococcus pyogenes* which cross-react with human tissues

Structural component of *S. pyogenes*	Human tissue with which it cross-reacts
Capsular hyaluronic acid	Synovial fluid
Cell wall protein	Myocardium
Cell wall carbohydrate	Cardiac valves
Cytoplasmic membrane	Vascular intima
Peptidoglycan	Skin antigens

cardiac valves, vascular intima and skin antigens respectively (Table 20.2).

Toxins and enzymes

S. pyogenes produces several exotoxins and enzymes which contribute to its pathogenicity and identification.

Erythrogenic toxin (streptococcal pyrogenic exotoxin)

There are three antigenically distinct erythrogenic toxins A, B and C (streptococcal pyrogenic exotoxins; SPE A, SPE B and SPE C). Type A toxin is encoded by bacteriophage gene *speA*, type B toxin by chromosomal gene *speB* and toxin C by bacteriophage gene *speC*. **These exotoxins are superantigens** and have been associated with streptococcal toxic shock syndrome and scarlet fever.

Dick test: When 0.2 ml of suitably diluted toxin is injected intradermally in the susceptible children, it causes localized erythematous reaction at least 1 cm in diameter in 12–24 hours. This indicates susceptibility to the toxin and thus to scarlet fever. This test is known as Dick test. This toxin is antigenic. It is neutralized by antibodies found in convalescent sera.

Schultz–Charlton test: When the patient serum contains demonstrable antitoxin, the skin test becomes negative and an injection of homologous antitoxin intradermally in a patient of scarlet fever causes local blanching of the rash. This is known as Schultz-Charlton test.

Haemolysins

S. pyogenes produces two types of haemolysins. One of these is oxygen-labile hence designated as streptolysin O (SLO) and the other is oxygen-stable and soluble in serum hence designated as streptolysin S (SLS).

Streptolysin O: It is a heat-labile protein with a molecular weight of 50,000–75,000 daltons. It binds to the cholesterol containing erythrocyte membrane and produces large holes in it, leading to complete lysis. On blood agar, SLO activity is seen only in pour plates and in anaerobic cultures. It is inactive in oxidised form, but may be reactivated by treatment with reducing agents. It is irreversibly inactivated by cholesterol. It is lethal on intravenous injection into animals and has particularly toxic effect on the heart and leucocytes.

SLO is strongly antigenic. It induces brisk antibody response, usually within 10–14 days. **Antistreptolysin O (ASO)** may be demonstrated, *in vitro*, by its capacity to inhibit the haemolytic action of the toxin. It provides a very important tool for determining a recent group A streptococcal infection. Such information is an important aid in the diagnosis of the late complications of streptococcal infections, which usually occur after the organisms have been eliminated from the host.

Streptolysin S: It is a small polypeptide with a molecular weight of less than 20,000 daltons. It is nonantigenic. It is oxygen-stable, so it is responsible for haemolysis around the surface colonies. In addition to causing β-haemolysis, it is able to inhibit chemotaxis and phagocytosis.

Streptokinase

Streptococci of groups A, C and G produce a substance called streptokinase which is actively fibrinolytic for human fibrin (blood clot) and can be recovered in streptococcal culture filtrates. It is an antigenic protein and neutralizing antibodies appear in convalescent sera. It acts on plasminogen, a factor present in normal plasma, which is converted into plasmin, an active proteolytic enzyme that lyses fibrin. It is thought to be at least partially responsible for the rapid spread of streptococcal infection by preventing the formation of a fibrin barrier around the infected site. It is given intravenously for the treatment of early myocardial infarction and other thromboembolic disorders.

Deoxyribonucleases (streptodornases)

S. pyogenes also elaborates enzymes that degrade DNA. Four immunologically and electrophoretically different types (A, B, C and D) of deoxyribonucleases have been found in streptococcal culture filtrates. Of these, B is most antigenic in man and demonstration of **anti-deoxyribonuclease B** is useful in the retrospective diagnosis particularly of skin infections, where ASO titre may be low. One or more of these enzymes are produced by all strains of *S. pyogenes*. They are capable of depolymerizing the highly viscous DNA which accumulates in thick pus as a result of disintegration of polymorphonuclear leucocytes. Thus these enzymes are probably responsible for serous character of streptococcal pus. Mixtures of streptokinase and streptodornase have been used therapeutically for breaking down blood clots, thick pus and fibrinous exudates in closed spaces such as joints or pleural cavity.

Hyaluronidase (spreading factor)

It is an enzyme which splits hyaluronic acid binding tissue cells together and also that of streptococcal capsules, consequently strains which produce large amounts of hyaluronidase produce little hyaluronic acid capsule. This enzyme is expected to play a part in the virulence of *S. pyogenes* by facilitating its spread. It is antigenic and antibodies to the enzyme are formed after infection. Hyaluronidase is produced by strains of group A, B, C and G streptococci.

Serum opacity factor (SOF)

SOF is an enzyme, lipoproteinase. It exists both as cell-bound and released from it. It produces opacity when applied to agar gel containing horse or swine serum. It is produced by group A streptococci of certain M types. It thus provides a means of classifying group A streptococci into two categories – SOF-producing and non-SOF-producing strains.

Pathogenicity

S. pyogenes is intrinsically a much more dangerous organism than *S. aureus* and has a much greater tendency to spread in the tissues, therefore, it is more likely to give rise to septicaemia. Various strains of *S. pyogenes* are carried normally in the respiratory tract, mouth and the skin of about 5% of general population. The carrier rate is generally higher in children between 1–15 years of age. Carriers and patients with acute infections are the sources of infection which is acquired by respiratory droplets or by direct or indirect contact. *S. pyogenes* causes:

   I. Suppurative diseases

  II. Non-suppurative sequelae

I. Suppurative diseases

1. Tonsillitis and pharyngitis

The main site of streptococcal infection is the throat where purulent tonsillitis is the most typical lesion. This condition characteristically occurs in older children and adults where it may constitute 30–40% of all cases of sore throat. In younger children, the infection is more diffuse (pharyngitis rather than tonsillitis) and less acute in character. The more acute localized lesion of older persons is believed to depend on a previous acquired allergy.

Occasionally, a peritonsillar or retropharyngeal abscess is produced and infrequently diffuse cellulitis of the floor of the mouth, known as **Ludwig's angina**, develops. From the throat, the organism may also involve the meninges leading to meningitis and the lungs leading to pneumonia. The latter is usually a complication of other infections involving respiratory tract such as influenza and measles. Epidemiological studies have revealed that, commonly, a school child brings the infection home and spreads it within the family.

2. Scarlet fever

Scarlet fever may be caused by any type of group A *Streptococcus* that produces erythrogenic toxin. The disease consists of a combination of a streptococcal sore throat and a generalized erythema, although occasionally the rash can accompany a streptococcal wound infection. The rash consists of widespread erythema with punctate spots. The skin of the face is generally clear. Whether the rash is secondary to a direct action of the circulating toxin or to a generalized cutaneous hypersensitivity reaction is not known. In the favour of the latter possibility is the observation that infants under the age of two years rarely develop the disease and do not show positive Dick test. Due to unknown reasons, scarlet fever has become very uncommon in recent decades.

3. Impetigo

This is caused predominantly by *S. pyogenes*. It may also be caused by group C and G streptococci and by *S. aureus*. Impetigo is a skin infection that occurs most often in young children, particularly those living in crowded, low socioeconomic conditions. Streptococcal impetigo is characterized by occurrence on the skin of a superficial discrete crusted spot seldom exceeding an inch in diameter, which lasts for 1–2 weeks and heals spontaneously without leaving a scar.

4. Erysipelas

This is an acute, spreading, intensely erythematous skin lesion with a sharply demarcated but irregular edge and sometimes with superficial vesicles and bullae.

5. Other group A streptococcal infections

S. pyogenes is the most important cause of **puerperal sepsis**. In this condition, the organisms are almost invariably derived from attendant nurses or doctors or from contaminated instruments. It may also cause wound and burn infections.

II. Non-suppurative sequelae

There is a considerable evidence that *S. pyogenes* is in some way the cause of acute rheumatic fever (ARF) involving the heart and joints, and acute glomerulonephritis (AGN) involving the kidneys. These conditions differ from suppurative infections in that:

(a) These conditions appear only between 2–3 weeks after infection with *S. pyogenes*. *S. pyogenes* is no longer detectable when the complications set in.

(b) Many cases are not preceded by overt streptococcal infection but in many of these, high titres of antibodies to streptococcal extracellular antigens, particularly to streptolysin O, are frequently demonstrable.

(c) Streptococci are not directly demonstrable in the lesions in these conditions.

Differentiating features between acute rheumatic fever and acute glomerulonephritis are given in Table 20.3.

Table 20.3. Differentiating features between acute rheumatic fever and acute glomerulonephritis

	Acute rheumatic fever	*Acute glomerulo-nephritis*
Primary site of infection	Throat	Skin/throat
Serotypes involved	Any	Pyoderma strains 49, 53–55 and 59–61 and pharyngitis strains 1 and 12
Immune response	Marked	Moderate
Complement level	Unaffected	Lowered
Repeated attacks	Common	Absent
Penicillin prophylaxis	Essential	Not indicated
Course	Progressive or static	Spontaneous resolution
Prognosis	Variable	Good

Acute rheumatic fever (ARF)

ARF develops in a small percentage (roughly 3%) of individuals, 2–3 weeks after the onset of acute streptococcal pharyngitis caused by any type of group A streptococci. It is characterized by fever, migrating polyarthritis, and carditis, and is frequently associated with subcutaneous nodules. Recovery from ARF occurs without residual injury to the joints, but permanent damage to the heart may occur. The mechanism by which streptococci produce rheumatic fever is still obscure.

There have been reports that a common cross-reacting antigen exists in some group A streptococci and the heart. In this case, antibodies synthesized in response to the streptococcal infection could react with antigens in the heart, causing cellular destruction and permanent damage. This theory is supported by the observation that following a streptococcal epidemic, most patients who develop ARF have higher titre of anti-streptococcal antibodies in their sera than do those who escape the disease. Circulating immune complexes have also been found in serum of the patients with ARF.

Acute glomerulonephritis (AGN)

AGN is less frequently a consequence of streptococcal infection than is ARF. In contrast to ARF, which occurs only after pharyngitis, AGN may be seen after either a pharyngeal or a cutaneous infection. Most cases of AGN occur 2–3 weeks following skin infection or pharyngitis caused by pyodermal (M types 1 and 12) and pharyngeal (M types 49, 53–55 and 59–61) strains of *S. pyogenes*. These strains are known as nephritogenic strains.

Poststreptococcal AGN probably develops because some components of glomerular basement membrane are antigenically similar to the cell membranes of nephritogenic β-haemolytic streptococci. Therefore, antibodies which are produced by the host against the latter cross-react with the former. Alternatively, streptococcal antigen-antibody complexes may lodge in the glomeruli. In either case, the activation of the C3 and C5 components of complement leads to tissue destruction. This is supported by the detection of C3 as well as γ-globulin and streptococcal antigens in the glomerular lesion.

Laboratory diagnosis
(Flowcharts 20.1 and 20.2)

In acute infections, diagnosis is established by identification of β-haemolytic streptococci that have been isolated from the patient, while in non-suppurative complications, diagnosis is based on the demonstration of rising titre of antibody to one or more streptococcal antigens.

Specimens

Throat and nasal swabs from cases of sore throat or from suspected carriers, high vaginal swabs from cases of puerperal sepsis, pus or pus swabs from

Flowchart 20.1. Laboratory diagnosis of suppurative sequelae of *Streptococcus pyogenes*

Specimens
(Throat and nasal swabs, high vaginal swab, pus, blood)

Gram staining
(Gram-positive cocci
arranged in chains)

Direct fluorescent
antibody technique

Culture

Inoculate blood agar plate

Incubate at 37°C for 24 hours

Look for small (0.5–1 mm) colonies surrounded
by a wide zone of β-haemolysis

In case of bacteriological examination
of skin lesions, selective media
(crystal violet blood agar and PNF medium)
may by used

Lancefield grouping

If the isolate belongs to group A, perform M typing and/or
sensitivity to bacitracin (Maxted's observation)

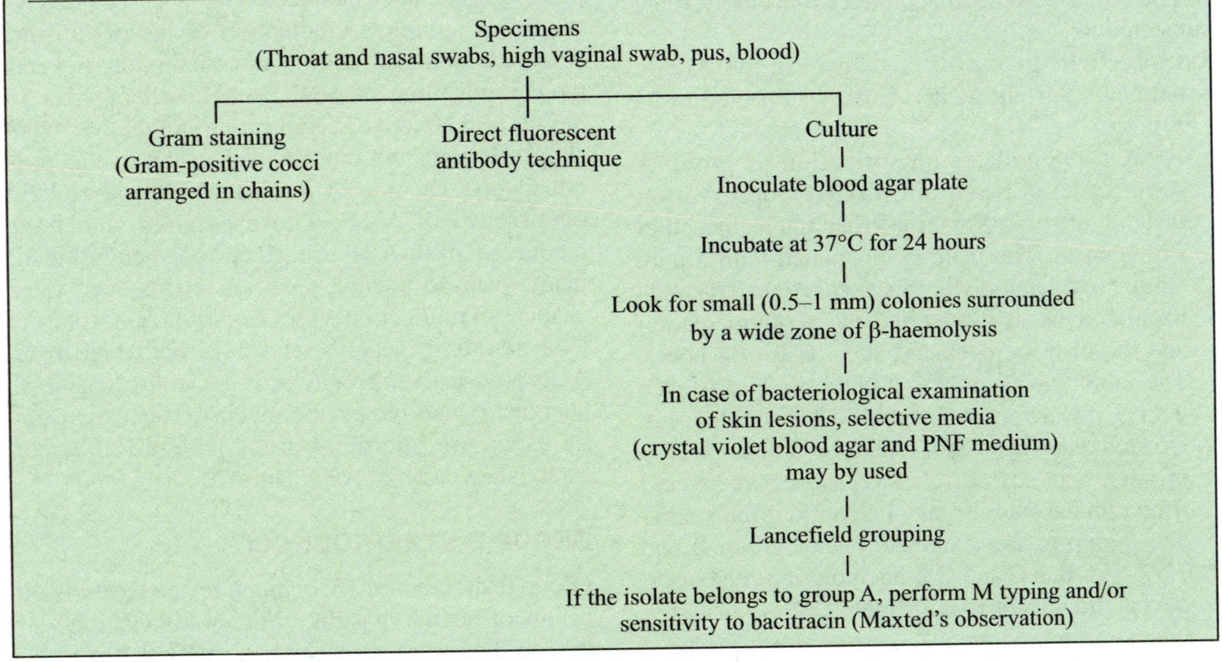

Flowchart 20.2. Laboratory diagnosis of non-suppurative sequelae of *Streptococcus pyogenes*

Specimen
(Serum, preferably paired sera)

Antistreptolysin O test
(titres higher than
200 Todd units/ml
are significant)

Antideoxyribonuclease
B test
(titres higher than
300 or 350 are significant)

Streptozyme
test

Antistreptokinase
test

Antihyaluronidase
test

Anti-
NADase

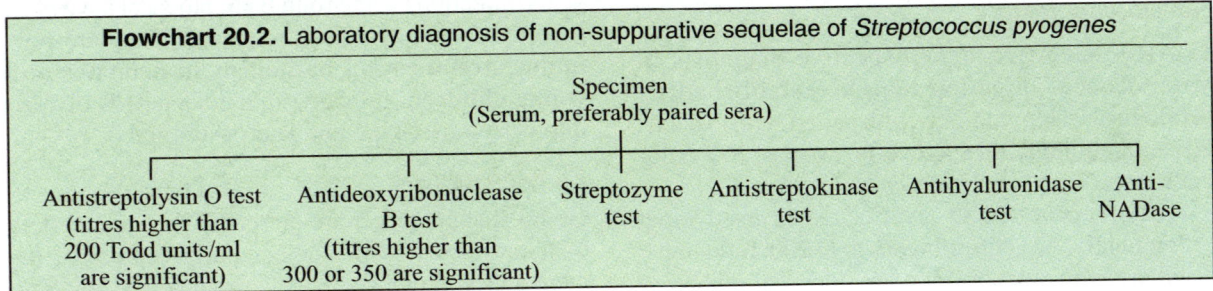

suppurative infections, and blood from cases of systemic infections are the usual specimens collected.

Gram staining

The observation of typical Gram-positive cocci arranged in chains on microscopic examination of smear of pus or CSF may indicate the likelihood of the presence of streptococci.

Fluorescent antibody technique

The examination of throat swab by the direct fluorescent antibody technique may be used for rapid identification of group A streptococci.

Culture

Inoculate pus or swab on blood agar plate immediately. Incubate it at 37°C for 24 hours and look for β-haemolytic colonies of streptococci. If there is likely to be delay, swab should be sent to the laboratory in Pike's medium (blood agar containing 1 in 1,000,000 crystal violet and 1 in 16,000 sodium azide distributed as for stab cultures in tubes). In case of bacteriological examination of skin lesions, crystal violet blood agar and PNF medium are useful selective media that inhibit many commensal organisms.

Identification

Streptococcal colonies that produce β-haemolysis are subjected to:

- **Lancefield grouping** and in case the isolate belongs to group A, it is further subjected to **M typing**.
- A rapid method for identification of group A streptococci is based on **Maxted's observation** that they are more sensitive to bacitracin than other streptococci. The plate is inoculated with a pure culture of β-haemolytic *Streptococcus*, a 0.04 units bacitracin disc is placed in the area of inoculation and the plate is incubated at 37°C for 24 hours. The inhibition of growth around the disc is seen with *S. pyogenes* but not with other streptococci. However, this test is not totally reliable as 5–15% of bacitracin-susceptible streptococci recovered from clinical sources may belong to groups other than group A. For example, 6% of group B and 7.5% of group C and G β-haemolytic streptococci are bacitracin-sensitive. About 7.5% of α-haemolytic streptococci are also bacitracin-sensitive.

Serological tests

In ARF and AGN, a retrospective diagnosis of streptococcal infection may be established by serological tests, preferably with paired sera, to detect a rise in antibody titre to one or more of the extracellular products of *S. pyogenes*.

- **Antistreptolysin O** (ASO) test is used most frequently. ASO titres higher than 200 Todd units/ml are indicative of prior streptococcal infection.
- **Antideoxyribonuclease B** (anti-DNase B) estimation is also commonly employed. Titres higher than 300 or 350 are taken as significant.
- Other tests, only occasionally used, are antistreptokinase, antihyaluronidase and anti-NADase.
- **Streptozyme test**, which is a passive slide haemagglutination test using erythrocytes sensitized with a crude preparation of extracellular antigens of streptococci, is a convenient, sensitive and specific screening test.

Treatment

Penicillin is highly effective in the treatment of all acute infections and penicillin resistance has not yet been observed in *S. pyogenes*. Therapeutic levels of penicillin should be maintained for at least 8–10 days to ensure complete eradication of the organisms. Adequate treatment during acute infection prevents the complications of ARF. Penicillin therapy for 10 days is also effective in eradicating streptococci from skin infections, but unfortunately, such treatment is not always capable of preventing the subsequent occurrence of AGN. Those persons who have recovered from ARF are given oral penicillin for many years to prevent recurrence. However, since chances of reinfection with a nephritogenic strain are low, therefore, persons who have recovered from AGN are not given prophylactic penicillin. In patients allergic to penicillin, erythromycin or cephalexin may be used. Antimicrobial drugs have no effect on established cases of AGN and ARF.

GROUP B STREPTOCOCCI

Group B streptococci (*S. agalactiae*) are the etiologic agents of bovine mastitis and their association with human disease was recognized in 1930s. In recent years, infections with group B streptococci have been reported with increasing frequency. They are now **major streptococcal pathogens in neonates and young children**. Infection in the neonate is divided into early-onset-type and late-onset-type.

Early-onset-type

Group B streptococci are present in the vaginal flora of about 25% of all women. Early rupture of the membranes, prolonged labour, prematurity, low birth weight and heavy colonization of mother's vagina by group B streptococci lead to early-onset-type infection. Within first five days of life the neonate develops septicaemia and pneumonia, and in spite of the intensive antibiotic therapy, such infections carry a mortality rate of 50–70%. Meningitis may also develop.

The serotype of group B streptococci isolated from the anterior nares, external auditory meatus, umbilicus and rectum of the neonate, with or without infection, in almost all the cases, is similar to that isolated from the cervicovaginal canal, urethra or rectum of the mother. The fact that some babies delivered by caesarean section become infected indicates that direct spread of the organism to the uterus may take place.

Late-onset- type

This type of infection develops between second to fourth weeks of life. Baby acquires infection from the hospital personnel during nursing procedures. Baby to baby spread may also occur. The infecting organism is rarely found in the mother's vagina. This type of infection is not as severe as early-onset-type, but has a high incidence of residual effects often of a neurological nature.

Group B streptococci may also cause adult infections, including septicaemia, endocarditis, meningitis, and local septic lesions in the female genital tract, the urinary tract, surgical wounds and skin. Occasionally, they may lead to pneumonia, empyema, arthritis and osteomyelitis.

S. agalactiae possesses the enzyme hippuricase, which hydrolyzes sodium hippurate. Another test to identify group B streptococci is the CAMP reaction (Christie, Atkins and Munch-Peterson), which can be demonstrated as an accentuated zone of haemolysis (butterfly appearance) when *S. agalactiae* is inoculated perpendicular to a streak of *S. aureus* grown on blood agar (Fig. 20.3). Occasional strains are bacitracin sensitive.

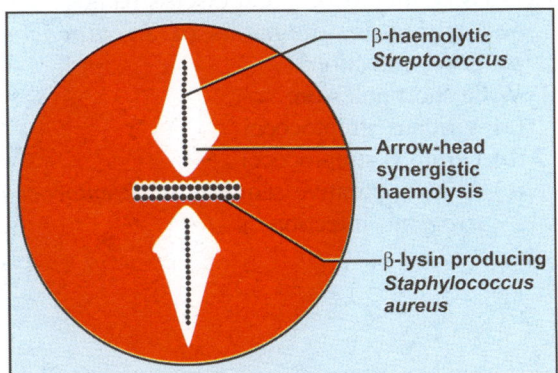

Fig. 20.3. CAMP test.

GROUP C STREPTOCOCCI

Group C streptococci comprise four species – *S. equi, S. equisimilis, S. dysgalactiae* and *S. zooepidemicus*. They produce wide zones of β-haemolysis and can cause sore throat, skin and wound infections, post-partum sepsis, pneumonia, septicaemia, meningitis, endocarditis and AGN.

GROUP G STREPTOCOCCI

These organisms are part of the normal flora of skin, particularly at damp sites, and of gut, pharynx and vagina. These may cause sore throat, pneumonia, septicaemia, endocarditis, and bone, joint, skin and wound infections.

GROUP D STREPTOCOCCI

The Group D streptococci include *S. bovis* and *S. equinus*. Until the mid-1980s, the group D streptococci were divided into the enterococcal and nonenterococcal groups. Those found in the intestinal tract were part of the enterococcal group and have now been placed in a new genus, *Enterococcus*, but nonenterococcal group remains part of the group D streptococci. Both *Enterococcus* and group D streptococci can grow in the presence of 40% bile and also hydrolyze aesculin to aesculetin and glucose.

The species most commonly associated with human disease is *E. faecalis*, but infections caused by *E. faecium, E. durans, E. avium* and other enterococci also occur. Identification of various species of *Enterococcus* is made on biochemical grounds. *E. faecalis* ferments mannitol with gas production. It is VP-positive and can grow on blood tellurite agar producing black colonies.

Enterococci may cause urinary tract infection, wound infection, infective endocarditis, biliary tract infection, peritonitis, suppurative abdominal lesions and septicaemia.

VIRIDANS STREPTOCOCCI (ORAL STREPTOCOCCI)

Viridans streptococci are heterogenous group of α-haemolytic and nonhaemolytic streptococci. Most isolates of viridans streptococci do not possess a group-specific carbohydrate; hence they cannot be classified under Lancefield classification of streptococci. They are constantly present as commensals in the mouth and oropharynx.

At least five species of viridans streptococci have been recognized. These include *S. salivarius, S. sanguis, S. mutans, S. mitior (mitis)* and *S. milleri*. Viridans streptococci, chiefly *S. mutans* and to a lesser extent *S. sanguis*, are involved in the production of **dental caries**. They break down dietary sucrose, producing acid and a tough adhesive dextran. The acid damages dentine and the dextran bind together food debris, epithelial cells, mucus and bacteria to form **dental plaques** which lead to caries.

In persons with predisposing factors, such as valvular disease of heart, viridans streptococci may cause **infective endocarditis** (IE). *S. sanguis* is the most common causative agent of infective endo-carditis. Tooth extraction and injury of the oral cavity in such persons is dangerous, because from oral cavity they may enter into the blood stream and cause IE. Tooth extraction in such individuals should be done under antibiotic cover. Other organisms which may also cause IE include *E. faecalis* and other enterococci, *S. aureus*, coagulase-negative staphylo-cocci, *Coxiella burnetii* and some fungi.

Diagnosis of IE is established by repeated blood cultures. Viridans streptococci can be recognized by their α-haemolytic colonies on blood agar, their failure to grow on MacConkey medium and their sensitivity to penicillin. When isolated from mouth, throat and respiratory tract, they are regarded as harmless commensals and when isolated from blood or a closed lesion they are likely to be pathogenic. These streptococci are generally susceptible to penicillin, though some strains may be resistant. Therefore, antibiotic sensitivity of these organisms should also be carried out.

STREPTOCOCCUS MG

This belongs to group F streptococci. It has been isolated from the sputum of normal individuals and those suffering from primary atypical pneumonia. These patients frequently have in their sera agglutinins to *Streptococcus* MG.

KEY FACTS

- Streptococci are Gram-positive, non-motile, catalase-negative cocci. They are ovoid to spherical in shape and occur in chains (*Streptococcus pyogenes*) or pairs (*Streptococcus pneumoniae*)
- Because of their complex nutritional requirements, **blood-enriched medium** is generally used for their isolation. The diseases caused by this group of organisms are diverse, some of the most prevalent being, for example, acute infections of the throat and skin, caused by group A streptococci (*Streptococcus pyogenes*), genital tract colonization by group B streptococci (*Streptococcus agalactiae*), and endocarditis caused by viridans group of streptococci
- There is a considerable evidence that *Streptococcus pyogenes* is in some way the cause of **acute rheumatic fever** and **acute glomerulonephritis**

IMPORTANT QUESTIONS

1. Classify streptococci and discuss pathogenicity and laboratory diagnosis of *Streptococcus pyogenes* infection.
2. Write short notes on:
   (a) Viridans streptococci
   (b) Group B streptococci
   (c) Non-suppurative sequelae of *Streptococcus pyogenes* infection.

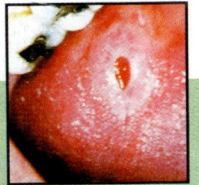

Chapter 21

Streptococcus Pneumoniae (Pneumococcus)

Pneumococcus was first identified in 1881 by Louis Pasteur and Sternberg independently. This organism carries historical importance in that the research work with pneumococcal transformations provided the initial proof that **DNA alone is the carrier of genetic information**.

Morphology

The pneumococcus is a non-motile, non-sporing, Gram-positive coccus. In the material taken from the body, it occurs characteristically in pairs of **flame-shaped** cocci about 1 μm in diameter, the rounded ends of the cocci being adjacent to each other (Figs. 21.1 and 21.2). The cell wall of pneumococcus contains an antigen, referred to as **C substance**, that is similar to the carbohydrate antigens contained in the cell wall of β-haemolytic streptococci. In cultures they usually appear in chains like streptococci. The pneumococcus is capsulated. The capsule encloses each pair and it is best seen in the material taken directly from the exudates and may be lost on repeated cultivation. Pneumococcal capsule can be demonstrated by following methods:

- As a clear halo in India ink preparation.
- By direct special staining techniques.
- It can also be seen and typed by treatment with homologous type-specific antibody which

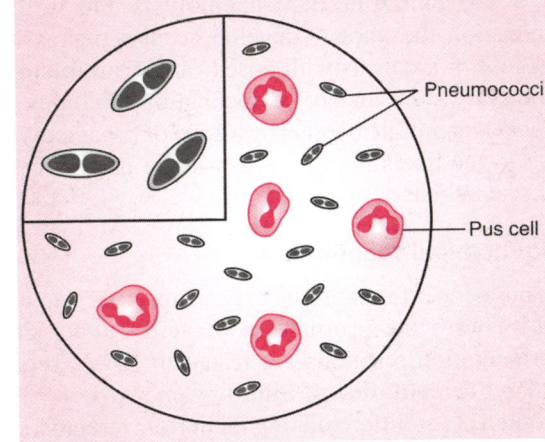

Fig. 21.1. Pneumococci in pus. Inset: enlarged view.

combines with the capsular polysaccharide and renders it refractile – **Quellung reaction**.

Cultural characteristics

Aerobe and facultative anaerobe, may need 5–10% CO_2 for primary isolation. Optimum temperature 37°C (range 25–40°C), pH 7.8 (range 6.5–8.3) and grows only on enriched media.

On **blood agar**, after 18–24 hour incubation at 37°C, virulent strains with abundant capsular polysaccharide produce small (0.5–1 mm in diameter),

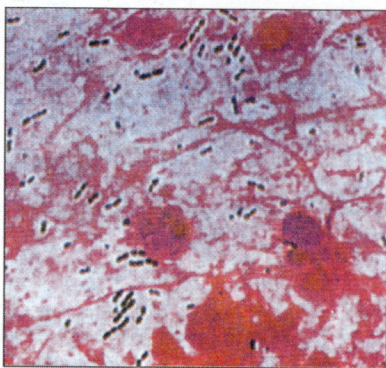

Fig. 21.2. Gram-stained sputum smear showing Gram-positive, encapsulated, extracellular diplococci from a patient of pneumococcal pneumonia.

round, dome-shaped, translucent colonies surrounded by a 2–3 mm zone of α-haemolysis. On further incubation, the colonies develop a central depression because of autolysis with raised rim (**draughtsman colony**). Under anaerobic incubation, colonies on blood agar are surrounded by a zone of β-haemolysis due to the liberation of oxygen-labile pneumolysin by pneumococci.

Biochemical reactions

Pneumococci ferment glucose, sucrose, lactose and inulin with the production of acid but no gas. Fermentation reactions are tested in Hiss's serum water. **Fermentation of inulin** by pneumococci is a useful test for differentiating them from streptococci which do not ferment it. They are catalase and oxidase-negative.

Bile solubility test

Pneumococci are bile-soluble while viridans and other streptococci are not. Bile salts, (sodium deoxycholate and sodium taurocholate) lyse pneumococci when added to actively growing cultures in an artificial culture medium. Pneumococci produce autolytic enzymes leading to autolysis in older cultures. The addition of bile salts is thought to accelerate this process.

For bile solubility test, inoculate the test organism in 5 ml serum digest broth or infusion broth, incubate it at 37°C for 18 hours. While still warm, add 0.5 ml of 10% sodium deoxycholate solution and reincubate

at 37°C. Within 15 minutes initially turbid culture becomes clear and transparent due to the lysis of pneumococci. Alternatively, touch a suspected pneumococcal colony on blood agar plate with a loopful of 2% sodium deoxycholate solution at pH 7. Incubate the plate at 37°C for 30 minutes. The colony disappears, leaving an area of α-haemolysis.

Sensitivity to physical and chemical agents

Pneumococci are delicate organisms. They can be killed by moist heat at 55°C in 10 minutes and readily by most disinfectants. They are sensitive to a wide range of antimicrobial drugs including benzyl-penicillin, other penicillins, cephalosporins, erythromycin, tetracycline, clindamycin and co-trimoxazole. Some strains resistant to β-lactam antibiotics and erythromycin have been reported.

Optochin sensitivity test

Pneumococci are highly sensitive to killing by optochin (ethyl hydrocuprein hydrochloride). Optochin sensitivity test is used for identification of pneumococci and distinguishing them from viridans streptococci, both of which produce α-haemolysis on blood agar. Optochin is a quinine derivative that inhibits the growth of pneumococci but not of viridans streptococci. For testing, a filter paper disc containing 5 μg of optochin is applied to the surface of a blood agar plate streaked with a lawn of pure culture. Plate is incubated at 37°C in air with 5–10% CO_2. Pneumococcus shows a zone of inhibition of 14 mm or more around the 6 mm optochin disc or 16 mm or more if 10 mm disc is used. Viridans streptococci grow right up to the disc. The differences between *S. pneumoniae* and viridans streptococci are given in Table 21.1.

Antigenic structure

1. Capsular antigen

The most important of pneumococcal antigens is the capsular polysaccharide on the basis of which the pneumococci are divided into more than 90 serologic types named 1, 2, 3, etc. As this polysaccharide diffuses into the culture medium or infective exudates and tissues, it is also known as **specific soluble substance** (SSS).

Table 21.1. Differences between *Streptococcus pneumoniae* and viridans streptococci

	S. pneumoniae	Viridans streptococci
1. Morphology		
• Shape	Flame-shaped cocci	Round or oval cocci
• Arrangement	In pairs	In chains
• Capsule	Present	Absent
2. Cultural characteristics		
• On blood agar medium	After 24 hour incubation, colonies are small (0.5–1 mm), round, dome-shaped, translucent and surrounded by 2–3 mm zone of α-haemolysis. On further incubation, the colonies develop a central depression with raised rim (draughtsman colonies)	After 24 hour incubation, colonies are dome-shaped, opaque and surrounded by a narrow zone (1–2 mm in diameter) of α-haemolysis
• In liquid medium	Uniform turbidity	Granular turbidity, powdery deposit
3. Bile solubility	Positive	Negative
4. Inulin fermentation	Positive	Negative
5. Optochin sensitivity	Positive	Negative
6. Animal pathogenicity (intraperitoneal inoculation in mice)	Fatal, death of mice in 1–3 days	Non-pathogenic

The capsule of the pneumococcus is essential for virulence, its role being to protect the organism from phagocytosis. Only smooth encapsulated (S) strains are pathogenic for man and most laboratory animals. Active or passive immunization against a specific polysaccharide produces a high level of resistance to infection with pneumococci of homologous type. Laboratory strains that have lost the ability to produce a capsule are nonpathogenic.

The typing of individual isolates can be performed by:

• **Quellung reaction** in which the capsules of pneumococci are made more easily visible when acted upon by specific antisera. It is performed by mixing equal quantities of specimen (sputum, pus or sediment of CSF) or light suspension of the test organisms with type-specific pneumococcal antiserum. After waiting for 15–30 minutes, for the reaction to occur, the mixture is examined microscopically using a 100X objective. If Quellung reaction is positive, the capsule of the pneumococci will appear quite prominent as compared with those in the same specimen mixed with saline solution as a control. The increased prominence of the capsule or swelling is apparently due to an alteration of its refractive index after reacting with the antiserum. Pooled sera may be tested first and then in turn the individual type-specific antisera until one of them is found to give positive result.

• **Agglutination** of the cocci with the type-specific antiserum.

• **Precipitation** of SSS with the specific antiserum.

2. Somatic antigen

Pneumococcal cell wall contains a species-specific carbohydrate hapten. It is referred to as pneumococcal C substance. This appears to be analogous to (though antigenically different from) the group-specific C antigens of β-haemolytic streptococci.

3. M protein

Type-specific protein antigens analogous to the M protein of *Streptococcus pyogenes*, but immunologically distinct, are present in pneumococci. Antibodies to the pneumococcal M protein do not inhibit phagocytosis and are, therefore, not protective.

4. C-reactive protein (CRP)

CRP is an abnormal protein (β-globulin). It appears in acute phase sera of cases of pneumonia but disappears during convalescence. It also appears in some other pathological conditions. It is known as C-reactive protein because it precipitates with C antigen of pneumococci. It is not an antibody. Its production is stimulated by bacterial infection, inflammation, malignancy and tissue destruction. It disappears when inflammation subsides. It is used as an index of response to treatment in rheumatic fever and certain other conditions. It is tested by:

- capillary precipitation of patient serum with antiserum prepared in rabbits against purified CRP, and
- passive agglutination using latex particles coated with anti-CRP antibody.

Genetic variation

Repeated subcultures of *S. pneumoniae* may result in smooth to rough (S → R) variation. In R form, the organisms are noncapsulated, autoagglutinable, avirulent and form rough colonies. R forms arise as a result of mutation. Rough pneumococci derived from capsulated organisms of one type can be permanently transformed into capsulated organisms of a different or same type by treatment with DNA derived from different or same serotype of pneumococci. This **transformation** is of considerable historical interest since its discovery by Griffith was the first indication that the **genetic material could be transferred from one microorganism to another**.

Toxin production

S. pneumoniae produces an oxygen-labile haemolysin (pneumolysin) and a leucocidin. But both these are weak toxins and there is no conclusive evidence that they play an important role in infection.

Pathogenicity

Between 5–70% of normal human adults carry one or more serological types of *S. pneumoniae* in their throats, yet epidemics of pneumococcal pneumonia are rare and morbidity low. This is due to following reasons:

- Many of the commensal pneumococci are noncapsulated and avirulent.
- Bacterial antagonism, primarily with α-haemolytic streptococci, tends to limit the growth of pneumococci in the pharynx.
- Normal epiglottal reflex, mucociliary escalator and cough reflex.

Therefore, pneumococcal pneumonia is rarely a primary infection and results only when the normal defence barriers of the respiratory tract are disturbed. Chilling, general anaesthesia, convulsions, cerebrovascular accidents, epilepsy, morphine, alcoholic intoxication and head injury predispose to pneumococcal pneumonia. These factors impair epiglottal reflex, mucociliary escalator and cough reflex, thus facilitating aspiration of pneumococci in the infected secretions from the upper respiratory tract into lower respiratory tract.

Viral infections of upper respiratory tract are a major contributory cause of pneumococcal pneumonia. Pneumococci present in the nasopharynx proliferate in the viral-modified environment and are carried down into the alveoli by the thin bronchial secretions. Aspiration of small quantities of oropharyngeal secretions can also be demonstrated in the healthy individuals during sleep. Person to person spread, by droplet infection, is uncommon.

In adults, most of the pneumococcal infections are caused by types 1–8 and 18. In children, commoner prevalent types are 6, 14, 19 and 23. The most important disease caused by *S. pneumoniae* is **pneumonia, either a lobar pneumonia or a bronchopneumonia**. The latter is characteristically a disease of young children and older adults over 50 years, while lobar pneumonia is almost exclusively a disease of the age group 10–50 years. Other pneumococcal lesions are acute bronchitis, sinusitis, otitis media, mastoiditis, meningitis, endocarditis, suppurative arthritis and peritonitis.

S. pneumoniae is the etiologic agent in about half of the children with otitis media. *S. pneumoniae* is a common cause of **bacterial meningitis** that affects patients of all ages. Pneumococcal meningitis is most often seen in children and the elderly. Pneumococcal meningitis may occur as a complication of otitis media or lobar pneumonia. Sometimes it is a consequence of fracture of skull with tearing of meninges. Bacteraemia may complicate pneumococcal pneumonia in about 15% of patients.

Laboratory diagnosis (Flowchart 21.1)

The diagnosis is carried out by demonstration of pneumococci in sputum (Fig. 21.2), exudate, blood

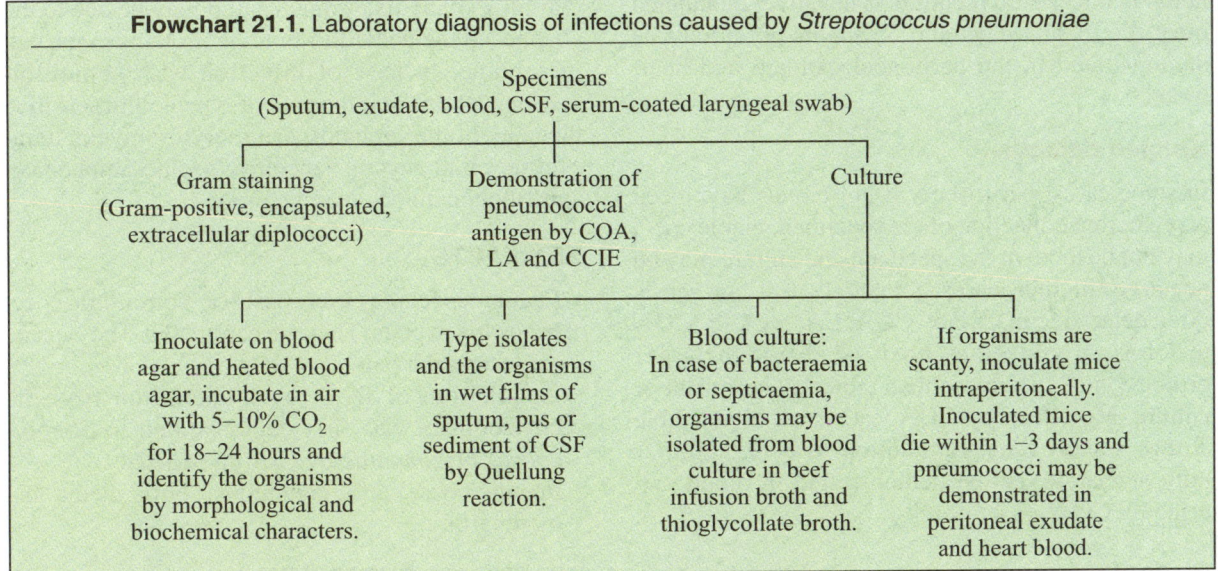

Flowchart 21.1. Laboratory diagnosis of infections caused by *Streptococcus pneumoniae*

Specimens
(Sputum, exudate, blood, CSF, serum-coated laryngeal swab)

Gram staining
(Gram-positive, encapsulated,
extracellular diplococci)

Demonstration of
pneumococcal
antigen by COA,
LA and CCIE

Culture

Inoculate on blood
agar and heated blood
agar, incubate in air
with 5–10% CO_2
for 18–24 hours and
identify the organisms
by morphological and
biochemical characters.

Type isolates
and the organisms
in wet films of
sputum, pus or
sediment of CSF
by Quellung
reaction.

Blood culture:
In case of bacteraemia
or septicaemia,
organisms may be
isolated from blood
culture in beef
infusion broth and
thioglycollate broth.

If organisms are
scanty, inoculate mice
intraperitoneally.
Inoculated mice
die within 1–3 days and
pneumococci may be
demonstrated in
peritoneal exudate
and heart blood.

and cerebrospinal fluid (CSF) by Gram staining, culture and by demonstration of pneumococcal antigen by coagglutination (COA), latex agglutination (LA) and countercurrent immunoelectrophoresis (CCIE).

Microscopy

The sputum is homogenized by agitating the specimen for 30 minutes in a mechanical shaker with an equal quantity of distilled water and a small number of glass beads. Gram-stained smears are prepared from homogenized sputum and examined. In acute otitis media, *S. pneumoniae* may be demonstrated in fluid aspirated from the middle ear. In meningitis, the presumptive diagnosis may be made from Gram-stained films of centrifuged deposit of CSF.

Culture

The sputum, after homogenisation, if necessary, is inoculated onto blood agar and heated blood agar media and incubated in air with 5–10% CO_2 for 18–24 hours. If the sputum is unobtainable, as in young children, a serum-coated laryngeal swab is taken and processed. The organisms isolated are identified by their morphological and biochemical characters.

The growth of *S. pneumoniae* may be typed with appropriate antisera. Typing can also be done by

Quellung reaction in wet films of sputum, pus or sediment of CSF.

Blood culture

Since many healthy individuals carry pneumococci in their throats, therefore, demonstration of organisms in sputum or throat culture is not necessarily indicative of pneumococcal disease. Many pneumococcal infections are associated with a bacteraemia or septicaemia. Therefore, if pneumococci are isolated from patient's blood, the diagnosis of a severe pneumococcal infection can be made with certainty. In all cases of suspected acute bacterial pneumonia sample of blood obtained by venipuncture, prior to administration of antimicrobial drugs, should be cultured immediately in beef infusion broth and thioglycollate broth.

Cerebrospinal fluid

In case of suspected meningitis, a centrifuged deposit of CSF should be examined immediately in a Gram film, cultured on blood agar and heated blood agar and incubated in air with 5–10% CO_2 for 18–24 hours.

Mouse inoculation

In specimens where the organisms are scanty, isolation may be obtained by intraperitoneal inoculation in mice, even if culture is negative. Inoculated mice die in 1–3 days and *S. pneumoniae* may be demonstrated in the peritoneal exudate and heart blood.

Antigen detection

In some cases, particularly if antibiotics have been given before collection of the specimen, viable cocci may not be there in the specimen and culture may be negative. In such cases, pneumococcal antigen is often detectable in CSF by COA, LA or CCIE. COA test for antigen gives positive result in larger proportion of specimens than either a Gram film or culture. Moreover, by COA test, result is available within a short time. In addition to CSF, capsular polysaccharide can be demonstrated in blood and urine by CCIE.

Chemotherapy

Treatment with penicillin should be started as soon as pneumococcal pneumonia is suspected. Penicillin-resistant pneumococci do not form penicillinase. The available evidence suggests that the resistance is chromosomally determined and it may be due to the changes in the penicillin-binding proteins in the cell membrane. In case of infection with penicillin-resistant strains or if the patient is penicillin sensitive then any of the cephalosporins, erythromycin, tetracycline, clindamycin, vancomycin, chloramphenicol and sulphonamides may be used.

KEY FACTS

- Pneumococci are Gram-positive, non-motile cocci occurring in pairs. They are capsulated. The capsule encloses each pair
- Acquisition of DNA by a bacterium from its environment was first demonstrated in *Streptococcus pneumoniae* by Griffith in 1928
- Pneumococci cause pneumonia, otitis media and meningitis

IMPORTANT QUESTIONS

1. Tabulate differences between viridans streptococci and *Streptococcus pneumoniae*.
2. Describe pathogenicity and laboratory diagnosis of *Streptococcus pneumoniae* infection.

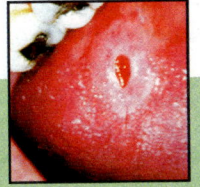

Chapter 22

Neisseria

The genus *Neisseria* has Gram-negative cocci with adjacent sides flattened. Important species of the genus *Neisseria* are *N. meningitidis*, *N. gonorrhoeae*, *N. flavescens*, *N. subflava*, *N. sicca*, *N. mucosa*, *N. lactamica* and *N. polysacchareae*. **N. gonorrhoeae and N. meningitidis are the primary human pathogens of the genus.** *N. gonorrhoeae* is always pathogenic, but *N. meningitidis* may be found as a commensal inhabitant of the upper respiratory tract of carriers. Other species are commonly found as commensals in the upper respiratory tract. However, *N. flavescens*, *N. subflava* and *N. lactamica* may rarely cause meningitis in man. Pathogenic *Neisseria* species are fastidious organisms, requiring enriched media for optimal recovery.

NEISSERIA MENINGITIDIS (MENINGOCOCCUS)

Morphology

They are Gram-negative cocci, 0.6–0.8 µm in diameter. They usually occur in pairs with adjacent sides flattened or concave and long axes parallel. They are typically seen in large numbers inside polymorphonuclear leucocytes (Fig. 22.1). Fresh isolates of most *N. meningitidis* serogroups are encapsulated. They are non-sporing and non-motile.

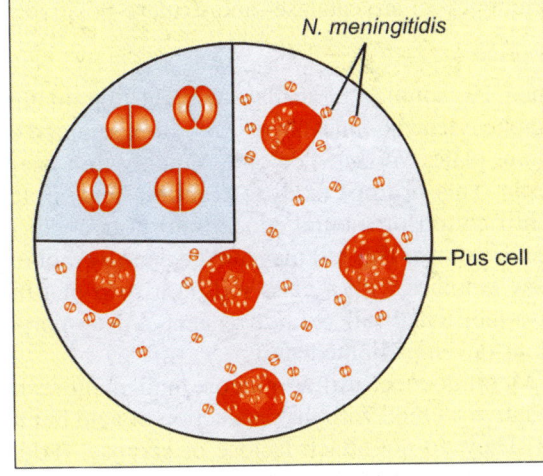

Fig. 22.1. *Neisseria meningitidis* in CSF. Inset: enlarged view showing adjacent sides flattened or concave and long axes parallel.

Cultural characteristics

Meningococci have exacting growth requirements and do not grow on ordinary media. Growth occurs on media enriched with blood or serum. These substances are believed to promote growth by neutralizing certain inhibitory substances found in culture media rather than by providing additional nutrients. However, they grow well on trypticase-soy agar and Mueller-Hinton medium without the addition of blood or serum. They are strict aerobes, no growth occurring anaerobically. The growth is facilitated by 5–10% CO_2 and high humidity. The optimum temperature and pH for the growth of meningococci are 35–36°C and 7.0–7.4 respectively.

- On **blood agar**, after 24 hour incubation, the colonies of meningococci are small about 1 mm in diameter, round, convex, grey, non-haemolytic and translucent. After 48 hours incubation, colonies are larger with an opaque raised centre and thin transparent margins which may be crenated.
- On **heated blood agar** (**chocolate agar**), colonies of meningococci are slightly larger than those on ordinary blood agar.

Biochemical characters

Meningococci are catalase- and oxidase-positive.

Oxidase test

When 1% solution of oxidase reagent (tetramethyl paraphenylenediamine dihydrochloride) is poured on culture plate, *Neisseria* colonies quickly turn deep-purple. This **prompt oxidase reaction** helps in the identification of meningococci and gonococci in mixed cultures. This test may also be done by rubbing a few colonies with a glass rod on a strip of filter paper moistened with oxidase reagent. A deep-purple colour develops immediately.

Meningococci utilize glucose and maltose by oxidative method with the production of acid but no gas. They do not attack lactose or sucrose. Indole and hydrogen sulphide are not produced and nitrates are not reduced.

Sensitivity to physical and chemical agents

In culture, meningococci die out in a few days. They are killed by heating at 55°C in 5 minutes or less. They are highly susceptible to desiccation and oxidation, death occurring usually within an hour or two. Weak disinfectants such as 1% phenol or 1% mercuric chloride kill them in 1–2 minutes.

Antigenic structure

N. meningitidis possesses a polysaccharide capsule and on the basis of immunologic specificity of capsular polysaccharide it has been subdivided into 12 serogroups – A, B, C, X, Y, Z, 29E, W-135, H, I, K and L. With the exception of group D, the capsular polysaccharide of these groups have all been chemically characterized. Most meningococcal infections are caused by strains of groups A, B and C with a small proportion of infections being due to strains of groups Y and W-135. Groups X, Z and 29E are only rarely associated with some form of immune deficiency. Serogroups H, I, K and L have been isolated from carriers and have not been associated with disease.

Pathogenicity

Meningococci are normally carried in nasopharynx of 5–10% of healthy individuals. During epidemics the carrier rate of the epidemic strains may range from 20–90%. **An increase in carrier rate heralds the onset of an epidemic.** The carrier state may last for a few days to months. The average carriage in a nonepidemic setting is 10 months. The carrier rate is higher in the members of the household of a patient with meningococcal disease. **The meningococcal carrier is important in the transmission of meningococci and provides reservoir of infection.** Human resistance to meningococcal disease is relatively high and the incidence of healthy carriers is invariably higher than that of the cases of the disease.

Like most of the respiratory infections, meningo-coccal meningitis is disseminated by droplet infection, direct contact and less often by fomites. Infection is spread by patients and convalescents to a limited extent, but the healthy carriers of meningo-cocci are of primary importance. The meningococcal disease can be divided into three stages:

1. First stage

The organisms appear in nasopharynx leading to **nasopharyngeal infection**, which is usually asymptomatic but might result in a minor inflammation. This state may last for days to months and will induce the formation of protective antibodies within a week, even though the infection remains asymptomatic.

2. Second stage

In a small percentage of cases, the meningococci may enter the blood stream from posterior nasopharynx, probably by way of the cervical lymph nodes. This stage is known as **meningococcaemia**. The patient develops **fever, malaise and petechial skin lesions** due to foci of infection in the capillaries. The organisms may also cause lesions in the joints and lungs and, rarely, may cause massive bilateral haemorrhages in the adrenals. This is known as **Waterhouse-Friderichsen syndrome**.

The haemorrhagic lesions occurring in both the skin and internal organs, particularly the adrenals, are believed to be due to the release of endotoxin. Meningococci possess pili, which probably allow intimate contact with host cells, and the organisms appear to release endotoxin. Meningococci may also result in a condition known as **disseminated intravascular coagulation (DIC)**. In such situations, blood clots may block circulation to the extremities, necessitating amputation.

3. Third stage

Meningococci infect the meninges causing the major symptoms of severe headache, stiff neck and vomiting accompanied by delirium and confusion. The route of spread of meningococcus from the nasopharynx to the meninges is controversial. The organisms may spread along the perineural sheaths of the olfactory nerves, passing through the cribriform plate may reach the subarachnoid space or it may set up a preliminary sinusitis and reach the brain either via lymphatics or direct extension through the bone. Others believe that the meningococci reach the CNS via blood stream through a preliminary bacteraemia. In the favour of the latter are:

- the frequent positive blood cultures in the early stages of infection;
- the purpuric rash in many cases with the isolation of meningococci from the skin lesions; and
- the occurrence, particularly during epidemics of meningococcal septicaemia with rash but no clinical meningitis.

Meningococci may occasionally cause acute urethritis, epididymitis, vulvovaginitis and cervicitis. In the absence of complete laboratory identification of the etiologic agent these conditions would be labelled as gonococcal infections.

Laboratory diagnosis (Flowchart 22.1)

Specimens

CSF, blood, aspirate from skin lesions, pus from infected joint and throat, nasopharyngeal and in some cases genital swabs. Swabs should be transported in Stuart's transport medium. All specimens where meningococcal infection is suspected must be submitted to the laboratory immediately.

Cerebrospinal fluid

In meningococcal meningitis, CSF is under pressure and is turbid due to a large number of poly-morphonuclear leucocytes present in a typical case. For bacteriological examination, the CSF is divided into three portions.

One portion is centrifuged and Gram-stained smears are prepared from the deposit. Meningococci will be seen mainly inside polymorphs, but often extracellularly also. Strains causing meningitis are usually encapsulated and may show a distinct pink halo surrounding the cells. The capsule may also make the cells more resistant to decolourization and they may appear Gram-positive. When present in small numbers, meningococci may be detected by immunofluorescent technique. The supernatant contains meningococcal antigen, which may be demonstrated by precipitation test with polyvalent or monovalent antimeningococcal serum. Counter-immunoelectrophoresis provides a rapid and sensitive method for demonstration of meningococcal antigen.

Second portion of CSF is inoculated on blood agar or chocolate agar and incubated at 35–36°C under 5–10% CO_2. Colonies appear after 18–24 hours which may be identified by morphological and biochemical reactions. The meningococcus isolated may be typed by agglutination with polyvalent or monovalent antimeningococcal serum.

Third portion of CSF is incubated for 18–24 hours, either as such or after adding an equal volume of glucose broth and then subcultured on blood agar or chocolate agar. This method may sometimes succeed where direct plating fails.

Blood culture

Blood culture is often positive in meningococcaemia and in early cases of meningitis. Specimen of blood is inoculated into blood culture bottle of trypticase-

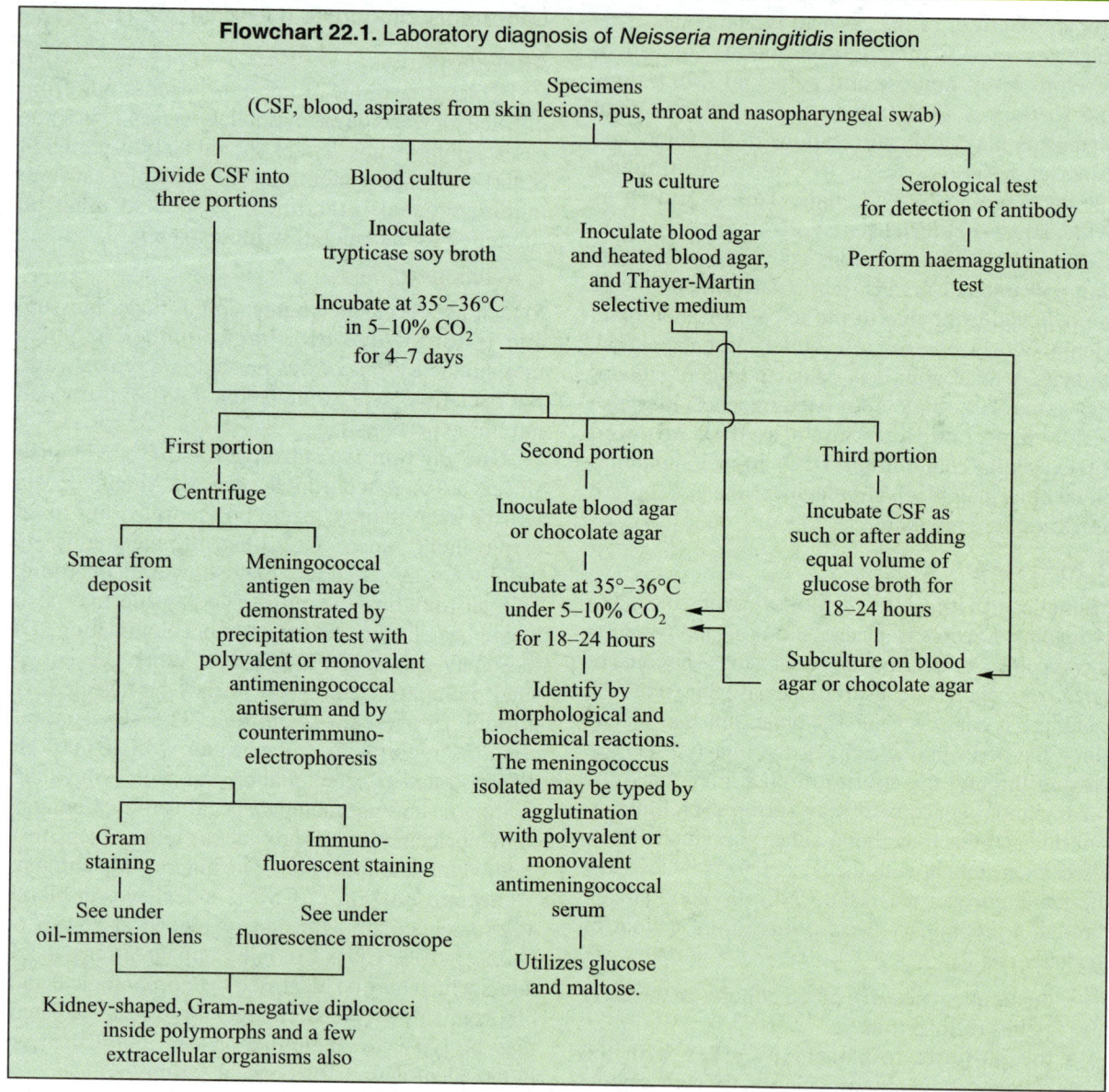

Flowchart 22.1. Laboratory diagnosis of *Neisseria meningitidis* infection

Specimens
(CSF, blood, aspirates from skin lesions, pus, throat and nasopharyngeal swab)

Divide CSF into three portions

Blood culture
|
Inoculate trypticase soy broth
|
Incubate at 35°–36°C in 5–10% CO_2 for 4–7 days

Pus culture
|
Inoculate blood agar and heated blood agar, and Thayer-Martin selective medium

Serological test for detection of antibody
|
Perform haemagglutination test

First portion
|
Centrifuge

Smear from deposit

Meningococcal antigen may be demonstrated by precipitation test with polyvalent or monovalent antimeningococcal antiserum and by counterimmuno-electrophoresis

Gram staining
|
See under oil-immersion lens

Immuno-fluorescent staining
|
See under fluorescence microscope

Kidney-shaped, Gram-negative diplococci inside polymorphs and a few extracellular organisms also

Second portion
|
Inoculate blood agar or chocolate agar
|
Incubate at 35°–36°C under 5–10% CO_2 for 18–24 hours
|
Identify by morphological and biochemical reactions. The meningococcus isolated may be typed by agglutination with polyvalent or monovalent antimeningococcal serum
|
Utilizes glucose and maltose.

Third portion
|
Incubate CSF as such or after adding equal volume of glucose broth for 18–24 hours
|
Subculture on blood agar or chocolate agar

soy broth. It should be incubated at 35–36°C in 5–10% CO_2 for 4–7 days, with daily subcultures on blood agar. Look for oxidase-positive colonies of Gram-negative diplococci as above.

Pus aspiration and swabs

In addition to blood agar and heated blood agar, **Thayer-Martin selective medium** is used for the culture of materials expected to yield a mixture of organisms. These include pus, aspirates, and throat, nasopharyngeal and genital swabs. Vancomycin, colistin and nystatin which are present in Thayer-Martin medium inhibit Gram-positive bacteria, Gram-negative bacteria and yeast contaminants respectively, while allowing the growth of pathogenic *Neisseria*. Meningococci may sometimes be demonstrated in petechial lesions by microscopy and culture.

Serological diagnosis

This may be attempted in cases of chronic meningo-coccal septicaemia where no organisms have been isolated. Specific antibodies to capsular poly-saccharide may be demonstrated by haemaggluti-nation test.

Polymerase chain reaction (PCR)

Meningococcal DNA in CSF or blood can be amplified and detected by PCR.

Treatment

Almost all clinical isolates of *N. meningitidis* are sensitive to penicillin. Penicillin G in high doses, given intravenously or intrathecally, if necessary, is the treatment of choice. In penicillin sensitive individuals, chloramphenicol has been regarded as an alternative to penicillin therapy for meningococcal meningitis but recent studies show that cefotaxime or ceftriaxone are at least as effective and avoid the possibility of blood dyscrasia. All these drugs have the advantage of being effective against *Haemophilus influenzae* and *Streptococcus pneumoniae*, the other two principal causes of meningitis in childhood after neonatal period.

At the end of a course of therapy with penicillin, it is important to give eradicative treatment with rifampin or ciprofloxacin, because penicillin does not eradicate *N. meningitidis* from the nasopharynx and a patient returning home as a carrier may infect others. This probably does not apply to cefotaxime or ceftriaxone.

Prophylaxis

Chemoprophylaxis

Outbreaks of disease may be controlled by chemo-prophylaxis alone.
- **Rifampin** is recommended for chemoprophylaxis in children although it is effective in eradicating meningococcal carriage in only 80–90% of the population treated. After prophylaxis, rifampin-resistant strains may be found in a small number of patients and may on rare occasions give rise to disease in contacts.
- **Ciprofloxacin** is widely used as a prophylactic for adolescents and adults as a single oral dose.

All household and intimate contacts of a case should be given a chemoprophylaxis as a routine.

Vaccines

Vaccines containing group-specific capsular poly-saccharides of meningococci of groups A, C, Y and W-135 are available and are good immunogens. Vaccines containing all four polysaccharides are used in some countries for immunization of military recruits. For civilian purposes, a vaccine containing A and C polysaccharides alone is adequate. The protection provided by the vaccine is group-specific and lasts for at least three years but does not prevent meningococcal carriage. At present, no vaccine is available against group B meningococci because capsular polysaccharide of this group is a poor immunogen.

NEISSERIA GONORRHOEAE (GONOCOCCUS)

Morphology

Morphology and staining characteristics of *N. gonorrhoeae* are similar to those of *N. meningitidis*.

Cultural characteristics

Gonococci are more difficult to grow than meningo-cocci. They are aerobes, but may grow anaerobically also. Addition of 5–10% CO_2 is essential for primary isolation. Growth occurs best at pH 7.0–7.4 and at a temperature of 35–36°C. They can be isolated on media enriched with blood, either partially lysed by heat (chocolate agar) or completely lysed by saponin.

Heated blood agar may be made selective for the isolation of pathogenic neisseriae by the addition of vancomycin, colistin and nystatin. This selective medium (**Thayer-Martin medium**) is valuable in isolating gonococci from heavily contaminated specimens. Trimethoprim may be added to Thayer-Martin medium to inhibit swarming *Proteus* species that are occasionally present in cervicovaginal and rectal specimens. This chocolate agar medium containing vancomycin, colistin, nystatin and trimethoprim is known as **modified Thayer-Martin medium**.

- On **heated blood agar**, after 24 hour incubation, colonies are small about 1 mm in diameter, grey, convex and translucent. After 48 hour incubation, colonies are larger 1.5–2.5 mm in diameter, sometimes with an opaque raised centre and thin transparent margins which may be crenated.
- On **Thayer-Martin medium** growth is slower, although colonies are similar to those on heated blood agar.

On the basis of colonial appearance, auto-agglutinability and virulence, Kellogg divided gono-cocci into four types (T1–T4). Type T1 and T2 form brown colonies, bear numerous pili and are designated as P+ and P++ respectively. They are auto-agglutinable and virulent. Types T3 and T4 form larger, granular, non-pigmented colonies, are non-piliated (P−), form smooth suspensions and are avirulent.

Biochemical reactions

N. gonorrhoeae resembles *N. meningitidis* with the exception that the former can utilize only glucose and the latter glucose and maltose with the production of acid only.

Antigenic structure

N. gonorrhoeae is antigenically heterogeneous. Surface structures include the following:

1. Pili: Pili are nonflagellar surface appendages. These are hair-like structures, several micrometers in length, 7 nm in diameter and are seen on the surface of gonococci of types T1 and T2. These play an important role in attachment of gonococci to the cell. Furthermore, the pili are antiphagocytic. Removal of pili from cells by treatment with trypsin results in their phagocytosis and destruction.

2. Outer membrane proteins: Gonococci possess three major outer membrane proteins named proteins I, II and III. Protein II appears to be associated with the adherence of the gonococci to the host cells.

3. Lipooligosaccharide (LOS): It differs in its chemical structure from lipopolysaccharide (LPS) of Gram-negative bacilli. It does not have long O antigenic side chains. Toxicity in gonococcal infections is largely due to the endotoxic effect of LOS.

Antigenic variation

N. gonorrhoeae and *N. meningitidis* are among several organisms whose surface structures are known to change antigenically from generation to generation during growth of a single strain. The mechanism involved has been more extensively studied in gonococci but appears to be similar in both the species. The antigenic structures of major interest are pili, protein II and LOS, for which there is evidence of antigenic variation both *in vitro* and *in vivo*.

Sensitivity to physical and chemical agents

N. gonorrhoeae is a very delicate organism. It is readily killed by heat, drying and antiseptics. It may remain viable for a day or so in pus contaminating linen or other fabrics. In cultures, gonococci die in 3–4 days at room temperature. Freeze-drying is the most reliable method for long-term storage of gonococci.

Pathogenesis

N. gonorrhoeae causes **gonorrhoea**. It is a sexually transmitted disease that, with few exceptions, is acquired through sexual contact with an infected individual. *N. gonorrhoeae* is **exclusively a human pathogen** although chimpanzees have been infected by artificial inoculation. It is never found as a commensal although a proportion of those infected, particularly women, may remain asymptomatic. These may develop systemic or ascending infection at a later stage.

Gonococci ordinarily enter the body through the mucous membrane of the genitourinary tract, apparently penetrating between columnar epithelial cells. Stratified squamous epithelium is relatively resistant to infection. After an incubation period of 2–7 days, the organism evokes an acute inflammatory response in the subepithelial tissue giving rise to the purulent urethral or vaginal discharge, dysuria and frequency of micturition. In male, the acute urethritis may extend to the prostate, testes, seminal vesicles, epididymis and sometimes the periurethral tissue. If untreated it is often followed by fibrosis and stricture.

In women, the endocervix is the primary site of infection. The urethra may also become infected. **In** adult women, the vagina usually escapes because of the acidic pH of the vaginal secretions, but severe vulvovaginitis can occur in prepubertal girls. The primary infection may spread from urethra, vagina and cervix to Bartholin's glands, uterus, fallopian tubes, ovaries and pelvic peritoneum causing a pelvic inflammatory disease resulting in sterility. Bacteraemia may occur in fulminating cases, in both men and women, and is occasionally complicated by endocarditis, acute purulent arthritis or both.

- Babies born to infected women may contract serious gonococcal infection of the eye (**ophthalmia neonatorum**) during passage through infected birth canal.
- **Anorectal infection** occurs in both sexes. In men this follows homosexual rectal intercourse. In women, it can follow rectal intercourse, but may also arise as a result of autoinoculation of rectal mucosa with infected vaginal discharge (direct contagious spread).

- **Gonococcal pharyngitis** may follow orogenital contact in either sex.
- **Conjunctivitis** may occur usually by auto-inoculation with fingers.

Laboratory diagnosis (Flowchart 22.2)

Specimen swab is collected from urethra, endocervix, anal canal, vagina (in case of paediatric patient), Bartholin's glands, oropharynx and conjunctival swab. Disinfectants should not be used when preparing the patient for collection of specimen because small amounts of these may be toxic and impede the recovery of the organisms in culture. Calcium alginate and some cotton swabs have been shown to be inhibitory to *N. gonorrhoeae*, so Dacron or rayon swabs are preferred. These swabs should be either inoculated directly onto growth medium or transported to the laboratory in a transport medium such as Amies medium with charcoal and plated within 6 hours.

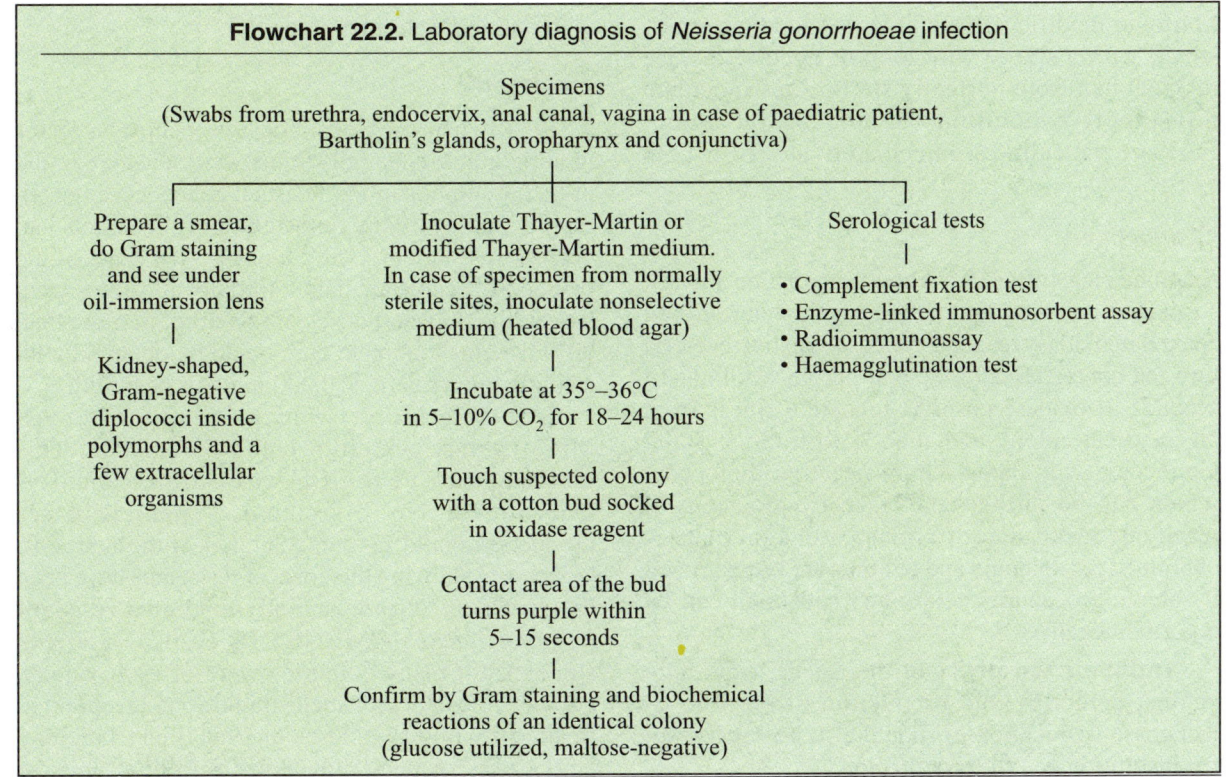

Flowchart 22.2. Laboratory diagnosis of *Neisseria gonorrhoeae* infection

Specimens
(Swabs from urethra, endocervix, anal canal, vagina in case of paediatric patient, Bartholin's glands, oropharynx and conjunctiva)

Prepare a smear, do Gram staining and see under oil-immersion lens
↓
Kidney-shaped, Gram-negative diplococci inside polymorphs and a few extracellular organisms

Inoculate Thayer-Martin or modified Thayer-Martin medium. In case of specimen from normally sterile sites, inoculate nonselective medium (heated blood agar)
↓
Incubate at 35°–36°C in 5–10% CO_2 for 18–24 hours
↓
Touch suspected colony with a cotton bud socked in oxidase reagent
↓
Contact area of the bud turns purple within 5–15 seconds
↓
Confirm by Gram staining and biochemical reactions of an identical colony (glucose utilized, maltose-negative)

Serological tests
↓
- Complement fixation test
- Enzyme-linked immunosorbent assay
- Radioimmunoassay
- Haemagglutination test

Microscopy

Prepare smear by rolling the swab gently over the surface of a glass slide in one direction only. Do not rub swab, it may distort microscopic morphology. Do the Gram staining and see under oil-immersion lens. The observation of characteristic kidney-shaped Gram-negative diplococci lying within polymorpho-nuclear leucocytes with a few extracellular organisms from a symptomatic male with discharge correlates at a rate of 95% with culture and presumptive evidence of gonococcal infection. If no organisms are visible on Gram staining, report the smear as negative.

Culture

All specimens received in the laboratory for recovery of *Neisseria* species should be held at room temperature and plated as soon as possible. Media should be warmed to room temperature before inoculation, because *Neisseria* species are susceptible to cold. Roll specimen swab firmly in a 'Z' pattern onto selective medium (Thayer-Martin or modified Thayer-Martin) and then cross-streak with a sterile wire loop or needle. In case of specimen from normally sterile sites inoculate nonselective medium (heated blood agar). Incubate the cultures immediately at 35–36°C in 5–10% CO_2.

Observation

Examine plates after 18–24 hours incubation and test suspected colonies by touching with a cotton bud soaked in oxidase reagent. Oxidase-positive bacteria turn the contact area of the bud purple within 5–15 seconds. If oxidase-positive, prepare a smear from an identical colony and stain it with Gram stain. Gonococci will appear Gram-negative diplococci which can be further confirmed by biochemical reactions. Incubation of primary isolation plate is continued for 48 hours and cultures are re-examined by above procedures before any specimen can be reported negative.

Antibiotic sensitivity of the isolate, especially against penicillin and production of enzyme β-lactamase (penicillinase) should also be carried out for instituting an effective therapy.

Serology

From some chronic cases or from some patients with metastatic lesions such as arthritis, it may not be possible to isolate gonococci in culture media. Serological tests may be of value in such cases. Antibodies of the IgG, IgM and IgA classes are produced during gonococcal infection. Complement fixation tests with suspensions or crude extracts of gonococci have been used for many years. These are not very sensitive and may also give non-specific results. Defined gonococcal antigens including pilar and outer membrane protein antigens, have been used in radioimmunoassay, ELISA andhaemagglutination tests.

Many of these new methods are much more sensitive than the original complement fixation test and may give useful results in high-risk groups. However, these tests may remain positive for months and years after the disease has been cured. Therefore, they do not distinguish present from past infections and give an appreciable proportion of false positive results. Some of these may be due to cross-reactions with antibodies to meningococci.

Treatment

In 1935, when sulphonamides were introduced for treating gonorrhoea, all strains were sensitive to the drug, but sulphonamide-resistant gonococci emerged rapidly and by 1946, almost 90% of the strains had become resistant in some countries. At the same time penicillin became available. Initially all strains were susceptible to small doses of this drug. In more than 90% patients complete cure could be obtained with a single injection of 150,000 units of penicillin.

By 1958, gonococci with reduced sensitivity (high MIC) against penicillin could be isolated. This resistance to penicillin was chromosomally-determined. No β-lactamase (penicillinase) production could be demonstrated in these strains. Gonococci showing this form of resistance have been designated as '**chromosomally-mediated resistant N. gonorrhoeae**' (**CMRNG**). By 1970, over 50% of strains from many countries were of such variety. Patients infected with such strains do not respond to treatment with usual doses of penicillin. Therefore, large doses of penicillin, 2.4–4.8 million units of aqueous procaine penicillin G intramuscularly, preceded by probenecid 1 gram orally is recommended. Ampicillin 3.5 gram + probenecid 1 gram is an effective oral alternative. However, ampicillin is not effective for the treatment of pharyngeal and anorectal gonorrhoea.

In 1976, **penicillinase-producing** *N. gonorrhoeae* (**PPNG**) were isolated from widely separated areas in the United States and in England. Such strains have since been found to be very prevalent in the Philippines, Singapore, Thailand and West Africa. Penicillinase production, in gonococci, is plasmid-mediated. Penicillin is ineffective in patients infected with such strains. Alternative drugs in PPNG infected cases include tetracycline and certain cephalosporins (cefoxitin, cefotaxime and ceftriaxone) in combination with probenecid.

Gonococcal ophthalmia neonatorum can be prevented by local application of 0.5% erythromycin or 1% tetracycline ophthalmic ointment to the conjunctiva of newborn.

Prophylaxis

Control of gonorrhoea consists of early detection of cases particularly those infected females who have asymptomatic infections. These cases should be treated. Because the incubation period of symptomatic gonorrhoea is short, tracing and treating the recent sexual contacts lessens the spread of the disease. Greater mobility and greater sexual freedom has contributed to the acquisition of gonorrhoea. Use of condom and health education can help in the control of the disease to a great extent.

KEY FACTS

- The genus *Neisseria* consists of **Gram-negative cocci**, usually arranged in pairs, and are **oxidase-positive**
- Two *Neisseria* species are pathogenic for humans—*Neisseria gonorrhoeae* (gonococcus), the causal agent of **gonorrhoea**; and *Neisseria meningitidis* (meningococcus), a frequent cause of **meningitis**
- Gonococci and meningococci are non-motile and usually occur in **pairs** with adjacent sides flattened or concave and long axes parallel. They are typically seen in large numbers **inside polymorphonuclear leucocytes**. They cannot be differentiated from each other under microscope. However, they can be differentiated in the laboratory by their **sugar utilization patterns**, and by the **sites of their primary infections**

IMPORTANT QUESTION

Discuss pathogenesis and laboratory diagnosis of:

(a) Meningococcal meningitis
(b) Gonorrhoea

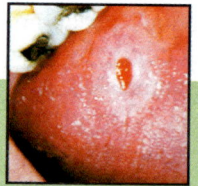

Chapter 23

Corynebacterium Diphtheriae

Corynebacteria are pleomorphic, club-shaped, Gram-positive bacilli arranged in V forms or palisades. The most important member of the genus *Coryne-bacterium* is *C. diphtheriae*. It was first observed and described by Klebs (1883) but was first cultured by Loeffler (1884). Therefore, it is known as the **Klebs-Loeffler bacillus**.

CORYNEBACTERIUM DIPHTHERIAE

Morphology

They are thin, slender, non-sporing, non-capsulated, non-motile, non-acid-fast, Gram-positive bacilli of varying lengths with an average size of 3 × 0.3 μm. They frequently possess club-shaped swellings at one or both ends, a characteristic feature which is responsible for the name of the genus (*coryne* means club). When dividing, the bacilli snap and bend abruptly and appear as angled pairs resembling letters V or L or parallel rows of 3–4 bacilli (palisades) which resemble Chinese letters (*Chinese letter arrangement* or *Cuneiform arrangement*) (Figs. 23.1 and 23.2).

Although Gram-positive, *C. diphtheriae* is readily decolourized. Another characteristic of this organism is its granular and uneven staining. When stained with methylene blue or toluidine blue, the granules in the cell stain metachromatically (i.e., granules that stain

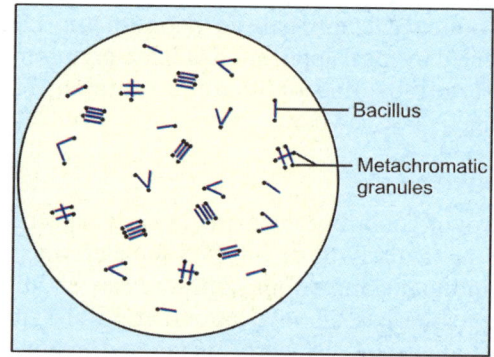

Fig. 23.1. *Corynebacterium diphtheriae* showing meta-chromatic granules and Chinese letter arrangement.

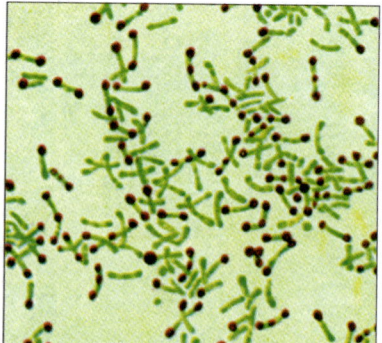

Fig. 23.2. *Corynebacterium diphtheriae* showing meta-chromatic granules.

a colour different from the primary dye colour) reddish-purple. Most cells contain 2 or 3 of these, and they tend to be on the poles. The granules consist of long-chain inorganic polyphosphates. These granules are known as **metachromatic granules** or **volutin granules** or **Babes-Ernst bodies**. In unstained wet preparations, they appear as round refractile bodies within the bacterial cytoplasm.

With Albert stain, the granules stain bluish-black and the cytoplasm green. The granules are not seen during active growth, but start to appear towards the end of the logarithmic growth period. The granule formation is best seen on Loeffler's serum slope. It appears that they represent storage depots for materials needed to form high-energy phosphate bonds. Their presence in thin slender bacilli helps to distinguish *C. diphtheriae* from short, thick, plumpy, non-pathogenic diphtheroids which lack them.

Cultural characteristics

Diphtheria bacillus is an aerobe and facultative anaerobe, has an optimum temperature for growth of 37°C (range 15–40°C). It can grow on ordinary nutrient agar, but its growth is improved by the presence of animal proteins such as serum or blood. Two media are useful for this purpose:

1. **Loeffler's serum slope:** Diphtheria bacilli grow rapidly on Loeffler's serum slope, and colonies can be seen in 6–8 hours, long before other bacteria grow. The colonies are at first small, white, opaque discs, but on continued incubation increase in size and may acquire a yellow tint.

2. **Blood tellurite agar (BTA):** The addition of 0.03–0.04% potassium tellurite (K_2TeO_3) makes the medium selective for corynebacteria by inhibiting most other pathogenic and commensal bacteria. It may retard the growth even of corynebacteria so that colonies may be very small after 24 hours, therefore, incubation should be continued for 48 hours. On this medium, colonies of *C. diphtheriae* become grey to black because tellurite or tellurous ions are able to diffuse through the cell wall and membrane and are reduced to tellurium metal, which is precipitated inside the cell.

On the basis of colonial morphology on BTA, diphtheria bacilli can be divided into three biotypes – mitis, intermedius and gravis (Table 23.1). These names were originally proposed to relate to the clinical severity of the disease produced by the three biotypes. Mitis, intermedius and gravis biotypes produce disease of mild, intermediate and severe variety respectively. However, this association is not constant. In general, biotype mitis is predominant in endemic areas, while intermedius and gravis tend to be epidemic.

Biochemical reactions

C. diphtheriae ferments glucose, maltose and on rare occasions sucrose with the production of acid without gas. It does not ferment lactose, mannitol and trehalose. For biochemical differentiation of three biotypes of *C. diphtheriae*, starch and glycogen are used. Gravis strains ferment both but intermedius and mitis strains ferment neither.

The fermentation tests are usually done by culture for 24 hours at 37°C in **Hiss's serum peptone water medium**. Calf or rabbit serum should be used in the medium, because some batches of ox and sheep sera contain a saccharolytic enzyme that gives rise to false positive results. *C. diphtheriae* is H_2S-positive and reduces nitrate to nitrite. It does not liquefy gelatin or hydrolyze urea.

Most strains of the biotype mitis show β-haemolysis on sheep, rabbit or horse blood, gravis strains are often weakly haemolytic, but intermedius strains are non-haemolytic (Table 23.1).

Susceptibility to physical and chemical agents

C. diphtheriae is readily killed by moist heat at 58°C in 10 minutes, and by the commonly used disinfectants. It is, however, relatively resistant to drying and may remain alive for weeks in dust and on fomites when dry and protected from sunlight.

Toxin production

Toxigenic strains of *C. diphtheriae* produce a potent exotoxin which is an iron-free, crystalline, heat-labile protein. Its molecular weight is 61,150 daltons and is made up of two parts – A and B with molecular

Table 23.1. Differentiation of three biotypes of *Corynebacterium diphtheriae*

Character	Gravis	Intermedius	Mitis
1. Morphology	Uniformly stained short rods. Some degree of pleomorphism with irregularly barred tear-drop forms. Few or no granules.	Long, irregularly barred cigar-shaped rods, highly pleomorphic. Poor granulation.	Long, curved, pleomorphic, wispy rods with terminal swellings. Prominent granulation.
2. Colony characters on blood tellurite agar after 18–24 hours incubation	Dull greyish black, opaque colonies, 1.5–2.5 mm in diameter. In 2–3 days, 3–5 mm in diameter flat colony with raised dark centre, radially striated periphery and crenated edge – 'daisy-head' colony.	Small (0.5–0.75 mm in diameter), grey colony with a darker centre and a shining surface – 'frog's egg' colony. There is little change in size after 48 hours incubation.	Grey, opaque colonies, 1.5–2.0 mm in diameter with regular margins and glossy smooth surface. On further incubation the colony becomes flat with central elevation and regular margins – 'poached egg' colony.
3. Haemolysis of sheep, rabbit and horse blood	Weakly haemolytic	Non-haemolytic	β-haemolytic
4. Growth in broth	Surface pellicle, granular deposit and little or no turbidity	Uniform turbidity with fine granular deposit	Uniform turbidity with pellicle later
5. Fermentation of starch and glycogen	+	–	–
6. Serotypes	13	4	40
7. Toxigenic strains	Almost 100%	95–99%	80–85%
8. Predominant strains in	Epidemic areas	Epidemic areas	Endemic areas

weights of 21,150 and 40,000 daltons respectively. Fragment B is required for transport of fragment A into the cell where it inhibits polypeptide chain elongation at the ribosome. Inhibition of protein synthesis is probably responsible for both the necrotic and neurotoxic effects of the toxin. When the toxin is treated with formalin it is converted into toxoid.

Almost all strains of gravis, 95–99% of intermedius and 80–85% of mitis produce this toxin. However, toxin produced by different biotypes is antigenically similar. The classic **Park-Williams strain (PW8)** of *C. diphtheriae* isolated in 1896, is still used as a source of toxin for preparation of diphtheria toxoid (vaccine).

Lysogeny and toxin production

Only those strains of *C. diphtheriae* which are lysogenic for β phage or related temperate phages produce diphtheria toxin. Non-toxigenic strains may be rendered toxigenic by infecting them with β phage.

This is known as **lysogenic** or **phage conversion**. The toxigenicity remains only as long as the bacillus is lysogenic. When the bacillus is cured of its phage, as by growing it in the presence of antiphage serum, it loses the toxigenicity. The structural gene (*tox* gene) for diphtheria toxin resides on phage genome and is expressed under certain nutritional conditions.

Iron concentration and toxin production

Diphtheria toxin is produced most actively, *in vitro*, when iron concentration is decreased, although other factors such as osmotic pressure, amino acid concentrations and pH also have a role. Optimum iron concentration for toxin production is 0.1 mg per litre of the medium. Toxin production stops at 0.5 mg per litre of the medium. Reason for this is not known. The repressor of the *tox* gene appears to be an iron containing protein. When sufficient iron is present suppressor is formed which inhibits toxin production.

Pathogenicity

C. diphtheriae causes natural infection only in man. Experimental infection can, however, be produced in various laboratory animals. Infection spreads directly from person to person via nasopharyngeal secretions. Spread is facilitated by intimate contact. Most clinical infections are probably contracted from carriers rather than symptomatic patients. Nasal carriers are particularly dangerous because they shed large number of bacilli which may survive for many weeks in dust and on dry fomites. Children are susceptible after the age of 3–6 months when passive immunity derived from maternal antibodies has disappeared. Incidence is highest among young children, but outbreaks also occur among teenagers and young adults.

Incubation period is 3–4 days, however, it may be as short as 1 day. When toxigenic diphtheria bacilli become lodged in the throat of a susceptible individual, they first multiply rapidly on epithelial cells and produce an exotoxin (diphtheria toxin) that causes local tissue necrosis. The organisms then multiply in cell debris, produce more toxin leading to enlargement of the lesion. The combination of cell necrosis and an exudative inflammatory response of tissue leads to an accumulation of necrotic cellular material, erythrocytes, fibrin and bacteria, which forms a characteristic **diphtheritic pseudomembrane** (in Latin *diphtheria* means pseudomembrane) varying in colour from white to grey to yellow. Since epithelial cells of the mucosa are incorporated in the pseudomembrane, therefore, attempts to remove it produce bleeding.

Diphtheritic pseudomembrane usually appears first on tonsils or posterior pharyngeal wall. The infection may then spread either upwards into nasal passages or downwards into the larynx and trachea. In laryngeal diphtheria, mechanical obstruction may cause suffocation unless the airway is restored by intubation or tracheostomy.

Diphtheria bacilli do not, as a rule, penetrate deeply in the underlying tissues, or the blood, but they produce a powerful exotoxin. Toxin is absorbed into the blood stream from the site of infection and causes toxaemia and various systemic complications. The toxin has a **special affinity for certain tissues, notably heart muscles, nerve endings and adrenal glands**. Death often results from cardiac failure, but necrotic and often haemorrhagic lesions are usually seen in many organs at necropsy, and in laryngeal diphtheria death is due to suffocation caused by mechanical obstruction.

Although diphtheria is usually a disease of the upper respiratory tract, primary or secondary lesions may occur in other parts of body. The most common nonrespiratory site is the skin (**cutaneous diphtheria**). In cutaneous diphtheria, lesions usually appear at the site of minor abrasions as chronic, spreading, nonhealing ulcers covered by greyish membrane. Rarely, diphtherial infections of conjunctiva, cornea, vagina and ear may occur. These are almost always secondary to pharyngeal or skin infection.

The degree of toxaemia is influenced by the site of infection and the size of the local lesion. Toxin is more readily absorbed from the nasopharyngeal mucosa than from laryngotracheal lesions, and lesions of skin differ from those elsewhere in being associated with lower degree of toxaemia.

Laboratory diagnosis (Flowchart 23.1)

Because early administration of antitoxin is of paramount importance, specific treatment should be instituted immediately on suspicion of diphtheria, without waiting for laboratory confirmation. The disease runs a quick course and any delay may be fatal. Laboratory confirmation of diphtheria is necessary for the initiation of control measures and for epidemiological purposes. Diagnosis of diphtheria is based on isolating *C. diphtheriae* from the infected area and demonstrating its toxin-producing ability.

Specimens

Two swabs are taken from the local lesion which is usually in the throat but may also be in the nose, larynx, ear, conjunctiva, vagina and skin or from the nose and throat of contacts or suspected carriers. No antiseptics, in the form of gargles, etc., must have been applied within 12 hours. The swabs should be rubbed over the affected area and pseudomembrane, if formed, should be scraped with swab stick or where there is no definitely localized lesion the swabs

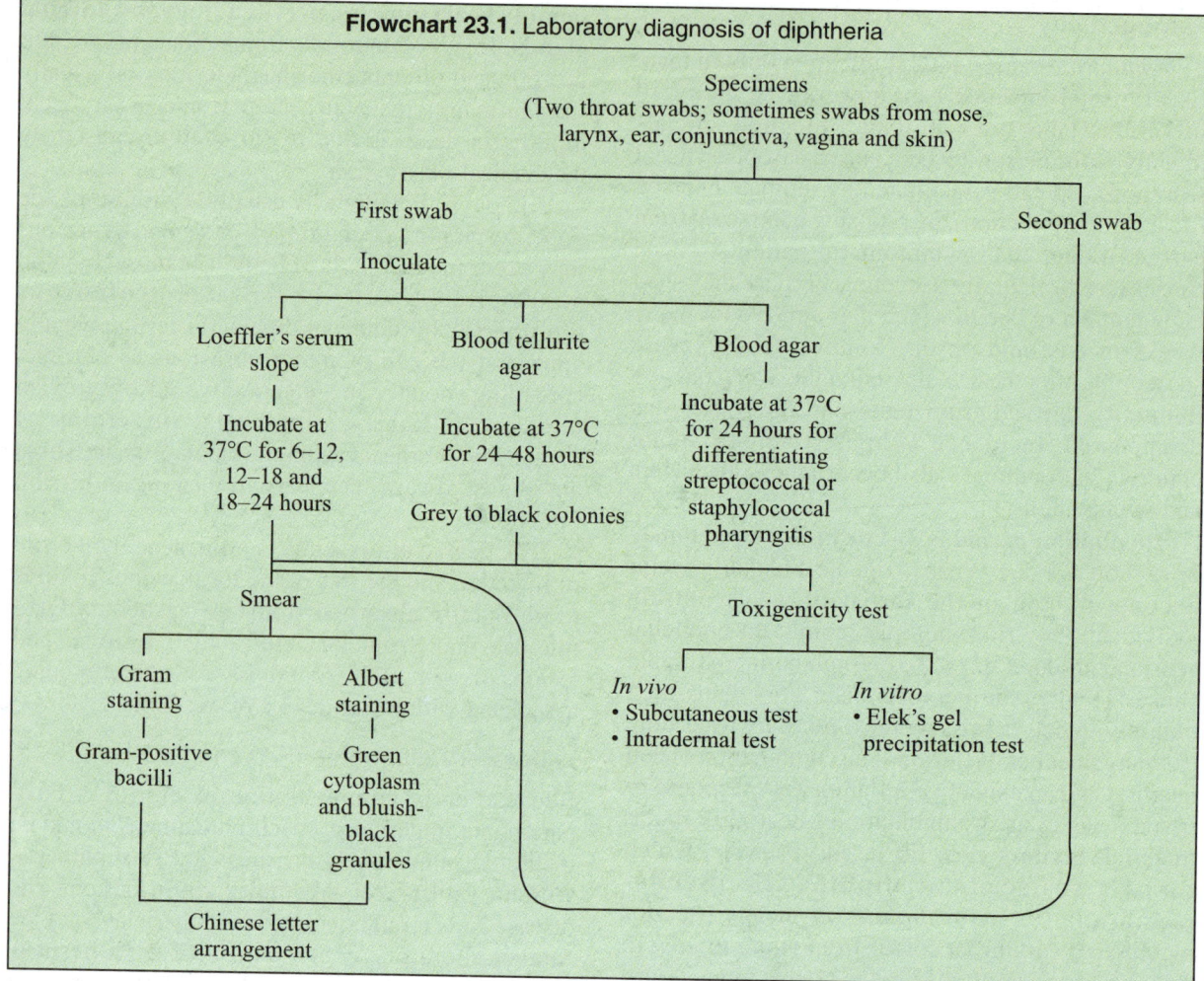

Flowchart 23.1. Laboratory diagnosis of diphtheria

should be rubbed over the mucous membrane of posterior pharyngeal wall and tonsils.

Microscopy and culture

One swab should be inoculated on Loeffler's serum slope, blood tellurite agar and a plate of ordinary blood agar, the last for differentiating streptococcal or staphylococcal pharyngitis, which may simulate diphtheria. All these media are incubated at 37°C. Loeffler's serum slope is examined after 12–18 hours. If an early result is urgently required then culture may be examined after 6–12 hours, but if it is negative the examination must be repeated after 18–24 hours.

The resultant growth is mixed by emulsifying it with a wire loop in the condensation fluid and from this smears are made and stained by Gram and Albert methods. Blood tellurite agar is examined after 24 hours, and after 48 hours if no growth is obtained after 24 hours. The growth is identified by colonial morphology, Gram staining, Albert staining and biochemical reactions (Table 23.1).

With the **second swab, two smears** are prepared and stained by Gram and Albert methods, but only in a small proportion of cases can positive results be obtained in this way and cultures should always be made as a routine procedure, irrespective of direct examination. Smear from Loeffler's serum slope may be the first indication of the presence of diphtheria bacillus.

Toxigenicity or virulence tests of C. diphtheriae

The identification of an isolate as *C. diphtheriae* does not mean that the patient has diphtheria. Diagnosis of diphtheria depends on showing that the isolate produces diphtheria toxin. This can be done by either *in vivo* or *in vitro* testing. *In vivo* testing is rarely done because the *in vitro* method is reliable, less expensive, and free from the need to use animal.

1. *In vivo*
   - Subcutaneous test
   - Intradermal test
2. *In vitro*
   - Elek's gel precipitation test

Subcutaneous test

Emulsify the growth from an overnight culture on Loeffler's serum slope in 2–4 ml broth and inject 0.8 ml of the emulsion subcutaneously into two guinea pigs, one of which has been protected with intramuscular injection of 500 units of diphtheria antitoxin 18–24 hours previously. If the strain is virulent, the unprotected animal will die within four days.

Perform autopsy on any of the animals dying within this period. If the isolate is toxigenic then the unprotected animal shows:

- Gelatinous haemorrhagic oedema at the site of inoculation.
- Blood-stained pleural and peritoneal exudate.
- Haemorrhagic inflammation of adrenal glands.

If neither animal dies, the culture is non-toxigenic. If both animals die, the culture is virulent or toxigenic, but not *C. diphtheriae*. This method is usually not employed because the animal is sacrificed.

Intradermal test

Inoculate one colony of suspected *C. diphtheriae* isolate from BTA on a moist Loeffler's serum slope. Incubate at 37°C for 24 hours. Prepare a dense suspension of culture on this medium in 3 ml broth and inject 0.1 ml of this intradermally into the shaved side of a guinea-pig or rabbit. After four hours, the animal is injected intraperitoneally with 500 units of antitoxin. Thirty minutes later a second sample of the test suspension is injected intradermally on the opposite side.

Non-specific inflammatory reaction may occur at both sites within 24–48 hours, but if toxigenic bacilli are present, only the site injected before the antitoxin was administered will progress to form a characteristic necrotic lesion in 48–72 hours. With this test first injection acts as test and second as control and about five strains (10 injections) can be tested on each animal. Moreover, the animal does not die. Therefore, intradermal test is better than subcutaneous test.

Elek's gel precipitation test

This is a gel precipitation test. Pipette 10 ml of nutrient agar that has been cooled to 55°C in a water bath and 2 ml sterile calf serum in a petri dish and rotate 20 times to mix. Before the medium solidifies, place a 1 cm × 8 cm filter paper strip that has been soaked in the diphtheria antitoxin 500–1,000 units/ml across the middle of the plate on the surface of the agar. Allow the medium to solidify and then place the plate in the incubator with the lid ajar to allow the surface moisture to evaporate.

Inoculate the plate within 2 hours after drying by streaking a heavy inoculum of the culture to be tested across the plate at right angles to the antitoxin strip. Parallel to this streak, at a distance of about 15 mm from it, streak a known toxigenic strain of *C. diphtheriae* on one side of the test strain and streak a non-toxigenic strain on the other side. Incubate the plate at 37°C and examine after 24 and 48 hours. Look for **white lines of precipitation** a few mm from the paper strip, that extend out from the line of bacterial growth, forming an angle of about 45°.

These white precipitin lines form where the toxin from pathogenic strains of *C. diphtheriae* combines with the antitoxin in optimum concentration from the paper strip, thus identifying the strains of *C. diphtheriae* that produce the toxin. At 24 hours, the line is best seen with the help of a hand lens, at 48 hours it is more obvious. Look for continuity between the line from unknown culture and that from the known toxigenic culture (Fig. 23.3). This test is very convenient and economical.

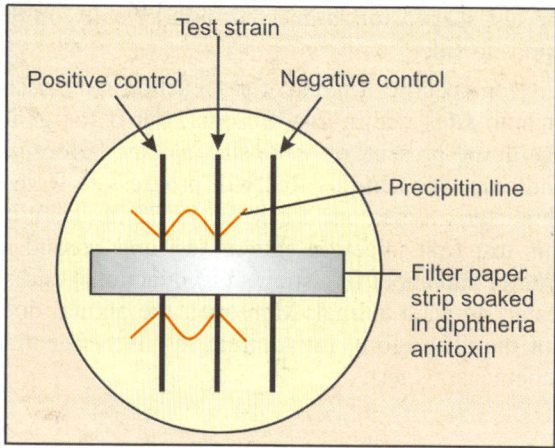

Fig. 23.3. Elek's test.

Epidemiology

Extensive use of toxoid against diphtheria has resulted in almost disappearance of this disease from the developed countries. With active immunization not only number of cases has been brought down to negligible level, the prevalence of toxigenic strains has also reduced considerably. However, diphtheria is endemic in many developing countries. The disease is commoner in rural than in urban areas. It is typically a disease of schools and institutions where children of the susceptible age are herded together. Humans are the only natural hosts of *C. diphtheriae* and, thus the only significant reservoir of infection. Asymptomatic carriers and persons in the incubation stage of the disease are the major sources of most infections.

Prophylaxis

Because only man appears to be an important reservoir of *C. diphtheriae*, and because all strains elaborate the same antigenic type of toxin, it is possible to eradicate diphtheria by immunization. In fact, by immunization the disease has been virtually eradicated from most advanced countries. The purpose of immunization is to increase protective levels of antitoxin in circulation. Early in the development of diphtheria prophylaxis, immunizing agents were scarce and were not free from risk. It was, therefore, customary to test the susceptibility of the individual before active immunization was

given. The susceptibility test used was Schick test which was introduced in 1913. This test is no longer used now. For details, the first edition of this book may be consulted. The methods of immunization available are active, passive or combined.

Active immunization

This can be carried out by single and combined vaccines:

Single preparations: These include toxin-antitoxin mixture, formol toxoid, alum-precipitated toxoid, purified toxoid and aluminium phosphate precipitate.

Combined preparations: These consist of diphtheria toxoid in combination with tetanus toxoid (DT) only or tetanus toxoid and killed suspension of pertussis bacilli (DPT or triple vaccine). The component antigens of DPT can be given separately also, but giving them together not only minimizes the number of injections, but also improves immune response because the **pertussis vaccine acts as an adjuvant for the toxoids**. A quadruple preparation incorporating, in addition, inactivated polio vaccine, has also been used.

DPT and oral polio vaccines are given at the age of 6 weeks, 10 weeks, 14 weeks and 16–24 months followed by DT at the age of 5–6 years.

Diphtheria vaccine is highly effective. Fully immunized individuals may become infected with *C. diphtheriae*, because the antibodies are directed against the toxin, but the disease is mild. Serious infection and death occur only in unimmunized or incompletely immunized individuals.

Passive immunization

This is an emergency measure, to be employed when susceptible (non-immunized) individuals are exposed to infection. It consists of subcutaneous administration of 500–1,000 units of antitoxin or anti-diphtheritic serum (ADS). Contacts immunized within the previous 5 years should receive a booster dose of toxoid.

Combined immunization

Since protection conferred by passive immunization is of short duration, therefore, ADS should be administered on one arm and first dose of diphtheria toxoid on the other arm, to be continued by the full course of active immunization.

Treatment

Treatment of diphtheria consists of antitoxic and antibiotic therapy. The antitoxin should be administered promptly, as soon as clinical diagnosis is made to neutralize the toxin being produced, because antitoxin is ineffective if given after the toxin is bound to cell receptor sites. Therefore, for antitoxic therapy, one should not wait for bacteriological confirmation of the diagnosis. The dosage recommended is 20,000 units intramuscularly for moderate cases and 50,000–100,000 units for serious cases, half the dose being given intravenously.

C. diphtheriae is sensitive to penicillin, erythromycin, rifampin and many other antibiotics, but the antibiotics do not neutralize circulating toxin and, therefore, are of value only when used concurrently with antitoxin. By killing diphtheria bacilli they prevent further toxin production. Diphtheria cases are generally treated with penicillin or erythromycin in addition to antitoxin. Penicillin-sensitive individuals can be given erythromycin. Erythromycin is more active than penicillin in the treatment of carriers.

DIPHTHEROIDS

Corynebacteria resembling *C. diphtheriae*, occur as normal commensals in the throat, skin and other areas. These may be mistaken for diphtheria bacilli and are known as diphtheroids. They stain more uniformly than diphtheria bacilli, are arranged in V forms or palisades rather than Chinese letter arrangement and possess few or no metachromatic granules. They can be differentiated from *C. diphtheriae* on the basis of biochemical characters and toxigenicity tests. The common diphtheroids are *C. pseudodiphtheriticum* and *C. xerosis*.

KEY FACTS

- *Corynebacterium diphtheriae* (diphtheria bacilli) are thin, slender, Gram-positive bacilli occurring in angled pairs, or parallel rows of 3–4 bacilli which resemble *Chinese letters*
- *Toxigenic* strains of *Corynebacterium diphtheriae* are responsible for **diphtheria**, the sometimes fatal upper respiratory tract infection of childhood
- The **diphtheria toxin is toxoidable**, and is a **component of the triple (DPT) vaccine**

IMPORTANT QUESTIONS

1. Discuss pathogenesis and laboratory diagnosis of diphtheria.
2. Write short notes on:
   (a) Diphtheria toxin
   (b) Prophylaxis of diphtheria

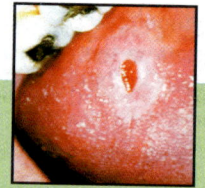

Chapter 24

Clostridium (Gas Gangrene, Food-Poisoning & Tetanus)

Anaerobic, Gram-positive, spore-bearing bacilli belong to the genus *Clostridium*. Spores are refractile, oval or spherical and usually wider (bulging) than the parent cell. They may be terminal, subterminal or central in the cell. Most clostridia possess flagella and are motile, but *C. perfringens* and *C. tetani* type VI are not. The motility is slow, and has been described as 'stately'. *C. perfringens* and *C. butyricum* are capsulated, while others are not. Filamentous forms are common. In 48 hour cultures, many of the bacilli may be Gram-negative.

Clostridia vary in their relationship to oxygen. Certain clostridia like *C. tetani* are obligate anaerobes. On the other hand, *C. perfringens* is much less fastidious. Natural habitat of the clostridia is soil, water, intestinal tract of animals and man, and decomposing plant and animal matter. A few species are opportunistic pathogens and can produce diseases like **gas gangrene** (*C. perfringens*), **tetanus** (*C. tetani*), **botulism** (*C. botulinum*), **food-poisoning** (*C. perfringens*) and **pseudomembranous colitis** (*C. difficile*).

The pathogenicity of these organisms depends on the release of highly destructive enzymes or powerful toxins. The toxins produced by *C. tetani* and *C. botulinum* attack nervous pathways and are referred to as **neurotoxins**, while toxins and aggressins produced by *C. perfringens* attack soft tissues and are referred to as **histotoxins**.

CLOSTRIDIUM PERFRINGENS (CLOSTRIDIUM WELCHII)

Morphology

They are large, Gram-positive, spore-bearing bacilli, measuring 4–6 × 1 µm with parallel sides and truncated or slightly rounded ends. They occur singly, in pairs or in small bundles. They are non-motile and form capsules in animal body. Spores are oval, subterminal or central and non-bulging (Fig. 24.1A). They are formed under natural conditions, e.g., in the bowel. They are only rarely seen in direct smears from wounds or cultures but can be demonstrated on growth in special media such as Ellner's medium.

Cultural characteristics

It is an anaerobe, but can grow under microaerophilic conditions. Optimum temperature for growth is 37°C. It grows best on media containing carbohydrate such as **glucose blood agar** and forms two main types of colonies. One is round, 2–4 mm in diameter, smooth, regular, convex, amorphous, greyish-yellow and slightly opaque. Other is umbonate with an opaque brownish centre and a lighter, translucent, radially striated periphery with a crenated edge.

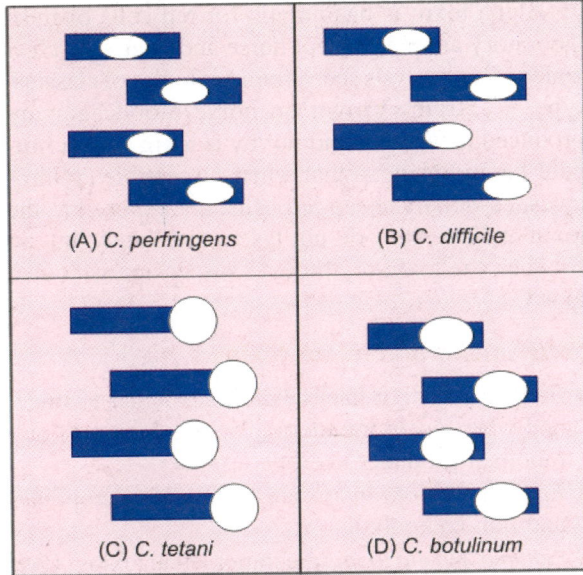

(A) *C. perfringens* (B) *C. difficile*

(C) *C. tetani* (D) *C. botulinum*

Fig. 24.1. Types of spores

On **horse blood agar**, colonies are usually surrounded by a zone of β-haemolysis and commonly also by an outer wider zone of incomplete haemolysis owing to the action of θ and α toxins respectively (**double zone haemolysis**).

Biochemical reactions

It is actively saccharolytic and ferments glucose, maltose, sucrose, lactose and starch with the production of acid and gas.

- In **litmus milk medium**, it ferments lactose and produces acid and gas. The acid clots the milk and the gas breaks up the clot resulting in **stormy clot reaction**. Production of acid is also indicated by change in the colour of the litmus from **blue to red**. The culture has sour butyric acid odour. It is indole-negative, MR-positive, VP-negative and H_2S-positive.

- **Gelatin is liquefied** but coagulated serum is usually not liquefied.

- In **cooked meat broth** (CMB), meat turns pink and is not digested. It produces phospholipase-C which gives opalescence around the colonies on egg-yolk containing medium.

Resistance to physical and chemical agents

Vegetative cells of *C. perfringens* are very sensitive to heat and disinfectants. However, spores generally resist routinely used antiseptics and disinfectants except formaldehyde and glutaraldehyde. Spores of type A2 food-poisoning strains and certain type C strains are markedly heat-resistant whereas those of type A1 do not survive boiling for more than a few minutes.

Toxins

C. perfringens produces **four major lethal, eight minor lethal or non-lethal toxins, and enterotoxin**. Major lethal toxins include α (alpha), β (beta), ε (epsilon) and ι (iota) and minor lethal toxins include γ (gamma), δ (delta), κ (kappa), λ (lambda), μ (mu), η (nu), θ (theta) and ν (eta).

On the basis of four major toxins, *C. perfringens* can be divided into **five types, A to E** (Table 24.1). Typing is done by neutralization tests with specific antitoxins by intracutaneous injection in guinea-pigs or intravenous injection in mice. Strains of *C. perfringens* type A that produce enterotoxin are associated with a mild form of food-poisoning. Typical food-poisoning strains (type A2) are non-haemolytic or feebly haemolytic on horse blood agar and have markedly heat-resistant spores but classical (type A1) strains are β-haemolytic and have relatively heat-sensitive spores.

Table 24.1. Typing of *Clostridium perfringens*

Type	Toxin produced			
	α	β	ε	τ
A	+	−	−	−
B	+	+	+	−
C	+	+	−	−
D	+	−	+	−
E	+	−	−	+

Alpha toxin

It is produced by all types of *C. perfringens* but most abundantly by type A strains. It is the most important toxin and is responsible for the profound toxaemia of gas gangrene. It is thermostable, lethal for mice, guinea-pigs, rabbits, pigeons and sheep, and when given intradermally, produces a necrotic lesion. It is Ca^{++} or Mg^{++} dependent phospholipase (lecithinase-C). In the presence of free Ca^{++} or Mg^{++}, it produces opalescence in serum or egg-yolk containing media by splitting phospholipid complexes. This reaction can be inhibited by specific antitoxin. This is the basis of Nagler's reaction.

Nagler's reaction

A culture plate containing 6% agar, 5% peptic digest of sheep blood and 20% human serum or 5% egg-yolk is prepared. The plate is dried. On one half of the plate, 2–3 drops of *C. perfringens* antitoxin are spread and allowed to dry. The plate is then inoculated with the test organisms or the exudate under study and incubated anaerobically at 37°C for 18 hours. On the section containing no antitoxin, *C. perfringens* colonies show surrounding zone of opalescence, i.e., Nagler's reaction whereas colonies of the remainder half of the plate show no change (Fig. 24.2). It is because of specific neutralization of the alpha toxin. The incorporation of neomycin sulphate inhibits aerobic sporing organisms and coliform organisms. The complex medium of **Willis and Hobbs** (1959) also incorporates lactose and neutral red to indicate lactose-fermenting organisms, and milk to indicate proteolysis.

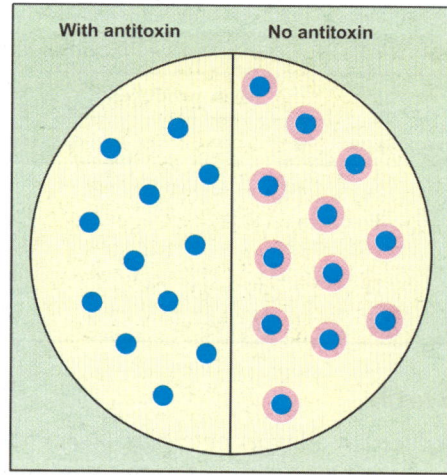

Fig. 24.2. Nagler's reaction.

Alpha toxin is haemolytic for red cells of most laboratory animals except horse and goat. The clear zones of haemolysis seen around colonies of classical type A1 strains grown on horse blood agar are produced by θ toxin and not by α toxin. It is a **hot-cold haemolysin**, so that when susceptible erythro-cytes, especially sheep red cells, are exposed to the toxin at 37°C, they do not lyse immediately, but do so when the toxin-erythrocyte suspension is cooled to 4°C.

Other major and minor toxins

- *Beta toxin* is not haemolytic, it is lethal to mice, and when given intradermally in guinea-pigs and rabbits it produces necrotic lesions.
- *Epsilon* and *iota toxins* are lethal and necrotizing, and non-haemolytic.
- *Gamma* and *eta toxins* are minor lethal toxins. They are neither necrotizing nor haemolytic.
- *Delta toxin* is lethal and actively haemolytic for the red cells of sheep, goat, pig and cattle.
- *Theta toxin* is oxygen-labile haemolysin anti-genically related to streptolysin O. It is moderately lethal.
- *Lambda toxin* is non-lethal, non-necrotizing proteinase and gelatinase.
- *Kappa*, *mu* and *nu* toxins are collagenase, hyaluronidase and deoxyribonuclease respectively.

Enterotoxin

C. perfringens type A strains produce a potent enterotoxin. It is a heat-labile, non-diffusible protein with a polypeptide chain and a molecular weight of 34,000–35,000 daltons. *It is formed in the intestine at the time of sporulation.*

Pathogenesis

C. perfringens may lead to following infections:

1. Wound infection

C. perfringens occurs normally in the soil, particularly that of manured and cultivated land, and animal and human excreta. The infection usually results from contamination of a wound with these. Wound may get contaminated with patient's own faeces during surgery or after accident. Clostridia may also be present on the normal skin, especially on the perineum and thigh. These may also cause infection.

The presence of devitalized or dead tissue due to crushing of tissues and the severing of arteries in accidental and war injuries, blood clots, extravasated fluid, foreign bodies (bullets, shell fragments and bits of clothing) and coincident infection with aerobic organisms reduce the oxygen tension. This leads to germination of clostridial spores followed by multiplication of vegetative forms with the production of exotoxins and enzymes into the surrounding environment causing more tissue destruction and resulting in a rapid and fulminating spread of the organism in the necrotic environment. In addition, carbohydrates may be fermented, resulting in production of large quantities of gas in the tissues.

The pressure resulting from gas formation may cause still more restriction of the blood supply to adjoining tissue and hence more necrosis. Hyaluronidase produced by *C. perfringens* breaks down intercellular cement substance and promotes the spread of the infection along tissue planes. Collagenase and proteinase produced by this organism break down tissues and virtually liquefy muscles. In the absence of surgical and antitoxic treatment, severe toxaemia and death frequently ensue. Three types of clostridial wound infections are recognized:

1. *Wound contamination:* Here one or more clostridia are present in the traumatized tissue without evidence of infection. Up to 80–90% isolates of *C. perfringens* from hospitalized patients represent simple saprophytic wound contamination.
2. *Clostridial cellulitis:* In this condition, infection is confined to local fascial planes in the absence of significant toxaemia. The infecting clostridia are of low invasive power and poor toxigenicity. There is a seropurulent discharge from the wound with an offensive odour and prognosis is good.
3. *Clostridial myonecrosis or gas gangrene :* In this condition, there is invasion of healthy muscle tissue and striking systemic intoxication as discussed above.

Monomicrobial gas gangrene is rare. It is almost always a polymicrobial infection, the infecting bacterial species commonly include a number of clostridial and non-clostridial anaerobes together with a variety of facultative anaerobes such as *Escherichia coli*, *Proteus* and *Staphylococcus*.

The **incubation period of gas gangrene** is 2–3 days. The disease develops with increasing pain, tenderness and oedema of the affected part along with systemic signs of toxaemia. There is a thin watery discharge from the wound, which later becomes profuse and serosanguinous. Accumulation of gas (predominantly hydrogen which is less soluble than carbon dioxide) makes the tissue crepitant.

2. Food-poisoning

Enterotoxin producing strains of *C. perfringens* are associated with a mild form of food-poisoning. **It is third most common etiologic agent of food-poisoning after *Salmonella* spp. and *S. aureus*.** Both heat-resistant (A2) and heat-sensitive (A1) strains of *C. perfringens* are capable of causing food-poisoning. The incriminated food is usually meat that has been cooked hours in advance and then cooled slowly, or even allowed to stand at room temperature for several hours before being served. Before cooking, the meat may get contaminated with heat-resistant spores from the animal's intestine at the abattoir or from soil and dust during transit to shops and then from shops to houses and catering establishments.

Heat-resistant spores may survive the whole cooking procedure and during cooling period they germinate in the anaerobic environment produced by the cooked meat and multiply. If spores of heat-sensitive strains contaminate uncooked meat, they are not likely to cause food-poisoning because they usually do not survive cooking. However, if dust containing heat-sensitive spores contaminates cooked meat, the spores germinate in the meat and multiply during the period of storage before serving.

Virtually 100% of healthy population carries classical β-haemolytic *C. perfringens* in their gut, and 2–30% carry heat-resistant *C. perfringens*. After ingestion of large number of vegetative cells in food, multiplication occurs in the intestine for a brief period followed by sporulation and the production of an **enterotoxin**. Patient develops abdominal cramps and diarrhoea with foamy and foul smelling stools 8–12 hours after ingestion of the contaminated food. It usually subsides within 24 hours. There is little vomiting or fever. No specific treatment is indicated.

3. Necrotizing jejunitis (Enteritis necroticans)

It is a severe and often fatal disease caused by *C. perfringens* type C. In addition, *C. perfringens* may also cause necrotizing colitis, gangrenous appendicitis, biliary tract infection, brain abscess and meningitis, panophthalmitis, thoracic infections, and urogenital infections.

Laboratory diagnosis
(Flowcharts 24.1 and 24.2)

The diagnosis of gas gangrene must primarily be made upon clinical grounds and initiation of treatment should not await full laboratory report. The function of laboratory is only to provide confirmation of clinical diagnosis.

Specimens

Specimens to be collected include (1) edges of affected muscles, (2) necrotic tissue, and (3) exudate from the depth of the lesion, where infection seems to be most pronounced, to be collected with a capillary pipette.

Microscopic examination

Gram smears are prepared. If gas gangrene exists, smear shows typical Gram-positive bacilli often with other bacteria. Thick, stubby, Gram-positive rods suggest *C. perfringens*.

Culture

Aerobic and anaerobic cultures are made on fresh blood agar and heated blood agar. To prevent swarming by some anaerobes, 5–6% agar in plates is used. A plate of human serum or egg-yolk agar with *C. perfringens* antitoxin spread on one half of the plate is used for Nagler's reaction.

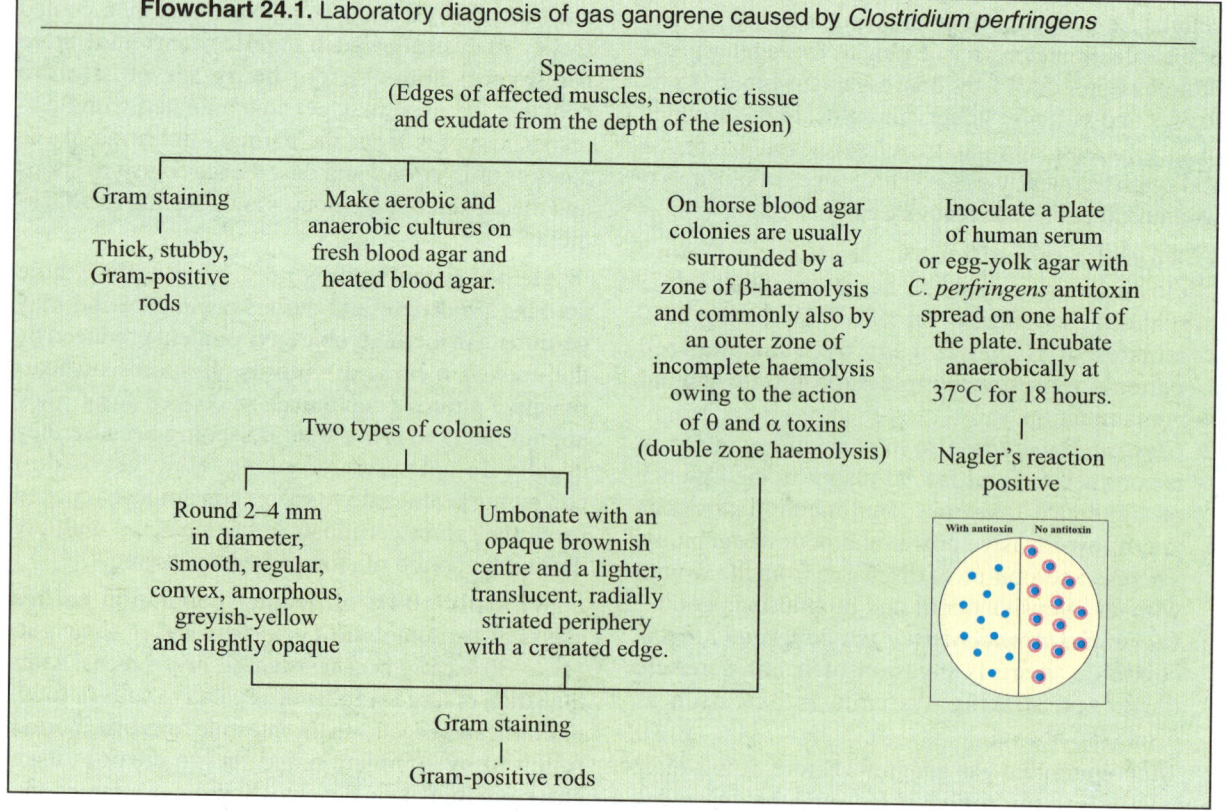

Flowchart 24.1. Laboratory diagnosis of gas gangrene caused by *Clostridium perfringens*

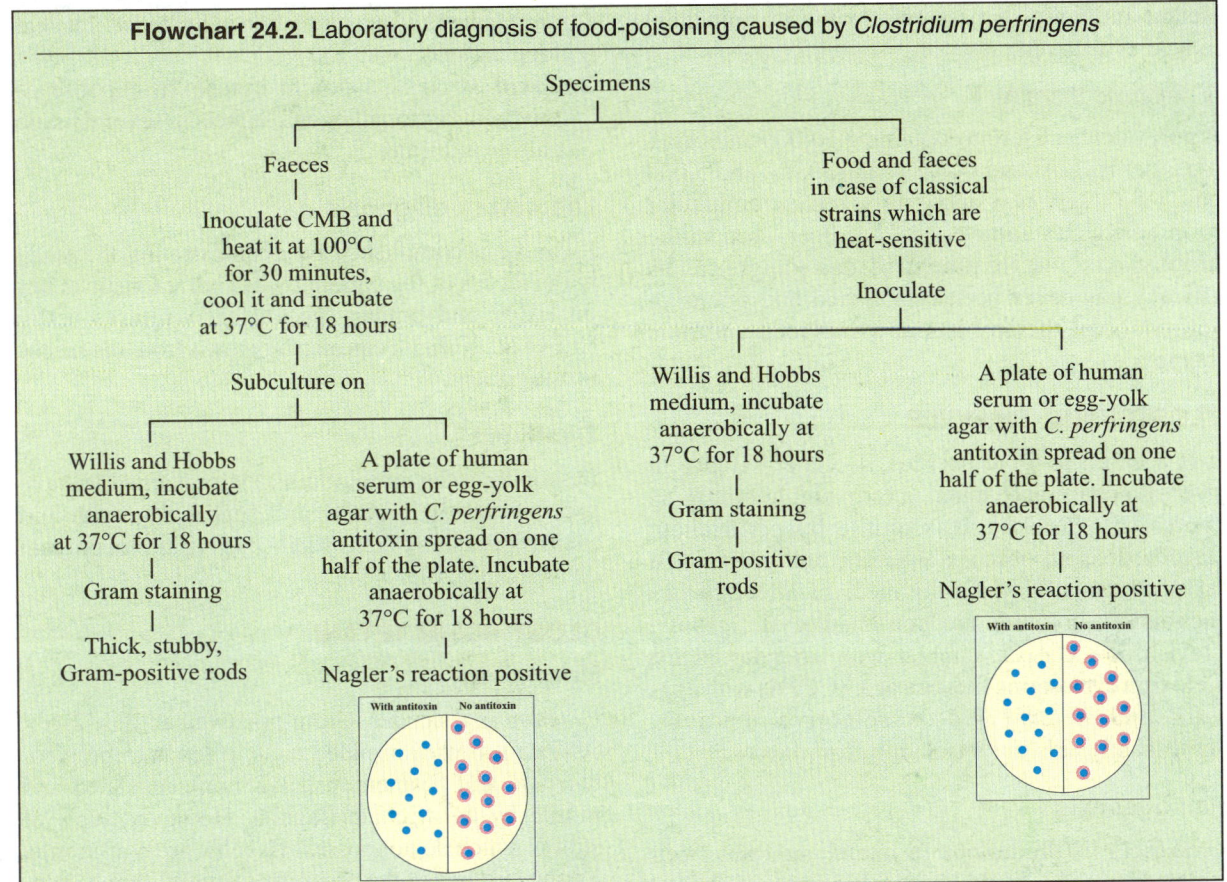

Flowchart 24.2. Laboratory diagnosis of food-poisoning caused by *Clostridium perfringens*

For isolation of *C. perfringens* from faeces, inoculate CMB and heat it at 100°C for 30 minutes, cool it and incubate it at 37°C for 18 hours. Subculture on Willis and Hobbs medium, incubate anaerobically at 37°C for 18 hours. Look for colonies of Gram-positive bacilli showing Nagler's reaction.

For isolation of classical strains which are heat-sensitive, stool specimen is inoculated on Willis and Hobbs medium with neomycin 70 μg/ml. Incubate and identify as above. For isolation of *C. perfringens* from food, process it as for the isolation of classical strains from stools.

Prophylaxis and treatment of gas gangrene

1. Toilet of the wound

The most important preventive measure against clostridial myonecrosis is early and adequate wound debridement and irrigation of the wound to remove blood clots, necrotic tissue and foreign material. This ensures elimination of the bulk of the contaminating organisms. Wound is not sutured but is left open after thorough cleansing and loosely packed. Hyperbaric oxygen chamber, in which an infected area is placed in a chamber containing pure oxygen under pressure, has been used with some success to stop the growth of the anaerobes.

2. Chemotherapy

Surgical toilet is combined with topical and parenteral antimicrobial therapy in high doses. This should be directed against clostridial element and likely coexistence of coliform organisms, Gram-positive and faecal anaerobes. Therefore, penicillin, metronidazole and an aminoglycoside may be given in combination. Clindamycin or a broad-spectrum β-lactam antibiotic such as cefotaxime or imipenem may also be given.

3. Antitoxic therapy

A polyvalent antiserum containing 10,000 units each of *C. perfringens* and *C. novyi* antitoxins, and 5,000 units of *C. septicum* antitoxin given intramuscular or in emergency intravenous, has been used in the prophylaxis and treatment of gas gangrene. Its efficacy has never been established and intensive antimicrobial therapy has now replaced antitoxic therapy.

CLOSTRIDIUM DIFFICILE

It is a Gram-positive bacillus, 4–8 × 0.5–1 μm in size with oval, subterminal or terminal, non-bulging spores (Fig. 24.1B). It is motile by peritrichate flagella. It is an obligate anaerobe and grows well on blood agar at 37°C. On this medium, after 24 hours incubation, colonies are non-haemolytic, glossy, greyish, low convex, circular with irregular edges. Cefoxitin cycloserine fructose agar (CCFA) with egg-yolk and neutral red, a selective medium, significantly aids in its isolation from faeces.

Pathogenesis

C. difficile is ubiquitous in nature, and has been isolated from soil, water, intestinal contents of various animals, vagina and urethra of humans, and faeces of 40–50% of neonates and only 3% of healthy adults. It has, however, been implicated as a causative agent of **antibiotic-associated diarrhoea** (AAD), **antibiotic-associated colitis** (AAC) and life threatening **pseudomembranous colitis** (PMC). These conditions have been associated with a number of antimicrobial agents particularly clindamycin and ampicillin. Use of these antibiotics leads to killing of antibiotic-sensitive organisms and overgrowth of *C. difficile* in the intestine leading to these conditions. Most of the cases of PMC are caused by *C. difficile* but infrequently it may also be caused by *S. aureus* and *C. perfringens*.

   C. difficile produces disease by the elaboration of two distinct exotoxins:

1. ***Toxin A:*** It is an enterotoxin that is primarily responsible for diarrhoea. It is capable of producing fluid accumulation in ligated rabbit ileal loop assay.

2. ***Toxin B:*** It is a potent cytotoxin capable of producing cytopathogenic effects in several tissue culture cell lines.

Laboratory diagnosis

It can be accomplished by demonstrating the toxin in the faeces of the patient by its characteristic effect on HEp2 and human diploid cell cultures or by ELISA. *C. difficile* can also be grown from the faeces of the patient.

Treatment

Discontinue the antibiotic that is presumed to have precipitated the disease, and suppress growth and toxin production of *C. difficile* by giving vancomycin or metronidazole.

CLOSTRIDIUM TETANI

Morphology

C. tetani is a slender, Gram-positive bacillus, 2–5 × 0.4–0.5 μm with rounded ends. It tends to be pleomorphic and filamentous. It is non-capsulated and motile by peritrichate flagella. However, type VI strains which do not possess flagella, are non-motile. Young cultures of the organisms usually stain Gram-positive but in older cultures and in smears made from the wounds, they are Gram-variable and even frank Gram-negative. The spores are spherical, terminal and twice the diameter of vegetative cells giving them typical **'drumstick' appearance** (Fig. 24.1C). The spores do not take up the Gram stain and appear as colourless round structures.

Cultural characteristics

C. tetani is an obligate anaerobe. The optimum temperature and pH for its growth are 37°C and 7.4 respectively. It can grow well on ordinary media, but its growth is improved by the addition of blood or serum.

- Colonies on **solid media** are irregularly round, 2–5 mm in diameter with fine branching projections. Some strains form colonies with thicker, translucent, yellow brown centre and thin, translucent, colourless periphery. Isolated colonies of *C. tetani* may not be obtained because of the tendency of the organism to swarm over the surface of the medium. However, non-motile variants may produce isolated colonies.

- On **horse blood agar**, the colonies of *C. tetani* are surrounded by a zone of α-haemolysis, which subsequently develops into β-haemolysis owing to the production of an oxygen-labile haemolysin known as tetanolysin.
- On **egg-yolk agar**, it does not produce opalescence or pearly layer.
- It grows well in **CMB**. The meat is not digested but shows slight blackening on prolonged incubation.

Biochemical reactions

C. tetani has slight proteolytic and no saccharolytic activity. Gelatin is slowly liquefied. Coagulated serum is rendered more transparent and softened but not liquefied. It is indole-positive and MR-, VP-, H_2S- and nitrate reduction-negative.

Sensitivity to physical and chemical agents

Spores of some strains of *C. tetani* are killed by boiling for 10–15 minutes, but some resist boiling for up to 3 hours and dry heat at 160°C for 1 hour. They can, however, be killed by autoclaving at 121°C for 15 minutes. They are inactivated by exposure to iodine (1% aqueous solution), hydrogen peroxide (10 volumes) and glutaraldehyde (2%) within a few hours. In the soil, spores of *C. tetani* can survive for years.

Antigenic structure

Flagellar (H), somatic (O) and spore antigens have been demonstrated in *C. tetani*. Spore antigens are different from H and O antigens. On the basis of agglutination and complement fixation tests, the strains of the organism have been divided into 10 (I–X) types of which type I and III are the commonest. This typing is on the basis of their H antigens. Type VI consists of non-flagellate strains. All the strains carry same O antigen. This permits identification of the organism by use of fluorescein-labelled antisera. Toxins formed by all types are pharmacologically and antigenically identical and are neutralized by antitoxin prepared

against any one type. However, within the same type some strains may be toxigenic and others non-toxigenic.

Tetanus toxins

C. tetani produces an oxygen-labile haemolysin (tetanolysin) but all the symptoms in tetanus are attributable to a potent neurotoxin (tetanospasmin). Different strains vary from completely non-toxigenic to very highly toxigenic.

1. Tetanospasmin

It is a heat-labile protein that may be inactivated by heating at 60°C for 20 minutes. **It is an extremely powerful toxin second in potency only to the exotoxin of *C. botulinum*.** It has a minimum lethal dose, for a mouse, of 50–75 ng. It gets toxoided spontaneously or in the presence of low concentrations of formaldehyde. It is a good antigen and is specifically neutralized by the antitoxin. The structural gene for toxin production is located on a 75-kilobase plasmid.

2. Tetanolysin

In addition to its neurotoxin, *C. tetani* produces an oxygen-labile haemolysin, antigenically related to streptolysin O and θ toxin of *C. perfringens*. There is no evidence that it plays a significant role in pathogenesis.

Pathogenesis

The spores of *C. tetani* are ubiquitous. They occur in the gastrointestinal tracts of man and animals. They are also present in the soil especially in manured soil. Tetanus develops following the contamination of wound with *C. tetani* spores. The source of infection may be soil, dirty clothing or faeces. Spores of *C. tetani* may be embedded in surgical catgut (prepared from cattle and sheep gut). Germination of spores is dependent upon the reduced oxygen tension occurring in devitalized tissue.

Infection strictly remains localized in the wound and the disease is due to the effect of a potent diffusible exotoxin (tetanospasmin). Conditions that favour the germination of spores and the multiplication of the organisms in the tissues are similar to those of *C. perfringens*. However, tetanus may also develop following superficial abrasion, septic abortion, thorn prick, and cleansing of auditory meatus with a small stick. **Tetanus neonatorum** follows infection of umbilical wound of newborn infants. **Postoperative tetanus** may be due to imperfectly sterilized catgut, intestinal contents during abdominal surgery and air of the operation theatre containing spore-bearing dust.

C. tetani remains localized at the site of initial infection and produces tetanus toxin. It is absorbed from the site of its production and ascends to the central nervous system via motor nerves. However, some toxin may be delivered from the site of infection via the blood to all nerves in the body and the subsequent transmission to the central nervous system depends upon uptake through neuromuscular nerve endings and intra-axonal transport. Therefore, the first symptoms in human tetanus appear in head and neck because of the shorter length of the cranial nerves.

Tetanospasmin resembles strychnine in its effect. It appears to act by interfering with the normal inhibition of motor impulses exercised by the upper motor neuron over the lower. This results in sustained muscle spasm and characteristic signs of spasm of jaw muscles (**lock jaw**, **trismus**) and facial muscles (**risus sardonicus**), and arching of the body (**opisthotonicus**).

The **incubation period** of tetanus varies from 2 days to several weeks but commonly it is 6–12 days. Tetanus is a serious disease with a high mortality rate of 80–90% without proper treatment and even with proper treatment it is 15–50%. Tetanus neonatorum and uterine tetanus have very high fatality rates (70–100%). **In rural India, it is fourth commonest cause of death.**

Laboratory diagnosis (Flowchart 24.3)

The diagnosis is usually based on clinical findings alone because the isolation of the organism can occur in the absence of the disease, and it is also possible to have tetanus and never isolate the organism.

Microscopy

Collect pus or necrotic material from the wound, prepare a smear and stain it by Gram's method. Examine under microscope for typical 'drumstick'

bacilli. But only a minority of specimens will show these. Direct immunofluorescence microscopy can also be employed for the demonstration of *C. tetani*.

Culture

Diagnosis by culture is more dependable. Pus or wound scrapings or excised bits of tissue from the necrotic depths of wound should be plated on one half of a blood agar plate and 3 bottles of CMB. Blood agar plate is incubated anaerobically at 37°C. *C. tetani* produces swarming growth which may be detected on opposite half of the plate after 1–2 days. Of the 3 inoculated CMB bottles, one should be incubated unheated, second is heated in a water bath at 80°C for 5 minutes and third for 20 minutes. The purpose of heating for different periods is to kill non-sporing bacilli, while leaving tetanus spores undamaged, which vary widely in heat-resistance. The heated bottles are also incubated anaerobically at 37°C.

Subcultures from all these bottles are made on half of a blood agar plate daily for 4 days. The plates are incubated anaerobically at 37°C and examined for the swarming edge of *C. tetani*. Incorporation of polymyxin B, to which clostridia are resistant, makes the medium selective. A blood agar plate containing 4% agar, to minimize swarming, is divided into 2 halves. One half is smeared with tetanus antitoxin. Both halves are then inoculated with growth assumed to be *C. tetani* and incubated anaerobically for 2 days. Colonies haemolytic on the untreated half, but not on the antitoxin half, are of *C. tetani*.

Toxigenicity test

The toxigenicity of the organisms is confirmed by demonstrating the production of tetanospasmin. Two mice, one unprotected and other protected, by giving 1,000 units of tetanus antitoxin intraperitoneally 1 hour before the test, are challenged with an intra-muscular injection in the hind leg of 0.1 ml of a 48 hour CMB culture supernate of the isolate. The protected mouse remains well. Signs of ascending tetanus develop in the unprotected animal after several hours, they begin in the inoculated leg and extend to the tail, then the other hind limb is affected and then generalized signs appear. The animal dies within 2 days.

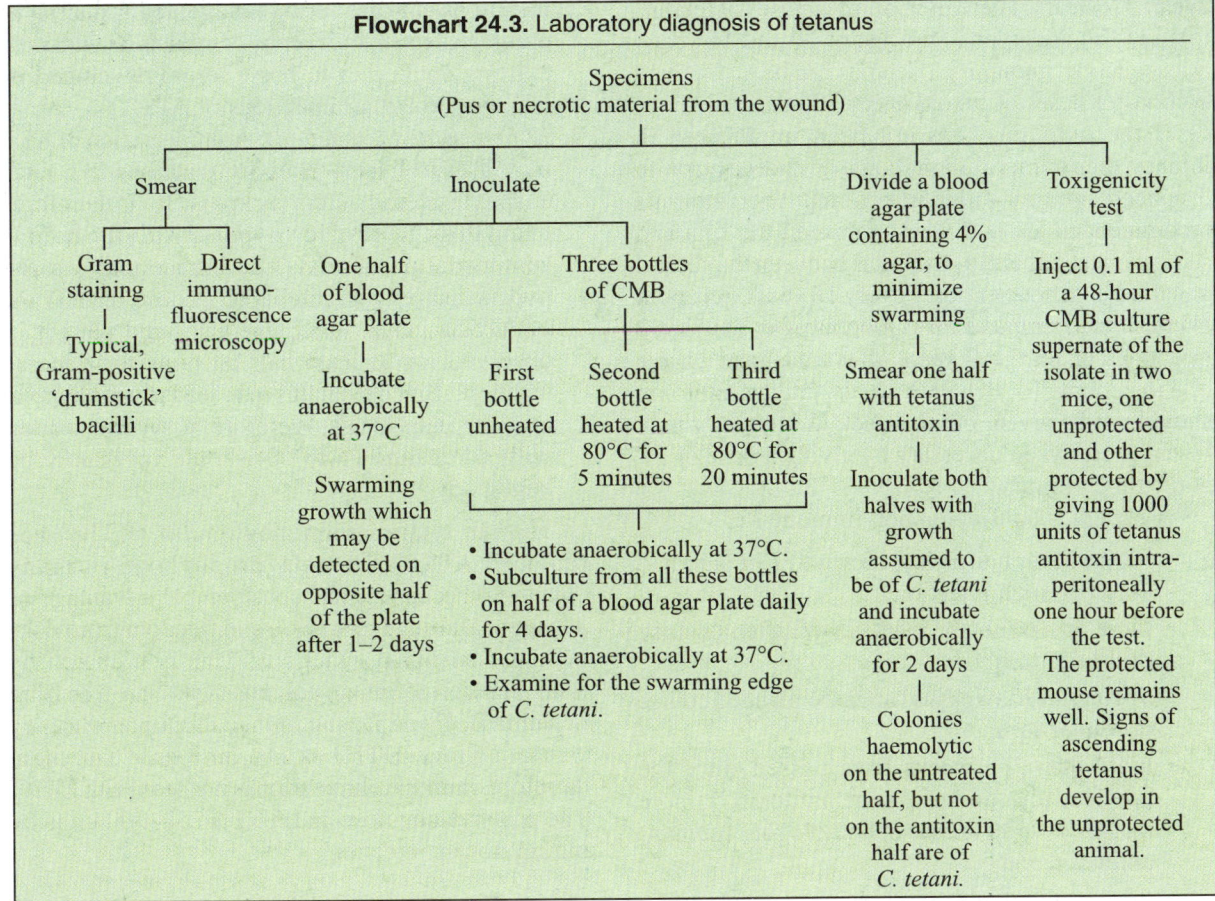

Flowchart 24.3. Laboratory diagnosis of tetanus

Prophylaxis

It is of 3 types:

1. Surgical prophylaxis

This includes prompt and adequate wound debridement, removal of foreign material, necrotic tissue and blood clots. This ensures elimination of the bulk of the contaminating organisms and an anaerobic environment for the growth of *C. tetani* is not provided. Clean superficial wounds that receive prompt attention may not require specific protection against tetanus.

2. Antibiotic prophylaxis

This includes prompt administration of antibiotics to destroy or inhibit *C. tetani* and pyogenic bacteria in the wound, so that the production of the toxin can be prevented. A long-acting penicillin or one tablet of erythromycin 500 mg twice daily for 5 days may be given preferably before the wound toilet. However, antibiotics have no effect on the toxin, therefore, antibiotic prophylaxis does not replace immunoprophylaxis.

3. Immunoprophylaxis

It includes 3 types of immunization:

(i) Active immunization

All persons should be actively immunized against tetanus in infancy and their immunity maintained by booster doses. Diphtheria-pertussis-tetanus (DPT) and oral polio vaccines are given at the age of 6 weeks, 10 weeks, 14 weeks and 16–24 months followed by diphtheria-tetanus (DT) vaccine at the age of 5–6 years. Thereafter, booster doses of tetanus toxoid (TT) are given at the age of 10 and 16 years. Subsequently, immunity to tetanus can be maintained by booster doses of toxoid every 10 years.

If the individual has not been immunized in infancy, then immunization should be carried out with 3 spaced intramuscular injections. The intervals recommended are 6–8 weeks between the first and second injections and 4–6 months between the second and third, and booster doses every 10 years. A patient is considered immune for 6 months after the first 2 injections or for 5–10 years after a planned course of 3 injections. To such individuals, tetanus antitoxin should not be given, but their active immunity may be enhanced when necessary by giving a dose of TT at the time of injury.

A patient is considered non-immune if:

- he has never had an injection of TT or if he had only one such injection;
- more than 6 months have passed after a course of 2 injections;
- 5–10 years have passed after the planned course of 3 injections;
- more than 2–3 weeks have passed since the previous injection of equine antitoxin or more than 6–8 weeks in case of homologous (human) antitoxin; and
- there is any doubt about his immunization.

Such individuals are considered for passive immunization.

(ii) Passive immunization

Tetanus antitoxin often called antitetanus serum (ATS) can be obtained by immunizing horses with TT. This serum is of value if given immediately after wounding. The usual prophylactic dose is 1,500 international units given intramuscularly or subcutaneously as soon as possible after injury. The injection may be repeated at a weekly interval till the danger of tetanus persists. Larger initial dose of 3,000–10,000 international units may be given when the wound is severe.

Disadvantages of ATS:

1. *Immune elimination:* The half life of ATS in man is about 7 days, and in persons who have had prior injections of horse serum (antigenic for man) it is eliminated much quicker by combination with pre-existing antibodies to horse serum developed in response to earlier injections of ATS.

2. *Hypersensitivity reactions:* Administration of ATS may lead to hypersensitivity reactions like fatal anaphylaxis and serum sickness. It is, therefore, mandatory to test for hypersensitivity before administration of ATS. The intradermal test for hypersensitivity is unreliable. A dose of 0.05 ml of ATS is given subcutaneously and patient is observed for at least half an hour for general reactions. Since even this may lead to anaphylaxis in some individuals, therefore, a syringe loaded with adrenaline (1/1,000) should invariably be kept ready.

Human tetanus immunoglobulin (HTIG) has replaced ATS for tetanus prophylaxis in many countries, because it has considerable advantage of a longer half life (3–5 weeks) and freedom from risks of hypersensitivity reactions. This is prepared by immunization of human volunteers who are free from hepatitis B, C and D, and human immunodeficiency viruses. Since HTIG is not antigenic for man, therefore, immune elimination is not seen with HTIG. The prophylactic dose of HTIG is 250–500 units by intramuscular injection.

(iii) Combined immunization

It consists of administering to a non-immune person ATS or HTIG at one site, along with the first dose of TT at another site, followed by second and third doses of TT at appropriate intervals.

CLOSTRIDIUM BOTULINUM

Morphology

C. botulinum is a straight or slightly curved Gram-positive bacillus with rounded ends. It measures about $5 \times 1\ \mu m$ (range $3.4–8.6 \times 0.5–1.3\ \mu m$) in size. It is non-capsulated and motile by peritrichate flagella. It produces heat-resistant spores that are oval, subterminal and bulging (Fig. 24.1D).

Cultural characteristics

It is an obligate anaerobe. Optimum temperature for growth is 35°C, but some strains can grow and produce toxin at 1–5°C. It can grow well on routine culture media. Surface colonies are large, irregular, smooth, semitransparent with fimbriate border. On horse blood agar, all strains except those of type G are β-haemolytic. All types except G produce opalescence and a pearly effect on egg-yolk agar (EYA).

Biochemical reactions

It ferments glucose, fructose and maltose. Types A, B and F are proteolytic; they liquefy gelatin and coagulated serum and digest meat in cooked meat broth, blackening it and producing a foul smell. They produce hydrogen sulphide. Types C, D and E are essentially non-proteolytic or feebly so; they do not decompose meat and they do not produce hydrogen sulphide. All types are indole-negative and catalase-negative.

Susceptibility to physical and chemical agents

Spores of *C. botulinum* are highly resistant, surviving boiling for several hours and some strains can even survive autoclaving at 121°C for 20 minutes. However, spores of type E strains are usually much less resistant. They may be inactivated by heating at 80°C (wet heat) for 30 minutes. Insufficient heating in the process of preserving food is an important factor in the causation of botulism.

Antigenic types

On the basis of the type of toxin produced, *C. botulinum* has been divided into eight sero-logically distinct types, A, B, C_1, C_2, D, E, F and G. The toxins produced by different types are antigenically distinct but pharmacologically similar. Types A, B and E are the principal causes of human illness.

Properties of botulinum toxin

Botulinum toxin is probably the most toxic substance known to mankind. It is a small protein with 19 amino acids and a molecular weight of about 150,000 daltons. Minimum lethal dose, of this toxin, for a mouse, is 0.03 ng and that for humans may be 1 μg. It acts slowly taking several hours to kill. It is a

neurotoxin which apparently acts by inhibiting the release of acetylcholine from the motor nerve endings of the parasympathetic system. The toxin is relatively stable being inactivated at 80°C for 30–40 minutes and at 100°C for 10 minutes. It resists digestion in the intestine and is absorbed through intestinal mucosa in an active form. It can be toxoided. It is a good antigen and is specifically neutralized by the antitoxin.

Pathogenicity

C. botulinum is widely distributed in soil and decaying vegetation, thus, many foods, both vegetables and meats, may become contaminated with these organisms. It is non-invasive and its pathogenicity is entirely due to the toxin produced by it. The disease caused by this organism is known as **botulism**. It is of 3 types:

1. Food-borne botulism

It is due to the ingestion of preformed toxin. The causative organism, *C. botulinum*, multiplies in the food before it is consumed, and produces a powerful soluble toxin. The source of botulism is usually preserved food such as meat and meat products, fish, and vegetables. Food responsible for botulism is usually abnormal in appearance and odour. Bulging of tins and the presence of gas bubbles on opening suggest contamination with *C. botulinum*. However, at times food may look normal.

Symptoms usually begin 18–36 hours after ingestion of food and may include nausea, vomiting, thirst, constipation, double vision, difficulty in swallowing, speaking and breathing. This may be followed by muscular weakness, blurred vision, and death as a result of respiratory failure. Case fatality varies from 25–70%.

2. Wound botulism

C. botulinum has occasionally been isolated from wound in man. Toxin is produced at the site of infection and is absorbed. The symptoms are those of food-borne botulism except those of gastrointestinal system. Symptoms appear 4–14 days after injury, in persons with *C. botulinum* infection.

3. Infant botulism

This entity was recognized in 1976. Affected infants have ranged from 3 weeks to 9 months in age and both sexes have been affected equally. Older children and adults are not susceptible. The infants ingest spores, but not preformed toxin, from soil, household dust, honey, etc. About 10% of honey samples have been shown to contain type A and B spores of *C. botulinum.* **Within the intestine, *C. botulinum* multiplies and elaborates toxin.** After a period of normal development, the infant develops constipation, listlessness, difficulty in sucking and swallowing, weak or altered cry, muscle weakness, ptosis, and loss of head control. Eventually the baby appears 'floppy' (**floppy child syndrome**) and develops respiratory insufficiency or respiratory arrest. Patient excretes toxin and spores in the faeces. Management consists of supportive care and assisted feeding.

Laboratory diagnosis

Diagnosis may be made by demonstration of the bacillus or the toxin in suspected residual food or in faeces.

Demonstration of toxin

Botulinum toxin may be demonstrated in the food or faeces. The food is macerated in sterile saline, and the filtrate inoculated into mice or guinea pigs intraperitoneally. The test animal develops dyspnoea, flaccid paralysis and dies within 24 hours. Control animals protected by polyvalent antitoxin remain healthy. Toxin may also be demonstrated in patient serum.

Demonstration of the organism

Gram-positive sporing bacilli may be demonstrable in smears made from the residual food. For the isolation of *C. botulinum*, the specimen is inoculated on EYA, blood agar and three bottles of CMB. Hold one of these three bottles in a water bath at 80°C for 10 minutes and another for 20 minutes and third is unheated. This procedure selects heat-resistant spores and also allows heat-sensitive spores to grow in unheated CMB. The culture media are incubated anaerobically at 30°C for 3–5 days. Cultures in CMB

are screened at intervals for toxin production in mice and presence of the organisms may be detected by fluorescent antibody test. Absence of toxin production up to 5 days usually rules out botulism. Subculture toxin-positive CMB culture onto EYA and blood agar. Incubate anaerobically at 30°C for 48 hours. The growth on EYA and blood agar (direct as well as subculture) is identified by Gram staining, fluorescent antibody procedure, colonial morphology and biochemical characters.

Treatment

The toxin still remaining in the stomach should be removed by lavage with 2–5% bicarbonate solution because toxin is labile in alkaline pH. Saline enemas may be given to remove toxin from the colon. Polyvalent antitoxin against common types, i.e., A, B and E or monovalent when the type of intoxication is known should be given as soon as possible. The antitoxin cannot reverse the effect of toxin already affecting the nerves but will neutralize unfixed toxin. Intensive nursing care and the use of mechanical respirator, when necessary, is of great importance.

Prophylaxis

Since botulism follows consumption of inadequately canned or preserved food, it can be prevented by proper canning and preservation of food. The food that exhibits the signs of spoilage (inflated cans, gas bubbles on opening and abnormal odour) should not be consumed. When an outbreak occurs, a prophylactic dose of polyvalent antitoxin should be given intramuscularly to all those who have consumed that food. **Those who may be exposed to the hazards of intoxication in the laboratory or of deliberate intoxication, as in biological warfare, may be protected by injecting three doses of mixed toxoid at two month intervals.**

KEY FACTS

- Clostridia are *anaerobic, spore-bearing, Gram-positive bacilli*. They are anaerobic because they *cannot utilize molecular oxygen* (aerobic metabolism) for production of energy
- Clostridia are also, in varying degrees, *damaged by free oxygen*, which limits the condition under

which these organisms can colonize the human body or cause disease. These organisms synthesize some of the **most potent exotoxins** known. For example, the toxins of specific clostridial species cause **botulism, tetanus, gas gangrene** and **pseudomembranous colitis**

- **Tetanus** causes **sustained muscle spasm** and the characteristic signs of spasm of jaw muscles (lockjaw, **trismus**) and facial muscles (**risus sardonicus**), and arching of the body (**opisthotonicus**)
- Tetanus toxin (**tetanospasmin**) can be **attenuated to form a toxoid**. The latter is **a component of the DPT** (diphtheria-pertussis-tetanus) **vaccine**

IMPORTANT QUESTIONS

1. Discuss pathogenicity and laboratory diagnosis of:
   (a) Gas gangrene
   (b) Tetanus
2. Write short notes on:
   (a) Nagler's reaction
   (b) Botulism
   (c) *Clostridium difficile*

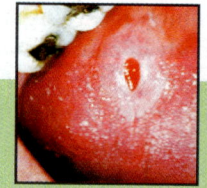

Chapter 25

Mycobacterium (Tuberculosis and Leprosy)

Mycobacteria are straight or slightly curved rods, however, coccobacillary, filamentous and branching forms also occur. The name *Mycobacterium* (fungus-like bacteria) was derived from the mold-like pellicle formed when members of this genus are grown in liquid media. This hydrophobic property is due to their thick, complex, lipid-rich, waxy cell walls. Due to their waxy cell walls they are difficult to stain, but once stained with hot carbol fuchsin, they resist decolourization with dilute mineral acids and alcohol. They are, therefore, known as **acid-fast bacilli** (AFB). Pathogenic and saprophytic mycobacteria are given in Table 25.1.

Most cases of human tuberculosis are caused by *M. tuberculosis* but some cases are due to *M. bovis*, which is the principal cause of tuberculosis in cattle and many other mammals. *M. africanum* includes a heterogeneous group of strains which have properties intermediate between *M. tuberculosis* and *M. bovis*. It also causes human tuberculosis.

MYCOBACTERIUM TUBERCULOSIS

Morphology

Tubercle bacilli are slender, straight or slightly curved rods with rounded ends. They measure $1–4 \times 0.2–0.8$ µm (average 3×0.3 µm) in size. In sputum and other clinical specimens they may occur singly or in small clumps. True branching is occasionally seen in old cultures and in smears from caseous lymph nodes. They are non-motile, non-sporing, non-capsulated and acid-fast.

The Ziehl-Neelsen acid-fast stain is useful in staining organisms from cultures or from clinical material. With this stain, the tubercle bacilli stain bright red, while the tissue cells and other organisms are stained blue (Fig. 25.1). Organisms in tissue and sputum smears often stain irregularly and have a beaded or barred appearance, presumably because of their vacuoles and polyphosphate content.

Tubercle bacilli may also be stained with auramine-rhodamine fluorescent stain and smears examined by fluorescence microscopy under low magnification. Tubercle bacilli are seen as yellow luminous organisms in dark field. When they have been detected under low power, the morphology of the bacilli is confirmed by observation with an oil-immersion objective. Tubercle bacilli are Gram-positive but it is difficult to stain them with the Gram stain. This is because of the failure of the dye to penetrate the cell wall.

Cultural characteristics

M. tuberculosis is an obligate aerobe while *M. bovis* is microaerophilic on primary isolation, becoming aerobic

Table 25.1. Pathogenic and saprophytic mycobacteria

MYCOBACTERIA CAUSING MAMMALIAN TUBERCULOSIS

- *M. tuberculosis* (human tubercle bacillus)
- *M. bovis* (bovine tubercle bacillus)
- *M. africanum* (intermediate between *M. tuberculosis* and *M. bovis*)
- *M. microti* (vole tubercle bacillus)

MYCOBACTERIA CAUSING LEPROSY

- *M. leprae* (human lepra bacillus)
- *M. lepraemurium* (rat lepra bacillus)

MYCOBACTERIA CAUSING JOHNE'S DISEASE

- *M. paratuberculosis*

MYCOBACTERIA CAUSING OPPORTUNISTIC INFECTIONS

Post-trauma abscesses
- *M. chelonae*
- *M. fortuitum*

Swimming pool granuloma
- *M. marinum*

Buruli ulcer
- *M. ulcerans*

Lymphadenopathy
- *M. avium-intracellulare*
- *M. scrofulaceum*

Pulmonary disease
- *M. avium-intracellulare*
- *M. kansasii*
- *M. xenopi*

Disseminated disease
- *M. avium-intracellulare*
- *M. chelonae*

MOTT BACILLI

- Photochromogens
- Scotochromogens
- Non-chromogens
- Rapid growers

SAPROPHYTIC MYCOBACTERIA

- *M. smegmatis*
- *M. phlei*

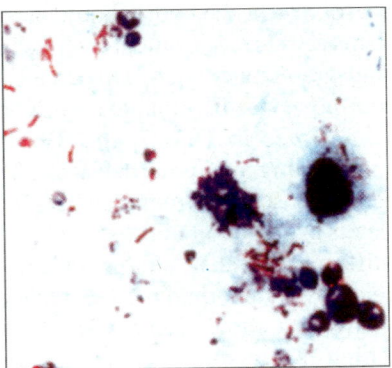

Fig. 25.1. Sputum smear showing acid-fast bacilli.

green and glycerol or sodium pyruvate, and solidified by heating (inspissation). **Malachite green inhibits the growth of organisms other than mycobacteria and provides a colour contrast against which colonies of mycobacteria can be easily seen.**

Lowenstein-Jensen glycerol medium is recommended for the isolation of human tubercle bacillus whose growth is enhanced by 0.75% glycerol, but glycerol at this concentration is inhibitory to *M. bovis* and so it may fail to grow on this medium. However, when the concentration of glycerol is reduced to 0.5%, it still improves the growth of *M. tuberculosis* but generally does not inhibit the growth of *M. bovis*. **Sodium pyruvate** improves the growth of both *M. tuberculosis* and *M. bovis*. Therefore, **Lowenstein-Jensen pyruvate medium** may be used for the isolation of the latter or both.

The average generation time of tubercle bacilli is about 14–15 hours, prolonged incubation is, therefore, necessary. *M. tuberculosis* grows well on LJ medium (**eugonic growth**). It produces visible growth on LJ glycerol medium, incubated at 37°C, in 2–8 weeks, although on primary isolation from clinical material from patients treated with antituberculous agents, colonies may take up to 12 weeks to appear. They grow as '**rough, tough and buff**' colonies – rough due to dry, irregular growth; tough due to difficulty in lifting the colony from the surface; and buff due to the pale yellow colour. On the other hand, *M. bovis* grows poorly on LJ glycerol medium (**dysgonic growth**) forming small, moist, smooth, flat and white colonies which easily break up when touched (Table 25.2). The growth of *M. bovis* is much better on LJ pyruvate medium.

on subculture. Optimum temperature for growth is 37°C (range 30–40°C) and optimum pH is 7.0 (range 6.0–7.6). Tubercle bacilli can grow on a wide range of enriched culture media but Lowenstein-Jensen (LJ) medium is most widely used. This medium consists of whole egg, asparagine, some mineral salts, malachite

In **glycerol broth**, the hydrophobic properties of the organisms cell surface result in a whitish wrinkled pellicle and granular deposit. Dispersed, uniform growth can, however, be obtained by subculturing them 2 or 3 times in **Dubos and Davis liquid medium** containing nonionic detergent Tween 80 (polyoxyethylene sorbitan monooleate). It wets the surface, deters aggregation of cells and permits them to grow diffusely. Virulent strains tend to grow as serpentine cords in the liquid media, while avirulent strains grow in a more dispersed fashion. The distinguishing features of *M. tuberculosis* and *M. bovis* are given in Table 25.2.

Sensitivity to physical and chemical agents

Tubercle bacilli are highly resistant to drying. When exposed to direct sunlight, organisms from culture are killed in 2 hours, but bacilli contained in sputum require an exposure of 20–30 hours. In dried sputum, protected from sunlight, they survive for as long as 6 months. The tubercle bacillus is generally more resistant to chemical disinfection than other non-spore-formers, especially when present in sputum. It can survive exposure to 5% phenol, 15% sulphuric acid, 3% nitric acid, 5% oxalic acid and 4% sodium hydroxide. It is destroyed by tincture of iodine in 5 minutes and by 80% ethanol in 2–10 minutes.

Cell wall

Cell wall consists of lipids, proteins and poly-saccharides. Lipid content accounts for 60% of the cell wall weight. Lipids of the cell wall, particularly the mycolic acid fraction, are responsible for:

- the hydrophobic character of the organisms, which tend to adhere to each other during growth in aqueous media and to float at the surface unless dispersed with detergents;
- relative impermeability to stains;
- acid-fastness;
- unusual resistance to killing by acids and alkalies;
- resistance to bactericidal action of antibodies and complement;
- slowness of growth by hindering permeation of nutrients into the cells; and
- cellular tissue reactions of the body.

The cell wall is made up of four layers. The innermost layer is peptidoglycan followed by arabino-galactan layer, mycolic acid layer and mycosides (Fig. 25.2).

Antigenic structure

Mycobacteria possess two types of antigens, cell wall (insoluble) and cytoplasmic (soluble) antigens. Cell wall antigens include arabinomannan, arabino-galactan and lipoarabinomannan. Cytoplasmic antigens, their molecular weights and chemical nature are given in Table 25.3. These include antigen 5, antigen 6, antigen 14, antigen 19, antigen 32, antigen 38 and antigen 60.

Table 25.2. Distinguishing features of Mycobacterium tuberculosis and M. bovis

Character	*M. tuberculosis*	*M. bovis*
1. Microscopic morphology	Slender, straight or slightly curved rods with barred or beaded appearance	Straight, stout, short uniformly stained rods
2. Colony morphology	Rough, tough and buff	Moist, smooth, flat, friable and white
3. Average duration of time for appearance of growth at 37°C	12–25 days. Growth is eugonic (luxuriant)	20–40 days. Growth is dysgonic
4. Effect of glycerol	In the concentration of 0.75% enhances the growth	In the concentration of 0.75% growth is inhibited. However, a concentration of 0.5% has no effect
5. Oxygen requirement	Obligate aerobe	Microaerophilic on primary isolation but becomes aerobic on subculture
6. Animal pathogenicity		
• Guinea-pig	+	+
• Rabbit	–	+

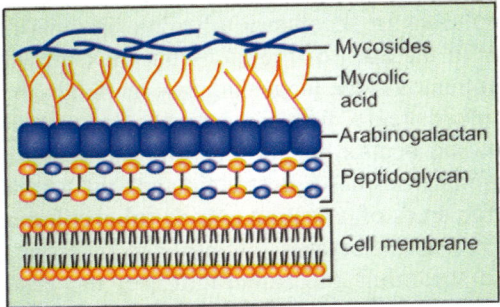

Fig. 25.2. Cell wall of *Mycobacterium tuberculosis*.

Table 25.3. Cytoplasmic (soluble) antigens of *Mycobacterium tuberculosis*

Antigen	Molecular weight in kilodaltons	Chemical nature
5	28.5–35	Protein
6	30	Protein
14	14	Protein
19	19	Protein
32	32	Protein
38	38	Protein
60	1,000-10,000	Lipopolysaccharide protein complex

Various serological tests like enzyme-linked immunosorbent assay (ELISA), radioimmunoassay (RIA) and latex agglutination have been tried for the serodiagnosis of tuberculosis. Of these tests, ELISA is considered to be the most sensitive and specific. ELISA test has been attempted using several antigenic materials such as antigen 5, antigen 6, antigen 60, purified mycobacterial glycolipids, unheated sterile culture filtrate of *M. tuberculosis* and purified protein derivative derived from *M. tuberculosis*.

Pathogenesis

Tuberculosis is the **leading cause of death** in the world from a bacterial infectious disease. According to WHO estimates one-third of the world's population has been infected. About 100 million individuals are infected annually, 8–10 million develop overt disease, 4–5 million become open or infectious cases and around 3 million die. In India, each year about 2 million develop active disease and about half a million die. It implies that every minute a death occurs due to tuberculosis in India. The situation is further compounded by the large scale increase of new cases associated with increasing HIV infection. **AIDS and tuberculosis form a lethal combination, each speeding up the other's progress.**

Humans become infected with *M. tuberculosis* most frequently by inhaling infective droplets coughed or sneezed into air by a patient with tuberculosis. Bovine tuberculosis is spread from animal to animal, and sometimes to human attendants, in moist cough spray. About 1% of infected cows develop lesions in the udder and bacilli are excreted in the milk which can then infect people who drink it raw. Thus, primary human tuberculosis due to *M. bovis* usually involves cervical or mesenteric lymph nodes. In developed countries, control of *M. bovis* in dairy herds and pasteurization of milk have virtually eradicated this organism. *M. avium* and closely related *M. intracellulare* (*M. avium-intracellulare*) cause lymphadenitis, pulmonary lesions and disseminated disease in 15–24% of patients with AIDS. Human tuberculosis is divisible into primary and post-primary (secondary) forms.

Primary tuberculosis

This begins with inhalation of the mycobacteria and ends with a T cell-mediated immune response that induces hypersensitivity to the organisms and controls 95% of infections. Inhaled tubercle bacilli are engulfed by alveolar macrophages in which they replicate to form the initial lesion or **Ghon focus**. It consists of a parenchymal subpleural lesion, often just above or just below the interlobar fissure between the upper and the lower lobes.

Some bacilli are transported by macrophages to the hilar lymph nodes. The Ghon focus together with the enlarged hilar lymph nodes forms the **primary complex**. In addition, the bacilli may be seeded by further lymphatic and haematogenous dissemination in many organs and tissues, including other parts of the lung. In case of *M. bovis* which enters the mouth, as in milk-borne bovine tuberculosis, the primary complexes involve the tonsil and cervical lymph nodes or the intestine, often the ileocaecal region, and the mesenteric lymph nodes.

Naive macrophages are unable to kill the mycobacteria, the latter multiply, lyse the host cell, infect other macrophages and sometimes disseminate through the blood to other parts of the lung and elsewhere in the body. Within about 10 days of infection, clones of antigen-specific T lymphocytes (CD4+ helper T cells and CD8+ suppressor T cells) are produced interacting with macrophages in two ways:

1. CD4+ helper T cells secrete interferon-gamma, which activates macrophages to kill intracellular mycobacteria. These activated macrophages are termed epithelioid cells from their microscopical resemblance to epithelial cells. These form a compact cluster or **epithelioid cell granuloma** around the foci of infection. Some of them fuse to form multinucleated giant cells.

2. CD8+ suppressor T cells kill macrophages that are infected with mycobacteria, resulting in the formation of **caseating granulomas** (delayed-type hypersensitivity reaction). Direct toxicity of the mycobacteria to the macrophages may also contribute to the necrotic centre. Activated macrophages in the granuloma are metabolically very active. They consume oxygen and the resulting anoxia and acidosis in the centre of the lesion probably kills most of the tubercle bacilli. Therefore, granuloma formation is usually sufficient to limit the primary infection.

Surrounding fibroblasts produce dense scar tissue which may become calcified. Not all bacilli are destroyed, some remain in a dormant form as **persisters**, which when reactivated cause post-primary disease. If a focus ruptures into a blood vessel, bacilli are disseminated throughout the body with the formation of numerous granulomas. From the millet seed-like appearance of the lesions, this is known as **miliary tuberculosis**.

Post-primary (secondary) tuberculosis

It is caused by reactivation of the primary lesion (endogenous), or by exogenous reinfection. Reactivation tuberculosis is particularly likely to occur in immunocompromised individuals including the elderly, transplant recipients and those who are infected with human immunodeficiency virus (HIV).

Granulomas of secondary tuberculosis most often occur in the apex of the lungs but may be widely disseminated in the lungs, kidneys, meninges, bones and other organs. The same process of granuloma formation occurs but the necrotic element of the reaction causes tissue destruction and the formation of large areas of caseation termed **tuberculomas**.

Proteases liberated by activated macrophages cause softening and liquefaction of the caseous material. Two special features of secondary tuberculosis are the presence of caseous necrosis and of cavities, which may rupture into blood vessels, spreading mycobacteria throughout the body, and break into airways, releasing infectious mycobacteria in aerosols and sputum (**open tuberculosis**).

Oral manifestations

The lesions of oral mucosa, in tuberculosis, are generally secondary to pulmonary disease. The organisms are carried in the sputum and enter the mucosal tissue through a small break in the surface. These may also be carried to the oral tissues by haematogenous route, to be deposited in the submucosa and subsequently proliferate and ulcerate the overlying mucosa. Lesions may occur at any site on the oral mucous membrane, but the tongue is most commonly affected (Fig. 25.3), followed by the palate, lips, buccal mucosa, gingiva and frenula.

The usual tuberculous lesion is an irregular, superficial or deep, painful ulcer which tends to increase slowly in size. Occasional mucosal lesions show swelling or fissuring, but no obvious clinical

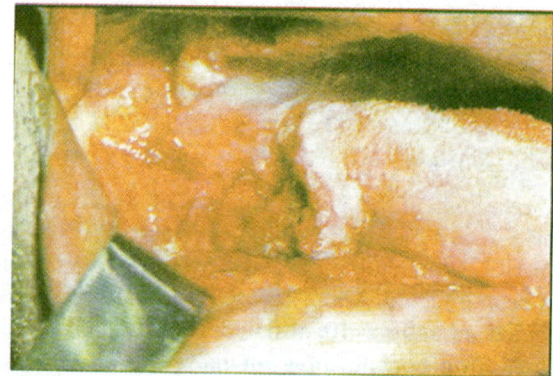

Fig. 25.3. A painful, deep and ragged-edged tuberculous ulcer of the tongue.

ulceration. Tuberculous gingivitis is an unusual form of tuberculosis which may appear as a diffuse, hyperaemic, nodular or papillary proliferation of the gingival tissues. Diffuse involvement of the maxilla or mandible may also occur, usually by haematogenous spread of infection, but sometimes by direct extension or even after tooth extraction. Tuberculous osteomyelitis frequently occurs in the later stages of the disease.

Immunity and hypersensitivity

Two immunologic responses, **antituberculous immunity and tuberculin hypersensitivity**, develop simultaneously in naturally infected host. Both these are mediated by T-cells sensitized to bacterial antigen. Humoral immunity appears to be of no relevance in tuberculosis and antibodies do not influence the course of disease. In the non-immune host, the bacilli are able to multiply inside phagocytes and lyse the host cells, while in immune host CD4+ helper T cells and CD8+ suppressor T cells are produced. The former secrete interferon-gamma which activates macrophages to kill intracellular mycobacteria and the latter kill the macrophages that are infected with mycobacteria.

Koch's phenomenon

The tuberculin reactivity was first demonstrated in guinea-pigs by Robert Koch (1890, 1891). The experiment that led to the demonstration of this reactivity is known as Koch's phenomenon. When a healthy guinea-pig is inoculated subcutaneously with a pure culture of tubercle bacilli, the puncture site heals quickly and there is no immediate visible reaction. But after 10–14 days a hard nodule appears which soon breaks down to form an ulcer that persists till the animal dies of progressive tuberculosis. The regional lymph nodes are enlarged and caseous.

But something totally different develops when a guinea-pig already ill with tuberculosis is inoculated. It is best to use animals that have been successfully inoculated 4–6 weeks previously. An indurated lesion appears at the site of second inoculation in a day or two which undergoes necrosis in another day to form a shallow ulcer that heals rapidly without involvement of the regional lymph nodes or other tissues. **Koch's phenomenon is a combination of hypersensitivity and immunity** and has three components:

1. A local reaction of induration and necrosis.
2. A focal response in which there occurs acute congestion and even haemorrhage around tuberculous foci in tissues.
3. A systemic response of fever which may sometimes be fatal.

Delayed (Type IV) hypersensitivity can be induced by live attenuated and killed bacilli, bacillary products and tuberculoprotein with a purified wax extract of bacilli. For the demonstration of hypersensitivity, live or killed bacilli or tuberculoprotein (tuberculin) may be employed. This hypersensitivity can be passively transferred by cells (cell-mediated) but not by serum.

Tuberculin test

Principle

Delayed, type IV or cell-mediated hypersensitivity.

Reagents

1. *Old tuberculin (OT):* It was originally described by Robert Koch. It is prepared by autoclaving or boiling a culture of tubercle bacilli, concentrating it 10-fold on a steam bath, filtering off the debris, and adding glycerol as preservative. OT is a crude product and different batches vary in their activity. The active constituent in this crude product is a protein which is remarkable for its heat stability. Stock solutions retain full potency for years when stored at 5°C. It has been replaced by purified protein derivative.
2. *Purified protein derivative (PPD):* A slightly more refined tuberculin called purified protein derivative was prepared by Seibert by growing *M. tuberculosis* in a semisynthetic medium, autoclaving, removing debris by filtration, concentrating the filtrate by ultrafiltration and precipitating several times with 50% saturated ammonium sulphate. The product is mostly a mixture of small proteins (average molecular weight 10,000).

The dosage of PPD is expressed in tuberculin units (TU). One large batch of PPD made by Seibert in 1939, PPD-S, was recognised by WHO as the international standard PPD-tuberculin and arbitrarily designated it to contain 50,000 TU per mg, 1 TU equal to 0.01 ml of OT or 0.00002 mg of PPD-S.

Method

1. *Mantoux test:* 0.1 ml of PPD containing 5 TU is injected intracutaneously into the skin of the volar aspect of the forearm. Those suspected of having tuberculosis, and therefore likely to react strongly, may first be tested with 1 TU. The site of inoculation is palpated 72 hours later. The development of an area of palpable, firm induration 10 mm or more in diameter is recorded as positive, and those between 5 and 9 mm in diameter as doubtful. The extent of the accompanying erythema is irrelevant and should be ignored. If the reaction is completely negative, the test may be repeated by giving an injection of 100 TU.

2. *Heaf test:* This test is done with a multiple puncture apparatus with 6 needles that prick 1–2 mm deep into the skin. A drop of undiluted PPD is spread on the area of skin selected for inoculation. The multiple puncture apparatus is pressed against this area of skin and needles are released. The test is read after 72 hours. Erythema and induration around at least 4 of the punctures is regarded as positive. The equipment must be adequately sterilized between each use to prevent transmission of hepatitis and AIDS.

Uses of tuberculin test

1. To diagnose active infection in infants and young children.
2. To measure prevalence of infection in a community.
3. To select susceptibles for BCG vaccination.
4. Indication of successful BCG vaccination.

False negative (tuberculin anergy)

1. Early tuberculosis.
2. Advanced tuberculosis.
3. Miliary tuberculosis.
4. In patients with measles and other exanthematous reactions.
5. Occasionally after chemotherapy and removal of lung lesion.
6. Advanced age.
7. Immunosuppressive therapy and defective CMI.
8. Lymphoreticular malignancy.
9. Sarcoidosis.
10. Severe malnutrition.

False positive

False positive reactions may be seen in patients with infection by related mycobacteria (atypical mycobacteria). These are usually low grade reactions and can be differentiated by testing with tuberculin prepared from these mycobacteria.

Laboratory diagnosis

It can be carried out by direct and indirect methods (Table 25.4). Bacteriological diagnosis can be established by demonstration of tubercle bacilli in clinical specimens by microscopy and cultural techniques. Only up to 50% of pulmonary and 25% of extrapulmonary tuberculosis can be diagnosed by smear examination.

Table 25.4. Laboratory diagnosis of tuberculosis

DIRECT METHODS
Bacteriological methods
- Direct microscopy
- Concentration of specimens
  - Petroff's method
  - Other methods
- Culture methods
  - Traditional
  - Radiometric

Molecular methods
- Polymerase chain reaction
- Ligase chain reaction

INDIRECT METHODS
- Serology
  - ELISA
  - Latex agglutination

Collection of specimen

- The specimen most commonly collected is **sputum** which consists of pus and mucus secretions coughed up from the lung. Patient is instructed to cough up the sputum into a clean wide-mouthed container. Disposable waxed cardboard containers are ideal. A morning specimen may be collected.
- If sputum is scanty, a 24 hour specimen may be collected. If no sputum is produced, **laryngeal swab** or **bronchial washings** are examined. In children, stomach washings may be examined as they tend to swallow sputum.

- Depending upon the site of involvement, **cerebrospinal fluid, pleural fluid, urine and aspirated fluid from bone and joint** are centrifuged and the deposits are examined.
- **Tissue biopsies** are homogenized and examined by microscopy and culture.
- In pulmonary and renal tuberculosis, three consecutive specimens of **sputum and urine** should be examined respectively.

Direct microscopy

Pour the sputum in a petri dish and examine. For preparation of smear, select **blood-tinged part** of the sputum, if it is not there then **purulent part** should be selected. The smear is stained by Ziehl-Neelsen technique and examined under oil-immersion lens. Acid-fast bacilli stain bright red against a blue background (Fig. 25.1.). To be detected microscopically, there must be 50,000–100,000 bacilli per ml of sputum. A negative report should not be given till at least 300 fields have been examined, taking about 10 minutes.

Concentration of specimens

Mycobacteria in a specimen can be decontaminated and concentrated into a small volume without inactivation. Such concentrate can be used for microscopy, culture and animal inoculation. Several methods are in use:

Petroff's method

It is a simple and widely used technique. Equal volumes of sputum and 4% sodium hydroxide are mixed and incubated at 37°C with frequent shaking till it gets liquefied and becomes clear. On the average, it takes 20–30 minutes. It is then centrifuged at 3,000 rpm for 30 minutes. The supernatant fluid is pipetted off and the deposit is neutralized by adding 8% hydrochloric acid in the presence of a drop of phenol red indicator.

Other methods

Instead of alkali, homogenization can be carried out by treatment with dilute acids (5% oxalic acid, 3% hydrochloric acid or 6% sulphuric acid) or mucolytic agents such as N-acetyl-L-cysteine with sodium hydroxide and pancreatin.

Culture

It is very sensitive for detection of tubercle bacilli. It may be positive with as few as 10–100 bacilli per ml of sputum and it is necessary for antimicrobial drug sensitivity testing. **Concentrate of sputum** is inoculated on two slopes of LJ medium. In case of **laryngeal swab**, add enough 5% oxalic acid to the tube to cover the swab and leave it at room temperature for 30 minutes to kill non-acid-fast contaminants. Squeeze the swab against the side of the tube to remove excess fluid and rub it over the surface of two slopes of LJ medium.

In case of **gastric washings**, 15 ml of the specimen is collected in a 25 ml bottle containing 5 ml of 15% trisodium phosphate, which will neutralize the acid. Then cap and shake the bottle. In the laboratory, homogenize and decontaminate the specimen by Petroff's method. Centrifuge and examine the deposit by Ziehl-Neelsen staining and culture on LJ medium.

In case of **renal tuberculosis**, three early morning specimens of urine should be collected. Twenty four hours collection is unsatisfactory due to increased bacterial contamination and lower recovery rate as compared with a single voided specimen. Each specimen should consist of 50–100 ml. It is centrifuged at 1500 g for 30 minutes and treat the deposit by Petroff's method. Prepare a smear and stain by Ziehl-Neelsen staining and inoculate on two slopes of LJ medium.

Tubercle bacilli are usually scanty in **pleural and peritoneal fluids**. Therefore, at least 50–100 ml of either of these should be collected. Centrifuge these fluids and treat the deposits by Petroff's method as above. In case of **CSF**, 3–4 ml is collected and centrifuged. The deposit is used for the smear and culture. **Pus** is directly used for smear and culture.

The inoculated media are incubated at 37°C. The cultures are examined weekly for 12 weeks. Growth of most strains of *M. tuberculosis* may appear in 2–8 weeks. But cultures should not be discarded as negative until they have been observed for 12 weeks. Longer incubation is necessary for strains originating from patients treated with antituberculous agents. However, by **radiometric method** the growth may be detected in about a week by using ^{14}C labelled substrates and measuring $^{14}CO_2$ evolved due to bacterial metabolism. The sensitivity of radiometric method is slightly more than that of traditional culture method.

Molecular methods

Polymerase chain reaction and ligase chain reaction are used as diagnostic techniques.

Serodiagnostic techniques

(a) Enzyme-linked immunosorbent assay (ELISA)

ELISA techniques employing various mycobacterial antigens, e.g., glycolipids from *M. bovis* BCG, antigens 5 and 6 from *M. tuberculosis*, 64 kDa protein of *M. bovis* BCG, 32 kDa protein antigen called P32 and antigen 60 of *M. bovis* BCG have been attempted for rapid diagnosis of different clinical forms of tuberculosis by estimating specific IgM, IgA and IgG antibodies in the sera of the patients. The sensitivity and specificity of ELISA test, when combined IgA and IgG antibody titres are considered, are 91.6% and 90.0% respectively.

(b) Latex agglutination

Latex particles coated with rabbit antibody to *M. tuberculosis* has been found giving an overall sensitivity of 94.4% and specificity of 99.2% for the diagnosis of tubercular meningitis.

Prophylaxis

Protection from tuberculosis may be afforded by public health measures, BCG vaccination and by chemoprophylaxis. General measures such as adequate nutrition, good housing and health education are important.

BCG vaccine

It is a live attenuated vaccine introduced by Calmette and Guerin (1921). This is a strain of *M. bovis* attenuated by repeated subcultures, every 3 weeks, for 239 subcultures on slices of potato soaked in auto-claved bile containing glycerol (5%) over a period of 13 years (1908–1921). This species was selected for vaccine preparation in preference to *M. tuber-culosis* because of the false assumption that it was of limited virulence in man. Injection of BCG in guinea-pig leads to dissemination and multiplication of the bacilli in different organs with the production of small tubercles. The lesions disappear slowly.

BCG vaccine is available in liquid form and freeze-dried (lyophilized) form. The latter is commonly used. The lyophilized vaccine supplied by BCG vaccine laboratory, Chennai, is reconstituted in sterile physiological saline to make a final concentration of 0.1 mg (moist weight) in 0.1 ml of the vaccine. Once reconstituted, vaccine should be utilized within 3–6 hours. Following injection of 0.1 ml of vaccine intradermally, the organisms grow to a limited extent in the tissues. Immunizing capability of the vaccine depends on this. Dead vaccine or tuberculin is not effective. BCG vaccine should be administered soon after birth failing which it may be given at any time during the first year of life.

A **small nodule** develops at the site of inoculation 2–3 weeks after injection. It increases slowly in size and by about 5 weeks it attains a diameter of 4–8 mm. It then subsides or breaks into a **shallow ulcer** which heals by scarring. Such individuals become **tuberculin-positive** after 4–6 weeks. A few cases have been recorded where BCG has given rise to progressive tuberculosis.

The protective efficacy of BCG vaccine has been determined in a number of vaccine trials. The results have varied from 80% efficacy to a total absence of protection. The immunity has been reported to last for about 10 years. The consensus of opinion at present is that BCG does protect from tuberculosis. The disease runs a milder course in immunized children. It is also believed to prevent meningeal, skeletal and miliary form of tuberculosis to a large extent. BCG vaccine stimulates T lymphocytes which reportedly offer some protection against leprosy and leukaemia also.

Complications of BCG vaccination

1. *Local:*
   - Abscess
   - Indolent ulcer
   - Keloid
   - Tuberculids (small satellite BCG tubercles developing in the neighbourhood of the site of vaccination).

2. *Regional:*
   • Lymphadenitis.
3. *Systemic:*
   • Fever
   • Erythema nodosum
   • Otitis media.

Contraindications of BCG

BCG vaccination is contraindicated in patients of tuberculosis, AIDS, measles, pertussis and eczema, and patients on steroids, and tuberculin-positive individuals.

Chemoprophylaxis

Chemoprophylaxis is advocated in:

• Unavoidable contact with a patient with open tuberculosis, e.g., a baby born to a mother with the disease.
• Tuberculin-positive but radiologically clear unvaccinated children.
• Older persons with radiological evidence of quiescent disease.

   Such individuals are given isoniazid alone with the assumption that bacillary load is small and the chance of emergence of a drug-resistant mutant is remote.

Chemotherapy

The antituberculous drugs include rifampin, isoniazid, pyrazinamide, streptomycin, ethambutol and thiacetazone. The first 4 of these are bactericidal and the others are bacteriostatic. Other less often used drugs include ethionamide, cycloserine, capreo-mycin, kanamycin and *p*-aminosalicylic acid.

   In clinical practice, mutational resistance is of great importance in tuberculosis. If patient is treated with only one antituberculous drug, initially the bacilli die in large numbers but, soon resistant mutants appear and multiply unchecked. Therefore, generally three drugs are given simultaneously. Initially prolonged treatment for two or more years used to be given. But with the advent of actively bactericidal drugs like rifampin, short course regimens of about 6 months have been found adequate in many cases.

   Tubercle bacilli resistant to a number of anti-tuberculous drugs (**multidrug-resistant tuber-culosis**, **MDR-TB**) is a growing problem. Prevalence of MDR-TB cases is on the high in India. MDR-TB cases threaten the effectiveness of chemotherapy for both the treatment and control of tuberculosis and require the use of second-line drugs that are more expensive, toxic and less effective than first-line antituberculous drugs.

ATYPICAL MYCOBACTERIA

Mycobacteria other than tubercle and leprosy bacilli, that normally exist as saprophytes of soil and water (environment) and occasionally cause opportunistic disease in man resembling tuberculosis are known as atypical, environmental, opportunistic, tuberculoid mycobacteria or MOTT (mycobacteria other than typical tubercle) bacilli. The names 'environmental' or 'opportunistic' mycobacteria are better suited as their natural habitat is soil or water and they cause opportunistic infections in human beings. Infection caused by these organisms is known as **myco-bacteriosis**. Atypical mycobacteria are:

• Acid-fast and alcohol-fast and may resemble or differ in morphology from tubercle bacilli.
• They may be longer and even filamentous.
• They can grow at 25°C and 37°C. Some of them (*M. xenopi*, *M. phlei* and *M. smegmatis*) can grow at 44°C.
• Some of them are rapid growers. They produce visible growth on LJ medium within one week.
• Some of them produce a bright yellow or orange pigment.
• They are resistant to antituberculous drugs such as streptomycin, isoniazid and *p*-aminosalicylic acid. All of them are resistant to at least one of these drugs. However, many strains are sensitive to rifampin.
• They are niacin and neutral red reactions negative.
• They produce enzyme arylsulphatase.
• They are non-pathogenic for guinea-pig but pathogenic for mouse.
• They occasionally cause opportunistic disease, resembling tuberculosis in man.

Classification

On the basis of production of bright yellow or orange pigment and rate of growth, Runyon (1959) classified atypical mycobacteria into four groups (Table 25.5). Atypical mycobacteria can grow on LJ medium. All strains of groups I, II and III grow slowly and form colonies in 2–8 weeks. However, group IV (rapid growers) produce colonies within one week.

Table 25.5. Atypical mycobacteria

Runyon group	Name	Species
I	Photo-chromogens	*Mycobacterium kansasii, M. marinum, M. simiae*
II	Scoto-chromogens	*M. scrofulaceum, M. gordonae, M. szulgai*
III	Non-chromogens	*M. avium, M. intracellulare, M. xenopi, M. ulcerans, M. malmoense, M. terrae, M. triviale, M. nonchromo-genicum*
IV	Rapid growers	*M. smegmatis, M. phlei, M. chelonae, M. fortuitum*

I. Photochromogens

They form colourless colonies when incubated in the dark, but when the young culture is exposed to light for one hour in the presence of air (cap of the culture bottle loosened) and re-incubated for 24–48 hours, they develop a bright yellow or orange pigment (beta-carotene).

This group contains three species – *M. kansasii, M. marinum* and *M. simiae*.

- *M. kansasii* causes chronic pulmonary disease resembling tuberculosis, particularly in old persons with pre-existing lung disease. It has been isolated on several occasions from piped water supplies. It grows well at 37°C on LJ medium yielding a good growth within two weeks and reduces nitrate to nitrite. The bacterial cells are usually elongated and have a distinct beaded appearance. It is usually sensitive to rifampin and several other anti-tuberculous drugs.
- *M. simiae* was originally isolated from monkeys. Like *M. kansasii*, it grows well at 37°C and causes pulmonary disease. It synthesizes niacin in significant amounts and may thus be falsely identified as *M. tuberculosis*.

- *M. marinum* was originally isolated from fish. It grows poorly or not at all at 37°C. It grows well at 33°C. It causes superficial granulomatous skin disease of man known as **swimming pool granuloma** or **fish tank granuloma**. It resembles *M. kansasii* in colonial and microscopic appearance. *M. marinum* may however be distinguished from *M. kansasii* by its:
  – poor or no growth at 37°C;
  – failure to reduce nitrate to nitrite and failure to produce catalase; and
  – ability to hydrolyze pyrazinamide.

II. Scotochromogens

These organisms form bright yellow or orange pigment in cultures incubated in the dark, though the intensity of the colour may increase on exposure to light.

- *M. scrofulaceum* is an important member of this group which may cause **scrofula** (cervical lymphadenitis) in children. The bacilli may be short or long and filamentous. It is resistant to isoniazid and sensitive to cycloserine and ethionamide.
- *M. gordonae* is often found in water. It is a frequent contaminant of clinical specimens and a rare cause of pulmonary disease.
- *M. szulgai* is a scotochromogen when incubated at 37°C and photochromogen at 25°C. It may occasionally cause pulmonary disease and bursitis.

III. Non-chromogens

They do not form pigment even on exposure to light. Medically important species include *M. intra-cellulare, M. avium, M. xenopi, M. ulcerans* and *M. malmoense*.

- *M. intracellulare* was formerly known as Battey bacillus as it was first detected in Battey State Hospital for tuberculosis in Georgia, USA. The infection with this organism is common in the Southeast USA, where the organism occurs in soil and water. It causes chronic pulmonary disease indistinguishable from tuberculosis.
- *M. avium* causes tuberculosis in fowls and sometimes in pigs. It is similar in reactions to *M. intracellulare*. It can grow at 45°C. *M. avium* and

M. intracellulare are the **commonest atypical mycobacteria** causing opportunistic infections in man. Colonies of both these species are smooth, non-pigmented and easily emulsifiable.

Because there is no clear-cut division between *M. avium* and *M. intracellulare*, therefore, they are usually grouped together as *M. avium-intracellulare* (MAI) or *M. avium* complex (MAC). This complex possesses 28 agglutination serotypes. Types 1, 2 and 3 are regarded as *M. avium* and the others as *M. intracellulare*. In man, MAC causes pulmonary disease indistinguishable from tuberculosis, lymphadenitis and disseminated disease, particularly in patients with AIDS.

- *M. xenopi* was first isolated from a skin lesion in a South African toad (*Xenopus laevis*). It is a thermophile and grows well at 45°C. It may cause pulmonary lesions in man. It has a limited geographical distribution. Most of the cases of pulmonary lesions, due to *M. xenopi* have been reported from South London.

- *M. ulcerans*, causative agent of **Buruli ulcer**, was originally isolated from ulcerative skin lesions in Australia in 1948. The name Buruli ulcer is derived from the Buruli district of Uganda where a large outbreak of the disease was extensively investigated. *M. ulcerans* grows slowly at 31–34°C but not at all at 37°C in primary culture. It produces an exotoxin which has been characterized as a high molecular weight phospholipoprotein-lipopolysaccharide complex, which when inoculated intradermally in the guinea-pig, causes inflammation, tissue necrosis and histopathological changes similar to those seen in human lesions. Therefore, this exotoxin may be involved in the pathogenesis of the disease.

- *M. malmoense* causes pulmonary disease and lymphadenitis. It was first isolated from patients from Malmo in Sweden. It is a very slow-growing species. On primary isolation, colonies may not be visible until after 10 weeks incubation. It causes pulmonary disease and lymphadenitis. It is resistant to isoniazid and rifampin and sometimes also to streptomycin and ethambutol.

- *M. terrae*, *M. triviale* and *M. nonchromogenicum* are rare pathogens which belong to Runyon group III (non-chromogens). They are sometimes grouped as the *Mycobacterium-terrae-trivialenon-chromogenicum* group.

IV. Rapid growers

Rapid growers which may be photo-, scoto- or non-chromogens, produce visible growth on LJ medium within one week, usually in 2–3 days. All the chromogenic rapid growers, e.g., *M. smegmatis* and *M. phlei* are saprophytes.

- *M. smegmatis* forms rough colonies, white to buff in colour. The bacilli are slender rods, which may be curved and beaded. Since it is normally present in smegma, a whitish secretion around the orifice of urethra, it is a frequent contaminant of urine specimens. Some strains of *M. smegmatis* are acid-fast but not alcohol-fast, therefore, they are not seen in a Ziehl-Neelsen smear if acid-alcohol is used as decolourizer. Other strains are both acid- and alcohol-fast. In such cases, rapid growth on LJ medium and guinea-pig inoculation distinguishes it from *M. tuberculosis*. *M. smegmatis* has been implicated in rare cases of pulmonary, skin, soft tissue, and bone infections.

- *M. phlei* is rarely encountered and is non-pathogenic. It grows as rough colonies that at first are buff coloured and later become yellow to orange. It can be differentiated from *M. smegmatis* by its ability to grow at 52°C and survive heating at 60°C for 4 hours.

Only two of the rapid growers, *M. chelonae* and *M. fortuitum* are human pathogens. Both these are coccoid to filamentous and form white to cream-coloured colonies. The former grows better at 25°C than at 37°C. *M. fortuitum* can further be differentiated from *M. chelonae* in reducing nitrate and assimilation of iron from ferric ammonium citrate. *M. chelonae* was originally identified as turtle and *M. fortuitum* as frog tubercle bacilli. They are found in soil and infection usually follows some injury and can lead to chronic abscess formation. They occasionally cause pulmonary or disseminated disease.

MYCOBACTERIUM LEPRAE

Morphology

Lepra bacilli are straight or slightly curved slender bacilli about the same size as tubercle bacilli (average size: 3 × 0.3 μm). They have pointed, rounded or club-shaped ends. They are non-motile and non-sporing. They are Gram-positive and stain more readily than *M. tuberculosis*. With Ziehl-Neelsen stain, they are less acid-fast than tubercle bacilli, so 5% sulphuric acid instead of 20% is employed for decolourization after staining with carbol fuchsin.

The bacilli are seen singly and in groups, intracellularly and lying free outside the cell. Inside the cells they are usually present in parallel bundles of 50 or more organisms bound together by a lipid-like substance, the **glia**. These masses of bacteria are known as **globi** which are seen inside the histiocytes which have a foamy appearance. These are known as **lepra cells** (Fig. 25.4).

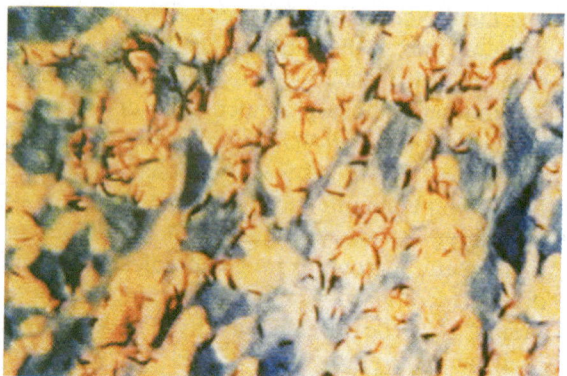

Fig. 25.4. Lepromatous leprosy showing acid-fast bacilli in macrophages.

Live bacilli in the smear appear solid and uniformly stained, while dead or dying forms appear fragmented, beaded and granular. The percentage of uniformly stained bacilli in the tissues is known as **morphological index (MI)**. This provides a method for assessing the progress of patients on chemo-therapy and is more meaningful than the old criterion, the **bacteriological index (BI)**. Poorly stained bacilli are probably dead. A continuing fall in the MI is encouraging and a fall succeeded by a rise indicates development of **drug resistance** in the bacteria. Bacteriological index of a smear is the total number of acid-fast bacilli in an oil-immersion field. It can be expressed from 1+ to 6+ by Ridley's scale (Table 25.6).

Table 25.6. Bacteriological index (Ridley's scale)

Bacteriological index	Number of acid-fast bacilli
6+	More than 1000 per oil-immersion field
5+	100–1000 per oil-immersion field
4+	10–100 per oil-immersion field
3+	1–10 per oil-immersion field
2+	1–10 per 10 oil-immersion fields
1+	1–10 per 100 oil-immersion fields

Cultivation

A large number of attempts at cultivation of *M. leprae*, in artificial culture media and in tissue culture, have been made and success has been claimed from time to time, but none has been confirmed so far. One of the best known of such reports came from Indian Cancer Research Centre (ICRC), Bombay (now Mumbai) (1962), where an acid-fast bacillus was isolated from a leprosy patient, employing human foetal spinal ganglion cell culture. This is known as **ICRC bacillus.** It has been adapted for growth on LJ medium.

There have been many attempts to transmit leprosy to various experimental animals. But the first breakthrough was achieved by Shepard (1960) when he reported a limited localized multiplication of *M. leprae* in the **footpad of mouse** in 1–6 months.

Nine-banded armadillo (*Dasypus novem-cinctus*) (Fig. 25.5) is highly susceptible to leprosy. This is presumably due to low body temperature. When inoculated with *M. leprae*, about 40% armadillos develop generalized infection with extensive multiplication of *M. leprae*.

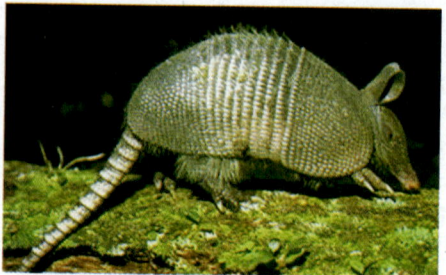

Fig. 25.5. Nine-banded armadillo.

Pathogenesis

Leprosy is an exclusively human disease and the only source of infection is the patient. The exact mode of infection is not clear. Very large number of bacilli are shed in nasal secretions (over 10^8 organisms per ml) and in discharges from superficial lesions of the cases of lepromatous leprosy. Organisms may be acquired by a susceptible person by way of skin to skin contact or through respiratory tract. It has also been suggested that insect vectors may have a role in transmission of leprosy.

Once worldwide in distribution, leprosy is now confined mainly, but not exclusively, to the under-developed areas of tropics and southern hemisphere. There has been a considerable decline in the number of cases, from 12 million in 1980s to less than two million in 1996, partly as a result of control programmes.

India has the maximum prevalence, with about a third of the global total. Leprosy is present in all states and territories of India, but with marked regional variations – Orissa and Bihar having the highest prevalence (> 5 per 1000 population) and Haryana the least (< 0.1 per 1000 population).

M. leprae causes **chronic granulomatous lesions** closely resembling those of tuberculosis with epithelioid cells and giant cells but **without caseation**. The organisms in the lesion are predominantly intracellular and like tubercle bacilli can proliferate in macrophages. The organism has predilection for skin, nerves and nasal mucosa though it is capable of affecting any tissue or organ.

In **cutaneous form** of the disease, large, firm nodules are distributed widely and on the face they create a characteristic **leonine appearance**.

In **the neural form**, segments of peripheral nerves are involved leading to **localized patches of anaesthesia**. The loss of sensations in fingers and toes increases the frequency of minor trauma, leading to secondary infection and mutilating injuries. Both forms may be present in the same patient.

Oral manifestations

Oral lesions consist of small tumour-like masses called **lepromas**, which develop on the tongue, lip or hard palate. These nodules show a tendency to break down and ulcerate. Gingival hyperplasia with loosening of the teeth has also been described.

Spectrum of leprosy

On the basis of clinical, histopathologic and immuno-logic findings, Ridley and Joplings (1966) introduced a scale for classifying the spectrum of leprosy into 5 types with hyperreactive tuberculoid (TT) leprosy at one pole and anergic lepromatous (LL) leprosy at the other.

Tuberculoid type: It is seen in patients with high degree of resistance where cell-mediated immunity is intact. The skin lesions are few and consist of non elevated hypo-or hyperpigmented macular anaesthetic patches involving the face, trunk and limbs. There are very few acid-fast bacilli (AFB) so that they are generally not seen microscopically (**paucibacillary disease**) and numerous epithelioid cells, giant cells and lymphocytes as in tuberculosis. The local nerves are involved in the early stage and gradually the infection extends into the bigger nerve trunks which are thickened, hard and tender. This leads to deformities of hands, and feet. In tuberculoid leprosy, lepromin test is positive due to intact CMI. Antimycobacterial and autoantibodies are rarely produced.

Lepromatous type: It is the generalized form of the disease and is found in individuals where the host resistance is low. Patient develops numerous nodular skin lesions (**lepromata**) on face, ear lobes, hands, feet and less commonly trunk. Skin lesions contain many macrophages, often seen as large foamy cells packed with AFB (Fig. 25.4). In advanced cases, there may be 10^9 *M. leprae*/g of skin (**multibacillary disease**). Cooler parts of the body, such as ear lobes, are particularly infiltrated by bacilli. Blood stream may be invaded, with resulting foci in the liver, spleen, adrenals, testicles and bone marrow and excretion of the organisms in milk. In addition, there is heavy infection of upper respiratory tract, particularly the nasal mucosa, from which the organisms are shed.

There is slow and symmetric thickening of nerves and anaesthesia. Nodular skin lesions ulcerate due to repeated trauma as a result of loss of sensation. The ulcerated nodules become secondarily infected that leads to distortion and mutilation of extremities.

Lepromatous leprosy is more infectious than other types and has a poor prognosis. Because of deficient CMI, lepromin test is negative. Humoral antibodies against mycobacterial antigens are produced in high concentrations which play no protective role. **Autoantibodies are also produced.**

Borderline or dimorphous type: Many patients occupy an intermediate position on the spectrum and are classified as **borderline tuberculoid (BT), mid-borderline or borderline borderline (BB) and borderline lepromatous (BL)**. The characteristics of these five types are shown in Table 25.7.

Table 25.7. Characteristics of 5 types of leprosy					
	TT	BT	BB	BL	LL
1. AFB in the skin	–	+/–	+	+++	++++
2. AFB in nasal secretions	–	–	–	+	++++
3. Granuloma formation	++++	+++	+	–	–
4. Lepromin reaction	++++	+	+/–	–	–
5. Antibodies to *M. leprae*	+/–	+/–	+	+++	++++

In all types of leprosy, *M. leprae* organisms invade both sensory and motor nerves and destroy nerve fibres. **No other bacterial species has the capacity to enter nerves.** *M. leprae* invades dermal nerves and nerve trunks, but the most vulnerable sites are parts of the body that either tend to remain cool or are subject to trauma. The organisms are present in Schwann and perineural cells. The nasal bones are also involved in leprosy and their destruction may lead to **collapse of the nose**. The eye is frequently damaged by direct bacillary invasion or corneal infection secondary to paralysis of the eyelids leading to blindness.

Immunity

There seems to exist a high degree of innate immunity in man, therefore, only a minority of the contacts develop clinical manifestations of disease and many others develop a localized lesion that heals spontaneously. Infection with *M. leprae* induces both antibody-mediated and cell-mediated immunity (CMI). Of these, only CMI is protective. The type of leprosy

in an individual is determined by the status of CMI in him. When it is adequate, the lesions are of tuberculoid type and when it is inadequate, these are of lepromatous type. Patients with tuberculoid leprosy exhibit a strong delayed type hypersensitivity to lepromin. The macrophages phagocytose the bacilli and destroy them. Specific humoral antibodies are not prominent. There is no increase in immunoglobulin levels and the albumin globulin ratio in the serum is not altered.

Patients at the lepromatous pole of the spectrum exhibit negative lepromin test. Antibodies to *M. leprae* that cross-react with other mycobacteria may be detected in the sera of 75–95% of the patients. The albumin globulin ratio in the serum is reversed. The macrophages are able to phagocytose the bacilli, but instead of being destroyed, the bacilli proliferate in these cells. This is because of suppression of CMI in these patients.

Lepromin test

This reaction was first described by Mitsuda in Japan in 1919.

Lepromins

The lepromins used as antigen in lepromin test may be of human origin (lepromin-H) or of armadillo origin (lepromin-A) and are of two types:

1. **Integral lepromin (Mitsuda lepromin):** This was developed by Mitsuda in 1919 by boiling human lepromatous tissue rich in *M. leprae*. Standard Mitsuda lepromin contains 4.0×10^7 *M. leprae*/ml and has a shelf life of 2 years at 4°C. Mitsuda lepromin is increasingly being prepared from armadillo-derived *M. leprae* (lepromin-A).
2. **Bacillary lepromin:** This contains more of bacillary components and less of tissue. An important example of bacillary lepromin is Dharmendra antigen which is prepared by floating out the bacilli from finely ground lepromatous tissue with chloroform, evaporating it dry and removing the lipids by washing with ether. The antigen is made up in phenol saline for use.

Procedure

The test is carried out by the intradermal injection of 0.1 ml of lepromin. The response to this is biphasic:

1. **Early or Fernandez reaction:** It is characterized by an acute localized area of inflammation with congestion and oedema, more than 10 mm in diameter, appearing usually in 24–48 hours and tending to disappear in 3–4 days. Histologically, it consists of serous exudate with lymphocytic infiltration.

2. **Late or Mitsuda reaction:** It appears 1–2 weeks after the injection, reaching peak in 4 weeks. The reaction appears in the form of a nodule that may undergo central necrosis and ulceration. It takes several weeks to heal. Histologically, there is infiltration with lymphocytes, epithelioid cells and giant cells.

Fernandez reaction is like tuberculin reaction, a delayed type hypersensitivity (DTH). This reaction indicates that the patient has been infected at some time in the past. On the other hand, Mitsuda reaction is not a measure of pre-existing DTH, but is the **manifestation of cell-mediated immunity**, which the lepromin itself has induced. It thus discriminates between persons who are capable of responding to *M. leprae* and those who cannot.

Uses of lepromin reaction

1. To classify the lesions of leprosy patients. The reaction is positive in tuberculoid and negative in lepromatous leprosy patients.
2. To assess the prognosis and response to treatment. A positive reaction indicates a good prognosis and a negative one a bad prognosis. Conversion to lepromin positivity during treatment is the evidence of improvement.
3. To assess the resistance of an individual to leprosy.
4. For recruitment of persons to work in leprosy homes. Only lepromin-positive persons are recommended to be appointed.
5. To verify the identity of candidate *M. leprae*. Cultivable AFB, claimed to be *M. leprae*, should give matching results when tested in parallel with standard lepromin.

Laboratory diagnosis

As a routine, smears are made from affected parts of the skin and nasal mucous membrane. Material for smear is, however, sometimes taken from lymph nodes and affected nerves.

- In **lepromatous cases**, bacilli are always found in large numbers and about equally frequently in skin and nose. However, in the lepromatous cases under chemotherapy, nasal smears become negative earlier than the smears from skin lesions, consequently in cases under treatment, skin smears are more frequently positive than the nasal smears.

- In **tuberculoid cases**, as a rule, the bacilli are very few and found with great difficulty, or not at all. The characteristic histologic response in biopsy material is helpful in such cases and is essential for accurate classification of the disease within the disease spectrum.

Skin smears

The selection of site for taking smear is of great importance. Places where leprous lesions are most prominent, such as nodules, thick patches and areas of infiltration, should be selected. In case of patches, smears should be made from the thickened margins. In a patient with only diffuse infiltration, about 5–6 different areas of the skin should be sampled, including the skin over the ear lobes, buttocks, forehead, chin and cheeks. The specimen is obtained by **slit and scrape method**.

Thoroughly clean the selected portion of skin with spirit. This is necessary in order to remove any saprophytic acid-fast bacilli that may be present on the skin surface. Hold the skin pinched up and raised between the thumb and index finger of the left hand. This will squeeze out blood from the part and will minimize bleeding when the cut is made. With a small bladed-scalpel an incision, about 5 mm long and 3 mm deep, is made on the pinched skin. If any blood or lymph appears, wipe it away without releasing pressure on the held skin.

The blade of the scalpel is then turned at right angle to the cut (slit) and the bottom and sides of the slit are scraped with the point of the blade, several times in the same direction so that tissue fluid and pulp (not blood) collects on one side of the blade. This is gently smeared on glass slide.

Nasal scrapings

Smears from the nose are made by scraping a little material from the nasal septum, particularly from inferior turbinate bones, with a small-bladed knife.

When the smears dry, these are fixed by passing the slides twice or thrice over a flame with the surface carrying the smear uppermost. The smears are then stained by the Ziehl-Neelsen technique using 5%, instead of 20%, sulphuric acid for decolorization. Bacteriological and morphological indices (as already described) are also determined.

While examining smears from the nose, great care is needed because of the presence of weakly acid-fast diphtheroids in that site, which may be mistaken for acid-fast bacilli, especially when the smear is not properly decolourized. **Nasal smears are of great importance in deciding whether a leprosy patient is infectious or not.** They are positive in patients of leprosy of LL and BL type but are negative in all cases of BB, BT and TT. Furthermore, they disappear more rapidly from the nose as a result of chemo-therapy, than they do from skin lesions.

Skin and nerve biopsy

Skin biopsy is collected from active edge of the patches and nerve biopsy from thickened nerve for histological confirmation of tuberculoid leprosy when acid-fast bacilli cannot be demonstrated in direct smear. Skin biopsy is useful in the diagnosis and accurate classification of leprosy lesion but nerve biopsy is not required if a skin lesion is present.

Animal inoculation

- Injection of ground tissue from lepromatous nodules and nasal scraping from leprosy patient into the **footpad of mouse** produces typical granuloma at the site of inoculation in 1–6 months.
- **Nine-banded armadillo** is highly susceptible to leprosy. Such an animal, when inoculated with ground tissue from lepromatous nodules and nasal scrapings from leprosy patient, develops genera-lized infection with extensive multiplication of bacilli and the lesions produced resemble lepro-matous leprosy. The lesions which develop in the mouse and armadillo can be identified by histo-logical examination and Ziehl-Neelsen staining.

Lepromin test or Mitsuda reaction

It is not a diagnostic test but is a guide to the resistance of the patient to *M. leprae* infection.

Serological test

Serodiagnosis of leprosy may be carried out by detection of antiphenolic glycolipid 1 antibodies by latex agglutination, *M. leprae* particle agglutination and ELISA test.

Polymerase chain reaction (PCR)

PCR can be used for the diagnosis at an early stage before appearance of clinical symptoms. It is effective even in the diagnosis of paucibacillary leprosy, as **the detection limit of PCR is as low as one bacillus**. The PCR assay can be performed on biopsy specimens, skin scrapings and nasal secretions.

Treatment

Dapsone (4,4´-diaminodiphenyl sulphone, DDS) monotherapy was the standard treatment for all types of leprosy for a number of years. However, there is evidence that *M. leprae* is acquiring dapsone resistance. In view of this, multiple drug therapy is now recommended for the treatment of leprosy. Patients with paucibacillary lesions (TT, BT) are given rifampin 600 mg once a month and dapsone 100 mg daily for six months. For multibacillary lesions (BB, BL, LL), patient is administered rifampin 600 mg once a month, dapsone 100 mg daily and clofazimine 50 mg daily for 2 years.

Immunotherapy

Since lepromatous leprosy patients do not possess CMI, efforts are being made to induce effective CMI to *M. leprae* in these patients. Procedures for trying to achieve this objective include:

1. Intravenous injection of peripheral blood lympho-cytes obtained from patients with tuberculoid leprosy or from healthy donors possessing vigorous CMI and showing a strongly positive lepromin (Mitsuda) reaction.
2. Intravenous injection of transfer factor, an extract of lymphocytes, from patients suffering from tuberculoid leprosy. Sensitized lymphocytes secrete certain substances called lymphokines which stimulate the macrophages to ingest and kill the bacilli. If these substances are isolated and obtained from blood of patients with tuberculoid leprosy and injected into the lepromatous leprosy cases CMI can possibly be induced.
3. Intradermal injection of vaccine (see below).

Prevention

Measures for prevention of leprosy include:

- Early diagnosis and treatment.
- Surveillance of domestic contacts.
- Improvement of living conditions.
- Education.
- Vaccination.

Long-term chemoprophylaxis has given encouraging results in child contacts of infectious cases.

At present no effective vaccine against leprosy exists. A number of candidate vaccines (Table 25.8) have been tried and are still under trial. However, none of these has reached the stage for universal use. A candidate vaccine should be able to:

- induce upgrading in LL patients;
- bring about lepromin conversion both in the patients and healthy persons; and
- offer protection in animal models.

Table 25.8. Candidate anti-leprosy vaccines

First generation vaccines
- BCG
- Armadillo-derived killed *Mycobacterium leprae*
- BCG and killed *M. leprae*
- ICRC bacillus

Possible second generation vaccines
- Natural or recombinant form of 18, 31, 65 and 70 kDa proteins

KEY FACTS

- Mycobacteria are acid-fast beaded bacilli and resist decolourization with dilute mineral acids. Hence, a special stain, the Ziehl-Neelsen stain, is used to visualize them
- The above property is due to the high lipid content (40–60%) of the cell wall (mycolic acid), which is also an effective defence mechanism resisting phagocytosis
- *Mycobacterial infections are granulomatous and insidious*
- *Mycobacterium tuberculosis*, the causative agent of tuberculosis, is a long, slender, non-sporing, beaded bacillus. It grows slowly (up to 8–12 weeks) on Lowenstein-Jensen medium as 'rough, tough and buff' colonies
- *Multidrug-resistant tuberculosis (MDR-TB) is becoming an increasingly common problem, especially in the developing world*
- Mycobacteria other than typical tubercle (MOTT) bacilli is a collective name given to a group of mycobacteria of low human pathogenicity
- *Mycobacterium leprae* is less acid-fast than tubercle bacilli, so 5% sulphuric acid instead of 20% is employed for decolorization after staining with carbol fuchsin
- Leprosy, a disfiguring chronic illness, is caused by *M. leprae*

IMPORTANT QUESTIONS

1. Classify mycobacteria and discuss laboratory diagnosis of pulmonary tuberculosis.
2. Write short notes on:
   (a) Koch's phenomenon
   (b) Tuberculin test
   (c) BCG vaccine
3. Classify atypical mycobacteria and name diseases caused by them.
4. Write short notes on:
   (a) Photochromogens
   (b) Scotochromogens
   (c) Non-chromogens
   (d) *Mycobacterium avium* complex
   (e) Buruli ulcer
   (f) Swimming pool granuloma
5. Discuss pathogenesis and laboratory diagnosis of leprosy.
6. Write short notes on:
   (a) Lepromin test
   (b) Prevention of leprosy.

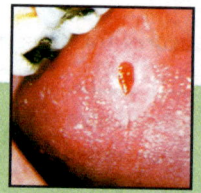

Chapter 26

Nonsporing Anaerobes

Nonsporing anaerobes constitute an important cause of human and animal infections. Many of these bacteria form commensal flora of man and animals in mouth and oropharynx, gastrointestinal tract and genitourinary tract. In the gut, the anaerobic bacteria outnumber the aerobes (*Escherichia coli*) by a ratio of 1000 : 1 and that of mouth, upper respiratory tract and female lower genital tract by 5 : 1 to 10 : 1. Some of these nonsporing anaerobes act as **opportunistic pathogens** when body resistance is lowered. They are particularly likely to set up infections in situations in which there is damaged and necrotic tissue. Anaerobic infections of the head, neck and respiratory tract are often associated with organisms found in the mouth, whilst infection in the abdominal and pelvic regions are more commonly associated with gut bacteria.

On the basis of morphology and staining characters, nonsporing anaerobes have been classified as under:

I. **Cocci**
   A. Gram-positive
      1. *Peptococcus*
      2. *Peptostreptococcus*
   B. Gram-negative
      • *Veillonella*

II. **Bacilli**
   A. Gram-positive
      1. *Lactobacillus*
      2. *Bifidobacterium*
      3. *Propionibacterium*
      4. *Actinomyces*
      5. *Mobiluncus*
      6. *Eubacterium*
   B. Gram-negative
      1. *Bacteroides*
      2. *Fusobacterium*
      3. *Leptotrichia*
      4. *Porphyromonas*
      5. *Prevotella*

III. **Spirochaetes**
      1. *Treponema*
      2. *Borrelia*

PEPTOCOCCUS

This genus has one species – *P. niger*. They are Gram-positive, non-sporing, anaerobic cocci with G + C content of DNA 50 mol %. They measure 0.4–1.2 μm in diameter and occur singly or in pairs or in clumps. They produce **black colonies on blood agar** after prolonged incubation and produce H_2S. They do not produce catalase and indole and do not reduce nitrate to nitrite.

They occur as normal flora of skin, gastro-intestinal tract and genitourinary tract. However, they may cause pyogenic infections of wounds, puerperal sepsis and urinary tract infection.

PEPTOSTREPTOCOCCUS

This genus has 9 species – *P. anaerobius*, *P. asaccharolyticus*, *P. prevotii*, *P. magnus*, *P. indolicus*, *P. micros*, *P. productus*, *P. heliotrinreducens* and *P. tetradius* (formerly *Gafficia anaerobia*). They are Gram-positive cocci occurring in pairs, chains or irregular masses. They are **obligate anaerobes**, measure 0.5–2 μm in diameter, non-haemolytic, catalase-variable, indole production and nitrate reduction variable. Some strains ferment carbo-hydrates but others are asaccharolytic.

They occur as normal flora of skin, mouth, gastrointestinal tract and genitourinary tract and are the **commonest anaerobic organisms** recovered from human infections like pleuropulmonary disease, chronic otitis media, brain abscess, puerperal sepsis and urinary tract infections.

P. anaerobius and *P. magnus* are the commonest anaerobic Gram-positive cocci isolated from wound infections.

P. anaerobius is the anaerobic coccus most commonly associated with puerperal infection.

VEILLONELLA

These are Gram-negative cocci occurring in pairs, short chains and clumps. They are obligate anaerobes, oxidase-negative, catalase-negative, non-motile and measure 0.3–2.5 μm in diameter. They are present as normal flora of the mouth, gastrointestinal and genital tracts. Colonies on blood agar, after 24 hours incubation are small, round, convex, shiny, opaque, light grey and non-haemolytic. In the broth culture, abundant gas is produced. *V. parvula* is isolated from clinical specimens, but little is known of its role in the production of infection.

LACTOBACILLUS

These are straight or curved rods that, like coryne-bacteria, frequently show bipolar bodies due to the presence of **metachromatic granules**. They are Gram-positive and non-sporing. Most strains are non-motile, while a few strains are motile by peritrichous flagella. The bacilli are of varying length and thickness with parallel sides. On an average they measure 1.5 × 1 μm in size and tend to occur singly or in chains. Occasionally, they may show filamentous forms.

Lactobacilli are normally present in mouth (*L. casei*, *L. fermentum*, *L. acidophilus* and *L. brevis*), gut (*L. acidophilus*, *L. fermentum* and *L. salivarius*) and in vagina (*L. acidophilus*, *L. fermentum*, *L. casei* and *L. cellobiosus*). In the mouth, they have been incriminated in the pathogenesis of **dental caries**. The mineral components of enamel and dentine are believed to be dissolved by the acid formed by the fermentation of sucrose and other dietary carbo-hydrates by lactobacilli. In the intestine, they synthesize vitamins such as biotin, vitamin B_{12} and vitamin K which may be absorbed by the host.

In the adult vagina, lactobacilli ferment glycogen which is deposited in the vaginal epithelial cells and form lactic acid, which accounts for the highly acidic pH of the vagina. This protects adult vagina from infection with gonococci. In prepubertal and post-menopausal vagina, lactobacilli are scanty. Lacto-bacilli occurring in vagina are collectively known as **Doderlein's bacilli.**

Lactobacilli are also found in plant materials such as silage and in food stuffs and agricultural products, particularly milk, cheese and fermented milk products and in fermented beverages such as wine and cider. In some of these products the multiplication of lactobacilli brings about desirable changes, in others it causes spoilage.

Lactobacilli grow best under microaerophilic conditions in the presence of 5% CO_2 and at pH 6. Better growth is obtained in media enriched with glucose or blood. Colonies on agar media are usually small, 1–3 mm in diameter, with entire margins. Some species form rough colonies. Selective media include Hadley's tomato juice agar (pH 5) and glucose yeast extract acetic acid agar of Rogosa et al., 1951.

Lactobacilli are non-pathogenic and different species are distinguished by the pattern of acidi-fication of various sugars and their requirement for vitamins.

BIFIDOBACTERIUM

They are non-motile, non-sporing and pleomorphic Gram-positive rods showing true and false branching. The name is derived from the frequent bifid Y-shaped cells. Most species are obligate anaerobes, but a few species, isolated from animals and bees, can grow in the presence of 90% air and 10% CO_2. Various bifidobacteria occur as normal flora in the mouth, gastrointestinal and genitourinary tracts. *B. bifidum* is common in the faeces of breast-fed and bottle-fed infants and in the faeces of adults and of animals. Bifidobacteria are non-pathogenic to man or laboratory animals.

PROPIONIBACTERIUM

Propionibacteria are pleomorphic, Gram-positive, coryneform rods, non-acid-fast and non-motile. They are aerotolerant, and growth may occasionally be obtained aerobically. Some species of *Propionibacterium* are found in milk and cheese and sometimes in other agricultural products. *P. acnes, P. granulosum* and *P. avidum* are normal inhabitants of human skin, mouth, gastrointestinal and genitourinary tracts. These are not normally regarded as pathogens but are found in **acne,** in some cases of **infective endocarditis** and in **infections associated with implanted prostheses.**

Genus *Actinomyces* is discussed in Chapter 28.

MOBILUNCUS

Mobiluncus is the generic name given by Spiegel and Roberts (1984) to a group of curved, motile Gram-variable, anaerobic, non-sporing rods isolated from human vagina in cases of bacterial vaginosis. This genus was tentatively placed in family Bacteroidaceae by them, but its taxonomic position is uncertain. Recent studies suggest that the genus *Mobiluncus* belongs to the order Actinomycetales and is closely related to the genus *Actinomyces*. This genus has two species: *M. curtisii* and *M. mulieris.*

Morphology

Both species are slightly curved rods and occur singly or in pairs. *M. curtisii* is short, 1.7 × 0.5 μm and Gram-variable while *M. mulieris* is long, 2.9 × 0.5 μm and Gram-negative. Both species are motile by means of multiple subpolar flagella.

Cultural characteristics

They are essentially anaerobes but can grow in an atmosphere of 5% O_2 and 95% N_2. They are fastidious and grow slowly at 33–37°C producing round, entire, low convex, smooth, translucent, colourless colonies, 2–3 mm in diameter, after anaerobic incubation on blood agar medium for five days. Addition of 10 μg/ml each of colistin and nalidixic acid to blood agar makes it selective for isolation of these organisms.

Biochemical reactions

They are oxidase- and catalase-negative. Small amounts of acetic acid and major amounts of succinic acid are produced in glycogen-containing media. Differentiating biochemical characters of both the species are given in Table 26.1.

Table 26.1. Differentiating characters of species of *Mobiluncus*

Character	*M. curtisii*	*M. mulieris*
1. Mean size of the bacterial cell	1.7 × 0.5 μm	2.9 × 0.5 μm
2. Gram staining reaction	Variable	Negative
3. Arginine hydrolysis	+	–
4. Hippurate hydrolysis	+	–
5. ONPG	+	–
6. Nitrate reduction	+	–

Pathogenicity

In association with *Bacteroides* species and *Gardnerella vaginalis, M. curtisii* and *M. mulieris* have been blamed to cause **bacterial vaginosis.** Of these, *Bacteroides* species constitute a major component. There is a foul-smelling (rotten fish smell) but non-purulent vaginal discharge. Rotten fish smell is accentuated when it is mixed with a drop of KOH solution. The vaginal pH is more than 4.5.

Laboratory diagnosis

Microscopic examination of fresh unstained smears of vaginal discharge show epithelial cells coated with bacteria (**'clue cells'**). *M. curtisii* and *M. mulieris* may be isolated from vaginal discharge by inoculation on blood agar and blood agar with colistin and nalidixic acid and identified as above.

Treatment

Mobiluncus species are susceptible to benzylpenicillin, clindamycin, erythromycin and gentamicin. For the treatment of infection by *Mobiluncus* species, penicillins are appropriate drugs. *M. mulieris* is more susceptible than *M. curtisii* to metronidazole.

EUBACTERIUM

Members of the genus *Eubacterium* are obligate anaerobic Gram-positive bacilli. They occur as normal flora of mouth and intestine. Some species (*E. brachy*, *E. timidum* and *E. nodatum*) are commonly seen in periodontitis. *E. lentum* is commonly isolated from non-oral clinical specimens.

BACTEROIDACEAE

Gram-negative, anaerobic, non-sporing and non-motile bacilli, ranging from short Gram-negative rods to filamentous and fusiform shapes, belong to family Bacteroidaceae. This family possesses five genera – (1) *Bacteroides*, (2) *Fusobacterium*, (3) *Leptotrichia*, (4) *Porphyromonas*, and (5) *Prevotella*. These anaerobes occur as commensals in the mouth, gastrointestinal and female genital tracts and are now recognized as **opportunistic pathogens** that may produce disease when the host resistance is lowered such as trauma, tissue necrosis, impaired circulation, administration of antibiotics, corticosteroids and cytotoxic agents, diabetes, malnutrition and malignancy.

The infections due to anaerobes are usually polymicrobial, more than one anaerobe being involved along with aerobic organisms. In anaerobic infections, the resultant pus is usually putrid (foulsmelling) and cellulitis is a frequent finding. Anaerobic infections of the head, neck and respiratory tract are often associated with organisms found in the mouth, whilst infections in the abdominal and pelvic regions are more commonly associated with gut bacteria.

BACTEROIDES

Bacteroides occur as commensals in the mouth, gastrointestinal and female genital tracts. This genus comprises the most common anaerobes isolated from clinical specimens. They are non-sporing, non-motile, Gram-negative bacilli. They are very pleomorphic, appearing as slender rods, branching forms or coccobacilli. They occur singly, in pairs or short chains. They grow readily in media such as brainheart-infusion agar in an anaerobic atmosphere containing 10% CO_2. They possess capsular polysaccharide which appears to be virulence factor. The capsule confers resistance to phagocytosis and intracellular killing.

They cause peritonitis following bowel injury, pelvic inflammatory disease, abdominal and brain abscesses, and empyema. Pus is often foul smelling. *B. fragilis* is the most frequent of the non-sporing anaerobes isolated from clinical specimens. *B. melaninogenica* forms black-pigmented or brown colonies on blood-containing media. The pigment is intracellular or cell-associated derivative of haemoglobulin (haemin). It has been isolated from lung or liver abscesses, mastoiditis, and lesions of intestine, mouth and gums.

FUSOBACTERIUM

Fusobacteria are Gram-negative, **strict anaerobic rods** of varied size and morphology. Some species of *Fusobacterium* produce long slender Gram-negative rods that are wide at the centre and taper towards the ends (fusiform), but others produce coccobacilli to very long and filamentous cells. They are usually non-motile and growth is often improved by 5–10% CO_2. They can be isolated on blood agar plates containing neomycin and vancomycin. After 48 hours incubation at 37°C, the colonies are striate or granular with irregular or crenated edge and a raised centre.

F. nucleatum is the most studied species. It may cause infections of head and neck region including dental and periodontal infections and cerebral abscess. *F. necrophorum* is an important animal pathogen. It may, however, sometimes cause infections in man similar to those caused by *F. nucleatum*.

LEPTOTRICHIA

This genus contains only one species, *L. buccalis* which is synonymous with *F. fusiforme*. They are anaerobic, non-sporing, non-motile, long, straight or slightly curved Gram-negative bacilli with considerable width and tapering ends. They measure 5–15 × 1–1.5 µm in size. They can be grown on blood agar at 37°C under anaerobic conditions with 5–10% CO_2. After 48 hours incubation, colonies are 2–3 mm in diameter, irregular and often striate. Many strains become aerotolerant after several subcultures.

L. buccalis is a normal flora of mouth and gastrointestinal tract. It is present in low proportions in **dental plaque**. However, in association with *Borrelia vincentii* it is believed to cause **acute ulcerative gingivitis** or **Vincent's angina**. It is seen in patients with malnutrition, debility and poor oral hygiene. It is characterized by pain, haemorrhage, foul odour, destruction of interdental papillae, inflammation of the gums and formation of a pseudomembrane. *L. buccalis* and *B. vincentii* are present in the exudate and pseudomembrane, and diagnosis is made by direct microscopy.

PORPHYROMONAS

Porphyromonas spp. are part of normal oral flora. *P. gingivalis* causes periodontal disease and *P. endodontalis* causes dental root canal infections.

PREVOTELLA

Prevotella contains *P. melaninogenica*, *P. buccalis*, *P. denticola* and other species. *P. melaninogenica* produces black or brown colonies on anaerobic blood agar. The colour is not due to the melanin pigment but is due to hemin derivative. It causes lung and liver abscess, mastoiditis, intestinal lesions and lesions of mouth and gums. Cultures of *P. melaninogenica* and dressings from wounds infected with the bacillus produce a characteristic red fluorescence when exposed to ultraviolet light.

Laboratory diagnosis

As anaerobic bacteria form part of the normal flora of the skin and mucous surfaces, their isolation from clinical specimens has to be interpreted cautiously. The mere presence of an anaerobe does not prove its causal role.

Specimen collection and transport

Specimens should be collected in such a manner as to avoid normal resident flora. For example, the sputum is unsatisfactory for culture from a suspected case of lung abscess; only material collected by aspiration is acceptable. In general, material for anaerobic culture is best obtained by tissue biopsy or by aspiration using a needle and syringe. Swabs are unsatisfactory specimens, but when they are to be used, they should be sent in Stuart's transport medium. Ideally, specimens should be placed in an anaerobic transport device that consists of an anaerobic tube or vial containing an anaerobic gas mixture substituted for air, which protects the organisms from oxygen exposure and drying during transport to the laboratory. Specimens should be delivered within 20 minutes for culture.

Direct microscopy

Examination of a Gram-stained smear shows numerous pus cells and a variety of organisms. In case of *P. melaninogenica* infection, examination of the specimen under ultraviolet light may show the bright red fluorescence.

Culture

Freshly prepared blood agar with neomycin, yeast extract, hemin and vitamin K is inoculated and incubated at 37°C in an anaerobic jar, with 10% CO_2. Anaerobiasis can also be maintained by GasPak system. Plates are examined after 24–48 hours. Some anaerobes, such as fusobacteria, require longer period of incubation. Parallel aerobic cultures should also be set up because in most anaerobic infections aerobic bacteria are also involved. Other anaerobic media, such as cooked meat broth and thioglycollate broth, may also be used for isolation of anaerobes.

Definitive identification of the anaerobes depends on colony morphology and various biochemical tests. Gas liquid chromatography is also useful to identify anaerobes in the specimens.

KEY FACTS

- Many nonsporing anaerobes form **commensal flora** of man and animals in **mouth and oropharynx**

- Lactobacilli have been incriminated in the pathogenesis of **dental caries**
- Moderately saccharolytic group of *Bacteroides* play an important role in the development of **dental plaque**, and in oral infections, including **periodontal disease**, **gingivitis**, **dental abscesses** and **maxillofacial sepsis**
- *B. gingivalis* is an aggressive **periodontal pathogen** in both humans and animals
- Fusobacteria inhabit **oral cavity**, **colon** and **female genital tract**
- *Fusobacterium nucleatum* and *F. periodonticum* are isolated mainly from **periodontal disease** sites and hence considered to be **periodontopathic bacteria**
- **Fusospirochaetal infections** caused by fusobacteria in combination with spirochaetes are **ulcerative gingivitis**, **Vincent's angina** and **cancrum oris** or **noma**

IMPORTANT QUESTION

Classify nonsporing anaerobes. Discuss pathogenicity and laboratory diagnosis of infections caused by them.

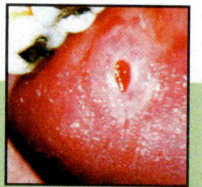

Chapter 27

Spirochaetes

The spirochaetes are elongated, motile, flexible bacteria twisted along the long axis. They have Gram-negative-type cell wall composed of an outer membrane, a peptidoglycan layer and a cytoplasmic membrane. They possess a varying number of fine fibrils which are attached subterminally at each pole of the cell and extend towards the opposite pole between outer membrane and peptidoglycan layer of the cell wall. Because of their similarity to other bacterial flagella they are known as **endoflagella**. The number of endoflagella per cell end is a morphologic characteristic of each species, in *Treponema*, that are pathogenic for humans, the number is 3 but occasionally 4, in most *Borrelia* it is 15–20 and in *Leptospira* it is one.

The spiral shape and serpentine motility of the spirochaetes depend upon the integrity of these endoflagella. Motility is of three types:

1. Flexion and extension.
2. Corkscrew-like rotatory movement.
3. Translatory motion.

Some are very actively motile while others are sluggish.

TREPONEMA

Treponemes (*trepos*, meaning to turn; and *nema*, meaning thread) are slender spirochaetes with fine spirals and pointed ends. Some of them are pathogenic for man, while others occur as commensals in mouth and genitalia. The pathogenic treponemes cannot be cultivated in laboratory media and are maintained by subculture in susceptible animals. *Treponema* species pathogenic for man include the causative agents of:

- venereal syphilis (*T. pallidum*),
- non-venereal treponematoses – yaws (*T. pertenue*),
- endemic syphilis (*T. endemicum*), and
- pinta (*T. carateum*).

TREPONEMA PALLIDUM

Morphology

It is a thin, delicate, long, motile, flexible organism which is twisted spirally round its long axis. It is 6–14 µm long. Its width is 0.13 µm in dried state, but is about 0.2 µm in the wet living state, which is just great enough for resolution with the light microscope. It has 6–12 coils which are remarkably evenly disposed at 1 µm intervals and the amplitude of spirals is 1–1.5 µm. They have tapering ends. It is actively motile exhibiting flexion and extension, translatory and corkscrew-like motility. As the spirochaete moves across the dark-field of the microscope, it often displays a **characteristic tendency** to bend at right angles near its midpoint. These secondary curves appear and disappear but its primary spirals remain unchanged.

Because of its weak refractility and slender thickness, about the limit of resolution by the light microscope, it is best seen in wet living preparation with the **dark-ground microscope**. In dried preparations, it needs to be thickened by **silver impregnation methods (Fontana's method is useful for staining films and Levaditi's for tissue sections)**. It cannot be stained by simple aniline dyes or by Gram's method. By prolonged Giemsa staining it stains pale pink. By **immunofluorescence method**, treponemes can be detected in tissues and body fluids.

Ultrastructurally, *T. pallidum* possesses usually three but occasionally four endoflagella attached subterminally at each end of the cell and extend towards the opposite pole between **outer membrane and peptidoglycan layer of the cell wall**. The endo-flagella from the two ends are more than half the length of the organism and interdigitate over the central portion of the organism, so that in transverse section there often appear to be 3 or 4 of them in section taken from terminal regions and 4–6 in sections from the central portion.

Cultivation

Pathogenic treponemes cannot be cultivated in artificial media and are maintained by subculture in susceptible animals. **Nichol's strain** of *T. pallidum* has been maintained, in rabbit testis, for several decades by serial testicular passage since it was isolated in 1913 from CSF of a patient with neuro-syphilis.

Cultivable treponemes such as *T. phagedenis* (**Reiter treponeme**) and *T. refringens* are non-pathogenic. They can be grown under strictly anaerobic conditions in Smith-Noguchi medium or in digest broth enriched with serum.

Sensitivity to physical and chemical agents

T. pallidum is a very delicate organism, therefore, syphilis is ordinarily acquired by sexual intercourse. It is readily inactivated by heating at 41.5°C for 1 hour. Susceptibility of *T. pallidum* was the basis of fever therapy of syphilis early this century. When infected blood is stored at 5°C in citrate anti-coagulant, infectivity is lost in 5 days or less. There-fore, transfusion syphilis can be prevented by storing blood for at least 5 days in the refrigerator before transfusion.

Treponemes from rabbit syphilomas of the testis preserved in the proper suspending fluids under anaerobic conditions remain actively motile for 2 days at 37°C and 4–7 days at 25°C. Frozen in a medium containing 15% glycerol at –70°C or below, they remain viable for years and provide a reliable source of antigens for immunological tests. **Lyophilization (freeze-drying) kills the organism.**

Antigenic structure

The antigenic structure of *T. pallidum* is poorly under-stood. Infection with these treponemes leads to the production of three types of antibodies. On the basis of these antibodies, the treponemal antigens may be divided into specific and non-specific antigens.

Specific antigens

1. Group-specific antigen

It is a protein antigen present in *T. pallidum* as well as in non-pathogenic treponemes, such as Reiter treponeme. Antibody to this antigen appears in serum of syphilitic patients. The antigen used in tests to detect group-specific antibodies is derived from the Reiter treponeme.

2. Species-specific treponemal antigen

It appears to be polysaccharide in nature. *T. pallidum* is used as antigen for detection of species-specific antibody.

Non-specific antigen

A non-specific antibody (reagin) appears in blood of syphilitic patients that reacts with a lipid hapten extracted from beef heart. The hapten is known as **cardiolipin** and is chemically a diphosphatidyl glycerol. It is not certain whether cardiolipin is an antigen contained in *T. pallidum* itself or a product of damaged tissue caused by infection.

Pathogenesis

T. pallidum is a **strict parasite** and its life outside the animal body is short. Most cases of syphilis are contracted during sexual intercourse. The trepo-nemes are present in the superficial genital lesions and pass from one partner to the other through **intact mucous membranes or through minor skin abrasions**. The disease may also be transmitted **congenitally**, by close contact with mucous membrane lesions as in **kissing** and through **blood transfusions**. Medical personnel are occasionally infected by an **accidental finger prick** with an infected needle.

In venereal syphilis, the treponemes penetrate mucosal surfaces or abraded skin and multiply at the site of entry and after an incubation period of about a month (range 10–90 days), the clinical disease sets in. The clinical manifestations fall into four stages – primary, secondary, latent and tertiary.

1. Primary syphilis

The primary lesion of syphilis is the **chancre** which is painless, relatively avascular, circumscribed, indurated, 1–2 cm in diameter. It ulcerates in the centre (Figs. 27.1 and 27.2). It is known as **hard chancre** to distinguish it from the non-indurated

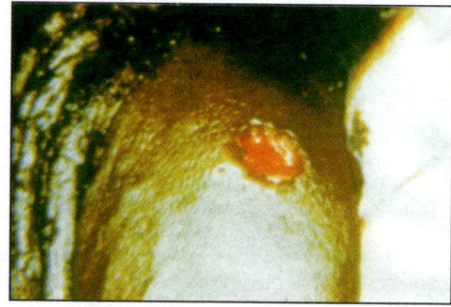

Fig. 27.1. A chancre of primary syphilis on the penis.

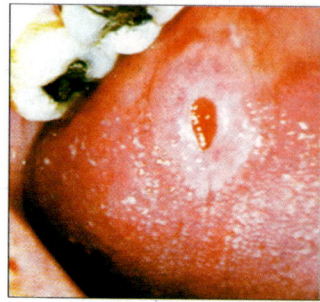

Fig. 27.2. A chancre of primary syphilis on the tongue.

lesion (**soft sore**) caused by *Haemophilus ducreyi*. The primary lesion of syphilis is also known as **Hunterian chancre**, after John Hunter who produced the lesions on himself experimentally. Histologically, it is oedematous and infiltrated predominantly with mononuclear cells.

Most frequently chancre appears on the external genitalia – prepuce, penis (Fig. 27.1), labia and vaginal wall. It may also occur on the cervix, perianal area, anal canal or on tongue (Fig. 27.2), and other oral mucous membranes. In some cases it may be on lips, cheeks and nipples (when it is acquired through kissing). Chancres usually occur singly but in immunocompromised individuals, such as those infected with human immunodeficiency virus, multiple chancres may develop.

A large number of treponemes are present in the primary lesion and in the serum that exudes from it. In the early days of infection, the spirochaetes invade the regional lymph nodes (inguinal in males and pelvic in females) and lead to **lymphadenitis**. The lymph nodes are swollen, discrete, rubbery and non tender. From lymph nodes treponemes enter into the blood stream in large numbers. *Chancre heals spontaneously in about 3–6 weeks even without treatment leaving a thin scar.*

2. Secondary syphilis

This sets in 2–6 months after the primary lesion heals during which period the patient is asymptomatic. The secondary lesions are due to widespread multi-plication of the treponemes and their dissemination through the blood. Patient develops marked consti-tutional symptoms, **diffuse erythematous cutaneous lesions**, particularly on the trunk and extremities, mucous patches in the oropharynx and **condylomata** at mucocutaneous junctions.

There may also be enlargement of the lymph nodes and sometimes involvement of the bones, joints, eyes and other organs. All the lesions of secondary syphilis, especially those involving mucous membranes on exposed surfaces discharge very large number of treponemes. Like the primary chancre, they constitute a very large reservoir of infection and they present a hazard to medical personnel who investigate and treat cases of syphilis.

Lesions of secondary syphilis undergo spontaneous healing in 4–5 years.

3. Latent syphilis

After the secondary lesions disappear, the disease becomes latent and can be detected only by serological tests. In many cases, this is followed by natural cure but in others, after several years, manifestations of tertiary syphilis appear.

4. Tertiary syphilis

Decades after the primary infection, patient may develop late or tertiary syphilis. It is a slowly progressive, destructive inflammatory disease that may affect any organ. It may lead to relatively benign ulcerating lesions of the skin, mucous membranes or bones, or **gummata** of the internal organs. More serious are lesions of heart and aorta that may lead to the formation of **aneurysms**, or of the central nervous system, of which **tabes dorsalis** and **general paralysis of the insane** are the most common.

The lesions of tertiary syphilis contain very few organisms and the remarkable severity of the lesions is attributed to an intense cellular immune response to the organisms and their products. Individuals with serologic evidence of AIDS appear to be at much higher risk of developing neurosyphilis. This may be due to the immunosuppression associated with AIDS.

Laboratory diagnosis (Flowchart 27.1)

The clinical diagnosis of syphilis is confirmed in the laboratory by:

A. Demonstration of *T. pallidum* by microscopy in the genital and rectal lesions of primary syphilis. Microscopy is not suitable for examining the dry skin rash of secondary syphilis, but treponemes are plentiful in the moist lesions at mucocutaneous junctions, such as mucous patches or condylomata. If primary chancre is healing, the microscopic examination of the exudate is often negative. At this stage, however, treponemes may be found in the fluid aspirated with a syringe from enlarged lymph nodes.

B. Demonstration of treponemes in tissues.

C. Demonstration of treponemal antigen in the lesion.

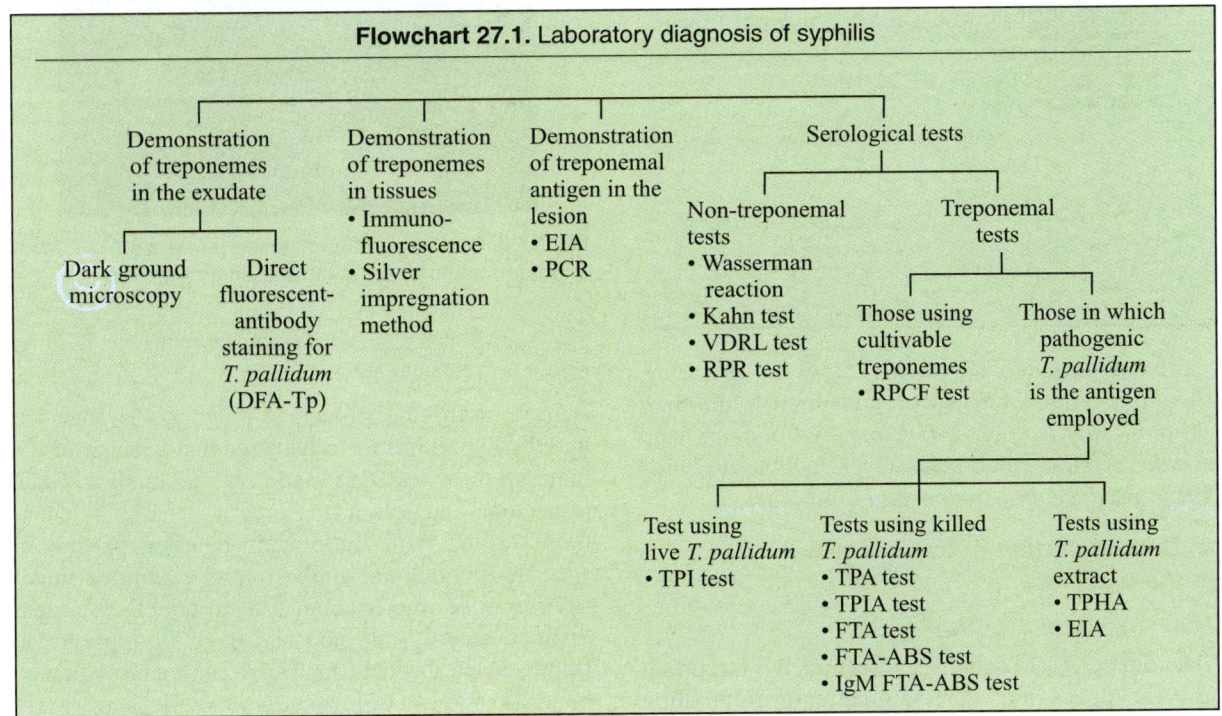

Flowchart 27.1. Laboratory diagnosis of syphilis

D. With the exception of very early stage of the disease, serological tests are the mainstay for the diagnosis of syphilis at all stages. These tests provide the sole means of detecting latent infection (Table 27.1).

Table 27.1. Methods of laboratory diagnosis of syphilis

A. **Demonstration of treponemes in the exudate**
  1. Dark-ground microscopy
  2. Direct fluorescent-antibody staining for *Treponema pallidum* (DFA-Tp)
B. **Demonstration of treponemes in tissues**
  • Immunofluorescence
  • Silver impregnation method
C. **Demonstration of treponemal antigen in the lesion**
  • EIA
  • PCR
D. **Serological diagnosis of syphilis**
  1. Nontreponemal tests
    (a) Wassermann reaction
    (b) Kahn test
    (c) VDRL test
    (d) RPR test
  2. Treponemal tests
    (a) Those using cultivable treponemes
      • RPCF test
    (b) Those in which pathogenic *T. pallidum* is the antigen employed
      I. Test using live *T. pallidum*
        • TPI test
      II. Tests using killed *T. pallidum*
        • TPA test
        • TPIA test
        • FTA, FTA-ABS, IgM FTA-ABS tests
      III. Tests using *T. pallidum* extract
        • TPHA
        • EIA

Every patient with positive syphilis serology, should be tested for HIV with the patient's informed consent and vice versa. HIV-infected patients who acquire syphilis run a more severe course and may fail to produce anti-treponemal antibodies.

A. Demonstration of treponemes in the exudate

1. Dark-ground microscopy

To avoid the risk of acquiring infection, it is important to wear gloves and exercise great care in handling the lesions. The surface of the lesion is cleansed carefully with a gauze swab soaked in warm normal saline and the margins are gently scrapped so that superficial epithelium is abraded. Gentle pressure is applied to the base of the lesion until serum exudes from its surface. If it is blood stained, it should be wiped away and process repeated until a clear fluid is obtained. The material is collected directly on a coverslip which is then placed on a glass slide and examined under dark-ground microscope.

T. pallidum is recognized by its slender structure, regularity of its spirals and slightly pointed ends (Fig. 27.3). Other spirochaetes are usually thicker and have rounded ends. It is motile with a to and fro drilling motion and occasional flexion of the body. Dark-ground microscopy is unsuitable for examining oral lesions because many of the non-pathogenic treponemes found there may be confused with *T. pallidum*.

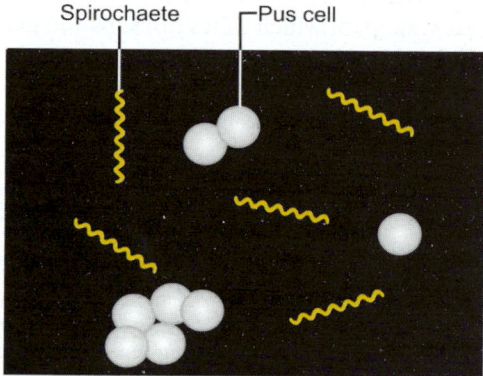

Fig. 27.3. Dark-ground illumination preparation of serous exudate from primary syphilitic chancre.

2. Direct fluorescent-antibody staining for T. pallidum (DFA-Tp)

A more definite approach to diagnosis is provided by DFA-Tp. It has the advantage that a smear of the material to be tested is made on a glass slide, fixed in acetone and sent to the laboratory. The smear is then stained with fluorescein-labelled pathogen-specific monoclonal antibody and examined under fluorescence microscope. The treponemes appear distinct, sharply outlined and have an apple-green fluorescence. Oral lesions which cannot be evaluated by dark-ground microscopy can be accurately examined by DFA-Tp. This test is 100% sensitive and specific, while dark-ground microscopy is 97% sensitive and 77% specific.

B. Demonstration of treponemes in tissues

Treponemes in the tissues can be demonstrated by immunofluorescence or silver impregnation method (Levaditi's stain).

C. Demonstration of treponemal antigen in the lesion

T. pallidum antigen in the lesion can be detected by enzyme immunoassay and polymerase chain reaction.

D. Serological diagnosis of syphilis

Depending upon the antigens used, serological tests for syphilis may be divided into the following:

1. **Nontreponemal tests** or **Standard tests for syphilis (STS)** in which cardiolipin or lipoidal antigen is used.
2. **Treponemal tests** in which treponemes are used as the antigen. These are of two types:

   (a) Those using cultivable treponemes, such as Reiter treponemes (*T. phagedenis*) as the antigen.

   (b) Those in which pathogenic *T. pallidum* is the antigen employed. These tests may further be classified according to whether the treponeme employed is live, killed or extracts of the treponemes.

Nontreponemal tests

Nontreponemal tests that can be employed are Wassermann, Kahn, Venereal Diseases Research Laboratory (VDRL) and the rapid plasma reagin (RPR) tests. The antigen used in these tests is an alcoholic extract of beef heart tissue (cardiolipin) to which lecithin and cholesterol are added. Wassermann reaction and Kahn test are complement fixation and tube flocculation tests respectively. Since Wassermann reaction offers no advantage over simple and rapid flocculation tests such as VDRL and RPR, therefore, World Health Organization (1982) recommended that its use should be discontinued. Similarly, Kahn test is rarely done these days.

VDRL test

VDRL test is performed as a slide test in which inactivated patient serum is mixed with a freshly prepared suspension of cardiolipin-lecithin-cholesterol antigen on a glass slide. The mixture is rotated, usually mechanically, for 4 minutes after which the flocculation (aggregation of antigen-antibody complexes in suspension) can be detected under a low power objective of a microscope.

VDRL test is used as a screening test and is positive in approximately 70% of primary and 99% of secondary syphilis. Antibody becomes detectable 7–10 days after the appearance of primary chancre. The titre of antibody may rise to 8 or 16 during primary syphilis and 16–128 during secondary syphilis. Titres decline beyond the secondary stage and around 30% of patients with late syphilis are non-reactive.

RPR test

In rapid plasma reagin test, VDRL antigen is adsorbed on finely divided carbon particles and suspended in choline chloride which blocks inhibitory factors in the serum thus eliminating the need to heat the serum before testing. The antigen is also stabilized with EDTA, allowing it to be used for up to 6 months when stored at 4–10°C. This test is performed by mixing one drop of patient serum or plasma (50 μl) with a drop of this modified antigen (20 μl), on a disposable plastic card (12.5 × 7 cm in size with 10 clearly defined test areas) using a disposable stick. The card is then rocked gently to and fro for 8 minutes and observed under strong source of light. In a positive test, the flocculation of carbon particles (black aggregates) is visible with naked eye. Black aggregates may be deposited at the periphery of the liquid. In a negative test, there is a complete absence of black aggregates with a uniform greyish background. Any specimen giving a positive reaction should then be tested quantitatively using doubling dilutions of serum (1 : 2, 1 : 4, 1 : 8, 1 : 16, 1 : 32, etc.).

Most laboratories use RPR test as a screening procedure for syphilis. The sensitivity and specificity of the RPR test are essentially the same as that of the VDRL test. The RPR is quick and easy to perform and serum sample does not need to be heat-inactivated. In addition, cards can be read macroscopically, in contrast to VDRL test which requires microscopic examination for interpretation. However, only disadvantage with the RPR test is that **it cannot be used to test cerebrospinal fluid, while VDRL remains the standard test for use with cerebrospinal fluid**.

Biological false-positive reactions

Antibodies against cardiolipin may be detected in the absence of *T. pallidum* infection and give what is known as biological false positive (BFP) reaction. In such cases, specific treponemal tests are negative and there is no history of present or past treponemal infection. BFP reactions may occur in 0.3–0.9% of all sera examined and are caused mainly by IgM antibody while reagin antibody in syphilis is mainly IgG. These reactions are of two types:

1. **Acute or transient BFP reaction** which may develop shortly after an acute febrile infectious disease and will disappear within a few weeks or months after the illness has subsided.
2. **Chronic BFP reactions** persist longer than 6 months. These may occur in a wide variety of infectious and noninfectious conditions associated with tissue damage. These include:
   – autoimmune diseases particularly systemic lupus erythematosus,
   – leprosy particularly lepromatous leprosy,
   – malaria,
   – relapsing fever,
   – infectious mononucleosis,
   – hepatitis, and
   – tropical eosinophilia.

Treponemal tests

(a) Those using cultivable treponemes

The antigen used to detect group-specific antibody is derived from *T. phagedenis* (Reiter treponeme). It is protein in nature, most probably derived from endoflagella and the test is known as **Reiter protein complement fixation (RPCF) test**. The principle of this test is the same as that of Wassermann test, but the antigen in RPCF test is extracted from *T. phagedenis*. This is less sensitive than cardiolipin tests in early syphilis but is more sensitive in late or latent syphilis. It is much more specific than cardiolipin tests, but false reactions still occur in a few cases. With the advent of newer treponemal tests such as *Treponema pallidum* haemagglutination assay, RPCF test is rarely done now a days. New ELISA tests based on purified endoflagella of *T. phagedenis* have been developed.

(b) Those in which pathogenic T. pallidum is the antigen employed

A number of specific tests are now available for the definite diagnosis of syphilis. All require live or killed or extracts of *T. pallidum* (Nichol's strain) grown in rabbit testes.

I. Test using live T. pallidum

- **Treponema pallidum immobilization (TPI) test:** This test determines the ability of patient serum to immobilize motile virulent *T. pallidum*. The test serum is incubated anaerobically with a suspension of the treponemes and complement. If antibodies are present, the treponemes will be found to be immobilized, when examined under dark-ground microscope. The test is considered reactive if more than 50% of the treponemes are immobilized, and non-reactive if less than 20% are immobilized. The test is doubtful if 20–50% treponemes are immobilized.

II. Tests using killed T. pallidum

- **Treponema pallidum agglutination (TPA) test:** In this test, a suspension of *T. pallidum*, inactivated by formalin, is mixed with test serum and incubated. The mixture is then examined under dark-ground microscope. In the presence of antibody, treponemes are found to be agglutinated. This test is not very specific and false positive reactions are common.
- **Treponema pallidum immune adherence (TPIA) test:** Suspension of inactivated treponemes is mixed with test serum, complement and fresh heparinised whole blood from a normal individual, and incubated. In the presence of antibodies, the treponemes will be found to adhere to the erythrocytes. In the absence of antibody, immune adherence does not take place. Both TPA and TPIA are not used in diagnostic laboratories, they serve primarily as research tools.

- **Fluorescent treponemal antibody (FTA) test:** It is an indirect immunofluorescence test. Smears of *T. pallidum* are prepared on slides and fixed with acetone. These slides can be stored in the deep freezer for several months. The patient serum is added on the smear and incubated for the antibody to react with the treponemes. The excess serum is then washed off and the antibodies that bind to the fixed organisms are detected by treating the smear with fluorescein-labelled antihuman immuno-globulin. After incubation and washing off the unfixed conjugate, slide is examined under fluorescence microscope. In a positive test, treponemes fluoresce.

Originally patient serum was used in a dilution of 1 in 5. At this dilution, the test has high sensitivity and poor specificity. Therefore, the dilution of the serum was raised to 1 in 200. In this test, called **FTA-200**, the specificity was improved but sensitivity was decreased. Therefore, this test was further modified to **fluorescent treponemal antibody absorption (FTA-ABS)** test. Here the patient serum is first absorbed with an extract of non-pathogenic *T. phagedenis* (Reiter treponemes) to remove group-reactive antibody. FTA-ABS test has high specificity and sensitivity. It is almost as specific as the more complicated TPI test. Therefore, it is the most widely used serologic test for detection of specific treponemal antibodies. **VDRL and FTA-ABS tests can also be performed on cerebrospinal fluid.** Antibodies do not reach from the blood stream but are probably formed in the CNS in response to treponemal infection.

FTA-ABS test becomes reactive around 3rd week of infection and is positive in 80%, 100% and 95% of primary, secondary and late syphilis respectively. Unlike VDRL test, its reactivity persists after successful therapy. However, occasionally the test may become non-reactive if treatment is given early in the disease. The specificity of this test ranges from 92–99%. **False positive reactions have been observed in patients with rheumatoid arthritis, lupus erythematosus, cirrhosis and hypergammaglobulinaemia and in 1% of normal persons.**

Another modification of this test, the **IgM FTA-ABS test, can detect IgM antibodies in congenital syphilis** thus distinguishing it from seropositivity due to passively transferred maternal antibodies which are IgG in nature. In addition, in the former repeated tests will show an increase in titre, whereas in the latter titre will fall.

III. Tests using T. pallidum extract

- **Treponema pallidum haemagglutination test (TPHA):** In this test, *T. pallidum* antigen is adsorbed onto the surface of red blood cells. When these red blood cells are mixed with patient serum, specific antibody, if present, causes haem-agglutination. As in FTA-ABS test patient serum is pre-absorbed with an extract of Reiter trepo-nemes to remove group-reactive antibody. TPHA reactivity may be detectable around the 4th week of infection. It is less sensitive than FTA-ABS in primary syphilis being positive in 65% of cases, but both give similar results for secondary and late syphilis. After treatment, TPHA invariably remains positive for life. **This test can also be used to detect localised production of anti-treponemal antibodies in cerebrospinal fluid, a marker of neurosyphilis.**

TPHA is very simple to perform, therefore, it was the first of the specific tests suitable for routine screening. Because of greater convenience and lower cost, TPHA may be performed in microtitre plates. This is referred to as **microtitre haem-agglutination-T. pallidum (MHA-TP) test.** Both these terms are used synonymously. Combination of a cardiolipin antigen test and TPHA is the most widely used screening procedure.

- **Enzyme immunoassay (EIA):** Ultrasonicate of *T. pallidum* antigen is coated on tubes or ferrous metal beads as a solid-phase carrier for antigen. Antibody in the patient serum is detected by enzyme immunoassay. Sensitivity and specificity of this test has been reported to be 90% and 98% respectively.

Prophylaxis

At present, there is no effective vaccine against syphilis. An infected individual may serve as a source of infection for 3–5 years during early syphilis. As transmission of the infection is by direct contact, it is possible to protect against syphilis by avoidance of sexual contact with an infected individual. The contacts are examined and given treatment. Other forms of prevention include:

1. The use of **mechanical barriers** such as condoms in which prevention of direct contact between infected mucous membranes is achieved.
2. The use of **antibiotic (penicillin) prophylaxis.** It, however, carries the danger that it may suppress the primary lesion without eliminating the infection.

Treatment

T. pallidum is sensitive to penicillin. So far there have been no reports of penicillin-resistance. In early cases, a single injection of 2.4 million units of benzathine penicillin is adequate. For late syphilis, this may be repeated weekly for 3 weeks. In patients allergic to penicillin, doxycycline may be used. Ceftriaxone is effective, particularly in neurosyphilis. *More aggressive and prolonged antibiotic therapy may be required in AIDS patients with syphilis due to impairment of immune function.* Antibiotic therapy of syphilitics, particularly with penicillin, may induce a systemic reaction known as **Jarisch-Herxheimer reaction.** This is believed to be due to the release of endotoxins following lysis of spirochaetes. This is characterized by rapid onset (1–2 hours) of fever, chills, myalgia, tachycardia, hyperventilation, vasodilation and hypotension. It is self-limiting and persists for only 12–24 hours.

BORRELIA VINCENTII

Borrelia vincentii is 7–18 μm long and 0.2–0.6 μm wide, with 3–8 loose, open coils of variable size. It is actively motile. It is easily stained with dilute carbol fuchsin, methyl violet, Giemsa and Leishman stains and is Gram-negative. It is an obligate anaerobe and can be cultured in sealed tubes containing digest broth enriched with ascitic fluid. *B. vincentii* is a normal commensal of mouth but may, under predisposing conditions such as malnutrition or viral infections, give rise to **ulcerative gingivostomatitis** or oropharyngitis (**Vincent's angina**).

In Vincent's angina, *B. vincentii* is often associated with 'fusiform bacillus' known as *Leptotrichia buccalis*. Vincent's angina is characterized by ulcerative lesions of mouth or tonsillar area. For the diagnosis, smears are made from the ulcerative lesions and are stained with dilute carbol fuchsin. A clinical diagnosis of Vincent's angina is confirmed when a large number of spirochaetes and fusiform bacilli are seen together with many pus cells.

KEY FACTS

- **Spirochaetes are long, slender,** coiled and highly **motile** bacteria that do not take up the Gram stain
- **Spirochaetes** comprise three genera – *Treponema, Borrelia* and *Leptospira*
- *Treponema pallidum,* the agent of **syphilis,** cannot be cultivated *in vitro* and is uniformly sensitive to **penicillin**
- Syphilis can be diagnosed by demonstration of treponemes, treponemal antigens and by serological tests

IMPORTANT QUESTIONS

1. Discuss laboratory diagnosis of syphilis.
2. Write short notes on:
   (a) VDRL test
   (b) Rapid plasma reagin test
   (c) Treponemal tests for serodiagnosis of syphilis.
   (d) *Treponema vincentii*
   (e) Lyme disease
   (f) Weil's disease
   (g) Leptospirosis

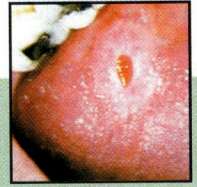

Chapter 28

Actinomycetes

Actinomycetes are Gram-positive bacteria varying from coccoid and pleomorphic forms to branched filaments. The colonial and microscopic morphology, and the types of infections caused, resemble those of the fungi, but these organisms are true bacteria. Like fungi they form delicate filaments called hyphae but, like bacteria, they are thin, possess cell wall containing muramic acid, have prokaryotic nuclei and are susceptible to antibacterial antibiotics. Human pathogenic actinomycetes belong to four genera (1) *Actinomyces*, (2) *Nocardia*, (3) *Streptomyces,* and (4) *Actinomadura*. *Actinomyces* is non-acid-fast and anaerobic or microaerophilic, *Nocardia* is aerobe and acid-fast (1% sulphuric acid), and *Streptomyces* and *Actinomadura* are aerobes and non-acid-fast.

ACTINOMYCES

Morphology

Actinomyces are Gram-positive, non-motile, non-sporing, non-acid-fast, 0.5–1 µm in diameter. They often grow in mycelial forms and break up into coccoid and bacillary forms. Most show true branching.

Cultural characteristics

They are facultative anaerobes. They grow best under anaerobic or microaerophilic conditions with the addition of 5–10% CO_2. The optimum temperature for growth is 35–37°C. They can be grown on brain-heart-infusion agar, heart-infusion agar supplemented with 5% defibrinated horse, rabbit or sheep blood. Suitable liquid media include brain-heart-infusion broth and thioglycollate broth which may be supplemented with 0.1–0.2% sterile rabbit serum. Most species show good growth after 3–4 days' incubation, however, *A. israelii* may take 7–14 days.

Pathogenesis

The *Actinomyces* causes the disease known as actinomycosis. In man, it is usually caused by *A. israelii*. The other species, *A. naeslundii*, *A. meyeri*, *A. odontolyticus* and *A. viscosus*, are very rare cause of actinomycosis. All these species are **commensals of the mouth**, therefore, **endogenous** cause of disease. In addition, *A. naeslundii*, *A. odontolyticus* and *A. viscosus* may cause **dental plaque** and **caries**. An association between root surface caries of teeth and *Actinomyces* has been described. A close relationship between *A. odontolyticus* and earliest stage of enamel demineralization, and the progression of small caries lesions have been reported.

Actinomycosis is a chronic suppurative disease characterized by peripheral spread to contiguous tissues, rare haematogenous spread, formation of sinus tracts which drain suppurative lesions and presence in the pus of colonies of *Actinomyces*. These colonies are 0.25–2 mm in diameter, white to yellowish and are known as '**sulphur granules**'. There are four important sites of primary infection in actinomycosis.

1. Cervicofacial

About two-thirds of cases of actinomycosis, in man, occur in the cervicofacial region. The primary lesion is usually in the mandible or maxilla and probably occurs by direct extension from a periodontal abscess, a traumatic lesion resulting from neglected carious or broken teeth, dental extraction or accidental fracture of jaw. Maxillary lesions may extend to the orbit, the cranial bones, the meninges and brain.

2. Thoracic

Thoracic actinomycosis commences in the lung probably as a result of aspiration of hyphal fragments of *Actinomyces* from tooth surfaces or dental caries or of *Actinomyces*-containing granules which commonly grow in tonsillar crypts without invading tonsillar tissue. The lesions in the lung may involve pleura and pericardium and spread outwards through the chest wall producing multiple draining sinuses.

3. Abdominal

Abdominal actinomycosis begins most often in appendix or rarely as a complication of perforating gastric ulcer or penetration of the mucosa of the colon by an object such as fish bone.

4. Pelvic

Pelvic actinomycosis occasionally occurs in women fitted with plastic intrauterine contraceptive devices.

Actinomycotic cholecystitis and actinomycosis of breast have also been reported by the authors.

Laboratory diagnosis

Specimens

Pus, sinus discharge, bronchial secretions, sputum or infected tissues are collected aseptically. These specimens may contain innumerable 'sulphur granules'. The granules may also be present on dressings removed from a draining sinus tract.

A. Microscopy

Pus from suspected cases is shaken with sterile water in a tube. '**Sulphur granules**' settle to the bottom. These are removed with a pasteur pipette. Granules are crushed between two slides and stained with Gram, and Ziehl-Neelsen staining using 1% sulphuric acid for decolourization. The granules are seen to consist of **Gram-positive hyphal fragments** 0.5–1 μm in diameter, sometimes remaining as intact hyphae several micrometers long and rarely with branches, surrounded by a peripheral zone of swollen radiating club-shaped structures presenting a **sun ray appearance**. These clubs are Gram-negative, weakly acid-fast and are believed to be **antigen-antibody complexes**. 'Sulphur granules' and mycelia in tissue sections can also be identified by direct fluorescence microscopy.

B. Culture

'Sulphur granules' are washed thoroughly in sterile normal saline in a petri dish or tube and crushed in a drop of saline with a glass rod. It is then inoculated on brain-heart-infusion agar, blood agar and in thioglycollate broth, and incubated both anaerobically and aerobically with 5–10% CO_2 at 35–37°C for up to 14 days. The colonies of *A. israelii* are 0.5–2 mm in diameter, white to grey-white, smooth, entire or lobulated resembling molar teeth (Fig. 28.1). The identity of the isolate may be confirmed by direct fluorescence microscopy and biochemical tests.

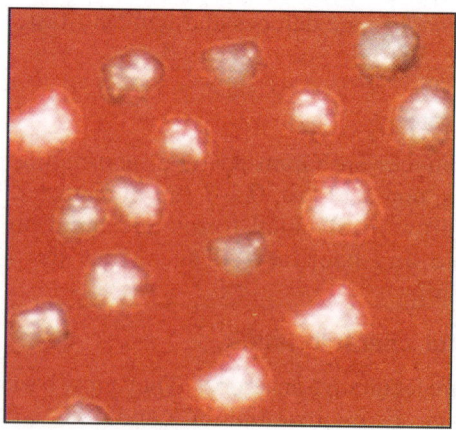

Fig. 28.1. Colonies of *Actinomyces israelii* on blood agar medium. These resemble molar teeth.

C. Biopsy

In haematoxylin and eosin stained sections, the 'sulphur granules' are deeply stained with haematoxylin except in the periphery which is stained by eosin, which shows short, radiate, club-like structures (Fig. 28.2). On Gram staining, the filaments are Gram-positive and periphery Gram-negative. The tissue reaction is a chronic suppurative, fibrosing, inflammatory process.

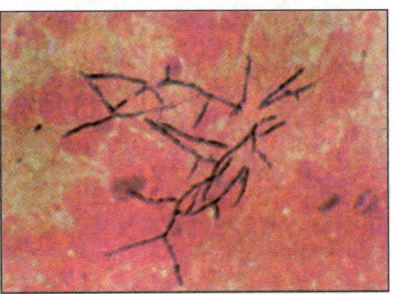

Fig. 28.3. Gram-stained sputum smear showing Gram-positive branched mycelia from a patient suffering from pulmonary nocardiosis.

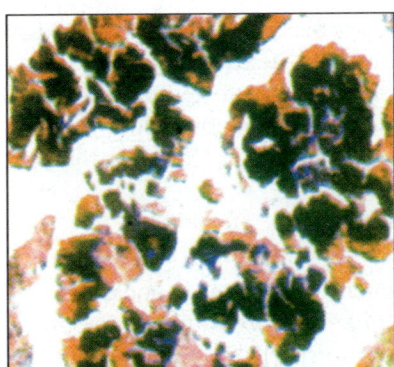

Fig. 28.2. Actinomycosis showing a grain of *Actinomyces israelii*. It is deeply stained with haematoxylin except in the periphery which is stained with eosin.

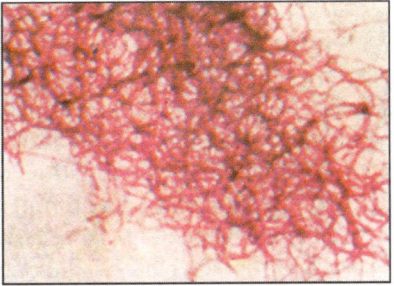

Fig. 28.4. Modified Ziehl-Neelsen staining showing acid-fast filaments of *Nocardia*.

Treatment

Surgical removal of affected tissues with large doses of penicillin, but prolonged courses up to 6 weeks are necessary for chronic infections. Tetracycline, because of its good bone penetration, may also be used.

NOCARDIA, STREPTOMYCES AND ACTINOMADURA

Morphology

Nocardiae are strictly aerobic, non-motile, Gram-positive bacteria (Fig. 28.3). They form hyphae that often fragment in situ or on mechanical disruption into rod-shaped or coccoid elements. They are acid-fast when decolourized with 1% sulphuric acid (Fig. 28.4). *N. madurae* which is non-acid-fast is now known as *Actinomadura madurae*. Unlike *Actinomyces*, nocardiae are environmental saprophytes with a broad temperature range of growth. *Streptomyces* and *Actinomadura* are strictly aerobic

and non-acid-fast. They produce an extensively branched substrate mycelium, with or without aerial hyphae. The latter do not fragment into rods and cocci.

Cultural characteristics

Nocardiae readily grow on nutrient agar, Sabouraud dextrose agar, brain-heart-infusion agar and yeast extract-malt extract agar. The inoculated plates should be incubated at 36°C for up to 3 weeks and examined both macroscopically and microscopically for growth every few days. Nocardiae form white, yellow, pink or brown colonies. *A. madurae* produces waxy, heaped, folded, membranous and tough colony. It may be white, tan, pale orange, pink or red in colour.

A. pelletieri produces heaped, irregular, waxy, and granular colony. It possesses areas of bright and dark red, sparse aerial hyphae. Colonies of *Streptomyces* are usually highly filamentous with dense aerial hyphae.

Pathogenicity

N. asteroides and sometimes *N. farcinica*, *N. nova*, *N. brasiliensis* and *N. otitidiscaviarum* produce opportunistic pulmonary disease known as nocardiosis in usually, but not always, immuno-compromised individuals including those receiving immunosuppressive therapy and those with AIDS. Soil and composting matter is known to be the natural habitat of *Nocardia*. It is, therefore, believed that man and animals acquire infection by inhalation of the organism from environmental sources.

Nocardiosis is a systemic bacterial disease. It generally originates as a pulmonary infection, varying in its course from mild and slowly progressive to fulminant and fatal. It may be characterized by single or multiple nodules, miliary pattern, scattered infiltrations, bronchopneumonia, abscesses, masses with central cavitation, pleural effusions and empyema. Dissemination from the primary focus of infection may occur through pleural extension, lymphohaematogenous spread or invasion of blood vessels with bacteraemia. Although every organ of the body may be affected, involvement of brain, meninges and spinal cord is said to be commoner than that of other parts such as skin, subcutaneous tissues, eye, liver, lymph node, etc. Infection with *Nocardia* organisms is serious.

Localized cutaneous and subcutaneous nocardiosis is encountered less frequently. Infection may occur through contaminated wound and by traumatic implantation. It usually involves feet and hands. The disease begins as a localized subcutaneous abscess that is invasive and quite destructive of the tissues and underlying bone. This lesion is known as **mycetoma**. It is characterized by swelling, draining, sinuses, and granules.

Laboratory diagnosis

Microscopy

Pus or purulent blood-flecked sputum is spread on a slide by crushing between two slides. The smears are stained by Gram and Ziehl-Neelsen techniques and examined under oil-immersion lens. Granules may be seen in specimens from cutaneous infection. Sampled tissue and pus from the draining sinuses are the specimens of choice for direct examination. The granules may be visualized by separating them from the pus with an inoculating needle and then washing in sterile saline. These may be crushed between two glass slides which are then used for Gram and Ziehl-Neelsen staining.

Culture

Pus, sputum or the granules are inoculated on nutrient agar, Sabouraud dextrose agar and brain-heart-infusion agar, and incubated at 36°C for 3 weeks. Culture media are examined both macroscopically and microscopically every few days for identification of the isolate.

Treatment

The treatment of choice of nocardial infection is sulphonamide with or without trimethoprim for 3 months or more. They are also susceptible to amikacin, imipenem, minocycline, tobramycin and vancomycin.

KEY FACTS

- *Actinomyces* spp. are **potentially pathogenic commensals** of the mouth in humans and animals. They are major component of **dental plaque**, particularly at proximal sites of teeth, and are known to increase in numbers in **gingivitis**

- An association between **root surface caries** of teeth and *Actinomyces* has been described

- *Actinomyces* spp. cause **cervicofacial**, **thoracic**, **abdominal** and **pelvic** actinomycosis, which are essentially **chronic granulomatous infections**

- The most important human pathogen is *A. israelii*

- **A prolonged course of antibiotics** (up to 6 weeks) may be necessary **to treat chronic actinomycosis**

IMPORTANT QUESTION

Discuss pathogenesis and laboratory diagnosis of actinomycosis.

SECTION D
Virology

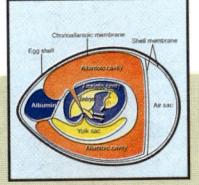

Chapter 29

General Properties of Viruses and Virus–Host Interactions

GENERAL PROPERTIES OF VIRUSES

Viruses are the **smallest infective agents**. They are perhaps the simplest form of life known. They are **obligate intracellular parasites**. Most forms of life – animals, plants and bacteria are susceptible to infection with appropriate viruses. Three main properties distinguish viruses from other micro-organisms:

1. Small size

Viruses are smaller than other organisms. They vary in size from 10–300 nm. Therefore, they can pass through bacterial filters and they cannot be seen by light microscope. However, the poxviruses which are the largest members of the virus family and are very similar in size to the smallest bacteria, are close to the resolution of light microscope. For visualization of all other viruses an electron microscope is necessary.

2. Genome

A virus carries its own genetic information in the form of either RNA or DNA, but not both. The genome may be single-stranded or double-stranded, circular or linear, and segmented or unsegmented. The type of nucleic acid, its strandedness, and its size are major characteristics used for classifying viruses into families.

3. Metabolically inert

Viruses have no metabolic activity outside susceptible host cells. They do not possess ribosomes or protein-synthesizing apparatus although some viruses contain one or more enzymes within their particles. Viruses, therefore, cannot multiply in inanimate media but only inside living cells. Inside the living cells the virus genome is capable of replicating new virus particles.

STRUCTURE OF THE VIRUSES

Viruses consist of nucleic acid core surrounded by a protein coat called **capsid**. The capsid is composed of repeating protein units called **capsomers**. The capsid with the enclosed nucleic acid is known as **nucleocapsid**.

Virus symmetry

Capsid of the virus particles shows three types of symmetry. It is determined by the arrangement of the capsomers around the nucleic acid.

1. *Icosahedral symmetry:* The capsomers are arranged as if they lay on the faces of an icosa-hedron which has 20 equilateral triangular faces and 12 corners or apices (Fig. 29.1). Viruses with icosahedral symmetry have a rigid structure and under the electron microscope have a charac-

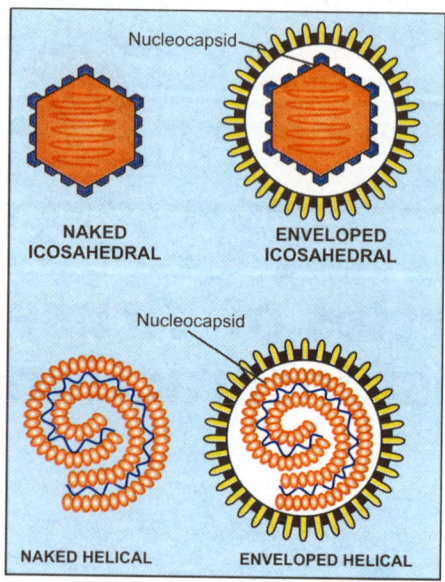

Fig. 29.1. Symmetry of viruses.

teristic hexagonal outline with triangular faces, but those less than 50 nm appear spherical.

2. *Helical symmetry:* The nucleic acid and the capsomers are wound together in the form of a helix or spiral.

3. *Complex symmetry:* Viruses (e.g., poxviruses) which do not show either icosahedral or helical symmetry due to complexity of their structure are referred to have complex symmetry.

Envelope

Generally, DNA viruses replicate and are assembled in the nucleus, and RNA viruses are assembled in the cytoplasm. The final assembly of some viruses occurs at the nuclear or cytoplasmic membrane. As the virus particle moves from the nucleus to the cytoplasm or passes from the cytoplasm to the extracellular space, an external lipid-containing envelope (host origin) with virus-coded polypeptides or virus-specified glycoproteins is added to the envelope. In mature virus particle the glycoproteins often appear as projecting spikes on the outer surface of the envelope. These are known as **peplomers**.

SUSCEPTIBILITY TO PHYSICAL AND CHEMICAL AGENTS

Outside the body and at room temperature many viruses, e.g., influenza, measles and mumps virus, are extremely labile and may survive for only a few hours. Other viruses such as polio and hepatitis A are much hardier and may survive under ordinary atmospheric conditions for many days, weeks or even months. Infectivity of most viruses, including human immunodeficiency viruses, is destroyed by moderate heat (55–60°C for 30 minutes), and heating clinical specimens in a water bath at 56°C for 30 minutes inactivates most viruses without impairing the sample for other assays. Some viruses are exceptionally thermostable. Hepatitis B virus resists heating at 60°C for one hour. 'Slow' viruses are highly heat-stable, e.g., some strains of scrapie resist autoclaving at 121°C for one hour.

The most efficient **disinfectants** for use against viruses are oxidizing agents such as H_2O_2, potassium permanganate, hypochlorite and organic iodine compounds. Formaldehyde and β-propiolactone are actively virucidal and are commonly employed for the preparation of killed viral vaccines. Most viruses are relatively resistant to phenol. Enveloped viruses which possess lipid-containing envelope are inactivated by **lipid solvents** such as ether, chloroform and detergents. **Chlorination** of drinking water kills most viruses, but its efficacy is greatly influenced by the presence of organic matter. Some viruses like hepatitis A and polio are relatively resistant to chlorination. **Antibacterial antibiotics** are ineffective against viruses. This property is made use of in eliminating bacteria from clinical specimens by antibiotic treatment before virus isolation.

REPLICATION OF VIRUSES

The genetic information necessary for viral multiplication is contained in the viral nucleic acid but the biosynthetic enzymes are lacking. They replicate by taking over the biochemical machinery of the host cell and redirecting it to the manufacture of virus components. The viral replication is divided into six stages.

1. Adsorption

The first event in the infection of a cell by a virus is the attachment of the virus particle to the cell surface. Virions come in contact with cells by random collision but adsorption or attachment is specific and is mediated by the binding of virion surface structures, known as ligands, to receptors on cell surface.

2. Entry into the host cells

Viruses enter the cells by the following mechanism:

After attachment, non-enveloped viruses are engulfed by a mechanism resembling phagocytosis, a process known as **viropexis**. In case of enveloped viruses, the envelope fuses with the plasma membrane of the host cell and releases the nucleocapsid into the cytoplasm.

Bacteria possess rigid cell walls. Bacteriophages, therefore, cannot penetrate into bacterial cells and only nucleic acid is introduced intracellularly by a complex mechanism.

3. Uncoating

This is the process of stripping the virus of its outer layers and capsid so that nucleic acid is released into the cell. With most viruses, uncoating is effected by the action of lysosomal enzymes of the host cells when the phagosome and lysosome fuse together.

4. Biosynthesis

This phase includes synthesis of:

- the viral nucleic acid;
- capsid protein;
- enzymes necessary in the various stages of viral synthesis, assembly and release; and
- certain regulatory proteins which serve to shut down the normal cellular metabolism and direct the sequential production of viral components.

Biosynthesis consists of following steps:

- Transcription of messenger RNA (mRNA) from viral nucleic acid.
- Translation of mRNA into '**early proteins**' or '**nonstructural proteins**'. These are enzymes and factors which initiate and maintain synthesis of virus components and induce shutdown of host protein and nucleic acid synthesis.
- Replication of viral nucleic acid.
- Synthesis of **late** or **structural proteins** which constitute daughter virion capsids.

5. Virion assembly

Assembly of the various viral components into virions occurs shortly after the replication of the viral nucleic acid and may take place in either the nucleus (herpes and adenoviruses) or cytoplasm (picorna and poxviruses). In case of enveloped viruses, the envelope is derived from the nuclear membrane if they assemble in the nucleus (herpesviruses) and from plasma membrane if they assemble in the cytoplasm of the host cell (orthomyxoviruses, paramyxoviruses and retroviruses). However, in this envelope virus-coded peplomers are also embedded.

6. Release

Release of completed viruses is the final step in virus multiplication. Viruses that exist as naked nucleocapsids may be released by:

- The lysis of the host cell (polioviruses) or they may be extruded by a process which may be called reverse phagocytosis.
- Enveloped viruses are released by a process of budding through special areas of host cell membrane (cytoplasmic or nuclear), where virus-specified transmembrane glycoproteins (peplomers) have been embedded.
- In case of bacterial viruses, the release of progeny virions takes place by the lysis of the infected bacterium.

VIRUS ISOLATION

As viruses are obligate intracellular parasites, they cannot be grown on any of the inanimate culture media. Most of the viruses can be cultivated in laboratory animals, chick embryos or cell cultures.

Laboratory animals

These animals have now almost disappeared from virus diagnostic laboratories, because simpler methods such as cell cultures are available. However, suckling mice, less than 24 hours old, are still used for the isolation of arboviruses, rabies virus, and some of the group A coxsackieviruses. These are inoculated intracerebrally and/or intraperitoneally, then observed for up to 2 weeks for the development of pathognomic signs before sacrificing for histologic examination of affected organs.

Chick embryos

Embryonated eggs offer several sites for the cultivation of viruses. Chorioallantoic membrane (CAM), allantoic cavity, amniotic cavity and yolk sac (Fig. 29.2) of 8–11 day old eggs are inoculated and incubated for 2–9 days. The duration of incubation depends on the virus type and route of inoculation. Viruses may kill the embryo or may produce visible lesions like pocks on CAM and haemagglutinating activity in the harvested amniotic and allantoic fluid. These effects help in the identification of the virus. Many viruses can be grown in eggs:

- Inoculation of **chorioallantoic membrane** produces visible lesions (pocks).
- Inoculation of **amniotic cavity** is used for primary isolation of influenza virus.
- Inoculation of **allantoic cavity** provides a rich yield of influenza and some paramyxoviruses.
- Inoculation of **yolk sac** is used for cultivation of some viruses, chlamydiae and rickettsiae.

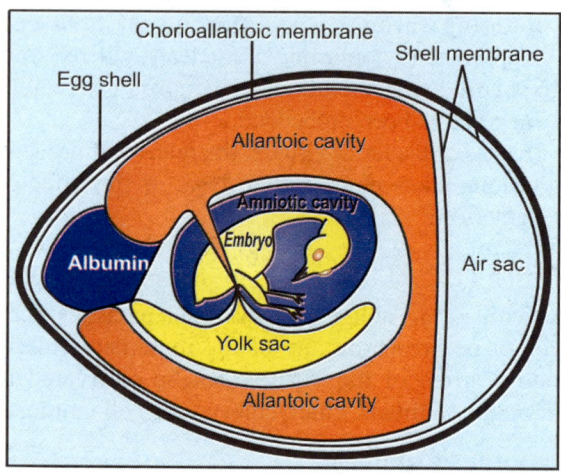

Fig. 29.2. Cross-section of an embryonated hen's egg.

Inoculation of allantoic cavity is employed for growing influenza virus for vaccine production. Other chick embryo vaccines are yellow fever (17D strain) and rabies (Flury strain) vaccines. Duck eggs are bigger than hen's eggs. Therefore, they provide a better yield of rabies virus and are used for the preparation of the inactivated nonneural rabies vaccines.

Cell culture

This is the type of culture routinely employed for diagnostic virology and for studying virus-cell interactions. Tissues are dissociated into component cells by the action of proteolytic enzymes such as trypsin or collagenase and mechanical shaking. The cells are washed, counted and suspended in a growth medium. The cell suspension is dispensed in glass or plastic bottles, tubes or petri dishes. The cells adhere to glass or plastic surface and on incubation, if culture conditions are suitable, they divide to form a confluent monolayer sheet of cells covering the surface within about a week. At this stage, cell division ceases due to contact inhibition. Cell culture is of three types (Table 29.1):

Table 29.1. Cell cultures in common use

1. **Primary cell culture**
   - Rhesus monkey kidney cell culture
   - Human amnion cell culture
   - Chick embryo fibroblast cell culture
2. **Semi-continuous (diploid) cell strains**
   - WI-38 Human embryonic lung cell strain
3. **Continuous cell lines**

• HeLa	Human carcinoma of cervix cell line
• HEp-2	Human epithelioma of larynx cell line
• KB	Human carcinoma of nasopharynx cell line
• McCoy	Human synovial carcinoma cell line
• Detroit 6	Sternal marrow cell line
• Chang C/I/L/K	Human conjunctiva, intestine, liver and kidney cell line
• Vero	African monkey kidney cell line
• BHK-21	Baby hamster kidney cell line

1. Primary cell culture

These are normal cells freshly taken from the body and cultured. They are capable of very limited growth *in vitro* perhaps 5–10 divisions at the most. Because these cells have a normal diploid chromosome complement, therefore, they are preferred for cultivating viruses meant for vaccine production. Important examples of primary cell cultures are rhesus monkey kidney cell culture, human amnion cell culture and chick embryo fibroblast cell culture.

2. Semi-continuous (diploid) cell strains

These are cells of a single type, usually fibroblasts, that retain their original diploid chromosome number and karyotype. They can be subcultured for about 50 passages (serial subcultures) before the cells die off. Diploid cells developed from human fibroblasts are susceptible to a wide range of human viruses. They are useful for isolation of some fastidious pathogens and for the production of viral vaccines, e.g., rabies vaccine is produced by cultivation of the fixed rabies virus in WI-38 human embryonic lung cell strain.

3. Continuous cell lines

These are cells of a single type that are capable of indefinite propagation *in vitro*. Therefore, they are known as continuous cell lines. They are usually derived from cancerous tissue but these cells have a heteroploid chromosome complement. Often they no longer bear any close resemblance to their cells of origin because of numerous sequential mutations during their long history in culture. Continuous cell lines such as HeLa, HEp-2 and KB derived from human carcinoma of cervix, human epithelioma of larynx, and human carcinoma of nasopharynx respectively, support the growth of a number of viruses. These cell lines have been used in the virus laboratories throughout the world for many years.

These cell lines may be maintained by serial subcultivation or stored at –70°C for use when necessary. Other cell lines (and their sources) in common use are McCoy (human synovial carcinoma cell line), Detroit 6 (sternal marrow cell line), Chang C/I/L/K (human conjunctiva, intestine, liver and kidney cell lines), Vero (African green monkey kidney cell line) and BHK-21 (baby hamster kidney cell line). The type of cell culture used for viral cultivation depends on the sensitivity of the cells to a particular virus.

Detection of virus growth in cell culture

Virus growth in cell culture can be detected by the following methods:

1. Cytopathic effect

Many viruses produce morphological changes in the cultured cells in which they grow. These changes are known as **cytopathic effects (CPE)** and viruses causing CPE are known as **cytopathogenic viruses**. Most CPE can be readily observed in unfixed and unstained monolayer of cells under low power of microscope. But fixation and staining of monolayer is essential in order to see details such as inclusion bodies and syncytia. Conventional haematoxylin and eosin is most suitable for this purpose. Fluorescent antibody staining is widely used to recognize viral antigens in such cultured cells. Following are the main types of CPE:

- **Rounding of cells:** Viral replication may lead to nuclear pyknosis, rounding, refractility, degeneration and eventually complete or partial detachment of infected cells from the glass. This is seen in picornaviruses.
- **Rounding and aggregation:** Some viruses may lead to cell rounding and aggregation into grape-like clusters which detach from the glass, leaving clear areas. It is seen in adenoviruses.
- **Syncytium formation:** Some viruses (measles, respiratory syncytial virus and HIV) lead to syncytium formation in which infected cells fuse with neighbouring infected or uninfected cells to form giant cells containing several (up to 100) nuclei.

2. Haemadsorption

Some orthomyxoviruses (influenza) and paramyxoviruses (parainfluenza, measles and mumps) code for red cell agglutinins which are incorporated into the cell membrane during infection, so that guinea-pig erythrocytes adhere to the infected cells. This adherence of erythrocytes to the infected cells is known as haemadsorption. It can be used to recognize infection with non-cytocidal viruses, as well as the early stage of cytocidal viruses. Sometimes virus can be detected by haemagglutination in the medium (culture fluid).

3. Interference

The multiplication of one virus in a cell usually inhibits the multiplication of a second virus, called **the challenge virus**, when it is added to the culture. This is because the first virus interferes with the replicative process of the challenge virus and is known as **interference challenge test**. This can be used for the detection of the growth of a non-cyto-pathogenic virus in cell culture.

A cell culture is inoculated with suspected clinical sample and incubated for several days. Then a standard dose of a known cytopathogenic challenge virus is introduced into the culture and after incubation, culture is observed for the CPE of challenge virus. If virus from original inoculum was replicating within the cells, replication of the challenge virus will be prevented and no CPE will be seen in the culture.

4. Transformation

Tumour-forming (oncogenic) viruses induce cell transformation and loss of normal contact inhibition, so that growth appears in a piled-up fashion producing **microtumours**. Some herpesviruses, adenoviruses, hepadnaviruses, papovaviruses and retroviruses (human T cell lymphotropic virus type 1) can transform cells.

5. Fluorescent antibody testing

Cells from virus infected cultures can be stained with fluorescein-conjugated antiserum and seen under fluorescence microscope for virus antigens. Both direct (DFA) and indirect fluorescent antibody (IFA) methods are useful in the identification of viral culture isolates. DFA testing is the most convenient method for identifying many viral isolates. It provides a complete identification in less than one hour.

6. Immunoperoxidase staining

Direct immunoperoxidase (DIP) staining method may also be used in identification of viruses isolated in cell culture.

7. Detection of enzymes

The virus isolate can be identified by detection of viral enzymes, such as reverse transcriptase in retro-viruses, in the culture fluid.

8. Electron microscopy

Viruses have distinctive appearances and can be detected by electron microscopy of ultra thin sections of infected cells.

NOMENCLATURE OF VIRUSES

The orders, families, subfamilies and genera of viruses are named with the suffix *virales, viridae,*

virinae and *virus* respectively. For example, the names of the order, family, subfamily and genus of measles virus are *Mononegavirales, Paramyxoviridae, Paramyxovirinae* and *Morbillivirus* respectively. Viral species are designated by vernacular terms, for example measles virus.

CLASSIFICATION OF VIRUSES

Viruses are classified into DNA and RNA viruses (Tables 29.2 and 29.3).

VIRUS-HOST INTERACTIONS

Different viruses may produce different effects ranging from no apparent cellular damage to rapid cell destruction. Some reactions of the host cell to viral infections are discussed below.

1. Inclusion bodies

A characteristic morphological change in cells infected by certain viruses is the formation of inclusion bodies (or inclusions) which can be seen by light microscope after fixation and staining. These may consist of aggregates of products of viral replication such as virus particles ready for release, overproduction of a particular viral protein or proteins or some aberrant cellular structure such as clumped chromatin. They may be present in the cytoplasm or in the nucleus or both of infected cells and may be acidophilic (stained by eosin) or basophilic (stained by haematoxylin), single or multiple, large or small and round or irregular. In general, those viruses that are assembled in the nucleus (usually DNA viruses) produce intranuclear inclusions, whereas cytoplasmic assembly (mainly RNA viruses) yields cytoplasmic inclusions.

- **Intracytoplasmic inclusion bodies** are found in cells infected with rabies virus (**Negri bodies**), vaccinia (**Guarnieri bodies**), fowlpox (**Bollinger bodies**), molluscum contagiosum (**molluscum bodies**), paramyxoviruses and reoviruses.
- **Intranuclear inclusion bodies** are found in cells infected with herpesviruses, adenoviruses and parvoviruses.
- **Both intranuclear and intracytoplasmic inclusion bodies:** Some viruses, for example, measles virus and cytomegalovirus may produce both intranuclear and intracytoplasmic inclusion bodies (Fig. 29.3).

Table 29.2. DNA viruses infecting humans

Family	Subfamily	Genus	Common members (species)
Poxviridae	Chordopoxvirinae	Orthopoxvirus	Variola, vaccinia, cowpox, monkeypox, ectromelia (mousepox) and rabbitpox viruses
		Parapoxvirus	Contagious pustular dermatitis virus of sheep (orf virus) and pseudocowpox (milker's node) virus
		Molluscipoxvirus	Molluscum contagiosum virus
		Yatapoxvirus	Yabapox, tanapox
Herpesviridae	Alphaherpesvirinae	Simplexvirus	Herpes simplex virus types 1 and 2
		Varicellovirus	Varicella-zoster virus
	Betaherpesvirinae	Cytomegalovirus	Human cytomegalovirus
		Roseolovirus	Human herpesvirus 6
	Gammaherpesvirinae	Lymphocryptovirus	Epstein-Barr virus
Adenoviridae	—	Mastadenovirus	47 serotypes of human adenovirus
Papovaviridae	—	Papillomavirus	Wart viruses
		Polyomavirus	Human polyomaviruses, murine polyoma virus and simian virus 40
Hepadnaviridae	—	Orthohepadnavirus	Hepatitis B virus of man, woodchuck and other animal hepatitis viruses
Parvoviridae	—	Dependovirus	Adeno-associated viruses (AAV)
		Erythrovirus	Parvovirus B19

2. Cytocidal infection

Viruses like enteroviruses and reoviruses kill their host cells by inhibition of protein, RNA and DNA synthesis.

3. Latent and persistent infections

Viruses have evolved mechanisms to continue to survive in the face of a strong host immune response. For example, herpes simplex types 1 and 2 and varicella-zoster viruses, following primary infection, travel up the peripheral nerves to the sensory ganglia. The viruses remain latent in the ganglia, to be reactivated periodically in some individuals causing recurrent lesions. Similarly, cytomegalovirus (CMV) and Epstein-Barr virus (EBV) are also known to establish latent infection. Some viruses like hepatitis B virus (HBV) may cause chronic infections which may remain clinically inapparent for many years. However, it may lead to more serious consequences, such as **cirrhosis or hepatocellular carcinoma**.

4. Cell transformation

Infection of cells with human T-cell lymphotropic virus type 1 (HTLV-1), HBV, hepatitis C virus (HCV), EBV and several papillomaviruses does not result in lytic infection and cell death, but leads to cell transformation. Viral (or proviral) DNA in transformed cells is **integrated into the cell DNA**. The transformed cells acquire a capacity to divide unrestrictedly leading to tumour production and these cells express distinctive antigens called **tumour-associated antigens**.

TRANSMISSION OF HUMAN VIRUS INFECTIONS

Viruses enter the body through the following routes (Table 29.4):

1. Respiratory tract

Many viruses enter the body through inhaled droplets expelled from the nose or mouth of infected persons

Table 29.3. RNA viruses infecting humans

Family	Subfamily	Genus	Common members (species)
Orthomyxoviridae	—	Influenzavirus A and B	Influenza A and B viruses
		Influenzavirus C	Influenza C virus
Paramyxoviridae	Paramyxovirinae	Paramyxovirus	Human parainfluenza virus types 1 and 3
		Rubulavirus	Human parainfluenza virus types 2, 4a and 4b, and mumps virus
		Morbillivirus	Measles virus
	Pneumovirinae	Pneumovirus	Human respiratory syncytial virus
Rhabdoviridae	—	Vesiculovirus	Vesicular stomatitis virus
		Lyssavirus	Rabies virus
Filoviridae		Filovirus	Marburg, Ebola and Reston viruses
Picornaviridae	• —	Enterovirus	Polioviruses (3), human echoviruses (32), coxsackieviruses (29) and a few other human enteroviruses
		Hepatovirus	Human hepatitis A virus
		Rhinovirus	Common cold rhinoviruses (over 100 serotypes)
Caliciviridae		Calicivirus	Human caliciviruses and hepatitis E virus
Reoviridae		Orthoreovirus	Human and animal reoviruses
		Rotavirus	Rotaviruses of man and animals
		Orbivirus	Tick-borne Kemerovo viruses of Siberia
		Coltivirus	Tick-borne agent causing Colorado tick fever in North America
Togaviridae	—	Alphavirus	Eastern, Western and Venezuelan equine encephalitis viruses, Ross River virus and chikungunya virus
		Rubivirus	Rubella virus
Flaviviridae	—	Flavivirus	Yellow fever, dengue, and St. Louis, Japanese, Murray Valley and Russian tick-borne encephalitis
		Hepatitis C	Hepatitis C virus
Coronaviridae	—	Coronavirus	Coronaviruses of mammals and birds
Arenaviridae	—	Arenavirus	Lymphocytic choriomeningitis virus, Lassa, Machupo, Junin and Guanarito viruses
Bunyaviridae	—	Phlebovirus	Sandfly fever virus and Rift Valley fever virus
		Bunyavirus	La Crosse and Oropouche viruses
		Nairovirus	Crimean-Congo haemorrhagic fever virus
		Hantavirus	Hantaan, Puumala, Belgrade, Seoul and Muerto Canyon viruses
Astroviridae	—	Astrovirus	Astroviruses
Retroviridae	Oncovirinae	BLV-HTLV retrovirus	HTLV-1 and HTLV-2
	Lentivirinae	Lentivirus	HIV-1 and HIV-2
	Spumavirinae	Spumavirus	Human foamy virus
—	—	Deltavirus	Hepatitis D virus

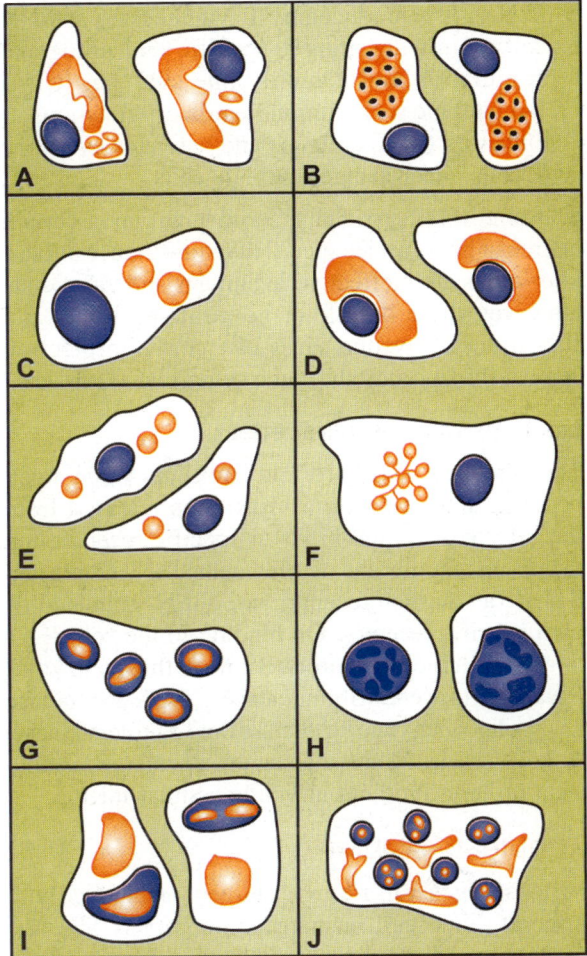

Fig. 29.3. Inclusion bodies in virus-infected cells. Intra-cytoplasmic (A–F): A, Vaccinia virus (Guarnieri bodies); B, Molluscipox virus (Molluscum body); C, Fowlpox virus (Bollinger bodies); D, Reovirus; E, Rabies virus (Negri bodies); F, Respiratory syncytial virus. Intranuclear (G–H): G, Herpes simplex virus; H, Adenovirus. Intracytoplasmic and intranuclear both (I–J): I, Cytomegalovirus; J, Measles virus.

Table 29.4. Transmission of human virus infections

Route of transmission	Viruses
Respiratory tract	**Respiratory viruses:** *Influenza A, B* and *C*, parainfluenza types 1–4, RSV, *Rhinovirus, Coronavirus*, adenovirus and coxsackievirus A
	Systemic viruses: Measles, mumps, rubella, varicella-zoster, CMV and EBV
Alimentary tract	Many enteroviruses including poliovirus types 1–3, HAV, HEV, adenoviruses, rotaviruses, Norwalk and related viruses, *Coronavirus, Astrovirus*, coxsackievirus A and B and echovirus
Skin	**Minor abrasions:** Papillomaviruses, molluscum contagiosum, cowpox, orf, milker's nodes viruses, herpes simplex viruses and HBV.
	Insect bite: Arboviruses
	Animal bite: Rabies virus, herpes B virus
	Injection: HBV, HCV, HIV-1, HIV-2, HTLV, CMV, EBV and Ebola virus
Genital tract	Papillomaviruses, herpes simplex viruses, HIV, HTLV, HBV, HCV
Conjunctiva	Some adenoviruses and a few entero-viruses

respiratory tract where they multiply and produce local disease. These are known as **respiratory viruses**. Other viruses, such as measles, mumps, rubella, varicella-zoster, CMV and EBV multiply locally to initiate a silent local infection which is followed by lymphatic or haematogenous spread to other parts of the body where more extensive multi-plication takes place before producing generalized disease.

2. Alimentary tract

Next to airborne infection, faecal-oral infection is the most important route of entry of viruses. They may be swallowed or infect cells in the oropharynx and then be carried to the intestinal tract. The viruses that initiate infection of humans via the alimentary tract are many enteroviruses including poliovirus types 1–3, HAV, hepatitis E virus (HEV), adenoviruses, rotaviruses, Norwalk and related viruses, coronavirus, astrovirus,

during talking, coughing or sneezing. This is the most important route of entry of viruses into the body. All viruses that infect the host via the respiratory tract probably do so by attaching to specific receptors on epithelial cells. Some viruses, such as influenza A, B and C, parainfluenza types 1–4, respiratory syncytial virus (RSV), rhinovirus, coronavirus, adenovirus and coxsackievirus A are restricted to coxsackie A and B and echovirus. These viruses can be transferred to the mouth of susceptible persons by contact of their fingers with the self-contaminated fingers of the infected persons. The latter may contaminate water supply or food and domestic flies may also convey virus from faeces to food.

3. Skin

Viruses may enter the body through minor abrasions (papillomaviruses, molluscum contagiosum, cowpox, orf, milker's nodes viruses, herpes simplex and HBV), insect bite (arboviruses), animal bite (rabies virus) or injection (HBV, HCV, HIV, HTLV, CMV, EBV and Ebola virus).

4. Genital tract

Papillomaviruses and herpes simplex viruses are sexually transmitted and produce lesions on the genitalia and perineum. HIV, HTLV, HBV and HCV are also sexually transmitted but do not produce local lesions.

5. Conjunctiva

It may also act as a portal of entry of some adeno-viruses and a few enteroviruses.

6. Congenital

Congenital infection may occur at any stage from the development of the ovum up to birth. In acute systemic infections, congenital infection usually leads to foetal death and abortion. Congenital infection with rubella and cytomegalovirus may result in a large variety of congenital abnormalities or death of the foetus.

INTERFERONS (IFN)

Interferons (IFNs) are a family of regulatory proteins induced by many viruses, by some bacteria and protozoa and by double-stranded nucleic acids. They are classified into three types:

1. **IFN-α:** It is induced by virus infection, produced by leucocytes and has 20 subtypes. It has antiviral activity by inhibiting protein synthesis.
2. **IFN-β:** It is induced by virus infection, produced by fibroblasts and epithelial cells and has only one subtype. It has antiviral activity by inhibiting protein synthesis.

3. **IFN-γ:** It is produced by T lymphocytes and NK cells following antigen-specific and mitogenic stimulation and has only one subtype. It is a lymphokine with immunoregulatory functions. It enhances MHC antigens and activates cytotoxic T cells, macrophages and NK cells.

Some IFNs especially β and γ display a certain degree of host species specificity, for instance, mouse interferons are ineffective in humans and vice versa. However, there is little or no viral specificity and IFN induced by one virus can confer protection against infection by the same or unrelated viruses.

Mechanism of antiviral effect

The synthesis of IFN (α and β) occurs when a cell becomes infected with a virus. It is released from the infected cell and binds to specific receptors on the plasma membrane of other cells. IFN-α and IFN-β share a common receptor while IFN-γ binds to its own specific receptor. On binding to the cell, IFNs α and β induce the production of three enzymes RNase L (an endoribonuclease), 2-5A synthetase (2′,5′-oligoadenylate synthetase) and a protein kinase. These enzymes inhibit translation of viral mRNA into viral proteins, without affecting cellular mRNA.

ACQUIRED IMMUNITY

Virions, in general, are good antigens and induce both antibody- and cell-mediated immunity (CMI), the primary mediators being, B and T lymphocytes respectively. The activities of both these cells are regulated by T helper (Th) and T suppressor (Ts) lymphocytes, lymphokines and monokines. For some diseases such as poxviruses, measles, herpes simplex virus and CMV infections, CMI appears to be the main immunospecific defence, for others, such as entero- and arbovirus infections, antibody production appears to be the main immunospecific defence.

Antibody-mediated immunity

IgG, IgM and IgA antibodies are produced in response to virus infection. IgG and IgM play a major role in blood and tissue spaces. IgA is a dimer, with four Fab fragments. Passing through epithelial cells, IgA acquires a "secretory component" to become secretory IgA (sIgA), which is secreted through mucosae into the respiratory, intestinal and urogenital tracts. It is more resistant to proteases than other immunoglobulins and it is the principal immuno-globulin on mucosal surfaces, and in milk and colostrum. Therefore, it is important in resistance to infection of the respiratory, intestinal and urogenital tracts. There are several ways in which antibody against viral components can protect the host:

1. Neutralization of infectious virus by preventing virus attachment, penetration or even subsequent events.
2. Opsonization of virions for phagocytosis and killing by macrophages.
3. Antibody may attach to viral antigens on the surface of the infected cells, rendering virus-infected cells prone to lysis by complement or destruction by phagocytes or killer (K) lympho-cytes.

Cell-mediated immunity

Antibody can neutralize free virions but once these agents get into cells, cell-mediated immunity operates. It prevents infection of target organs and promotes recovery from disease by destroying virus and virus-infected cells by any of the following four different processes:

1. Cytolysis by Tc cells.
2. Cytolysis by NK cells.
3. Antibody-complement-mediated cytotoxicity.
4. Antibody-dependent cell-mediated cytotoxicity (ADCC).

LABORATORY DIAGNOSIS OF VIRAL INFECTIONS

Indications for laboratory diagnosis

In spite of the fact that few effective chemo-therapeutic agents are available for the treatment of viral infections, following are the indications for laboratory diagnosis of viral infections:

1. Diseases caused by viruses for which antiviral chemotherapy is already available (herpesviruses) or is under clinical trials (HIV).
2. To detect emergence of drug-resistant mutants and for drug sensitivity testing.

3. Proper management of the patient, for example:
   - If rubella is diagnosed in the first trimester of pregnancy, abortion is recommended.
   - If a person is bitten by an animal, an early establishment of the diagnosis of rabies in the animal and postexposure immunization of the patient prevents the development of rabies.
   - If a woman has primary genital herpes at the time of delivery, caesarean section is indicated.
   - If a baby is born of an HBsAg-positive mother, immunization at birth is mandatory.
4. Screening of blood donors for HIV, hepatitis B and C helps to prevent spread of these viruses from symptomless carriers to others.
5. Early detection of dangerous epidemics like ebola, yellow fever, encephalitis, influenza, polio-myelitis, etc. is of vital importance in alerting authorities to initiate appropriate antimosquito control measures, immunization, quarantine or other forms of control.
6. To discover new viruses, for example, HIV was discovered in 1983.

Methods of laboratory diagnosis

Laboratory diagnosis of viral infections can be carried out by the following methods:

  I. Direct detection of virus, viral antigen or viral genome.
 II. Virus isolation.
III. Detection of specific antiviral antibodies.
 IV. Cytological or histological examination of cells from the site of infection.

I. Direct detection of virus, viral antigen or viral genome

1. Electron microscopy

Electron microscopy (EM) is one of the most useful tools for the direct demonstration of viruses in clinical specimens. On the basis of their distinctive appearances, most of the viruses can be assigned to the correct family. Viruses that are difficult to culture (*Rotavirus*, astroviruses) can be recognized by electron microscopy. The clinical material can be negatively stained with potassium phosphotungstate or uranyl acetate and scanned by EM. Clinical applications of electron microscopy include detection of *Rotavirus* and hepatitis A virus in faecal specimens, poxviruses in vesicle fluid and herpesvirus in brain biopsy tissue. This method can also be used for the identification of virus isolates in cell culture.

2. Immunoelectron microscopy

EM as a diagnostic tool has low sensitivity. For satisfactory results, the specimen should contain 10^7 virions per ml. The sensitivity of electron microscopy can be increased by mixing specific antibody to the specimen to aggregate the virus particles. These aggregates can be sedimented by centrifugation, negatively stained and observed under EM.

3. Fluorescence microscopy

Virions or viral antigens can be detected in frozen tissue sections, acetone-fixed cell smears, cells from virus infected cultures or vesicle fluid by direct or indirect fluorescent antibody technique. Fluorescence microscopy of brain biopsy can be used for the diagnosis of herpes simplex encephalitis and subacute sclerosing panencephalitis (a late sequelae of measles), and for the verification of rabies in the brain of animals suspected to be rabid. This method is also useful for the rapid diagnosis of respiratory infections caused by paramyxoviruses, orthomyxoviruses, adenoviruses and herpesviruses.

4. Light microscopy

Viral antigens in infected cells can be detected by immunoperoxidase staining. Tissue section or smear of infected cells is stained with antibody coupled to horseradish peroxidase. Hydrogen peroxide together with a benzidine derivative is then added. It forms a coloured insoluble precipitate which can be seen under ordinary light microscope (LM).

5. Viral antigens

These may be detected by direct and indirect ELISA, radioimmunoassay and latex agglutination.

6. Nucleic acid probes

- Enzyme-labelled or radiolabelled nucleic acid (DNA or RNA) sequences complementary to unique regions in nucleic acid sequences of most viruses are now manufactured commercially. These labelled complementary sequences are known as nucleic acid probes. Two strands of the target DNA molecule in the clinical specimens are first separated by boiling, then, following cooling, allowed to hybridize with a labelled single-stranded DNA or RNA probe present in excess. Depending on the type of label attached to the probe, hybridized-labelled probe can be detected by radiography, gamma-counting or a simple colourimetric evaluation (dot-blot hybridization).

- By use of nucleic acid probes cytomegalovirus, *Papillomavirus* and Epstein-Barr virus have been identified.

- **In situ hybridization** may be used to detect integrated or nonintegrated copies of viral genome in persistent infections or viral cancers.

- **Southern blot hybridization** and **northern blot hybridization** can be used for detection of DNA and RNA respectively.

7. Polymerase chain reaction (PCR)

It is a DNA amplification system that allows molecular biologists to produce microgram quantities of DNA from picogram amounts of starting material. It is based on repeated cycles of high temperature template denaturation, oligonucleotide primer annealing and polymerase mediated extension. With the revolutionary PCR technique, a target DNA sequence can be amplified at least 100,000 folds in just a few hours—a sharp contrast to the days required for conventional amplification methods (culture). Thus viral DNA extracted from a very small number of virions or infected cells can be amplified to the point where it can readily be identified using labelled probes in a hybridization assay. For the detection of viral RNA, it is first converted into DNA by reverse transcriptase.

PCR can be used for the diagnosis of infections caused by HIV-1, HIV-2, HTLV-1, cytomegalovirus, human *Papillomavirus*, herpes simplex viruses, HBV, HCV, HDV, HEV, rubella virus, Epstein-Barr virus, varicella-zoster virus, human herpes virus 6 and 7, *Parvovirus* B19, enteroviruses, coxsackieviruses, echoviruses, rhinoviruses, measles virus and *Rotavirus*.

II. Virus isolation

Most of the viruses can be cultivated in laboratory animals, chick embryos and cell cultures.

III. Detection of specific antiviral antibodies

Using panels of known antigens, a number of serological techniques may be used to detect specific viral antibodies. Paired sera should be collected from the patient, the "acute-phase" serum sample collected as early as possible in the illness and the "convalescent-phase" sample collected at least 2 weeks later. Antibodies in the serum samples can be detected by ELISA, RIA, western blot, latex agglutination, virus neutralization, haemagglutination inhibition, immunofluorescence, immunodiffusion and complement fixation tests.

IV. Cytological or histological examination of cells from the site of infection

Virus-induced histopathology (multinucleate giant cells and inclusion bodies) may be recognized by light microscopy. For example, demonstration of Negri bodies in the brain cells of animals is a useful method for presumptive diagnosis of rabies.

VIRAL VACCINES

Viral vaccines confer solid immunity and are, in general, more effective than bacterial vaccines. A number of viral vaccines have been outstandingly successful especially those directed against smallpox, yellow fever, poliomyelitis, measles and rubella. Smallpox vaccine has been used as a sole tool for global eradication of the disease. The World Health Organization is now determined on global eradication of poliomyelitis. No case of poliomyelitis has been reported from India after 11-02-2011. Viral vaccines are of three types:

I. Live-virus vaccines

These are prepared from:

- Attenuated strains that are almost or completely devoid of pathogenicity.
- Temperature sensitive (ts) and cold-adapted (ca) mutants.
- Recombinant live viral or bacterial vectors.

Advantages of live virus vaccines

1. A single dose is usually sufficient because they multiply in the human host and provide continuous antigenic stimulation over a period of time resulting in durable immunity.
2. They can be administered by the route of natural infection so that local immunity is induced.
3. They induce a wide spectrum of immunoglobulins including secretory IgA to whole range of viral antigens.
4. They also induce cell-mediated immunity.
5. They provide more effective long-lasting immunity than inactivated vaccines.
6. Some of them can be given as combined vaccines (measles-mumps-rubella vaccine).
7. Primary vaccine failures are uncommon and are usually the result of inadequate storage or administration.
8. They can, in general, be prepared more economically and more conveniently for mass immunization.

Disadvantages of live-virus vaccines

1. There is risk, however remote, of reversion of virulence.
2. The vaccine may be contaminated with potentially dangerous viruses such as oncogenic viruses.
3. Interference by pre-existing viruses may sometimes prevent a good immune response following live vaccination.
4. Live-virus vaccines are heat-labile and have to be preserved under strict refrigeration.
5. Some live-virus vaccines may cause local remote complications.

Currently available live-virus vaccines are oral polio, measles, mumps, rubella, yellow fever and varicella. Polyvalent measles-mumps-rubella (MMR) vaccine is also available.

II. Inactivated virus and virus subunit vaccines or non-replicating vaccines

Inactivated virus vaccines are prepared from virulent viruses by chemically destroying the infectivity while retaining the immunogenicity. Chemical agents used are β-propiolactone and formaldehyde. Subunit vaccines include purified viral proteins, purified proteins from cloned genes and synthetic peptides.

Advantages of non-replicating vaccines

1. Safety
2. Stability

Disadvantages of non-replicating vaccines

1. These vaccines need to be injected in large amounts. Primary course comprises of two or three injections. Thereafter, booster doses may be required at intervals over the succeeding years to revive waning immunity.
2. These vaccines have to be given by injections, therefore, local IgA immunoglobulins fail to develop.
3. Cell-mediated immunity is not induced.

   Currently available non-replicating viral vaccines include inactivated polio, rabies, influenza, hepatitis B, Japanese encephalitis and tick borne encephalitis.

III. Other vaccines

These include anti-idiotypic antibodies and viral DNA.

ANTIVIRAL THERAPY

As viruses are obligate intracellular parasites, they are absolutely dependent on the biosynthetic mechanisms of the host cell for their replication. Hence, most agents that block the replication of viruses are lethal to the cell. However, it is now known that viral replication may be checked at the level of attachment, penetration, transcription of viral nucleic acid, translation of viral mRNA and inhibition of viral DNA polymerase and reverse transcriptase and replication of viral nucleic acid (Table 29.5).

KEY FACTS

- **Viruses** are **obligate intracellular parasites**, which are metabolically inert, and can replicate only within living cells
- The virus **genome** has either **DNA** or **RNA** but **never both**
- The genome is protected by an **outer protein coat** (**capsid**) composed of **capsomers**; the **nucleocapsid** is the term given to the **protein and the viral genome** complex

Table 29.5. Major antiviral compounds used for treatment of viral infections

Drug	Viral spectrum
VIRAL POLYMERASE INHIBITORS	
Acyclovir	Herpes simplex, varicella-zoster
Cidofovir	Cytomegalovirus, herpes simplex
Foscarnet	Herperviruses, HIV-1, HBV
Ganciclovir	Cytomegalovirus
Valacyclovir	Herpesviruses
Vidarabine	Herpesviruses, vaccinia, HBV
BLOCKING OF VIRAL UNCOATING	
Amantadine	Influenzavirus A
HIV PROTEASE INHIBITORS	
Indinavir	HIV-1, HIV-2
Ritonavir	HIV-1, HIV-2
Saquinavir	HIV-1, HIV-2
REVERSE TRANSCRIPTASE INHIBITORS	
Lamivudine (deoxycytidine)	HIV-1, HIV-2, HBV
Nevirapine	HIV-1
Stavudine	HIV-1, HIV-2
Zidovudine (azidothymidine, AZT)	HIV-1, HIV-2, HBV
Zalcitabine (dideoxycytidine, ddC)	HIV-1, HIV-2, HBV
Didanosine (dideoxyinosine, ddI)	HIV-1, HIV-2
BLOCKING OF CAPPING OF mRNA	
Ribavirin	Respiratory syncytial virus, Influenzaviruses A and B, Lassa fever

- The nucleocapsid of viruses is arranged in one of three spatial configurations – **icosahedral**, **helical** or **complex symmetry**
- When a lipoprotein surrounds a virus it is called an envelope. **Nonenveloped viruses** are called **naked viruses**
- **Peplomers (spikes) are glycoprotein extensions** from the envelope, and play a role in the attachment of the virus to the target host cells
- Viruses are classified into families, genera & species
- The stages of **viral replication** are **adsorption, entry into host cells, uncoating, biosynthesis, virion assembly** and **release**

- **Viral vaccines confer solid immunity** and are, in general, more effective than bacterial vaccines

IMPORTANT QUESTION

Write short notes on:
(a) General properties of viruses
(b) Replication of viruses
(c) Virus isolation
(d) Detection of virus growth in cell culture
(e) Inclusion bodies
(f) Transmission of human virus infections
(g) Interferons
(h) Laboratory diagnosis of viral infections
(i) Viral vaccines

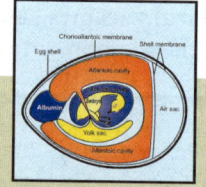

Chapter 30

Herpesviruses, Papillomaviruses, Adenoviruses, Mumps Virus, Measles Virus, Rubella Virus and Human Immunodeficiency Virus

HERPESVIRUSES

Herpesviruses belong to the family *Herpesviridae* which is divided into three subfamilies (Table 30.1).

Morphology

Herpesviruses are 120–200 nm in diameter. They comprise of four distinct structural elements – envelope, tegument, capsid and core (Fig. 30.1). Envelope is the outermost, it is composed of lipid with numerous small glycoprotein peplomers. Tegument is the electron-dense material present between envelope and capsid. It contains several proteins. Inner to the tegument is icosahedral capsid

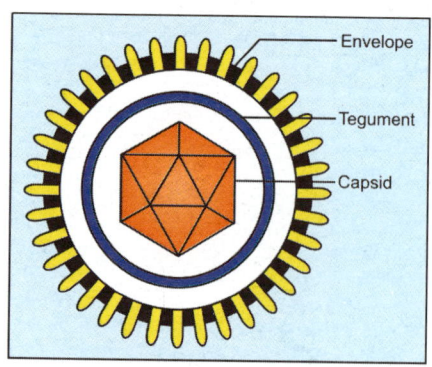

Fig. 30.1. Herpes virus.

Table 30.1. Human herpesviruses (HHV)

| Subfamily | Viruses | |
	Common name	Scientific name
Alpha-herpesvirinae	Herpes simplex virus type 1	Human herpesvirus 1
	Herpes simplex virus type 2	Human herpesvirus 2
	Varicella-zoster virus	Human herpesvirus 3
	Simian herpes B virus	Cercopithecine herpesvirus 1
Gamma-herpesvirinae	Epstein-Barr virus	Human herpesvirus 4
	Kaposi's sarcoma-associated herpesvirus	Human herpesvirus 8
Beta-herpesvirinae	Human cytomegalo-virus	Human herpesvirus 5
	—	Human herpesvirus 6
	—	Human herpesvirus 7

of 100 nm diameter. It has a total of 162 capsomers. Core, inside the capsid, consists of double-stranded, 124–235 kb DNA. With the exception of Epstein-Barr virus, members of the family *Herpesviridae* can be cultivated in cell cultures and produce giant cells and intranuclear inclusion bodies in infected cells.

HERPES SIMPLEX VIRUS (HSV)

There are two types of herpes simplex virus – type 1 virus (HSV-1) and type 2 virus (HSV-2). HSV-1 infects primarily the mouth, the eye and the central nervous system (regions of the body above the waist), but it is also responsible for a proportion of cases of genital herpes. HSV-2 infects genital and anal regions. The infections caused by herpes simplex viruses can be divided into primary infection, latent infection, and reactivation and recrudescence.

Primary infections

Infections caused by HSV-1

1. Acute gingivostomatitis
2. Herpetic whitlow
3. Keratoconjunctivitis
4. Eczema herpeticum
5. Encephalitis
6. Generalized infection

1. Acute gingivostomatitis

It is the most common primary lesion. It leads to acute and painful ulcers, coated with a greyish slough, inside the mouth on the buccal mucosa and on the gums (Fig. 30.2). The lesions may also involve the tonsils, pharynx or nose. Normally, the disease is self-limiting and lesions disappear in 2–3 weeks.

2. Herpetic whitlow

It is an occupational hazard of doctors and nurses,

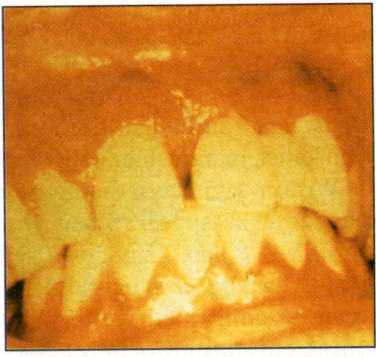

Fig. 30.2. Herpetic gingivostomatitis.

who acquire infection by implantation of virus from saliva and respiratory secretions of patients. Vesicles may also be produced on the skin of head and neck.

3. Keratoconjunctivitis

Infection of the eye by HSV-1 causes an extremely painful ulceration of cornea and vesiculation of the lids with associated conjunctivitis. In majority of the cases, the primary lesions heal in 2–3 weeks.

4. Eczema herpeticum

It is a superinfection of eczematous skin. It is mainly seen in young children. Crops of vesicles appear mainly on already eczematous areas with extensive ulceration.

5. Encephalitis

Both HSV-1 and HSV-2 can also infect central nervous system leading to herpes encephalitis.

6. Generalized infection

Rarely, primary infection with HSV-1 may lead to generalized disseminated infection. Patient develops acute gingivostomatitis, disseminated vesicular skin lesions, hepatitis and involvement of other organs.

Infections caused by HSV-2

1. Genital herpes
2. Aseptic meningitis
3. Neonatal infection

    It may rarely cause head and neck infections.

1. Genital herpes

HSV-2 causes one of the most prevalent forms of **sexually transmitted diseases**. It leads to the development of painful vesicles on the genitalia or anal regions with fever, malaise, and tender, swollen lymph nodes. In the females, lesions may occur on the perineum, vagina, cervix or vulva. In the males, the lesions may occur on the glans, prepuce or shaft of the penis. HSV-2 proctitis has been reported in homosexual men. Majority (80%) of cases of genital herpes are due to HSV-2 and remaining cases are due to HSV-1. These cases are possibly due to oro-genital sexual practices. HSV-2 may also be involved in oral infections. **It has also been blamed to cause cervical carcinoma.**

2. Aseptic meningitis

It may occur as a complication of HSV-2 genital infection.

3. Neonatal infection

It is acquired by the neonates usually from their mothers during passage through an infected birth canal, but in some cases it may be acquired in the immediate postnatal period from parents and nurses. Prenatally, a very few cases may acquire infection by viraemic transmission across the placenta or by ascending infection from the cervix. This may result in **abortions** or **congenital defects in the child**. If a woman has primary genital herpes at the time of delivery, the risk of neonatal herpes is 30–40%. Therefore, caesarean section is indicated in such mothers. Most of the cases of neonatal herpes are due to HSV-2, but those acquired postnatally may be due to HSV-1.

Neonatal herpes may present as:

- Disseminated disease, with a case fatality rate of 80%, most of the survivors being left with permanent neurologic or ocular sequelae.
- Encephalitis, with high mortality.
- Disease localized to mucocutaneous surfaces such as skin, eye and mouth.

Latent infection

During primary infection, the virus travels from the site of infection in the mouth to the trigeminal and probably other cranial and cervical ganglia. In genital herpes, HSV-2 travels to sacral ganglia. Within the sensory ganglia, viral DNA exists as a free circular episome perhaps about 20 copies per infected cells.

Reactivation and recrudescence

Reactivation of the virus is provoked by various stimuli such as common cold, fever, pneumonia, menstruation, exposure to sunlight, stress, etc. Infectious virions migrate along the nerve axon back to the nerve endings, where infection of epithelial cells may result in cluster of vesicles at the mucocutaneous junctions of the lips, in the nose, or eyes or on areas of skin that have experienced a primary infection. Reactivation recurs sporadically, sometimes often, throughout life.

Laboratory diagnosis

1. Specimens

Vesicle fluid, skin swab, saliva, conjunctival fluid, corneal scrapings, brain biopsy and CSF.

2. Microscopy

Diagnosis of HSV infection can be made by direct examination of clinical specimens by electron microscopy (EM), fluorescence microscopy (FM) and light microscopy (LM).

- Herpes virions may be demonstrated in the negatively stained smear of the specimen by EM.
- Viral antigens can be detected by FM in the cells scraped from the base of the lesions and tissue preparations stained by immunofluorescent staining.
- By LM, infected cell may be identified by characteristic changes, which include ballooning of cells, ground-glass nuclei, **eosinophilic intranuclear inclusions and multinucleated giant cells** (Figs. 29.3G and 30.3).

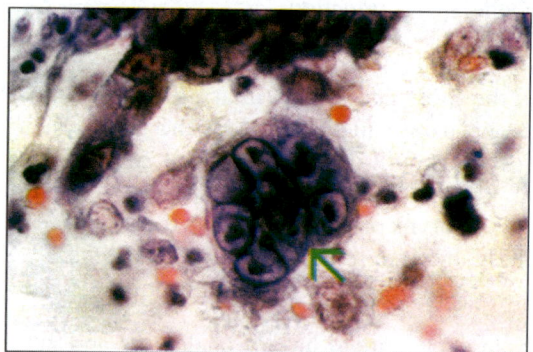

Fig. 30.3. Multinucleated giant cells with intranuclear inclusion bodies of herpes simplex virus.

3. Virus isolation

HSV can be isolated on human fibroblast or Vero cells although other mammalian cells also support its growth. Within 1–5 days distinctive foci of swollen, rounded cells appear. Some virus strains (particularly HSV-2 strains) may give rise to fusion of infected cells leading to **syncytium formation**. Diagnosis can be confirmed within 24 hours by **immunofluorescent staining** of infected cell culture. Differentiation of HSV-1 and HSV-2 can be made by use of monoclonal antibodies in immunofluore-scent staining or by **neutralization test** with specific antiserum.

4. Serology

Primary infections can be diagnosed serologically by detection of virus-specific IgM or of a rising IgG titre by complement fixation, neutralization, immunofluorescence, ELISA or RIA. However, serology is not widely used.

5. Polymerase chain reaction

Polymerase chain reaction may be used for detection of HSV DNA in CSF.

Chemotherapy

HSV infection can be successfully treated with acyclovir (acycloguanosine). It acts by interfering with viral DNA synthesis by inhibiting virus DNA-dependent DNA polymerase. For the treatment of ophthalmic herpes simplex infection, it may be used in the form of ointment. Oral acyclovir 200 mg 5 times daily for 10 days may be used for the treatment of primary herpes genitalis and orofacial herpes. For the treatment of herpes simplex encephalitis, neonatal herpes and disseminated infection in immuno-compromised patients, intravenous acyclovir (10 mg/kg, 3 times daily for 2–3 weeks) may be given.

VARICELLA-ZOSTER VIRUS (VZV)

VZV causes varicella (chickenpox) in children and herpes zoster (shingles) in adults and immuno-compromised patients. **Varicella follows primary infection in a nonimmune individual while herpes zoster is a reactivation of latent virus when immunity has fallen to ineffective levels.** A child can catch varicella from an elderly patient with herpes zoster, but the latter occurs only if the elderly or immunocompromised person had suffered from varicella in early part of his life.

VARICELLA

It is one of the common childhood exanthemata. Portal of entry of the virus is respiratory tract. Incubation period is about 2 weeks. The earliest mani-festation is a **maculopapular rash** that progresses

within a few hours to the vesicular stage. Vesicles characteristically are surrounded by a red rim. The lesions then rupture and crust or may become secondarily infected and pustular before healing.

Vesicles are centripetal in distribution, i.e., they are more profuse on the trunk followed by neck and proximal areas of limbs. Successive crops of vesicles appear over 2–5 days and as a result at any one time will have lesions at various stages of development on the same area of the skin. Some patients of vari-cella may develop viral pneumonitis, encephalitis, Guillain-Barré syndrome and Reye's syndrome. **Varicella tends to be more serious in pregnancy**, if the patient has not been infected during childhood. **VZV can cross the placenta following viraemia** in the pregnant woman and infect the foetus. A syndrome of **congenital malformations** with hypo-plasia of limbs, chorioretinitis and scarring of skin associated with maternal varicella in the first trimester may develop.

Oral manifestations

Small blister-like lesions occasionally involve the oral mucosa, chiefly the buccal mucosa, tongue, gingiva and palate as well as the mucosa of pharynx. The mucosal lesions, initially slightly raised vesicles with a surrounding erythema, rupture soon after formation and form small eroded ulcers with a red margin, closely resembling aphthous lesions. But these lesions are not painful.

HERPES ZOSTER

Herpes zoster or shingles is an **endogenous reacti-vation of virus** which has remained latent in one or more sensory ganglia following primary varicella many years earlier. Virus travels down sensory nerves to produce painful vesicles in the area of skin (dermatome) enervated from the affected ganglion. Thoracic nerves supplying the chest wall are most often affected. When the ophthalmic nerve of trigeminal ganglion is affected, the rash is distributed on the scalp and forehead. In about half the patients, the eye is affected leading to corneal ulceration, stromal keratitis and anterior uveitis.

The accompanying pain is often very severe for up to a few weeks, but herpetic neuralgia, which occurs in half of all patients over 60 years of age, may persist for months which may require surgical ablation of the ganglion. Zoster of the seventh cranial ganglion may lead to **Bell's palsy** and **Ramsay Hunt syndrome** which is characterized by facial nerve palsy with a rash on the tympanic membrane and the external auditory canal. Herpes zoster may also cause encephalitis. In immunocompromised and cancer patients, disseminated herpes zoster is sometimes seen.

Oral manifestations

Herpes zoster may involve the face by infection of the trigeminal nerve. This usually consists of unilateral involvement of skin areas supplied by ophthalmic, maxillary or mandibular nerves. Lesions of the oral mucosa are fairly common, and extremely painful vesicles may be found on the buccal mucosa, tongue, uvula, pharynx and larynx. These generally rupture to leave areas of erosion.

Laboratory diagnosis

1. Direct examination of vesicle fluid by **electron microscopy** may reveal herpes virus particles.
2. Stained smears from the base of the lesion or sections from biopsy tissue show **multinucleated giant cells containing acidophilic intranuclear inclusion bodies**.
3. Rapid diagnosis is possible by using **monoclonal fluorescent antibody technique**.
4. VZV antigens can be detected in vesicle fluid by **ELISA**.
5. DNA can be extracted from virions in vesicle fluid, amplified by **PCR** and detected by nucleic acid hybridization.
6. The virus can be **isolated** from vesicle fluid in human embryonic lung fibroblasts, human amnion, HeLa or Vero cells. Cytopathic effect is focal with refractile ballooned cells. It develops slowly over a period of 2 or more weeks. However, VZV antigen can be demonstrated in nuclear inclusions by immunofluorescence with monoclonal antibody before the end of first week.
7. Recent infection can be diagnosed by **ELISA** test for varicella-zoster specific IgM antibody in patient serum.

8. VZV DNA amplification by **PCR** is valuable for detection of VZV in CSF or aqueous humour.

Treatment

Acyclovir and vidarabine given intravenously are effective in the treatment of severe varicella and herpes zoster (e.g., in the immunocompromised patients).

EPSTEIN-BARR VIRUS (EBV)

EBV has been named after the virologists (Epstein and Barr) who first observed it under electron microscope in cultures of lymphoblasts from Burkitt's lymphoma. EBV replicates in epithelial cells of nasopharynx and salivary glands, especially the parotid, lysing them and releasing infectious virions into saliva. B lymphocytes appear to become infected when they infiltrate infected nasopharyngeal mucosa. Inside B cells, EBV normally fails to replicate but establishes lifelong latency.

Most shedding of virus takes place in the oral cavity, therefore, transmission of virus requires salivary contact, either through kissing or contaminated eating utensils. Most infections are symptomless, especially when acquired during childhood. However, in adolescents it may cause **infectious mononucleosis** or glandular fever, infections in immunocompromised hosts and when EBV exerts its oncogenic potential, it may cause **Burkitt's lymphoma**, **B cell lymphoma** and **nasopharyngeal carcinoma**.

Oral manifestations

At the onset the throat is painful and congested but exudate is absent. Clusters of fine petechial haemorrhages may be seen at the junction of hard and soft palates. Subsequently, a white pseudomembrane may develop on the tonsil and on other parts of the oral mucosa, and oral ulceration may occur. **It also causes oral hairy leucoplakia in HIV-infected patients** (Fig. 30.4).

Laboratory diagnosis

The clinical picture of infectious mononucleosis is so variable that laboratory confirmation is required. This can be carried out by:

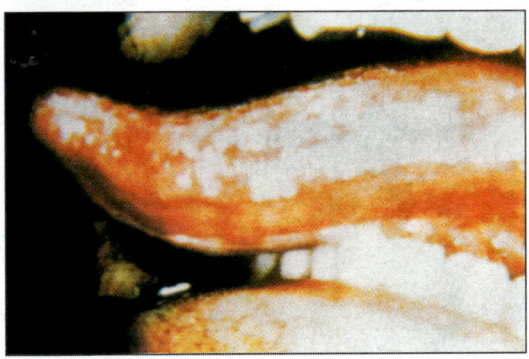

Fig. 30.4. Oral hairy leucoplakia.

1. Differential white blood cell count

By the second week of the illness patient develops leucocytosis (10,000–20,000/µl or more). Lymphocytes and monocytes account for 60–80%. Of these, 20% or more are "**atypical lymphocytes**". The latter are large pleomorphic blasts with deeply basophilic vacuolated cytoplasm and lobulated nuclei. They persist for 2 weeks to several months.

2. Paul-Bunnell heterophile antibodies

Infectious mononucleosis is accompanied by production of **heterophile agglutinins**. These are heterophile IgM antibodies elicited by EBV infection. These antibodies appear in 85–90% of patients sera during the acute phase of illness, reaching peak levels 2 weeks after the onset. Their titre decreases rapidly after fourth week and are not detectable after 3 months. Heterophile antibodies may be readily detected by a rapid slide agglutination test or Paul-Bunnell test. Agglutination of sheep or horse red cells by patient serum, adsorbed with guinea pig kidney cells to remove Forssman antibody, is the basis of this test.

3. EBV-specific antibodies

More reliable indicator of EBV infection is the demonstration of IgM antibody to the EBV viral capsid antigen by ELISA or indirect immunofluorescence. This antibody becomes detectable within 4 weeks and declines rapidly over the next 3 months or so.

4. Virus isolation

Saliva or throat washing and peripheral blood leucocytes can be inoculated onto umbilical cord lymphocytes. If specimen contains EBV, it leads to immortalization of the cells to produce a lymphoblastoid cell line.

5. PCR and DNA hybridization

EBV can also be detected by PCR and DNA hybridization.

CYTOMEGALOVIRUS (CMV)

CMV is the largest virus in the family *Herpesviridae*, being 150–200 nm in size. The virus exhibits strict host-specificity. *In vivo*, CMV replicates in epithelial cells in salivary glands, kidneys and respiratory epithelium. *In vitro*, they can be isolated in human fibroblast cells. An individual infected with CMV carries the virus for life and may shed it intermittently in saliva, urine, semen, cervical secretions and breast milk. The virus is found in 0.3–2.4% of populations that have been sampled throughout the world. Infection is transmitted by close contact between individuals, and blood transfusion. It may be acquired at any time, i.e., prenatal, perinatal and postnatal.

PRENATAL (INTRAUTERINE) INFECTION

CMV is the most common agent to cause intrauterine infection and prenatal damage to foetus leading to congenital abnormalities. Approximately 1% of all babies become infected in utero. Maternal viraemia following primary CMV infection or a reactivation during pregnancy may result in foetal infection. Majority (95%) of these are without obvious symptoms at the time of birth and 5% symptomatic infants have cytomegalic inclusion body disease. These infants show signs of growth retardation, hepatosplenomegaly, jaundice, thrombocytopenia, microcephaly, encephalitis and chorioretinitis. Of the remaining 95%, about 15% develop deafness and mental retardation.

PERINATAL INFECTION

This is acquired from infected maternal genital secretions or from breast feeding.

POSTNATAL INFECTION

This may be acquired by kissing (from saliva), sexual intercourse or artificial insemination (from semen), blood transfusion and organ transplantation.

Infections acquired after birth are generally sub-clinical. However, it may cause hepatitis in young children. In adults and older children, it may cause a syndrome resembling EBV infectious mono-nucleosis, but with a negative Paul-Bunnell test and no pharyngitis or lymphadenopathy. CMV may cause widely disseminated infection in immunocompromised individuals such as graft recipients and AIDS patients leading to interstitial pneumonia, chorioretinitis, hepatitis, arthritis, chronic gastrointestinal infection, encephalitis, Guillain-Barré syndrome and transverse myelitis.

Laboratory diagnosis

1. Specimens

CMV can be isolated from urine, saliva, stool, breast milk, semen, cervical secretions and blood leucocytes.

2. Demonstration of cytomegalic cells

Cytomegalic cells can be demonstrated in centrifuged deposits of urine or saliva.

3. Isolation of virus

The specimens are inoculated on cultured human fibroblasts. The virus replicates very slowly, therefore, characteristic CPE of foci of swollen refractile cells with cytoplasmic granules may take 2–3 weeks to appear. When stained, these cells are multi-nucleated giant cells containing acidophilic inclusions with perinuclear halo (owl's eye appearance) in the nuclei and cytoplasm (Figs. 29.3I and 30.5). For precise identification, the cell line may be stained by immunofluorescence or immuno-peroxidase technique using monoclonal antibody.

4. Polymerase chain reaction (PCR)

CMV DNA, in the specimen, can be amplified by PCR.

5. Serology

CMV-specific IgM can be detected in the patient serum by ELISA.

Treatment

For the treatment of severe CMV infections such as pneumonia, chorioretinitis and colitis in AIDS

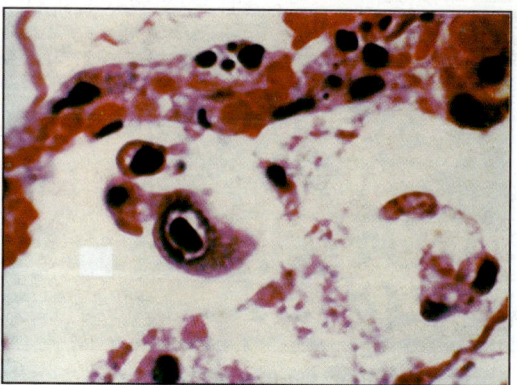

Fig. 30.5. Cytomegalovirus infection showing intra-nuclear inclusion bodies with perinuclear halo (owl's eye appearance).

patients or in other immunocompromised patients, ganciclovir is the drug of choice.

HUMAN HERPESVIRUS 6

Human herpesvirus 6 (HHV-6), with characteristic herpes group features, was discovered in human lymphocytes in 1986. It infects dividing CD4+ T lymphocytes. Infected T cells show ballooning with nuclear and/or cytoplasmic inclusions. Macrophages are also infected. These comprise an important reservoir of HHV-6. It can be isolated from saliva, thus suggesting that salivary glands may act as major reservoir and the saliva as main route of transmission. It can be cultured on transformed B lymphocytes, NK cells, glial cells, fibroblasts and epithelial cells.

Most HHV-6 infections appear to be symptom-less. They may, however, cause:

1. ***Exanthema subitum or Roseola infantum:*** This is a mild facial rash occurring commonly between 6 months and 3 years of age with sudden onset of fever.
2. ***Mononucleosis with cervical lymphadenopathy:*** This may occur in a few adults developing primary infection.

Laboratory diagnosis

1. Virus isolation

HHV-6 can be isolated from peripheral blood mono-nuclear cells in early febrile stage of the illness by co-cultivation with cord blood lymphocytes.

2. Immunofluorescence

Virus antigen can be detected in the infected cells by immunofluorescence using monoclonal antibodies.

3. Polymerase chain reaction (PCR)

Virus genome can be amplified by PCR.

4. Serology

Both virus antigen and antibodies can be detected, in patient serum by ELISA.

HUMAN HERPESVIRUS 7

Human herpesvirus 7 (HHV-7) was discovered in 1990. Like HHV-6, it may also cause roseola infantum. It is proposed that a new genus *Roseolovirus* may be created for HHV-6 and HHV-7, which belong to the subfamily *Betaherpesvirinae*. Like HHV 6, HHV 7 also appears to be widely distributed and transmitted through saliva. Both HHV-6 and HHV-7 infect T lymphocytes using the same CD4 receptors on these cells.

HUMAN HERPESVIRUS 8

Human herpesvirus 8 (HHV-8) was identified in 1994. It causes **Kaposi's sarcoma**, a vascular endothelial tumour common in HIV disease. DNA, amplification by PCR is the method of detection of HHV-8.

CERCOPITHECINE HERPES VIRUS 1

Cercopithecine herpesvirus 1 or simian herpes B virus or herpesvirus simiae is similar to herpes simplex virus. It commonly infects Old World (Asiatic) macaque monkeys causing a mild vesicular eruption on the tongue and buccal mucosa similar to primary herpetic stomatitis in humans.

Human infection with herpes B virus may be acquired from a bite or from handling infected animals. The typical lesions produced are vesicles on the buccal mucosa, which ulcerate shedding the virus and infecting contacts. Infection has also been transmitted in the laboratory from infected monkey kidney cell cultures.

After 5–20 days of exposure patient develops local inflammation at the site of entry, usually on the skin, accompanied by itching, numbness and vesicular lesions. It may be followed by fatal ascending myelitis. Diagnosis can be made by:

- Electron microscopy of vesicle fluid.
- Isolation of the virus from blood, vesicle fluid, conjunctival swab and CSF.
- DNA amplification by PCR.

PAPILLOMAVIRUSES

Papillomaviruses are 55 nm in diameter and have an icosahedral capsid composed of 72 capsomers. The genome is a supercoiled dsDNA molecule of 7.2–8.0 kilobase pairs. They are host species-specific and infect the squamous epithelia and mucous membranes of higher vertebrates, including man. There are over 100 types of human papillomaviruses (HPV). These are distinguished on the basis of the homology between their genomes. **Papillomaviruses cannot be grown in cell cultures.**

Pathogenesis

HPV are not only host species-specific but also display a predilection for the skin and certain mucous membranes. They cause cutaneous warts, genital warts, recurrent respiratory papillomatosis, oral papillomatosis and cancer. The infection is transmitted by indirect or direct contact including sexual contact.

ORAL PAPILLOMATOSIS

Infection is usually acquired by orogenital contact with infected sexual partner. It is caused by HPV types 6, 7, 11, 13, 16 and 32. Multiple papillomatous lesions may develop on the buccal mucosa, a condition known as oral florid papillomatosis. **Oral papillomas sometimes progress to malignancy.** HPV-16 DNA has been reported in a minority of oral carcinomas. HPV (and also Epstein-Barr virus) has also been blamed to cause **hairy leukoplakia** on the tongue in patients infected with human immunodeficiency virus.

Laboratory diagnosis

It can be carried out by:

1. Histopathology and cytopathology

These reveal characteristic features of HPV infection.

2. Electron microscopy

Papillomavirus particles can be readily seen by electron microscopy in most warts but are less in number in genital warts.

3. Immunocytochemistry

The HPV capsid antigen in paraffin sections of tissues or in cell smears can be detected by an immuno-peroxidase test using a commercially available anti-serum prepared by immunization of rabbits with bovine *Papillomavirus* particles disrupted with sodium dodecyl sulphate. It detects all the genital HPV types. However, monoclonal antibodies that can differentiate the genital types have now been produced and may be used as diagnostic tools.

4. Detection of viral nucleic acid

Viral DNA in fresh tissues, fixed tissues and exfoliated cells can be detected by DNA hybridization and polymerase chain reaction.

ADENOVIRUSES

Adenoviruses belong to the family *Adenoviridae*. They are nonenveloped, icosahedral viruses (Fig. 30.6) containing linear double-stranded DNA that replicates in the nucleus of the infected cell. They

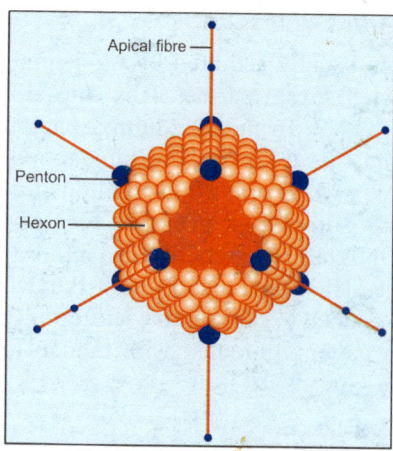

Fig. 30.6. Morphology of adenovirus.

measure 70–75 nm in diameter. The capsid is composed of 252 capsomers – 240 hexons make up the 20 triangular faces of icosahedron and 12 pentons form the vertices. From each penton projects an apical fibre, 9–31 nm in length, that serves to bind specifically to receptor sites on the host cell. The family *Adenoviridae* comprises of two distinct genera – *Mastadenovirus* and *Aviadenovirus*. They possess mammalian and avian adenoviruses respectively. There are 52 serotypes of human adenoviruses, which have been assigned to 7 (A–G) species (Table 30.2).

Table 30.2. Classification of human adenoviruses

Species	Serotype	Total
A	12, 18, 21	3
B1	3, 7, 16, 21, 50	5
B2	11, 14, 34, 35	4
C	1, 2, 5, 6	4
D	8–10, 13, 15, 17, 19, 20, 22–30, 32, 33, 36–39, 42–49, 51	32
E	4	1
F	40, 41	2
G	52	1
	Total	52

Cultivation

Human adenoviruses can be grown in monolayers of HeLa, HEp-2, KB and human embryo kidney cells. Cytopathic changes may take several days to develop and consist of **cell rounding and aggregation in grape-like clusters**. Infected cells swell and become ballooned and show characteristic **basophilic intranuclear inclusion bodies**.

Pathogenesis

Adenoviruses may infect via the conjunctiva or the nasal mucosa. Faecal-oral spread, particularly among children can also occur. They multiply initially in the conjunctiva, pharynx or small intestine and spread to preauricular, cervical and mesenteric lymph nodes. Most of the enteric and some of the respiratory infections are subclinical. In children, asymptomatic infection of tonsils and adenoids, leading to respiratory carriage, and Peyer's patches, leading to gut carriage, may persist for weeks or months.

Clinical syndromes

Incubation period is 5–8 days after which it may lead to:

I. Respiratory infections

1. *Pharyngitis* particularly in young children.
2. *Pneumonia* in infants and young children.
3. *Acute respiratory disease:* This syndrome is characterized by fever, chills, pharyngitis, cervical lymphadenitis, nonproductive cough and malaise.

II. Ocular infections

1. *Pharyngoconjunctival fever:* This syndrome of febrile pharyngitis and conjunctivitis occurs in outbreaks in children.
2. *Epidemic keratoconjunctivitis:* It is a severe and highly contagious infection involving all age groups. It often occurs in epidemic form and is characterized by follicular conjunctivitis and progresses to involve the cornea.

III. Genitourinary infections

1. *Cervicitis* and *urethritis*.
2. *Acute haemorrhagic cystitis:* It is mainly seen in infants and young children.

IV. Enteric infections

Adenoviruses may cause *infantile gastroenteritis* in up to 10% of the cases.

Laboratory diagnosis

1. Specimens

Throat swab, nasopharyngeal aspirate, transtracheal aspirate, bronchial lavage, conjunctival swab, corneal scraping, urine, anal swab, faecal swab, genital secretions, and biopsy and autopsy materials.

2. Microscopy

- Virus particles may be seen directly in stool extracts by **electron microscopy** and **immunoelectron microscopy**.
- Viral antigens in the cells from respiratory tract, eye, urine, biopsy or autopsy material and infected cell cultures may be demonstrated by **immunofluorescence** using polyclonal or monoclonal antibodies.

3. Serology

- Viral antigens in faeces and nasopharyngeal secretions may be detected by **ELISA** using monoclonal or polyclonal antibodies.
- Enteric adenoviruses may be detected by **latex agglutination** method using latex particles coated with specific antibody to each virus.

4. Detection of viral DNA

- Viral DNA in the faeces may be detected by **polyacrylamide gel electrophoresis**.

5. Virus isolation

- Virus from the clinical specimens, may be **isolated on** HeLa, HEp-2, KB and human embryo kidney cells.

6. DNA probes and polymerase chain reaction

- **DNA probe and polymerase chain reaction** are used to identify enteric adenovirus serotypes 40, 41 and 42 directly in stool specimens, which do not grow in cell cultures.

MUMPS AND MEASLES VIRUSES

Mumps and measles viruses are enveloped viruses 150–300 nm in diameter. They possess single-stranded, negative sense, RNA genome as a single piece and helical nucleocapsid. Mumps virus has a surface glycoprotein possessing both haemagglutinating and neuraminidase activity while measles virus has haemagglutinating and no neuraminidase activity.

MUMPS

Pathogenesis

Mumps is predominantly a disease of childhood. The mumps virus is transmitted by way of respiratory and oral secretions and respiratory tract is the portal of entry. It multiplies in the upper respiratory tract and in local lymph nodes. The virus then enters the blood stream and the infection spreads to many organs of the body. The major manifestation is

painful swelling of one or both parotid glands occurring 14–18 days after exposure. It may also cause meningoencephalitis, orchitis, oophoritis, pancreatitis, arthritis, myocarditis and renal dysfunction.

Laboratory diagnosis

1. Virus isolation

Virus can be isolated from saliva from affected gland, throat swab, CSF and urine on primary monkey kidney cells, H292 and HEp-2 cells. It produces little cytopathic effect but virus can be detected by immunofluorescence and haemadsorption (of guinea-pig or chicken red cells) which can be inhibited by specific antiserum.

2. Serology

For rapid diagnosis, ELISA is useful for detecting mumps-specific IgM antibodies in the serum.

3. Polymerase chain reaction (PCR)

Molecular diagnosis can be done using reverse transcriptase PCR in oral fluid, CSF, saliva and urine.

Prophylaxis

A live attenuated vaccine, derived by passage in chick fibroblasts, offers 95% protection which lasts for 12 years. It can be given by subcutaneous injection in combination with attenuated measles and rubella strains (MMR vaccine). This vaccine is administered to children of both sexes, aged 15 months.

MEASLES

Pathogenesis

Measles is the **commonest highly contagious childhood disease** spread by respiratory secretions. Virus gains access to the human body via the respiratory tract, where it multiplies locally. The infection then spreads to the regional lymphoid tissue, where further multiplication occurs. This leads to primary viraemia. It disseminates the virus, which then replicates in the reticuloendothelial system, followed by **second viraemia**. It seeds the epithelial surfaces of the body, including skin, respiratory tract, and conjunctiva where focal replication occurs. Measles virus can replicate in certain lymphocytes, which aids in dissemination throughout the body. **Multinucleated giant cells (Warthin–Finkeldey cells) with intranuclear inclusions are seen in lymphoid tissues throughout the body.**

After an incubation period of 10–12 days, patient develops upper respiratory tract infection with high fever, rhinitis, cough and conjunctivitis. **Koplik's spots**, which are small, 1–3 mm in diameter, bluish white spots surrounded by erythema can be seen on the buccal mucosa during this stage and are pathognomonic of measles. After 1–2 days, the acute symptoms decline with the appearance of characteristic maculopapular rash which appears first on the neck and then spreads to the rest of the body. **The rash is due to type IV hypersensitivity to viral antigens.** In next 10–14 days, rash fades with considerable desquamation and sometimes by discoloration of the skin. There is only one antigenic type of measles virus. Infection confers lifelong immunity.

Since measles decreases the resistance of the respiratory epithelium, therefore, patient may develop secondary bacterial infections like sinusitis, otitis media, bronchitis, bronchiolitis, croup and bronchopneumonia. Giant cell pneumonia may occur most frequently in those with impaired cell-mediated immunity. In addition, acute postinfectious encephalitis and subacute sclerosing panencephalitis (SSPE) may occur in 1 in 1000 and 1 in 300,000 cases of measles respectively.

Subacute sclerosing panencephalitis (SSPE) is a rare and late complication of measles infection. The disease begins insidiously 5–15 years after a case of measles. It is characterized by progressive mental deterioration, involuntary movements, muscular rigidity, and coma. It is invariably fatal. **Patients with SSPE exhibit high titres of measles antibody in cerebrospinal fluid and serum, and defective measles virus in brain cells.** With the widespread use of measles vaccine, SSPE has become less common.

Laboratory diagnosis

1. Specimens

Nasal secretions, throat washings, blood, urinary sediment, and CSF in SSPE.

2. Direct microscopy

Giemsa-stained smears of nasal secretions show multinucleated giant cells.

3. Immunofluorescence

The measles virus antigen can be detected in the cells of nasal secretions by immunofluorescence.

4. Virus isolation

The measles virus can be isolated, though with some difficulty, from throat washings, blood, urinary sediment, etc. on monkey kidney, primary human embryo kidney and human amnion cells. The appearance of multinucleated giant cells containing numerous acidophilic inclusions in cytoplasm and nuclei, in the cultured cells, suggests the presence of measles virus (Fig. 29.3J). Final confirmation is done by immunofluorescent staining with monoclonal antibody.

For rapid diagnosis, both multinucleated giant cells and viral antigens can be detected in the cells aspirated from nasopharynx.

5. Serological diagnosis

Measles antibody in the patient serum can be detected by IgM capture ELISA. Complement fixation test can be carried out on acute and convalescent sera. A rise in antibody titre is diagnostic. **Demonstration of high titres of measles antibody in the CSF is diagnostic of SSPE.**

6. Polymerase chain reaction (PCR)

Reverse transcriptase PCR is a sensitive and specific method of diagnosis.

Prophylaxis

Children of the age of 15 months are given MMR vaccine, followed by a booster at the age of 4–6 years.

RUBELLA VIRUS

Morphology

Rubella virus is a pleomorphic, roughly spherical, 50–70 nm in diameter, with a single-stranded RNA genome. It is surrounded by an envelope carrying haemagglutinin peplomers.

Pathogenesis

Rubella or German measles is primarily a mild childhood fever. It may be acquired congenitally or postnatally. It is not transmitted by arthropods.

POSTNATAL RUBELLA

Rubella virus is excreted in oropharyngeal secretions and infection is acquired by inhalation. Virus multiplies locally in the upper respiratory tract and in the cervical lymph nodes, followed by dissemination throughout the body by the way of the blood stream. After an **incubation period** of 2–3 weeks patient develops fever, fine, pink, discrete macules of the erythematous rash which first appear on the face, then spread to the trunk and limbs. Fever is usually inconspicuous but a characteristic is that postauricular, suboccipital and posterior cervical lymph nodes are enlarged and tender from very early in the illness.

The illness is of short duration and recovery is usually complete within 3–4 days after appearance of rash. Nearly half of infections in children are asymptomatic but asymptomatic rubella is less common in adults. Mild polyarthritis usually involving hands occurs in about 60% adult women. Complications like thrombocytopenic purpura, postinfectious encephalopathy and rubella panencephalitis though rare are sometimes observed.

CONGENITAL RUBELLA

Rubella virus can cross the placental barrier, particularly in early pregnancy, and infect the foetus, where it disseminates and grows in every foetal organ. It may result in a large variety of **congenital abnormalities or death of the foetus**. Congenital abnormalities may include total or partial neurosensory deafness, cataracts, glaucoma, microphthalmia or retinopathy leading to blindness, congenital heart disease especially patent ductus arteriosus, sometimes accompanied by septal defects and pulmonary artery stenosis, microcephaly with mental retardation, thrombocytopenic purpura and hepatosplenomegaly. This is known as **congenital rubella syndrome** (CRS).

About 20% of all infants infected in utero during the first trimester of pregnancy are born with severe and usually multiple congenital abnormalities and many of the remainder have milder defects. Severe congenital abnormalities may lead to intrauterine death with abortion or stillbirth. If rubella occurs in the fourth month of pregnancy, the risk reduces to approximately 5% and the only abnormality likely to be seen is neurosensory deafness. If infection occurs after fourth month of pregnancy, congenital abnormalities are very infrequent.

Laboratory diagnosis

1. Virus isolation

Rubella virus can be isolated from adult throat swab, and from the throat, urine, CSF or leucocytes of a newborn infant with CRS on RK13 (rabbit kidney), SIRC (rabbit cornea) and Vero cells. CPE is inconspicuous, therefore, rubella virus, in cell culture, is detected by **interference** with the CPE of a challenge virus (coxsackievirus A9) and by **immuno-fluorescence** or **immunoperoxidase staining** for detection of antigen in such cells.

2. Serology

Recent infection with rubella virus can be diagnosed by the demonstration of rubella IgM antibody in a single sample of blood, collected between 3 and 21 days after onset of rash, by ELISA, radioimmuno-assay and haemadsorption inhibition test. In case of rubella IgG antibody, four-fold or more rise in titre in paired sera has a diagnostic value. Antibodies of IgM class do not persist beyond 4–5 weeks after onset of illness, but IgG antibodies usually persist throughout life.

In a newborn baby, demonstration of rubella IgM antibody is diagnostic of congenital rubella as IgM antibodies do not cross the placenta. However, many babies have rubella IgG antibodies, acquired transplacentally.

Prophylaxis

A live attenuated MMR vaccine is recommended for all infants in the second year of life, followed by a booster at the age of 4–6 years.

RABIES VIRUS

Rabies virus is **bullet-shaped** 180 × 75 nm, with one end rounded or conical and the other plane or concave (Fig. 30.7).

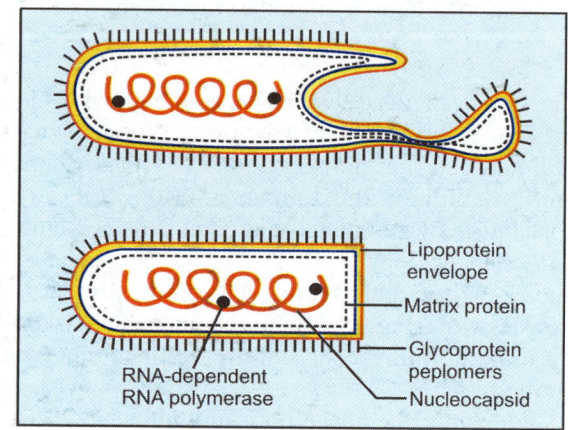

Fig. 30.7. Rabies virus

The core of the virion consists of a minus sense 11–12 kilobase, single-stranded RNA enclosed in a helically wound nucleocapsid. RNA-dependant RNA polymerase enzyme which is essential for the initiation of replication of the virus is enclosed within the virion in association with the ribonucleoprotein core. The latter is surrounded by matrix protein (viral membrane) which may be invaginated at the plain end. The matrix protein in turn is surrounded by a lipoprotein envelope which carries glycoprotein peplomers (spikes). These mediate the binding of the virus to acetylcholine receptors in neural tissues, induce haemagglutination-inhibiting antibodies, and stimulate cytotoxic T cell immunity. The spikes do not cover the plain end of the virion.

Pathogenesis

Rabies is a natural infection of dogs, foxes, wolves, skunks, cats and bats. Rabies virus is excreted in the saliva of affected animals. Man acquires infection by the bite of rabid dog or other animals. Infection by bite of rabid animal results in deposition of rabies-infected saliva deep in the striated muscles (Fig. 30.8). The virus replicates in the muscle cells or cells

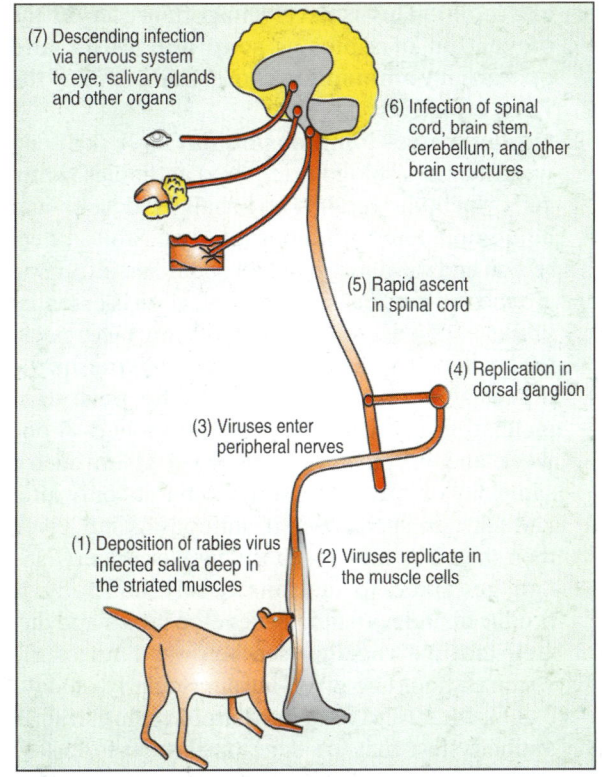

(7) Descending infection via nervous system to eye, salivary glands and other organs

(6) Infection of spinal cord, brain stem, cerebellum, and other brain structures

(5) Rapid ascent in spinal cord

(4) Replication in dorsal ganglion

(3) Viruses enter peripheral nerves

(1) Deposition of rabies virus infected saliva deep in the striated muscles

(2) Viruses replicate in the muscle cells

Fig. 30.8. Pathogenesis of rabies virus.

of the subepithelial tissues. After it reaches a sufficient concentration, it infects peripheral nerves in the muscle or skin.

Once within the nerve fibres, it is out of reach of any circulating antibody and it travels along the axon towards the central nervous system **at a speed of 3 mm per hour**. In the central nervous system, it multiplies and produces encephalitis. The virus then spreads outwards along the nerve trunks to various parts of the body including the salivary glands. **It multiplies in the salivary glands and is shed in the saliva.** There is little evidence that haematogenous or other modes of spread are involved.

Clinical features

Following the bite of a rabid animal, the **incubation period** is usually between 1–2 months. However, it may be as short as 9 days and rarely as long as a year or more. It is shorter in children than in adults and shorter in persons bitten on the face or head and

longer in those bitten on the legs. This is related to the distance the virus has to travel to reach the brain.

After a prodromal phase of malaise, headache, fever and paraesthesia at and around the site of bite, muscles become hypertonic and the patient becomes anxious, with episodes of hyperactivity, aggression and convulsions. **Patient develops difficulty in drinking, together with intense thirst. Patient may be able to swallow dry solids but not liquids.** Attempts to drink bring on painful spasm of pharynx and larynx producing choking and gagging. Thereafter, mere sight or sound of water precipitates distressing muscular spasm leading to **hydrophobia (fear of water)**. **The rabies in animals does not have this peculiar feature.**

The furious form of rabies, gradually subsides into delirium, convulsions, coma and death. Sometimes only the dumb form is seen, with symmetrical ascending paralysis followed by coma and death. The disease, once developed, is almost always fatal in 4–14 days. However, there are rare reports of survival after prolonged intensive treatment.

Laboratory diagnosis

1. Demonstration of Negri bodies

Sections or impression smears of brain stained by Seller's technique may reveal inclusion bodies, known as **Negri bodies**. These are intracytoplasmic, round or oval, eosinophilic with basophilic inner granules (Fig. 30.9). Negri bodies vary in size, from 3–27 μm in diameter and are seen mainly in the

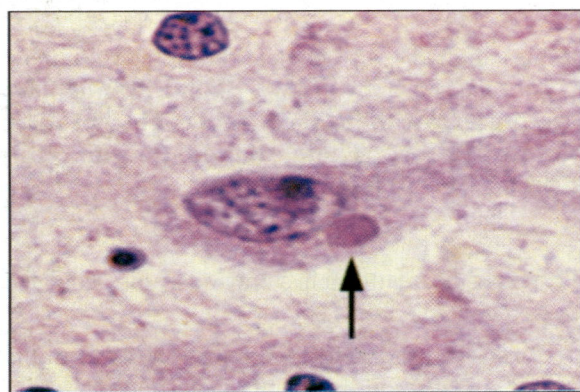

Fig. 30.9. Intracytoplasmic eosinophilic inclusion bodies in cells infected with rabies virus (Negri bodies).

pyramidal cells of Ammon's horn, in Purkinje cells of hippocampus, brain stem and cerebellum. Negri bodies may be absent in about 20% of the cases.

2. Demonstration of rabies antigen by direct immunofluorescence

- **Antemortem:**
  In salivary, corneal or conjunctival smears or skin biopsy from the nape of the neck.
- **Postmortem:**
  In impression smears of the cut surface of the salivary gland, hippocampus, brain stem or cerebellum.

3. Detection of genomic RNA and viral mRNA

It is carried out by PCR and dot-blot hybridization assay with ^{32}P-labelled cDNA probes on skin biopsy, corneal impression or saliva.

4. Virus isolation

- **Mouse inoculation:**
  Rabies virus can be isolated by inoculation of suckling mice. The animals die in 7–21 days. However, they may be killed after five days and brain smears stained with fluorescent antibody.
- **Isolation in cell culture:**
  Rabies virus can be grown in baby hamster kidney, human diploid lung fibroblasts, chick embryo fibroblasts and Vero monkey kidney cells. No cytopathic changes are observed but rabies antigen can be detected by fluorescent antibody staining 18–24 hours after inoculation.

5. Detection of rabies antibodies

Rabies antibodies can be detected in the serum and CSF of the patient by ELISA. **High titre antibodies are present in the CSF in rabies but not after immunization. Their demonstration can, therefore, be used for diagnosis.**

Postexposure treatment and prophylaxis

Postexposure treatment in a previously unvaccinated person consists of:

1. **First-aid treatment** to eliminate virus from the site of infection by prompt cleansing of wound with plenty of soap and water or solutions of quaternary ammonium compounds (such as cetavalon). This is a very important step in the prevention of rabies as **soap and water and quaternary ammonium compounds destroy the virus effectively.**

2. **Human rabies immunoglobulin** 20 IU/kg body weight or heterologous (equine) antirabies serum 40 IU/kg body weight – up to half the dose should be administered intramuscularly in the gluteal region and the remaining half should be infiltrated around the bite. Passive immunization is essential in cases of severe bites notably on face, neck, thorax and arms and in cases of licking of the mucous membranes because the period of incubation in such cases may be limited to one week and vaccination even when given on the same day of bite, offers solid immunity only after 2 weeks. In such cases if antibody is not given then the virus may reach the target organ (CNS) and get fixed to neurons before antibody is produced and patient may develop rabies and die.

3. **Cell culture vaccine** (see below): 1 ml of the vaccine should be given intramuscularly on days 0, 3, 7, 14, 30 and 90 in the **deltoid region**. Rabies antibody test may be done on day 30 to ensure that the patient has developed a satisfactory response.

4. Adequate tetanus prophylaxis should be ensured.

RABIES VACCINES

Rabies is the only human disease that can be prevented by active immunization after infection, because a long incubation period of the disease allows time for immunity to develop before the onset of symptoms.

I. Neural vaccines

Vaccination after exposure to rabies was introduced by Pasteur in 1885. He injected a young boy, bitten by a rabid dog, with ground-up spinal cords of rabies infected rabbits. The infected spinal cords had been dried for various lengths of time to partially inactivate the virus. After this came the vaccines (Table 30.3) which consisted of rabies-infected sheep brain in which virus was inactivated with phenol (Semple vaccine) or beta-propiolactone (BPL vaccines). The dose schedule of neural vaccines require repeated

Table 30.3. Rabies vaccines

I. Neural vaccines
 1. Semple vaccine
 2. Beta-propiolactone (BPL) vaccine
 3. Suckling mouse brain vaccine
II. Non-neural vaccines
 A. Duck egg vaccine
 B. Cell culture vaccines
  • Human diploid cell (HDC) vaccine
  • Purified chick embryo cell (PCEC) vaccine
  • Purified Vero cell (PVC) vaccine

and painful injections and their potency is low. Moreover myelin component of the neural vaccines sensitizes 1 in 500 vaccinees leading to neuroparalytic accidents.

Since the brain tissues of newborn animals contain little myelin and they provide high yields of virus, therefore, a vaccine prepared from suckling mouse brain and inactivated with beta-propiolactone was used, but was discontinued because of its poor immunogenicity.

II. Non-neural vaccines

A. Duck egg vaccine

Vaccine prepared from virus grown in duck embryos and inactivated with BPL was used for many years. It has been discontinued because of its poor immunogenicity.

B. Cell culture vaccines

(a) Human diploid cell (HDC) vaccine

This vaccine consists of fixed rabies virus grown on human diploid lung fibroblasts and inactivated with BPL or tris-n-butyl phosphate. It is highly antigenic and free from serious side effects but there may be local reaction in around 15% vaccinees. Because of the greater potency of HDC vaccine, quantity administered is much less than that of neural vaccines. Only five or six doses given intramuscularly in the **deltoid region** in 1.0 ml volumes on days 0, 3, 7, 14, 30 and 90 after exposure are recommended. The last dose is optional. *HDC vaccine should not be injected in gluteal region because high fat content in this region retards the absorption of vaccine.*

(b) Purified chick embryo cell (PCEC) vaccine and Purified Vero cell (PVC) vaccine

Because of its high cost, HDC vaccine is not available to majority of the patients in developing countries where rabies is a major public health problem. Therefore, to reduce the cost, a number of other cell culture vaccines have been developed using cells more easily grown in bulk than human diploid cells. This has allowed the cost of vaccine to be reduced. Rabies vaccines with a similar potency to HDC vaccine have been produced in chick embryo fibroblasts and Vero cells. The vaccines produced in these cell cultures are known as purified chick embryo cell vaccine (PCEC vaccine) and purified Vero cell (PVC) vaccine respectively. *No problems have arisen from a change of vaccine mid course and rabies antibody titres have been satisfactory in those people who were given more than one type of cell culture vaccine.*

HUMAN IMMUNODEFICIENCY VIRUS

Isolation of the aetiological agent of AIDS was first reported in May, 1983 by Luc Montagnier and colleagues from Pasteur Institute Paris. They isolated a retrovirus from a West African patient with persistent generalized lymphadenopathy and they called it lymphadenopathy associated virus (LAV). On this pioneering work, Luc Montagnier has been conferred Noble Prize in medicine in 2008. In March, 1984 Robert Gallo and colleagues from National Institute of Health, Bethesda (USA) reported isolation of a retrovirus and called it HTLV-3. In 1986 it was named as HIV, a member of family *Retroviridae*, subfamily *Orthoretrovirinae* and genus *Lentivirus*. Two antigenic types of HIV have been identified (Table 30.4). HIV-1 represents the original LAV/HTLV-3. HIV-2 was isolated from West Africa in 1986.

Morphology

HIV is a spherical enveloped virus, about 90–120 nm in diameter with a three layer structure (Fig. 30.10). In the centre are two identical copies of ssRNA (9.2 kb each) associated with reverse trans-

Table 30.4. Human retroviruses

Subfamily	Genus	Virus	Disease
Orthoretro-virinae	*Retro-virus*	HTLV-1	Adult T cell leukaemia/lymphoma
		HTLV-2	Prevalent in intra-venous drug users, not associated with disease
	Lenti-virus	HIV-1	AIDS
		HIV-2	AIDS
Spumaretro-virinae	*Spuma-virus*	Human foamy virus	Nil

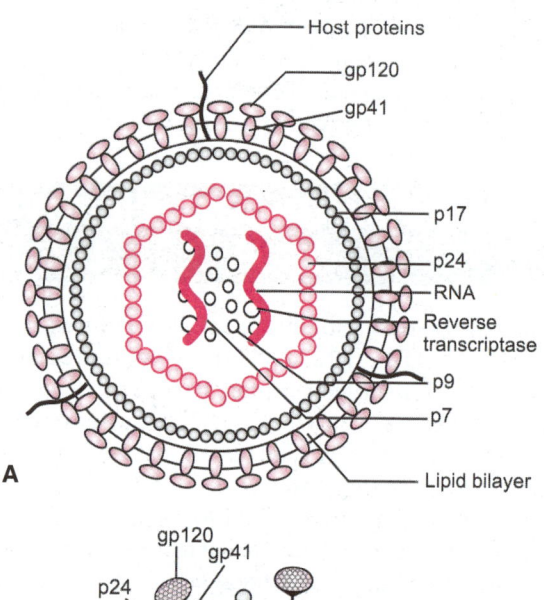

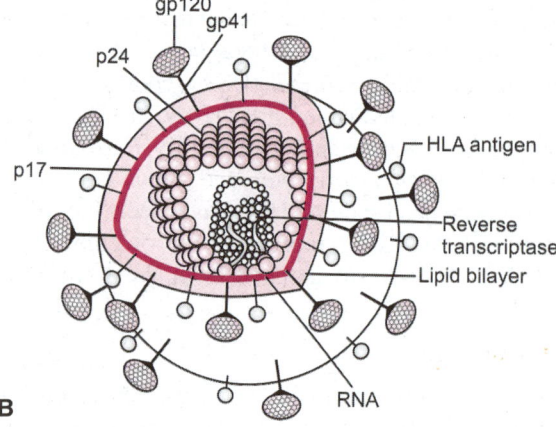

Fig. 30.10. Diagrammatic (A) and 3D (B) views of human immunodeficiency virus.

criptase and surrounded by an icosahedral capsid, which in turn is surrounded by a matrix protein followed by a host cell membrane-derived lipid bilayer envelope from which project 72 glycoprotein peplomers.

The genome of HIV contains three major genes, each coding for two or more polypeptides. The proteins (p) and glycoproteins (gp) are indicated by their molecular weight expressed in kilodaltdons.

1. The *gag* (group-specific antigen) gene encodes a precursor protein p55. It is cleaved into three proteins – p24 (core and capid protein), p15 and p17 (matrix protein).
2. The *env* gene determines the synthesis of envelop glycoprotein (gp160) which is cleaved into the two envelope components – gp120 which forms the suface spike and gp41 which is the trans-membrane anchoring protein.
3. The *pol* gene encodes polymerase reverse trans-criptase and other viral enzymes, such as protease and endonuclease. It is expressed as precursor protein which is cleaved into proteins p31, p51 and p66.

HIV-1 is divided into 3 groups – M, N and O. Group M (major) is responsible for global epidemic. Group O (outlier) is less common. It is mostly confined to West Africa. Group N (non-M, non-O) represents a few strains isolated from Cameroon. Group M has further been divided into nine subtypes or clades A, B, C, D, F, G, H, J and K. Subtype A is most prevalent being worldwide, while B is the most common in the Americas and Europe. **Subtype C is most prevalent in India and China.** The common types in Africa are A, C and D. In Asia, the common subtypes are B, C and E. HIV-2 is divided into six subtypes (A–F).

Resistance

HIV is a delicate virus. It is thermolabile, being inactivated at 56°C in 30 minutes and in seconds at 100°C. At room temperature, in dried blood, it may survive for up to seven days. It is susceptible to common disinfectants. It can be inactivated in 10 minutes by treatment with 35% isopropyl alcohol, 70% ethyl alcohol, 5% formaldehyde, 2% glutaraldehyde, 3% hydrogen peroxide, 0.5%

household bleach, 0.5% sodium hypochlorite and 2.5% Tween-20. For treatment of medical and dental instruments 2% solution of glutaraldehyde is useful.

Modes of transmission of the virus

There are three modes of transmission of HIV – **sexual, parenteral** and **perinatal**. Of these, sexual mode of transmission is the most important. AIDS in 80% of the patients is due to sexual mode of transmission and 10% each is due to parenteral and perinatal mode of transmission. During sexual intercourse virus gets transmitted from man to man, man to woman and woman to man. The risk of transmission is higher to the passive (receptive) partner and higher following anal intercourse (1% per episode) than vaginal intercourse (0.1% per episode) because mucosal tears are very frequent during anal intercourse and virus-laden lymphocytes in the semen can directly enter through these tears. Presence of another sexually transmitted disease enhances the risk of acquiring HIV infection especially if genital ulcers are present, as in syphilis or chancroid. Risk is also greatly enhanced if the sexual partners are more than one. It has been observed that 75% of HIV infections in India are occurring through heterosexual contact.

Parenteral transmission may occur through blood transfusion. Therefore, each unit of blood should be tested for AIDS and if found positive, it should be incinerated. Transmission of HIV has been recorded in a few recipients of blood transfusion even when blood was found to be negative for HIV antibodies. This occurs when blood is collected in the "**window period**", i.e., the interval between the time of exposure to the virus and development of detectable levels of antibodies.

Infection can also be transmitted by blood products like plasma, serum and cells from HIV-positive individuals and AIDS cases. It can also be transmitted from the donors of bone marrow, semen and organs like cornea, kidney, heart, etc. Therefore, donors of various fluids and organs should be screened for AIDS before they donate them. AIDS can also be transmitted by sharing blood contaminated syringes. Therefore, AIDS is more common in intravenous drug users who share syringes and needles, HIV can also be transmitted by the use of unsterile syringes and needles by doctors and health staff and through the barber's razor.

The third mode of transmission of infection is **perinatal**, i.e., **vertical transmission** from mother to the baby. Infection may be transmitted across the placenta before birth. Some of those who do not develop this infection before birth may develop it from the genital secretions during birth and from mother's milk after birth.

Replication of HIV

HIV attaches via its gp120 envelope glycoprotein (surface spike) to the CD4 antigen complex which is the primary HIV receptor on CD4+ (helper/inducer) T lymphocytes and cells of the macrophage lineage. The CD4 molecule has binding avidity for gp120 of HIV. Then by pinocytosis, the nucleocapsid of the virion enters into host cell. The envelope of the same does not enter into the cell. After entry into the cell, the nucleocapsid releases its RNA into the cytoplasm. The viral reverse transcriptase, acting as an RNA-dependent DNA-polymerase, makes a DNA copy of the genomic RNA. The ssDNA is made double-stranded by the same enzyme, now acting as a DNA-dependent DNA-polymerase.

This dsDNA moves to the nucleus, and several such molecules become integrated as provirus at random sites in the host cell chromosome causing a latent infection. The integrated provirus is transcribed by cellular RNA polymerase II either for the production of mRNAs which are translated into proteins or for the production of genomic RNA for insertion into progeny virions.

HIV establishes a latent infection with or without an initial productive phase. In this state, the integrated proviral DNA remains silent without transcription or expression of most viral proteins. Certain factors, however, can activate the virus and convert the latent state into productive HIV infection. During viral replication, naked virus buds from the surface of the infected cell and acquires a lipoprotein envelope which contains lipid derived from the host cell membrane and glycoproteins which are virus-coded.

Pathogenesis

AIDS is a unique sexually transmitted disease without local genital manifestations at any time during infection but with grave systemic manifestations. The first cells to become infected may be resident tissue macrophages or submucosal lymphocytes in the genital tract or rectum. The virus is then transported to the draining lymph nodes, where it replicates extensively.

Two or three weeks after infection, most patients develop viraemia, fall in CD4+ T lymphocytes and **glandular fever-like illness**. Since HIV infects cells expressing CD4 antigen, therefore, in the circulation the virus is found in CD4+ T lymphocytes and also in monocyte-macrophage cells, which may act as a reservoir for virus. Macrophages are also important in carrying the virus into the central nervous system across the blood-brain barrier.

Virus is also present in the plasma. It is probably derived from the lysis of activated lymphocytes. Within one month or so, viraemia declines to a near undetectable level and illness subsides. This is brought about by CD8+ cytotoxic T lymphocytes, natural killer (NK) cells and antibody-dependent cell-mediated cytotoxicity (ADCC).

This is followed by a **long asymptomatic period** of 1–15 years (average 10 years). During this period, only a small number of circulating CD4+ cells are producing virus and only low titres of virus are present in the blood. However, many infected cells can be detected in the lymph nodes. Follicular hyperplasia develops in these and other lymphoid organs. When CD4+ T cell count falls below 400/µl, a large number of virions spill over from the degenerating lymph nodes into the blood and opportunistic infections with various microorganisms may develop. Cause of death is the opportunistic infections, malignancy and cachexia-like state. Fall in CD4+ T cell count is due to:

1. Viral cytolysis of CD4+ T cells.
2. Infected CD4+ T cells can fuse, via gp120, with up to 100 uninfected CD4+ T cells forming a unit called syncytium. This will lead to the death of the entire unit.
3. Immune cytolysis of infected T cells by cytotoxic T cells, NK cells, ADCC and antibody/complement-mediated lysis.
4. HIV may also infect stem cells, so that there is no replacement.

5. AIDS may be an autoimmune disease, causing autoimmune destruction of infected CD4+ T cells.

Clinical features

The Centers for Disease Control in Atlanta, USA have classified the clinical course of HIV infection under various groups (Table 30.5).

Table 30.5. Classification of HIV infection and AIDS (Centers for Disease Control, USA)

Group I	Acute HIV infection or HIV seroconversion illness
Group II	Asymptomatic infection
Group III	Persistent generalized lymphadenopathy
Group IV	Symptomatic HIV infection
A	Constitutional disease
B	Neurological diseases
C	Secondary infectious diseases
C1	Specified infectious diseases listed in the CDC surveillance definition for AIDS, such as *Pneumocystis jirovecii* pneumonia, cryptosporidiosis, toxoplasmosis, generalized strongyloidiasis, cryptococcosis, CMV or herpes diseases
C2	Other specified secondary diseases, such as oral hairy leukoplakia, *Salmonella* bacteraemia, nocardiosis, tuberculosis, thrush
D	Secondary cancers such as Kaposi's sarcoma, lymphomas
E	Other conditions

I. Acute HIV infection

Two to three weeks after infection, most patients develop acute-onset fever with or without night-sweats, malaise, headache, myalgia, arthralgia, lethargy, diarrhoea, depression, sore throat, lymphadenopathy, skin rash, mucocutaneous ulcerations and sometimes meningoencephalopathy. Spontaneous resolution occurs within one month. There is a temporary fall in CD4+ and CD8+ T cells, followed by CD8+ lymphocytosis. Virus, viral nucleic acid or viral p24 antigen may be detected during this illness. Tests for HIV antibodies are usually negative at the onset of the illness but become positive during its course. Therefore, acute HIV infection is also known as **seroconversion illness**.

II. Asymptomatic infection

All persons infected with HIV, whether they develop seroconversion illness or not, pass through a long asymptomatic period of 1–15 years (average 10 years). They show positive HIV antibody tests during this phase and are infectious.

III. Persistent generalized lymphadenopathy (PGL)

Twenty five to thirty per cent of the patients who are otherwise asymptomatic develop enlarged lymph nodes, at least 1 cm in diameter, in two or more non-contiguous extrainguinal sites, that persists for at least three months. PGL must be distinguished from other causes of lymphadenopathy such as the lymphomas.

IV. Symptomatic HIV infection

Following features indicate disease progression:

1. Downward trend of CD4+ T cells in successive samples.
2. The ease of virus culture.
3. The presence of p24 antigen in the plasma.
4. The loss of antibody to p24 antigen.

When CD4+ T cell count falls below 400/µl, the patient may develop constitutional symptoms like fever, night sweats, diarrhoea, weight loss and opportunistic infections which generally are not life-threatening. The latter include infections of skin and mucous membranes such as oral hairy leukoplakia (Fig. 30.4), oral and oesophageal candidiasis, gingivitis, seborrhoeic dermatitis, bacterial folliculitis, chronic sinusitis, warts and molluscum contagiosum. Gastrointestinal infections caused by *Candida albicans* and *Cryptosporidium* and reactivation of herpes simplex and varicella-zoster infections also occur. In these patients, mycobacterial infections are also common.

When CD4+ T cells drop below 200/µl, their numbers generally begin to decline at an accelerated rate, the titre of virus in blood increases markedly and there is irreversible breakdown of immune defence mechanisms, leaving the patient a prey to progressive opportunistic infections and malignancies (Table 30.6). Most of the patients with HIV disease die of infections other than HIV. Tuberculosis is the commonest opportunistic infection.

Table 30.6. Opportunistic infections and malignancies commonly associated with HIV infection

I. Bacterial
  1. *M. avium* complex
  2. *Mycobacterium tuberculosis* – disseminated or extrapulmonary
  3. *Salmonella* – recurrent septicaemia

II. Viral
  1. Cytomegalovirus
  2. Herpes simplex virus
  3. Varicella-zoster virus
  4. Epstein-Barr virus
  5. Human herpesvirus 6
  6. Human herpesvirus 8

III. Fungal
  1. Candidiasis
  2. Cryptococcosis
  3. Aspergillosis
  4. *Pneumocystis jiroveci* pneumonia
  5. Histoplasmosis
  6. Coccidioidomycosis

IV. Parasitic
  1. Toxoplasmosis
  2. Cryptosporidiosis
  3. Isosporiasis
  4. Microsporidiosis
  5. Generalized strongyloidiasis

V. Malignancies
  1. Kaposi's sarcoma
  2. B cell lymphoma and non-Hodgkin's lymphoma

VI. Slim disease

Oral manifestations of AIDS

Oral lesions are a prominent and often early sign in patients with HIV disease (Table 30.7). Candidiasis is present in most patients, often as the first manifestation of immunodeficiency. Pseudomembranous candidiasis (thrush) in these patients is usually found on the palatal and buccal mucosae. White lesions of hyperplastic candidiasis are usually found on the posterior part of the buccal mucosa and sometimes on the palatal mucosa.

Other manifestations in patients with HIV disease include angular cheilitis (fissuring and ulceration at the corner of the mouth) and mucocutaneous candidiasis.

Patients with AIDS have an increased risk for other bacterial, fungal, and viral infections of the

Table 30.7. Oral manifestations of AIDS

Fungal
- Candidiasis
  - Pseudomembranous candidiasis (chronic thrush)
  - Hyperplastic
  - Erythematous
  - Angular cheilitis
  - Mucocutaneous

Bacterial
- Increased risk of dental caries and periodontitis
- Acute necrotizing ulcerative gingivitis
- Mycobacterial infection
  - *M. tuberculosis*
  - *M. avium-intracellulare*

Viral
- Herpetic stomatitis
- Hairy leukoplakia
- Herpes zoster
- Human papillomavirus (*Condyloma accuminatum*)

Tumours
- Kaposi's sarcoma
- Non-Hodgkin's lymphoma
- Squamous cell carcinoma

Miscellaneous
- Recurrent aphthous ulcers
- Delayed wound healing

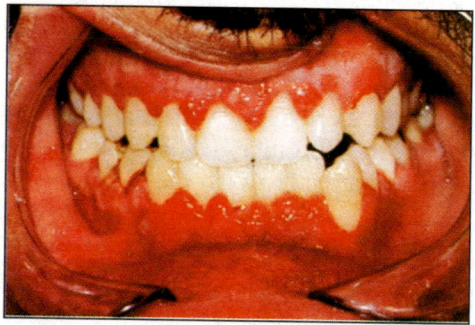

Fig. 30.11. Acute necrotizing gingivitis.

immune system has been compromised by HIV infection. The lesions are usually bilateral, soft, white, hairy excrescences on the lateral margins of the tongue. However, lesions can be unilateral, corrugated, or smooth, or occur elsewhere on the tongue or oral mucosa. A corrugated surface is more common than a hairy surface.

HIV transmission and dental care workers

There is no risk of HIV transmission by either saliva or blood in routine dental care. However, accidental injury via contaminated needles are associated with a very low risk of infection (0.5–1.0%). The disclosure of possible HIV transmission to five patients by an infected dentist, in Florida, USA, has raised important ethical, moral and legal issues pertaining to continued delivery of dental care by infected dental personnel. However, the dental transmission route has been questioned and it is believed that the patients acquired the infection from high-risk activities.

Laboratory diagnosis

Laboratory tests employed for the diagnosis of HIV infection may be classified into three groups (Table 30.8).

1. **Screening (E/R) tests:**
   These are serological tests which are used to screen antibodies against HIV. These tests are of two types.

   (a) *ELISA:* It is a highly sensitive and specific test and a standard procedure for diagnosing HIV infection. The sensitivity and specificity of ELISA is 99.7% and 95% or more respec-

mouth. **Dental caries** and **gingivitis** may be quite troublesome. **Acute necrotizing ulcerative gingivitis** should prompt the clinician to consider that the patient may have AIDS. It is painful bacterial infection of the gingiva caused primarily by the *Fusobacterium* species, probably in combination with oral spirochaetes. As the name implies, it is acute (a rapid onset); necrotizing (the interdental gingival papillae necrose into a crater-like shape); ulcerative (necrosis causes surface ulcerations); gingivitis (limited to gingiva without progressing beyond the mucogingival line) (Fig. 30.11).

The oral lesions of herpes simplex infections in patients with AIDS are often multiple, deeper, more painful and heal slower than the herpes simplex lesions in immunocompetent individuals.

Hairy leukoplakia (Fig. 30.4) is a common and early sign of immunodeficiency, particularly in HIV-infected male homosexuals. It appears to be induced by Epstein-Barr virus, possibly in combination with human papillomavirus or *Candida*, in patients whose

Table 30.8. Laboratory tests for the diagnosis of HIV infection

1. **Screening (E/R) tests**
   (a) ELISA
   (b) Rapid tests
       – Dot blot assays
       – Particle agglutination (gelatin, RBC, latex, microbeads)
       – Dip stick and comb tests (ELISA technology based)
       – Immunochromatography based tests
2. **Supplemental tests**
   (a) Western blot assay
   (b) Immunofluorescence test
3. **Confirmatory tests**
   (a) Virus isolation
   (b) Detection of p24 antigen
   (c) Detection of viral nucleic acid
       – In situ hybridization
       – Polymerase chain reaction

tively. If two ELISAs are used then accuracy is 99.93%. If one ELISA and western blot is used then accuracy is 99.99%. ELISA test usually takes 2–3 hours to yield result.

(b) *Rapid tests:* These tests have a total reaction time of less than 30 minutes.

2. **Supplemental tests:**

These tests also detect antibodies against HIV. These tests are recommended for validation of the positive results of the screening tests. Supplemental tests are often referred to as confirmatory tests which is not a correct nomenclature as these tests do not confirm the results of screening tests but provide additional information only. These include:

(a) *Western blot assay:* Western blot is highly specific and sensitive assay. In this assay, HIV proteins from detergent disrupted purified virions are separated according to their electrophoretic mobility and molecular weight by polyacrylamide gel electrophoresis, then blotted onto nitrocellulose membrane by standard blotting procedure. The membrane is then cut into strips having a full complement of viral proteins.

A serum sample found positive by screening test is reacted with the strip followed by washing. Antibodies which attach to separated viral antigens on the strip are detected by anti-human gammaglobulin antibody to which enzyme has been tagged. Enzyme substrate is subsequently added which indicates positive test. The substrate changes colour in the presence of enzyme and permanently stains the strip. The position of the band on the strip indicates the antigen with which the antibody has reacted.

(b) *Immunofluorescence test:* In this test, HIV infected cells are acetone fixed onto glass slides and then reacted with test serum followed by fluorescein conjugated anti-human gammaglobulin. A positive reaction appears as apple-green fluorescence of cell membrane under fluorescence microscope.

Many workers have shown that **saliva** is an acceptable and often favourable alternative to serum for HIV antibody testing. Blood of HIV-infected individuals is a hazardous substance that occasionally leads to HIV infection among healthcare workers. Saliva is safer medium than blood for 4 reasons:

1. HIV is rarely found in the saliva of HIV infected individuals;
2. when found in saliva the concentration of HIV tends to be very low;
3. there appear to be factors in saliva that inhibit viral infectivity; and
4. there is no possibility of needle stick injuries associated with specimen collection.

Saliva is specially useful for HIV testing among groups such as injectable drug users who may have collapsed blood vessels and those who refuse to give blood sample. ELISA test for saliva has sensitivity and specificity of 98% and 99.4% respectively.

3. **Confirmatory tests:**

These are the tests which confirm HIV infection in an individual who is either seropositive or has equivocal results from various serological tests. These include:

(a) *Virus isolation:* HIV can be isolated from patient's peripheral blood lymphocytes by cocultivation with normal healthy donor's lymphocytes in the presence of mitogens and T cell growth factor (interleukin-2). Isolation of the virus is a slow process taking 3–6 weeks and must be conducted under conditions of strict biocontainment. Therefore, virus isolation is carried out only in certain research and reference laboratories. The presence of the virus is detected by **assays for reverse transcriptase and p24 antigen in the culture fluid**. Less readily HIV can also be isolated from plasma, CSF, genital secretions and various organs such as brain and bone marrow.

(b) *Detection of p24 antigen:* p24 antigen can be detected in the serum by ELISA in 30% patients during 'window period', 10% of asymptomatic patients and 50–60% of AIDS patients. As the antibody response builds up, antigen tests become negative. Late in infection p24 antigen may reappear.

(c) *Detection of viral nucleic acid:* Viral nucleic acid can be detected by **in situ hybridization and polymerase chain reaction**. The latter is the most sensitive assay. It can detect a single copy of RNA or proviral DNA from infected cells.

Antiretroviral therapy

The care of the human immunodeficiency virus infected patient has changed dramatically in the last few years. Potent new antiretroviral drugs combined with updated treatment strategies have now achieved efficient inhibition of HIV replication in most patients. Classes of drugs include both nucleoside and nonnucleoside inhibitors of the viral enzyme reverse transcriptase, and inhibitors of the viral protease and integrase (Table 30.9). With the use of combination of drugs that target different proteins involved in HIV pathogenesis, a treatment strategy known as **highly active antiretroviral therapy (HAART)**, rates of death and illness have been dramatically reduced. Although the death rate due to AIDS in Europe and North America has fallen by 80% since HAART was introduced, relatively few people in poor countries have reaped these benefits.

Vaccines

The greatest challenge in AIDS research remains developing a vaccine that can either prevent the transmission of the virus, or failing that, halt progression

Table 30.9. Currently available antiretroviral agents

Nucleoside Reverse Transcriptase Inhibitors (NRTIs)		Nonnucleoside Reverse Transcriptase Inhibitors (NNRTIs)		Protease Inhibitors (PIs)	
Abacavir	– ABC licensed			Amprenavir	– APV Licensed, largely replaced by fosamprenavir
Didanosine	– ddI licensed	Delavirdine	– DLV licensed; rarely used		
Emtricitabine	– FTC licensed			Atazanavir	– ATV licensed
Lamivudine	– 3TC licensed	Efavirenz	– EFV licensed	Darunavir	– TMC114 licensed
Stavudine	– d4T licensed	Etravirine	– TMC125 Phase III trials	Fosamprenavir	– FPV licensed
Tenofovir	– TDF licensed			Indinavir	– IDV licensed
Zidovudine	– AZT, ZDV licensed	Nevirapine	– NVP licensed	Lopinavir	– LPV/RTV
				Nelfinavir	– NFV licensed
Fusion Inhibitors		**CCR5 Inhibitors**		Ritonavir	– RTV licensed; mostly used in low doses to boost other PIs
Enfuvirtide	– T-20 licensed	Maraviroc Selzentry	– Licensed in US		
		Vicriviroc	– Phase III trials		
Integrase Inhibitors				Saquinavir	– SQV licensed
Elvitegravir	– GS-9137 phase II trials	**Maturation Inhibitors**		Tipranavir	– TPV licensed
		Bevirimat	– PA-457 phase II trials		
Raltegravir	– 0518 Phase III				
Isentress MK	– Licensed				

to AIDS. Many different vaccine strategies, including viral and bacterial vectors, DNA vaccines, and peptide vaccines are being investigated. The effects of various adjuvants and different routes of administration are also being tested. Development of a vaccine is fraught with several problems unique to this virus. These include:

1. HIV can mutate rapidly and there is a possibility of recombination between different HIV strains. The prolonged asymptomatic period provides sufficient time for antigen drift to occur.
2. Antibody alone may be insufficient, CMI may also be necessary.
3. Virus normally enters by the mucosal route. Therefore, the vaccine should induce IgA antibody and submucosal lymphocytes.
4. HIV enters the body not only as free virions, neutralizable by antibody, but also as infected leucocytes in semen or blood, in which the virus or provirus is protected against antibody or T cell-mediated cytolysis.
5. Virus can spread from cell to cell by fusion to produce syncytia.
6. Virus readily establishes lifelong latent infection hiding from antibody.
7. HIV infects cells of immune system, notably CD4+ T lymphocytes and cells of monocyte/macrophage lineage.

Control

1. Do not have vaginal, anal or oral sex with prostitutes, male or female.
2. Reduce the number of your sex partners if you have more than one. Practice abstinence before marriage and fidelity after marriage. Mutual monogamy should be the objective of all heterosexual partners.
3. Men should always use condoms from start to finish and women should make sure their partners use them. Use of condom also protects from other sexually transmitted diseases and unwanted pregnancy.
4. Get all sexually transmitted diseases treated promptly.
5. Sexually promiscuous and parenteral drug users should not donate blood.
6. If you need blood transfusion, try to ensure that only screened blood is used.

7. Screening of donors of blood, blood products such as factor VIII, bone marrow, cornea, kidney, heart, semen and other organs and tissues should be carried out.
8. Avoid injections unless absolutely necessary, use presterilized disposable syringes and needles.
9. If you inject drugs, no matter what kind, never use anyone else's syringe.
10. HIV- or AIDS-positive individuals should not donate blood.
11. HIV- or AIDS-positive individuals should not allow anyone else to use their shaving kits.
12. Do not let the barber use a razor during your haircut.
13. Medical and laboratory personnel should follow strict standards of aseptic techniques in handling infectious material in the ward or laboratory.

KEY FACTS

- **Eight different types** of human **herpesviruses** (HHV) are described; they are **neurotropic** and **epitheliotropic**
- *Herpes simplex and **varicella-zoster** viruses cause **primary** and **reactivation** infection*
- *In general, **herpes simplex** viruses HSV types 1 and 2 cause infections **above and below the belt**, respectively (i.e., oral and genital infections)*
- *Herpetic gingivostomatitis is the primary infection and **herpes labialis** the **reactivation** infection caused by HSV-1*
- *Varicella-zoster (HSV-3) causes chickenpox (primary) and herpes zoster/shingles (reactivation) affecting well-defined dermatomes ('belt of roses from hell')*
- *Epstein-Barr virus (HHV-4) causes **infectious mononucleosis** or **glandular fever**, **oral hairy leucoplakia**, **nasopharyngeal carcinoma**, **Burkitt's lymphoma** and **B cell lymphoma***
- *Cytomegalovirus (HHV-5) causes **asymptomatic infection** in adults; if infection occurs during pregnancy, transplacental passage of the virus may cause serious **congenital defects***
- *Human herpesvirus 8 causes **Kaposi's sarcoma**, a vascular endothelial tumour common in HIV disease*

- *Mumps virus is the major agent of* **parotitis**
- *Measles is an acute febrile infection with an* **exanthematous rash***; prodromal symptoms of measles include* **Koplik's spots on the buccal mucosa**
- **Rubella** is a childhood fever resembling measles, except that it has a milder clinical course and shorter duration, however, if it is contracted in early pregnancy the virus can cause **severe congenital abnormalities and may cause the death of the foetus**
- **MMR** vaccine prevents **measles**, **mumps** & **rubella**
- HIV-1 M subtype C is more prevalent in India. However, western developed countries have HIV-1 subtype B as predominant subtype
- Subtype C is usually acquired by heterosexual contact and subtype B by homosexual contact
- In routine dental care, accidental injury via contaminated needles are associated with a very low (0.5–1%) risk of HIV infection.

- There are three modes of transmission of human immunodeficiency virus – **sexual**, **parenteral** and **perinatal**
- Patients with HIV disease during the course of their illness become a **microbial zoo** and **die of infections other than HIV itself**

IMPORTANT QUESTIONS

1. Discuss pathogenicity and laboratory diagnosis of herpes simplex virus types 1 and 2.
2. Write short notes on:
   (a) Varicella-zoster virus
   (b) Cytomegalovirus
   (c) Epstein-Barr virus
   (d) Rubella
   (e) Morphology and transmission of human immunodeficiency viruses
   (f) Oral manifestations of AIDS
   (g) Laboratory diagnosis of AIDS
   (h) HIV transmission and dental care workers

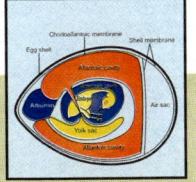

Chapter 31

Hepatitis Viruses

The term '**viral hepatitis**' is reserved for infection of the liver caused by a small (but growing) group of **hepatotropic viruses** (Table 31.1) named hepatitis A virus (HAV), hepatitis B virus (HBV), hepatitis C virus (HCV), hepatitis D virus (HDV), hepatitis E virus (HEV) and hepatitis G virus (HGV). Hepatitis F virus appeared briefly on the scene, but it proved to be a mutant of type B virus and not a separate entity. Therefore, it has been deleted from the list of hepatitis viruses.

HBV, HCV and HIV share common routes of transmission. Worldwide HBV accounts for an estimated 370 million chronic infections, HCV for an estimated 130 million, and HIV for an estimated 40–50 million.

HEPATITIS A VIRUS (HAV)

Hepatitis A virus (HAV) was previously classified as enterovirus type 72, but it has now been accorded the status of a separate genus, *Hepatovirus* of the family *Picornaviridae*.

Morphology

HAV is a nonenveloped 27 nm icosahedral virus containing linear, single-stranded RNA, 7.5 kb in length and of positive polarity (Table 31.1). It has only one serotype.

Resistance

HAV is one of the most stable viruses infecting humans. It can withstand heating at 60°C for one hour and treatment with 20% ether, acid (pH 1.0 for 2 hours) and many disinfectants. Inactivation of viral activity can be achieved by boiling for 1 minute, by contact with formaldehyde and chlorine, or by ultraviolet irradiation.

Cultivation

It can be transmitted to chimpanzees and several species of marmoset monkeys and can be grown in cell cultures of primate and human cells. **HAV is the only one of the human hepatitis viruses that can be cultivated in cell cultures.** It has also been cloned.

Pathogenesis

HAV is shed early in the stools of infected individuals, 1–2 weeks prior to the onset of symptoms, and persists for the first several days after the transaminase levels peak. There is very little virus in the serum and hardly any at all in other body fluids which explains the epidemiology of the disease as **faecal-oral enteric infection**. Transfusion-associated hepatitis A is exceedingly rare. It probably multiplies first in the intestinal epithelial cells and then spreads

Table 31.1. Hepatitis viruses

Feature	Hepatitis A virus	Hepatitis B virus	Hepatitis C virus	Hepatitis D virus	Hepatitis E virus	Hepatitis G virus
Year of identification	1973	1965	1989	1977	1980	1995
Family	*Picornaviridae*	*Hepadnaviridae*	*Flaviviridae*	Unclassified	*Caliciviridae*	*Flaviviridae*
Genus	*Hepatovirus*	*Orthohepadnavirus*	*Hepacivirus*	*Deltavirus*	Unnamed	*Hepacivirus*
Genome	ssRNA	dsDNA	ssRNA	ssRNA	ssRNA	ssRNA
Genome size	7.5 kb	3.2 kb	9.5 kb	1.7 kb	7.6 kb	9.4 kb
Virion	27 nm, icosahedral	42 nm, spherical	50–60 nm, spherical	36–38 nm, spherical	27–38 nm, icosahedral	?
Envelope	No	Yes (HBsAg)	Yes	Yes (HBsAg)	No	?
Stability	Heat- and acid-stable	Acid-stable	Ether- and acid-sensitive	Acid-sensitive	Heat-stable	?
Transmission	Faecal-oral	Parenteral, sexual	Parenteral, sexual	Parenteral, sexual	Faecal-oral	Parenteral, sexual
Vertical transmission						
• Intrauterine	No	Yes	Possible but rare	Possible but rare	Yes	?
• Perinatal	No	Yes	Yes	Yes	Yes	Yes
• Early postnatal infection	Possible but rare	Possible but rare	Possible	?	?	?
Incubation period	2–6 weeks	6 weeks–6 months	6–8 weeks	6 weeks–6 months	2–8 weeks	?
Onset	Acute	Insidious or acute	Insidious	Insidious or acute	Acute	?
Age preference	Children, young adults	Young adults, babies, toddlers	Any age but more common in adults	Any age	Young to middle-age adults	?
Antigens	HAV	HBsAg, HBcAg	HCV	HBsAg, HDAg	HEVAg	?
Antibodies	Anti-HAV	Anti-HBs, Anti-HBc, Anti-HBe	Anti-HCV	Anti-HBs, Anti-HD	Anti-HEV	?
Chronic carrier state	No	5–10%	50%	> 50%	No	?
Chronic hepatitis, cirrhosis	No	1–5%	20%	> 50%	No	?
Hepatocellular carcinoma	No	Yes	Yes	No	No	?

?, data not yet available.

to the liver via the blood. Viral antigens can be seen in the cytoplasm of hepatocytes.

Clinical features

Hepatitis A is an acute self-limiting disease with an incubation period of 2–6 weeks. The onset is abrupt with fever, malaise, anorexia, nausea and lethargy which comprise the prodromal (preicteric) stage. Hepatomegaly, due to cell necrosis, causes blockage of the biliary excretions resulting in jaundice. It may also produce pain in the right upper abdominal quadrant. The fulminant form of hepatitis A and liver failure can occur in less than 0.5% cases. Complete recovery occurs in 8–12 weeks.

In contrast to hepatitis B, hepatitis A infection does not produce extrahepatic manifestations, no carrier state and is not associated with cirrhosis or hepatocellular carcinoma.

Hepatitis A and dentistry

HAV is not a significant infection risk in dentistry as the route of transmission is faecal-oral. However, close contact with saliva may transmit infection as saliva may contain some HAV. Rarely infection may be transmitted by needle stick injury.

Laboratory diagnosis

Biochemical tests

Serum levels of both alanine and aspartate aminotransferase are markedly raised.

Immunoelectron microscopy

Virus particles can be demonstrated in faecal extracts by **immunoelectron microscopy**.

Serology

- Faecal HAV may be detected by ELISA.
- Detection of IgM anti-HAV by ELISA or RIA is the method of choice for the diagnosis of HAV infection. It is detectable in the serum for 2–6 months after the onset of symptoms. It is followed by the appearance of IgG anti-HAV which persists for many years and is a useful indicator of immunity.

Virus isolation

Virus, from the faeces, may be cultured on continuous cell lines of monkey kidney cells or human fibroblasts or hepatoma.

Polymerase chain reaction (PCR)

Trace amounts of HAV in food or water can be detected by PCR.

Prophylaxis

1. Proper collection, treatment and disposal of sewage.
2. Bathing and cultivation of shellfish for human consumption should not be allowed near sewerage outlets.
3. **Passive immunization** with normal human immunoglobulin (NIG) gives protection to seronegative individuals for a period of 4–6 months. It is recommended for the personnel travelling to highly endemic areas of the tropics and for the control of outbreaks in institutions such as homes for the mentally handicapped.

Hepatitis A vaccine consisting of formalin inactivated preparation of virions grown in human fibroblasts or monkey kidney cell lines, adsorbed to alum as an adjuvant, can be used for active immunization. Two doses injected one month apart with or without a booster after 6 months elicit a good immune response in 99% of vaccinees lasting for some years. Because of the low yield of virus from cultured cells the vaccine is costly. It may be given to high risk individuals like long-term visitors to countries in which HAV is endemic, sewage workers, sexually active homosexual men and intravenous drug users.

HEPATITIS B VIRUS (HBV)

Morphology

HBV or Dane particle is a complex 42 nm double shelled particle (Fig. 31.1 and Table 31.1). The outer surface or envelope contains **hepatitis B surface antigen (HBsAg)**. It is made up of lipid, protein and carbohydrate. It encloses an inner icosahedral 27 nm nucleocapsid (core) which contains **hepatitis B core antigen (HBcAg)**. Inside the core is the genome of HBV and a DNA-dependent DNA polymerase. The HBV genome consists of a 3.2 kilobase pair molecule of circular dsDNA of most unusual structure. The

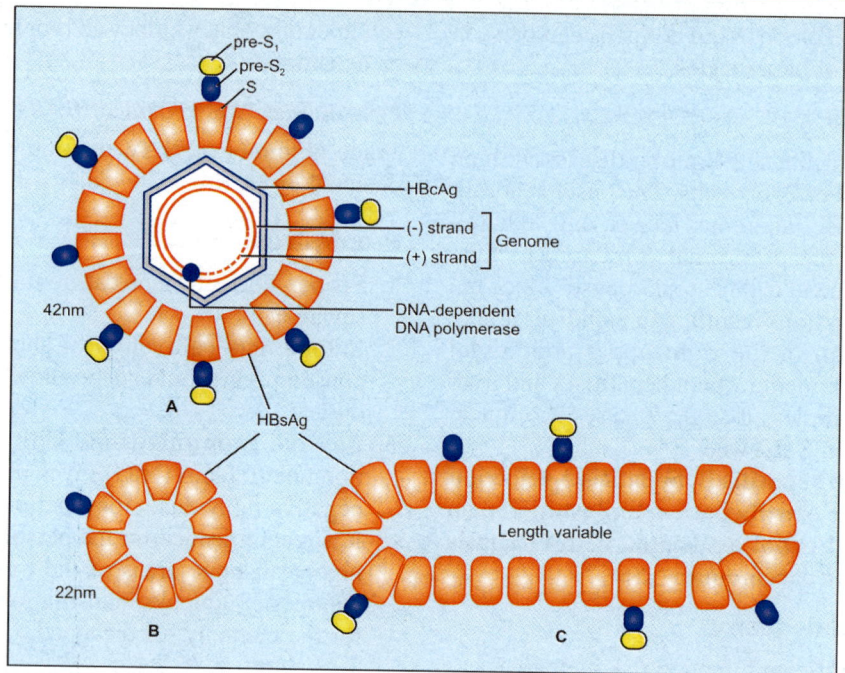

Fig. 31.1. Schematic diagram of hepatitis B virus particles: A, Dane particle; B, spherical particle; and C, tubular particle.

plus strand is incomplete leaving 15–50% of the molecule single-stranded. The minus strand is complete and contains four overlapping open reading frames (genes) coding for multiple proteins.

From the core protein is derived **hepatitis Be antigen (HBeAg)**. It is associated with the virion and is also found free in the plasma, especially when there is active viral replication.

Along with the mature virions, two subvirion morphological forms are formed in large excess (Fig. 31.1):

1. Spherical particles with a diameter of 22 nm.
2. Elongated tubules of similar diameter.

Both these pleomorphic structures are composed of HBsAg, are devoid of HBcAg and nucleic acid. They are not infectious and consist solely of surplus virion envelope. They normally occur in large (100- to 1,000-fold) excess over the mature 42 nm virions.

Cultivation and stability

HBV has not been cultivated in the laboratory. The chimpanzee is susceptible to experimental infection and can be used as a laboratory model. Experiments on chimpanzee inoculation reveal that the virus gets inactivated by heating at 60°C for 10 minutes and by treatment with hypochlorite (10,000 ppm available chlorine) and 2% glutaraldehyde in 10 minutes.

Pathogenesis

There are three important modes of transmission of HBV infection – parenteral, perinatal and sexual.

1. Parenteral transmission

HBV is present in the blood and in body fluids such as semen, vaginal secretions, menstrual discharge, saliva, colostrum and breast milk. The concentration of HBV in blood and body fluids is much greater than HIV. Less than 1 μl of blood contaminating a syringe or needle, can readily transmit hepatitis B from one individual to another. Transmission of infection may result from accidental inoculation of minute amounts of blood or fluid containing HBV during medical, surgical or dental procedures.

Needle stick injuries, use of contaminated needles and syringes, intravenous and percutaneous drug abuse, ear and nose piercing, tattooing, acupuncture, sharing of shaving razor and kissing can transmit HBV infection. HBsAg has been demonstrated in several species of mosquitoes and bedbugs, but transmission of infection by arthropods has not been authenticated. Professionals occupationally at risk include dentists, surgeons, pathologists, mortuary attendants and technicians working in serology, haematology, blood bank, biochemistry, micro-biology and haemodialysis units.

2. Perinatal transmission

HBV can be transmitted from carrier mothers to their babies during the perinatal period. Transmission probably occurs when maternal blood contaminates the mucous membranes of the newborn during birth. Infection may also result from **haematogenous transplacental transmission, breast-feeding and close postnatal contact** between infant and the infected parent.

3. Sexual transmission

Since HBV is present in semen and vaginal secretions, therefore, it can be transmitted by sexual contact. Sexually promiscuous individuals particularly male homosexuals are at very high risk. Most of the HBV infections are subclinical, particularly in childhood.

The course of acute HBV infection can be divided into three phases – preicteric, icteric and convalescent.

1. Preicteric (prodromal) phase

After an **incubation period** of 6 weeks to 6 months patient develops malaise, anorexia, weakness, myalgia, nausea, vomiting and pain in the right upper abdominal quadrant. A minority of patients develop arthralgia, urticarial or maculopapular rash, poly-arteritis nodosa and glomerulonephritis. These features may be related to circulating immune complexes.

2. Icteric phase

Two days to two weeks following the initial symptoms patient develops jaundice, pale stools and dark urine (bilirubinuria). Hepatocellular damage is detectable biochemically before the onset of jaundice and persists after it has resolved.

3. Convalescent phase

This phase is long and drawn out with malaise and fatigue lasting for several weeks. The duration of uncomplicated hepatitis is rarely more than 8–10 weeks, but mild symptoms may persist for more than one year.

HBV infection occurs virtually in every country of the world. **The carrier rate in India is estimated to be 5%.** Mild cases that do not result in jaundice are termed anicteric. Less than 1% of the icteric cases die of fulminant hepatitis, 90–95% recover with complete regeneration of the damaged liver within 2–3 months. The remaining patients progress to **chronic active hepatitis, cirrhosis and hepato-cellular carcinoma.** Hepatoma cells often contain HBV DNA, but the patient is usually negative for HBcAg and other indications of ongoing viral replication. Integration of HBV DNA fragments into the hepatocyte genome is a frequent event during HBV infection.

Hepatitis B and dentistry

A number of health care workers, including dental surgeons have been infected with HBV in clinical settings. In dentistry the risk of infection is greater among oral surgeons and periodontists than among general dental practitioners. The number of health care workers contracting infection reported since the introduction of the vaccine programme in 1987, especially in dentistry, has been small. However, there is an ever-present danger of hepatitis B trans-mission in dentistry if dental personnel are not vaccinated, or are vaccinated but with inadequate seroconversion.

Although the usual mode of transmission of hepatitis B is from the patient to the dentist, there are recorded outbreaks where dentists have transmitted the disease to the patient. Intraorally, the greatest concentration of HBV is at the gingival sulcus as a result of the continuous serum exudate, which is small in healthy people but greatly increased in diseased states, e.g., periodontitis.

Hepatitis B carriers

About 5–10% of HBV infections result in chronic carrier state. The latter may be defined as **persistence**

of HBsAg in the circulation for more than six months. Carriers are of two types:

1. *Super carriers:*
   They have HBeAg, high titres of HBsAg and DNA polymerase in their blood. HBV may also be demonstrable in their blood. Very minute amount of serum or blood from such carriers can transmit the infection.

2. *Simple carriers:*
   These are more common types of carriers who have low level of HBsAg, and no HBeAg, HBV and DNA polymerase in the blood. They transmit the infection only when large volumes of blood are transferred as in blood transfusion.

Laboratory diagnosis

Biochemical tests

Levels of serum transaminases (aminotransferases) are increased 5- to 100-fold. Both alanine amino-transferase and aspartate aminotransferase rise together late in the incubation period. Peak level is obtained about the time jaundice appears and reverts to normal in next 2 months. Serum bilirubin levels may rise up to 25-fold.

Detection of viral markers

Specific diagnosis of hepatitis B can be carried out by serological demonstration of viral markers (Table 31.2).

- **HBsAg** is the first marker to appear in blood after infection. It is detectable in blood even before elevation of transaminases and onset of clinical illness. Peak levels of HBsAg are seen in the preicteric phase of disease. It remains in circulation throughout the icteric or symptomatic course of the disease. It disappears with recovery from clinical disease in most patients, but may sometimes last for six months and even beyond. Antibody to HBsAg (anti-HBs) appears after disappearance of HBsAg and persists for very long periods. Anti-HBs is the protective antibody.

- **HBcAg** is not demonstrable in the serum because it is enclosed within the HBsAg coat. Anti-HBc antibody appears in serum a week or two after the appearance of HBsAg. It is the earliest antibody to appear in the blood. It persists lifelong, therefore, it serves as a useful indicator of prior infection with HBV, even after all viral markers become undetectable. Initially anti-HBc is predominantly IgM but after about six months, it is mainly IgG. Therefore, selective tests for IgM or IgG anti-HBc enable distinction between recent or remote infection respectively.

- **HBeAg** appears in blood along with HBsAg or soon afterwards. Circulating HBeAg is an indicator of active intrahepatic viral replication. **The presence in blood of DNA polymerase, HBV DNA and virions indicates high infectivity.** The disappearance of HBeAg coincides with the fall of transaminase levels in blood. It is followed by the appearance of anti-HBe.

- **Viral DNA polymerase** appears transiently during preicteric phase.

Table 31.2. Serological markers of hepatitis B infection

Clinical condition	Serological marker						
	HBsAg	HBeAg	Anti-HBs	Anti-HBe	Anti-HBc IgM	Anti-HBc IgG	HBV DNA
Incubation period	+	+	−	−	−	−	+
Acute hepatitis	+	+	−	−	+	+	+
Chronic active hepatitis	+	+	−	−	+	+	+
Asymptomatic carrier state	+	−	−	+	−	+	−
Past infection	−	−	+	−	−	+	−
Immunization without infection	−	−	+	−	−	−	−

Prophylaxis

Measures for the control of HBV infection are the same as those for HIV infection, i.e., screening of blood donors, use of sterile disposable syringes and needles by the medical personnel and parenteral drug users, reduction of the number of sexual partners, the use of condoms, etc. Medical personnel should wear gloves, gowns, masks and eye glasses to prevent exposure to blood and body fluids, avoidance of mouth-pipetting, eating or smoking in the place of work and proper hand washing after work. Blood spills should be cleaned up with 2% glutaraldehyde or 0.5% sodium hypochlorite. Disposable equipment should be incinerated and other equipment should be properly sterilized.

Passive immunization

Hepatitis B immune globulin (HBIG) is prepared from donors with high titres of anti-HBs. It can be given in the doses of 300–500 IU intramuscularly after accidental exposure, as may occur by needle stick injury or by splashing of blood from an HBsAg-positive patient. HBIG should be administered as early as possible after exposure and preferably within 48 hours. A second dose is usually given 4 weeks after the first. Passive immunization is also effective in reducing the risk of the carrier state in babies born to infectious mothers. HBIG must be given as early as possible but not later than 12 hours after birth. When this is repeated at monthly intervals for up to six months, the proportion of babies who become carriers can be reduced by about 70%.

Active immunization

Immunization against HBV is required for high risk individuals like:

- Health care personnel especially those in direct contact with blood and sharp instruments.
- Patients and health care personnel of institutions for the mentally retarded.
- Patients requiring repeated transfusion of blood and blood products.
- Patients on maintenance dialysis.
- Patients receiving prolonged inpatient treatment.
- Patients who require frequent tissue penetration.
- Parenteral drug users.
- Sexually promiscuous individuals and prostitutes.
- Spouses of those known to be infected with HBV.

Vaccines

Following vaccines are available:

1. **Plasma-derived hepatitis B vaccine:** It consists of purified 22 nm particles of HBsAg, prepared from the plasma of symptomless carriers. The particles are separated by ultracentrifugation and treated with proteinase, 8M urea and formaldehyde. The product is immunogenic, but becomes unacceptable because its source is human plasma, limited in availability and not totally free from possible risk of unknown pathogens.

2. **Recombinant yeast hepatitis B vaccine:** It is currently preferred vaccine. It is produced by cloning the *S* gene of HBV in yeasts *Saccharomyces cerevisae* and the HBsAg particles produced are extracted and purified for use as vaccine. This vaccine is safe, antigenic, free from side effects and as immunogenic as plasma-derived vaccine. It is adsorbed with aluminium hydroxide as adjuvant, stored in cold but not frozen and are injected intramuscularly into the **deltoid region** in a course of three doses given at 0, 1 and 6 months. Care should be taken to avoid injection into fat as this may produce poorer seroconversion rates.

3. **Recombinant chinese hamster ovary (CHO) cell hepatitis vaccine:** Expression system of CHO cells has been successfully used and the product is commercially available. This is the first vaccine using mammalian cell expression system.

4. **Synthetic peptide vaccines:** As the name indicates these are chemically synthesized polypeptide vaccines. These are safe and cheap. These are still under experimental stage.

Combined immunization

Greater protection is provided by combined passive and active immunization in postexposure prophylaxis. It is advisable to give the injections into different sites. Babies also respond to vaccine. The protective efficacy of the combined treatment is 90%.

HEPATITIS C VIRUS (HCV)

A virus of growing importance, hepatitis C virus (HCV), belongs to the genus *Hepacivirus* in the family *Flaviviridae*. The HCV viral particle is 50–60 nm in diameter and consists of an envelope derived from host membrane into which are inserted the virally encoded glycoproteins (E1 and E2) surrounding a nucleocapsid and a positive sense, single-stranded RNA genome of about 9,500 nucleotides.

The virus shows extensive genome heterogeneity and has been classified into six genotypes or clades (1–6) and more than 80 subtypes. Genotype 1 is the main HCV genotype prevalent worldwide and accounts for 40–80% of all isolates. Genotypes 2 and 3 are also found globally but to a lesser extent. HCV can be inactivated by exposure to chloroform, ether and other organic solvents and by detergents.

Cultivation

HCV has not been grown in culture, but has been cloned in *Escherichia coli*.

Pathogenesis

HCV transmission occurs by needle stick injuries or cuts with sharps, use of contaminated needles and syringes, transfusion of unscreened blood and sexual intercourse. HCV can be transmitted in utero, during parturition and by breast milk. Transmission by saliva and tears cannot be excluded. HCV transmission from a conjunctival blood splash has also been reported.

Incubation period of hepatitis C averages 6–8 weeks though it may range up to several months. About 75% infections are subclinical. The danger from hepatitis C is not the acute disease but the persistence of infection. As compared to hepatitis B, clinical infection with hepatitis C is generally less severe, has shorter preicteric period, milder symptoms, absent or less marked jaundice, somewhat lower serum alanine aminotransferase (ALT) levels and the case-fatality rate from fulminant hepatitis is 1% or less.

However, 85% or more of the acute HCV infections become chronic. The affected individuals have persistence of the virus in their blood, elevated ALT levels for at least a year or two or more and they are at risk, just as in hepatitis B, of developing **cirrhosis** and **hepatocellular carcinoma**.

Hepatitis C and dentistry

Oral manifestations of HCV infection include lichen planus, oral malignancy and salivary gland disease. Needle stick injuries are the most common way in which HCV is transmitted in clinical settings. The risk of HCV infection after a needle stick injury with HCV-contaminated blood may be 3–10% (approximately 10 times greater than for HIV).

Laboratory diagnosis

Diagnosis of HCV infection can be established by:
- detection of anti-HCV by ELISA,
- viral genome by PCR, and immunofluorescence, and
- in situ hybridization on biopsy and autopsy specimens.

In acute hepatitis C, there is peak increase in serum ALT and presence of antibody to HCV. In 30–40% of the patients, anti-HCV is not detectable until 2–8 weeks after onset of symptoms. However, HCV RNA is detectable during early acute phase. Chronic hepatitis C is characterized when anti-HCV is present and serum ALT levels remain elevated for more than 6 months. Antibodies to various HCV antigens are nearly universally present in patients who are chronically infected with HCV. Testing for HCV RNA by PCR confirms the diagnosis and documents that viraemia is present.

Prophylaxis

HCV infection can be prevented by screening of blood donors, avoidance of use of unsterile needles for intravenous drug abuse, tattooing and for medical and dental procedures. Many of the public health measures adopted to prevent transmission of human immunodeficiency virus and HBV by parenteral routes will assist efforts at controlling HCV.

HEPATITIS D VIRUS (HDV)

The HDV is a defective satellite virus requiring HBV as helper virus. It is spherical, 36–38 nm in diameter with HBsAg coat and HDAg nucleoprotein (Fig. 31.2). The genome consists of a single small circular molecule of minus sense RNA of 1.7 kilobase pairs (Table 31.1). It encodes its own nucleoprotein, the delta antigen or HDAg, but the outer capsid (HBsAg) of HDV virion is encoded by the genome of HBV coinfecting the same cell. Replication of HDV requires the concomitant expression of HBV gene products, therefore, HBV is necessary for the production of HDV virions. It belongs to the genus *Deltavirus*.

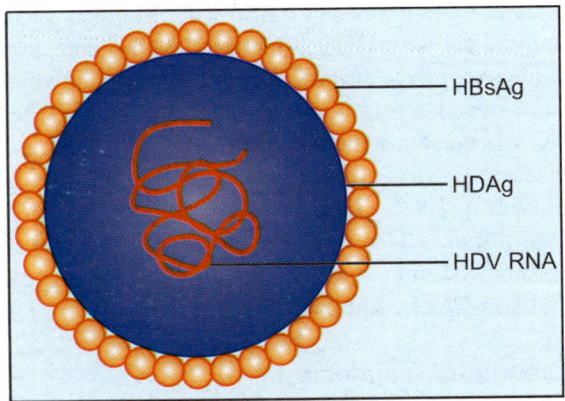

Fig. 31.2. Hepatitis D virus.

Pathogenesis

HDV is transmitted principally by blood and blood products, but also by sexual contact. Vertical transmission is also possible (Table 31.1). Two types of HDV infections are possible:

1. **Simultaneous coinfection with HBV and HDV in the same inoculum.** It most commonly results from parenteral transmission, for example, in intravenous drug users. The clinical and biochemical features of such infection resemble those of acute hepatitis B alone. However, coinfection with HBV and HDV may be more severe than the disease caused by HBV alone.
2. **Superinfection of an HBsAg carrier by HDV.** It is commoner and more serious because a large number of hepatocytes are already producing HBsAg, and HDV can replicate without delay with a relatively short incubation period. It leads to severe liver damage, fulminant HBsAg-positive hepatitis and elevated mortality (up to 20%).

In simultaneous acute HBV and HDV infections, IgM anti-HBc will be detectable, while in acute HDV infection superimposed on chronic HBV infections, anti-HBc will be of IgG class.

Hepatitis D and dentistry

There is at least one report of HDV transmission in dentistry in the USA, where up to 700 cases were recorded. At least four dentists were infected.

Laboratory diagnosis

The delta antigen is primarily expressed in liver cell nuclei where it can be demonstrated by immunofluorescence. In patients with HBV-HDV coinfection, shortly before the end of incubation period, HBsAg appears in the serum and towards the end of incubation period HDAg appears which can be detected by **ELISA** or **immunoblotting** and HDV RNA can be detected by **hybridization to a radiolabelled RNA probe**. Two or three weeks after infection, anti-HD IgM appears followed by anti-HD IgG. However, in chronic infection, the IgM antibody persists for years. It can be detected by **ELISA**.

Prophylaxis

HDV infection can be prevented by prevention of coinfection with HBV or of superinfection of HBV carriers and hence requires all the measures that apply to the prevention of HBV infection, including vaccination against HBV. HBV vaccine is effective, as HDV cannot infect persons immune to HBV.

HEPATITIS E VIRUS (HEV)

Hepatitis E virus belongs to the family *Caliciviridae*.

Morphology

Virions of HEV are spherical, nonenveloped and 27–38 nm in diameter. They possess single-stranded positive sense RNA genome of 7.6 kb which is surrounded by icosahedral capsid with characteristic surface depressions.

Pathogenesis

Infection is acquired by ingestion of faecally contaminated drinking water (**faecal-oral route**).

Incubation period of hepatitis E ranges from 2–8 weeks, with an average of 5–6 weeks. It occurs predominantly in the 15–40 years age group. Clinically, the disease closely resembles that of hepatitis A. However, bilirubin levels tend to be higher and jaundice deeper and more prolonged. The case-fatality rate is 0.5–3% but in infected pregnant women it varies from 10–20%. **Like hepatitis A, hepatitis E does not progress to chronic hepatitis, cirrhosis, cancer or carrier state.**

Hepatitis E and dentistry

Due to its mode of transmission, HEV does not pose a major risk of cross-infection in dentistry.

Laboratory diagnosis

1. **Exclusion of hepatitis A** by IgM serology and hepatitis B by absence of HBsAg and IgM anti-HBc.
2. **Immunoelectron microscopic examination** of patient faeces for aggregated calicivirus-like particles using monoclonal antibodies.
3. **ELISA** tests for IgM and IgG anti-HEV.
4. A **Western blot assay** for IgM and/or IgG anti-HEV.
5. **Polymerase chain reaction (PCR) assay** for the detection of HEV RNA (as cDNA) in patient faeces or in acute-phase sera.

Prophylaxis

Hepatitis E can be prevented by improved standards of sanitation and provision of chlorinated water throughout the developing world. During the epidemic, take boiled water and only cooked food. No vaccine or effective antiviral drugs exist.

HEPATITIS G VIRUS (HGV)

Hepatitis G virus (HGV) was first isolated from a patient with chronic hepatitis in 1996. Along with HCV it has been placed in family *Flaviviridae* genus *Hepacivirus*. The genome of HGV consists of 9.4 kb molecule of ssRNA of positive polarity. Its structure resembles that of HCV, but it has <25% homology with HCV. HGV replicates in peripheral blood cells, however, its replication in the liver is not known. The virus is transmitted parenterally (exposure to blood through transfusions, haemodialysis, or sharing equipment in injecting drug use), sexually, and from mother to child (Table 31.1). More than 30% of transfusion recipients and up to 80% of injecting drug users are HGV marker positive. HGV and human immunodeficiency virus (HIV) share same infection routes, and a significant proportion of HIV-infected subjects are HGV-coinfected.

The virus is present worldwide. Majority of the individuals with HGV infection have no detectable evidence of liver disease. There have been, however, cases of acute, fulminant and chronic hepatitis where HGV is presently the only explanation for their liver disease. There is no evidence of a causal relationship between HGV infection and hepatocellular carcinoma. HGV infection results frequently in chronic viraemia. It often subsides after several years and anti-HGenv antibody develops.

Laboratory diagnosis

HGV infection is mainly detected by reverse transcriptase polymerase chain reaction (RT-PCR). Recently, an immunoassay has been developed to detect anti-HGenv. Serum HGV RNA indicates viraemia, whereas anti-HGenv is associated with recovery. These can be found respectively in <2% and 9% of healthy blood donors. Prevalence increases in association with HCV or HBV infection.

Prophylaxis

HGV infection can be prevented by employing the same measures as for HBV, HCV and HIV.

Hepatitis G and dentistry

HGV RNA is present in whole saliva of infected individuals, but transmission through this route has not been determined. No data is available on the transmission of hepatitis G or the rate of HGV carriage in dental staff. No vaccine is available; implementation of universal infection control measures should be adequate to prevent transmission of this virus in dentistry.

KEY FACTS

- Viruses are by far the most important agents of hepatitis, and include hepatitis A, B, C, D, E and G. These **hepatotropic viruses** are classified into two groups depending on the route of transmission – the **faecal-oral route:** hepatitis A and hepatitis E (highly unlikely to be transmitted in dentistry); and the **parenteral route:** hepatitis B, C and D, and possibly hepatitis G (could be transmitted in dentistry)
- HAV is the only one of the human hepatitis viruses that can be cultivated in cell cultures
- Hepatitis A infection does not produce extrahepatic manifestations, no carrier state and is not associated with cirrhosis or hepatocellular carcinoma
- Hepatitis B is DNA virus while all other hepatitis viruses are RNA viruses
- The various types of viral hepatitis differ in severity of infection, morbidity, mortality rate, presence or absence of a carrier state, and frequency of long-term sequelae such as cirrhosis and cancer
- *Hepatitis A vaccine is safe and effective, and recommended for professionals working with institutionalized patients*
- **HBV** is transmitted by parenteral, perinatal and sexual routes
- *HBV vaccine is safe, effective and relatively long-lasting, and also protects against hepatitis D infection*
- *The number of dental care workers contracting hepatitis B since the introduction of the vaccine programme has been small, but there is ever-present danger of HBV transmission if personnel are not vaccinated or vaccinees do not seroconvert (up to 5%). Hence antibody levels should be ascertained after a vaccine course*

- *Intraorally, the greatest concentration of HBV is at the gingival sulcus as a result of the continuous serum exudate, which is small in health but greatly increased in diseased state*
- *Possible oral manifestations of* **HCV infection** *include* **lichen planus**, **oral malignancy** *and* **salivary gland disease**
- *Saliva of up to 50% of patients with acute and chronic hepatitis C infection may contain HCV RNA*
- *The risk of infection after a needle stick injury with HCV-contaminated blood may be 3–10% (compare 0.5 to 1.0% for HIV)*
- *The transmission and epidemiology of HDV infection are similar to HBV, and the virus is a major problem, especially in injecting drug users*
- **Hepatitis E virus** is transmitted by faecal-oral route, the main agent is contaminated drinking water
- Hepatitis G virus is present in saliva of infected individuals, common among injecting drug users and haemophilic patients; disease association has yet to be defined

IMPORTANT QUESTIONS

1. Discuss in detail hepatitis viruses and dentistry.
2. Write short notes on:
    - (a) Hepatitis A virus
    - (b) Hepatitis B virus
    - (c) Hepatitis C virus
    - (d) Hepatitis D virus
    - (e) Hepatitis E virus
    - (f) Hepatitis G virus

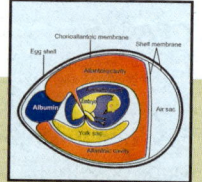

Chapter 32

Bacteriophage

Bacteriophages or simply phages are viruses that infect bacteria. Twort (1915) described an infectious agent that distorted the appearance of staphylococcal colonies and d'Herelle (1917) added filtrates of stools to young broth cultures of *Shigella* and after overnight incubation, some of the cultures were found to be clear and sterile. He suggested that the lytic agent was a virus and gave it the name bacteriophage (*phage*: to eat). Phages can readily be isolated from a wide range of environments such as sewage, soil and other natural sources of mixed bacterial growth.

Morphology

Bacteriophages that infect *Escherichia coli*, called T-even phages (T2, T4, T6), have been studied in great detail. They serve as the prototypes in describing the properties of bacteriophages. They are tadpole-shaped with a hexagonal head and a cylindrical tail.

Head: It consists of a tightly packed core of nucleic acid (double-stranded DNA) surrounded by a protein coat or capsid. The size of the head varies from 28–100 nm.

Tail: It consists of a long hollow core surrounded by a contractile sheath and a terminal base plate.

Attached to the base plate of the tail are six tail fibres and six tail pins. The virus uses the tail fibres

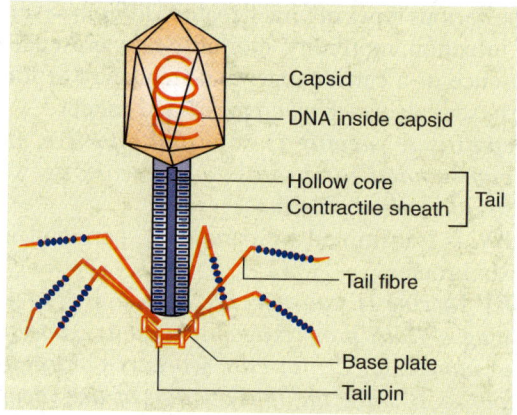

Fig. 32.1. Morphology of T4 phage particle.

to find a bacterium to infect and the tail pins on the base plate anchor the virus to the host-cell during infection. In contrast, phages T1, T5 and lambda of *E. coli* do not possess a contractile sheath and the tails of phages T3 and T7 of *E. coli* and P22 of *Salmonella* are short and non-contractile. Most of the phages possess double-stranded DNA, but single-stranded RNA or DNA and double-stranded RNA is present in some other phages.

Life cycle

Phages exhibit two different types of life cycle. In virulent or lytic cycle, there is intracellular multiplication of phages followed by lysis and release of progeny virions. In temperate or lysogenic cycle, the phage DNA either becomes integrated with the bacterial genome or exists as a free plasmid in the bacterial cell, replicating synchronously with it, causing no harm to the host cell.

1. Lytic cycle

The events between infection of a cell by a phage and its subsequent lysis to release daughter phage particles are similar for most phages. The lytic cycle of T-even phages is described below.

1. Adsorption

With the help of tail fibres and tail pins phage particles attach to virus-specific receptors on the host cell. Adsorption is a specific process and depends on the presence of complementary chemical groups on the receptor sites on the bacterial surface and on the terminal base plate of the phage. Infection cannot occur in the absence of adsorption. Therefore, most phages are highly specific for a limited number of bacterial hosts and this constitutes the basis of bacteriophage typing of bacteria.

2. Penetration

Following adsorption, six tail pins make contact with the host cell surface and firmly attach the phage plate to it. The contractile tail sheath then contracts forcing the hollow interior tail tube about 12 nm into the bacterial cell wall. The phage DNA then passes through the hollow interior tail tube. Penetration may be facilitated by the presence on the phage tail of lysozyme which produces a hole on the bacterial cell wall for the entry of phage core. After penetration, phages leave their empty capsids and tails outside the bacteria.

When bacteria are mixed with very large number of phages per bacterial cell, multiple holes are produced on the cell with consequent leakage of the cell contents. Bacterial lysis occurs without viral multiplication. This is known as **lysis from without**.

3. Synthesis

Immediately after penetration of the phage nucleic acid, synthesis of phage components is initiated. The first products to be synthesized are **early proteins**.

These are enzymes necessary for synthesis of phage components. Subsequently, **late proteins** appear, which are the protein subunits of the phage head and tail. During this period the synthesis of bacterial protein, DNA and RNA ceases.

4. Maturation

Phage DNA, head protein and tail protein are synthesized separately in the bacterial cell. The DNA is condensed into a compact polyhedron and **packaged** into the head and, finally, the tail structures are added. The assembly of phage components into the mature infective phage particles is known as maturation.

5. Release

The release of mature progeny phage particles occurs by a lysis of the bacterial cell. During replication of the phage, the bacterial cell wall is weakened and assumes a spherical shape. Phage enzymes act on the weakened cell wall causing it to burst or lyse, resulting in the release of mature daughter phages.

Eclipse phase: The interval between the entry of the phage nucleic acid into the bacterial cell and the appearance of the first infectious intracellular phage particles is known as the eclipse phase. It represents the time required for the synthesis of the phage components and their assembly into mature phage particles. The duration of eclipse phase is 15–30 minutes.

Latent period: The interval between the infection of a bacterial cell and the first release of infectious phage particles is known as latent phase.

2. Lysogenic cycle

Not all phage infections result in immediate progeny production and lysis of the host cell. There are many phages that, upon entering a sensitive cell, either undergo a lytic cycle like that described above or alternatively enter into a benign relationship with their hosts, called **lysogeny.** The phages that can develop both lytically and lysogenically are said to be **temperate phages.** In lysogenic state, the viral genome exists either inserted into the host chromosome or as a free plasmid in the bacterial cell. The phage genome in this state is known as **prophage**. It replicates along with the bacterial chromosome whether it is integrated or in plasmid form. A bacterium that carries a prophage is known as a **lysogenic bacterium** or **lysogen**.

The prophage confers certain new properties on the lysogenic bacterium. This is known as **lysogenic or phage conversion**. Following are the examples of lysogenic conversion:

Toxin production in *Corynebacterium diphtheriae* is determined by the presence in it of the prophage β. The elimination of this prophage abolishes the toxigenicity of the bacillus and nontoxigenic strains can be made toxigenic by lysogenization.

Clostridium botulinum types C and D produce toxin only if these are infected with phage CE β and DE β respectively.

A wide variety of temperate phages of *Salmonella* can **modify the antigenic properties** of somatic O antigen. The antigenic formula of *S.* Anatum is 3, 10: e, h: 1, 6 but when it is lysogenised by a temperate phage its antigenic formula becomes 3, 15: e, h: 1, 6 (*S.* Newington).

Occasionally, integrated prophage is excised from bacterial DNA, and phage multiplication and subsequent cell lysis ensues. This is known as **spontaneous induction of prophage**. It is a rare event but all lysogenic bacteria can be induced to shift to the lytic cycle by certain physical (UV rays) and chemical (nitrogen mustard) agents. A lysogenic bacterium is resistant to reinfection by the same or related phages. This is known as **superinfection immunity.**

Bacteriophages may act as **carriers of genes** from one bacterium to another. This is known as **transduction.** It has been discussed in the chapter on bacterial genetics and drug resistance.

Phage typing

The limited host range of many phages enables them to be used as an epidemiological marker to discriminate between bacterial strains that are biochemically or serologically indistinguishable. This method has been used to trace outbreaks of infection caused by *Staphylococcus aureus*, *S.* Typhi and *Vibrio*

cholerae. The strain to be typed is inoculated on a plate of nutrient agar to produce a lawn culture. After drying, the phages are applied over marked squares in a fixed dose (**routine test dose**). Routine test dose is the highest dilution of the phage preparation that produces confluent lysis. After overnight incubation, the culture will be observed to be lysed by some phages but not by others. The phage type of the strain is expressed by the designation of the phage/phages that lyse it. For example, if a strain of *S. aureus* is lysed by phages 50, 52A and 80, then the phage type is expressed as 50/52A/80.

Phage assay

When a phage is applied on the lawn culture of a susceptible bacterium, areas of clearing or lysis occur after incubation. Area of lysis caused by phage is known as **plaque**. Since a single phage particle is capable of producing one plaque, **plaque assay** can be employed for titrating the number of viable phages in a preparation.

KEY FACTS

- *Bacteriophages* are viruses that **infect bacteria**
- Bacteriophages play an important role in the transmission of *genetic information* from one bacterium to another by the process of *transduction*
- The phage genome may get integrated into the bacterial chromosome thus conferring, on the bacterium certain additional properties. This is known on **phage conversion**
- **Toxin production** in *Corynebacterium diphtheriae*, group A *Streptococcus* (erythrogenic toxin) and *Clostridium botulinum* types C and D is determined by bacteriophages
- The limited host range of many bacteriophages enables them to be used as an epidemiological marker (**phage type**)

IMPORTANT QUESTION

Write short notes on:
(a) Phage typing
(b) Lysogenic cycle of phages
(c) Lysogenic conversion

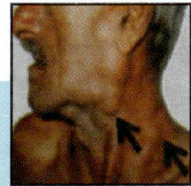

Chapter 33

Brief Introduction, Candidiasis and Systemic Mycoses Causing Oral Lesions

Fungi (singular, fungus) are a group of eukaryotic organisms which multiply both sexually and asexually by production of spores. The word '*fungus*' is derived from Latin meaning 'mushroom', which in turn is derived from Greek word '*spongos*' meaning 'sponge' which refers to the morphology of mushrooms. The term '*mycology*' is derived from Greek word '*mykes*' (mushroom) and '*logy*' (study) which means study of fungi. **Medical mycology** is the study of morphology, pathogenesis, diagnosis and treatment of fungal infections in human beings.

Fungi are eukaryotic, which means, each cell possesses well defined nucleus with nuclear membrane, mitochondria, Golgi apparatus and endoplasmic reticulum. They can be *distinguished from other eukaryotes* by a rigid cell wall composed of chitin, β-glucans, mannan, as well as other polysaccharides, proteins and lipids. Within the cell wall, the cytoplasm is bounded by a cytoplasmic membrane in which the predominant sterol is not cholesterol, as in humans, but **ergosterol**. Fungi differ from bacteria and other prokaryotes in many ways (Table 33.1).

Fungi are ubiquitous, capable of colonizing almost any environment, and generally play an invaluable part in the decomposition and recycling of organic matter. About 1.5 million species of fungi are known. Most of them are found as saprophytes in the soil and on decaying plant material, and about 600 species are known to cause human disease.

Fungi are now considered as significant cause of morbidity and mortality as they have emerged as important etiological agents of **opportunistic infections** in immunocompromised patients, which in turn is a result of emergence of AIDS, and inadvertent use of broad-spectrum antibiotics, steroids, and immunosuppressive agents.

MORPHOLOGY OF FUNGI

Broadly, fungi are divided into two morphological forms:

- Yeasts
- Molds

Yeasts are unicellular fungi reproducing asexually by budding (blastoconidia) or by formation of transverse septum known as fission. Fungal spores germinate to produce multicellular branching filamentous structures known as hyphae. All molds are composed of branching hyphae.

Although, all fungi exist in yeast or mold form but traditionally fungi are divided into four morphological groups:

1. Yeasts: Yeasts are round, oval or elongated unicellular fungi. These organisms remain in the yeast

311

Table 33.1. Distinguishing features of fungi and bacteria

Features	Fungi (Eukaryotic)	Bacteria (Prokaryotic)
Cell wall composition	Rigid, multi-layered, chitin, β-glucans, mannan, polysaccharides, proteins, lipids	*Gram-positive:* Peptidoglycan, teichoic acid *Gram-negative:* Lipopolysaccharides, proteins, lipoprotein and peptidoglycan *Acid-fast:* Lipids, proteins, polysaccharides
Cell membrane	Ergosterol (except in *Pneumocystis*)	Phospholipids, proteins
Cytoplasmic contents	Mitochondria, Golgi apparatus, endoplasmic reticulum	Lack mitochondria, Golgi apparatus, endoplasmic reticulum
Nucleus	True nucleus with nuclear membrane, and paired chromosome	Single, circular piece of DNA present in cytoplasm attached to mesosome, no nuclear membrane and nucleolus
Replication/Reproduction	Mitosis and meiosis	Binary fission
Spores	Method of *reproduction* (sexual and asexual)	Method of *preservation*; endospores
Morphology	*Yeast:* unicellular, *Mold:* multicellular	Coccal, bacillary, filamentous and spirochaetal forms

form at both room temperature (25°C) and body temperature (37°C). Most of them reproduce by an asexual process called budding in which the cell develops a protuberance which enlarges and eventually separates from the parent cell (Fig. 33.1A). Some reproduce by fission. They form moist or mucoid colonies. *Saccharomyces cerevisae* and *Cryptococcus neoformans* are the examples of nonpathogenic and pathogenic yeasts respectively.

2. Yeast-like: In some yeasts, like *Candida*, the bud remains attached to the mother cell and elongates, followed by repeated budding forming chains of elongated cells known as pseudohyphae. *C. albicans* and *C. stellatoidea* also produce germ tubes. **Germ tubes are the beginning of true hyphae** and appear as filaments that are not constricted at their points of origin on the parent cell. **If the filaments are constricted at their points of origin on the parent cell, they are pseudohyphae, not germ tubes** (Fig. 33.1B and C).

3. Molds: In molds, spores germinate to produce branching filaments called **hyphae** (singular, hypha). They are 2–10 μm in diameter. They may be septate or aseptate (coenocytic). Cells in septate hyphae communicate with each other through pores present in the septa, whereas in aseptate hyphae, the cells communicate freely as the protoplasm of the cells is

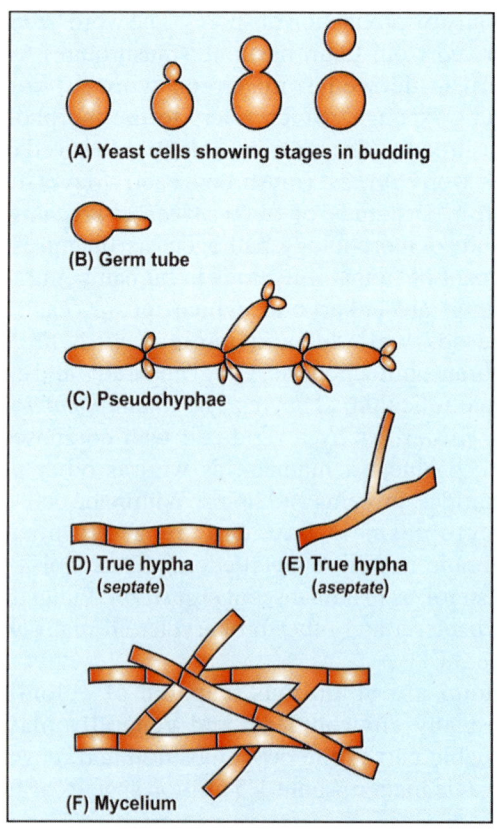

(A) Yeast cells showing stages in budding

(B) Germ tube

(C) Pseudohyphae

(D) True hypha (*septate*)

(E) True hypha (*aseptate*)

(F) Mycelium

Fig. 33.1. Basic fungal morphology.

continuous (Fig. 33.1D and E). The hyphae continue to grow (Fig. 33.1F) and branch to form tangled mass of growth called **mycelium** (plural, mycelia). In the culture medium, the part of the mycelium which projects above the surface is called **aerial mycelium** and the part growing in the medium is called **vegetative mycelium**. They reproduce by the formation of different types of sexual and asexual spores. Dermatophytes, *Aspergillus*, *Penicillium*, *Mucor* and *Rhizopus* are the examples of molds.

4. Dimorphic fungi: Many fungi pathogenic to man like *Histoplasma capsulatum*, *Sporothrix schenckii*, *Blastomyces dermatitidis*, *Coccidioides immitis*, *Paracoccidioides brasiliensis*, and *Penicillium marneffei* have a yeast form in the host tissue and *in vitro* at 37°C on enriched media, and hyphal (mycelial) form *in vitro* at 25°C.

If a single mycelium is capable of reproducing sexually, it is known as **homothallic**, *and if two mycelia are required to reproduce sexually, they are known as* **heterothallic** *fungi.*

CLASSIFICATION OF FUNGI

Robert H Whittaker, an American biologist, in 1969 grouped fungi in a separate kingdom in his Five-Kingdom System, i.e. Monera, Protista, Fungi, Plantae and Animalia. Kingdom Fungi includes terrestrial organisms like molds, yeasts and mushrooms, which do not have chlorophyll.

TAXONOMIC CLASSIFICATION

Fungi are divided into four classes – **Zygomycetes, Ascomycetes, Basidiomycetes** and **Deutromycetes (*Fungi Imperfecti*)**. The first three classes reproduce sexually and asexually, whereas the sexual state of Deutromycetes is not known and thus it is also known as 'Imperfect Fungi' or 'Mitosporic fungi'.

CLASSIFICATION OF MYCOSES

Infection caused by a fungus is known as **mycosis** (plural, mycoses). It can be divided into five categories:

I. **Superficial mycoses:** These are strictly surface infections involving skin, hair, nail and mucous membrane. These include:

- Infection of skin, hair and nail caused by dermatophytes.
- Infection of skin, nail and mucous membrane caused by *C. albicans*.
- Infection of skin caused by *Malassezia furfur* (pityriasis versicolor) and *Hortaea werneckii* (tinea nigra).
- Infection of hair caused by *Piedraia hortae* (black piedra) and *Trichosporon beigelii* (white piedra).

II. **Subcutaneous mycoses:** Mycoses of the skin, subcutaneous tissues and bones result from the inoculation of saprophytic fungi of the soil or decaying vegetation leading to progressive local disease with tissue destruction and sinus formation. The lesion may spread via lymphatics. These occur mainly in the tropics and subtropics. The principal subcutaneous mycoses are mycetoma, chromoblastomycosis, sporotrichosis and rhinosporidiosis.

III. **Systemic mycoses:** Systemic mycoses are caused by inhalation of airborne spores produced by the fungi which are present as saprophytes in soil and on plant material. From the lungs the fungus may disseminate to CNS, bone and other internal organs. Systemic mycoses include blastomycosis, histoplasmosis, coccidioidomycosis and paracoccidioidomycosis.

IV. **Opportunistic mycoses:** The opportunistic mycoses are infections attributable to fungi that are normally found as human commensals or in the environment. Virtually any fungus can serve as an opportunistic pathogen, and the list of those identified as such becomes longer each year. The most common opportunistic mycoses include aspergillosis, penicilliosis, mucormycosis, candidiasis, cryptococcosis and pneumocytosis.

V. **Miscellaneous mycoses:** These include penicilliosis, otomycosis and keratomycosis.

RHINOSPORIDIOSIS

Rhinosporidiosis is a chronic granulomatous disease characterized by the development of large polyps or wart-like lesions in the nose, conjunctiva and occasionally in ears, larynx, bronchus, penile urethra, vagina, rectum and skin. More than 90% of cases have been reported from India, Sri Lanka and South

America. In India, sporadic cases occur all over but endemic foci exist in parts of Orissa, Andhra Pradesh, Kerala, Chennai and Raipur (Chhattisgarh). Very rarely, there is haematogenous spread with metastatic lesions in the lungs, brain and bones.

It was thought to be caused by a fungus, *Rhinosporidium seeberi*, but all attempts at isolation from clinical material failed. On the basis of modern molecular based studies, it is now considered to be a **hydrophilic protistan**, hence called pseudofungal organism. It has not been cultured and animal inoculation is also not successful. Nothing definite is known about the mode of transmission of infection. However, it has been suggested that the organism is transmitted in dust or water. It is believed that fish may be the natural hosts of *R. seeberi*. Infection is more common in:

- persons bathing in muddy stagnant pools of water;
- those who dive into streams to collect sand from riverbeds;
- paddy cultivators; and
- in dry areas, after dust storm and eye injuries.

Pathogenesis

Rhinosporidiosis in upper respiratory sites is thought to be initiated by the implantation of endoconidia from the aquatic habitat into the respiratory mucosa, added by abrasions caused, for instance, by sand particles in river sand workers who dive into the water or by vigorous cleaning of the anterior nares with the fingers. Autoinoculation of the mucosa by endoconidia released from sporangia or after surgery may lead to satellite polyps in the adjacent regions. Polyps on the skin may result from implantation of endoconidia by scratching with contaminated fingers or through haematogenous dissemination from respiratory sites.

R. seeberi, as in the other mesomycetozoans, develops sporangia (cysts) with endoconidia. The endoconidia are subsequently released from mature sporangia in the infected host tissues and to the environment. Susceptible hosts may then acquire the infection after traumatic implantation of the resistant conidia. However, experimental infection in animals has so far been unsuccessful.

Laboratory diagnosis

Laboratory diagnosis depends on the histological examination of the lesion. *R. seeberi* can be identified in haematoxylin and eosin stained sections, but sometimes one may need special stains such as Gomori methenamine silver stain and periodic acid-Schiff stain to demonstrate the fungus. Surface epithelium is hyperplastic and beneath it is chronic inflammatory exudate. The epidermis and the stroma are riddled with sporangia (singular sporangium) 100–500 μm in diameter. These can be seen with the naked eye as small white dots. The sporangium contains hundreds of endoconidia 5–20 μm in diameter (Fig. 33.2). It develops a pore in its wall and ruptures at that site to scatter endoconidia into the stroma. New sporangia develop from these endoconidia.

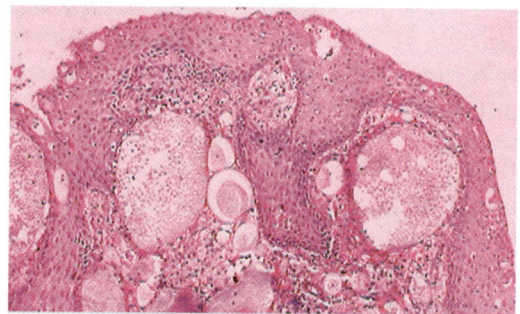

Fig. 33.2. Rhinosporidiosis showing sporangia and endoconidia.

Oral manifestations

Oronasopharyngeal lesions are often accompanied by a mucoid discharge and appear as soft red polypoid growth of a tumour-like nature which spread to pharynx and larynx. The lesions are vascular and bleed readily.

SPOROTRICHOSIS

Sporotrichosis is a chronic pyogenic granulomatous infection of the skin and subcutaneous tissues, although it may become disseminated by lymphatic spread. It is caused by *Sporothrix schenckii*, a dimorphic fungus. It occurs all over the world. The fungus is found in soil, decaying wood, thorns and on infected animals, including horses, cats, rats and dogs. The infection is due to the implantation of conidia through injured skin. It is more common in farmers and gardeners.

The initial lesion is a small ulcerated nodule commonly on the hand or the forearm. Nodules and abscesses occur along the draining lymphatics and the regional lymph nodes enlarge, suppurate and ulcerate. The primary lesion may remain localized or disseminate to involve the bones, joints, lungs and rarely CNS particularly in debilitated or immuno-suppressed individuals.

Laboratory diagnosis

In infected tissues, *S. schenckii* appears in the form of round, oval (4–6 µm) or elongated or cigar-shaped yeast-like cells with irregular budding (Fig. 33.3A). With ordinary stains, they are difficult to find. The use of PAS or methenamine silver stain and fluorescent antibody technique facilitates detection of these organisms.

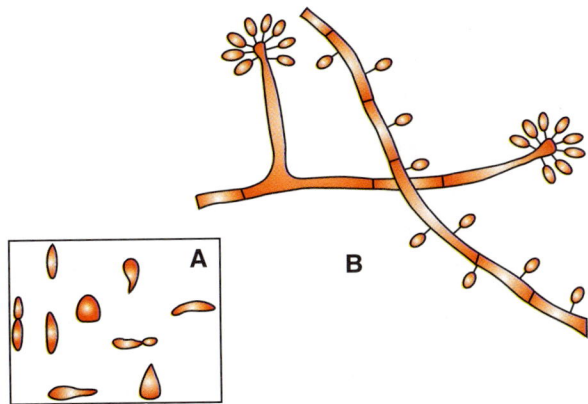

Fig. 33.3. Microscopic appearance of *Sporothrix schenckii* in the infected tissue (A) and in culture on Sabouraud dextrose agar at 25–30°C (B).

The abscesses may show the **asteroid body** (Fig. 33.4). This consists of central budding yeast cell with eosinophilic material radiating from it. In most human lesions very few yeast-like organisms can be seen. However, their number can be increased by inoculating pus from human sporotrichosis into an experimental animal such as mouse or rat.

The diagnosis is confirmed by isolation of the causative organism by culture of swabs from the

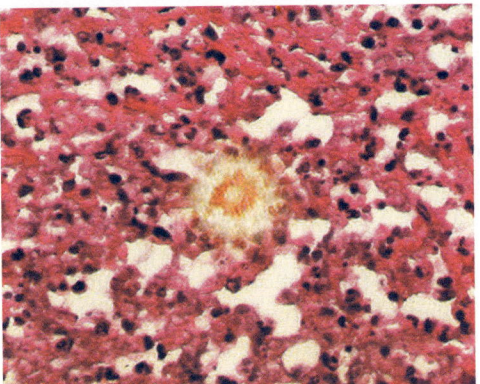

Fig. 33.4. Asteroid body with foreign body tissue reaction.

ulcerated lesions or pus aspirated from subcutaneous nodules or biopsy material. *S. schenckii* grows well on routine agar media, and at room temperature (25–30°C). Colonies appear within 3–5 days. These are cream-coloured initially, smooth and moist, gradually becoming dark brown or black and filamentous in texture. Some isolates are black from the beginning. Microscopical examination reveals thin (1–2 µm in diameter), septate and branching hyphae. The apex of the conidiophore is often slightly swollen and bears many small tear-shaped or round conidia (2–3 × 3–6 µm) on delicate threadlike denticles forming a "rosette-shaped" clusters in young cultures. Conidia also form singly along the hyphae (Fig. 33.3B).

To induce mycelial to yeast conversion, the fungus is inoculated on blood agar tubes and incubated at 37°C. The formation of yeast colonies may require several subcultures. Complete conversion seldom occurs, but a portion of the colony will develop cigar-shaped yeast-like cells.

A **latex agglutination test** for detection of antibodies against *S. schenckii* is available.

A **skin test** with sporotrichin antigen is positive in all patients with cutaneous sporotrichosis.

Oral manifestations

Nonspecific ulceration of the oral, nasal and pharyngeal mucosa also occurs in this disease, usually associated with regional lymphadenopathy. Lesions heal by soft, pliable scars even though the organisms may still be present in the tissues.

HISTOPLASMOSIS

Histoplasmosis is an intracellular mycosis of reticulo-endothelial system. It is caused by a dimorphic fungus, *Histoplasma capsulatum*. It is widely distributed throughout the world, occurring in some 60 temperate and tropical countries in the Americas, Africa and Australia. In India, it has been found to be endemic in West Bengal, and *H. capsulatum* has been isolated from the soil in Gangetic plain.

H. capsulatum grows in soil with high nitrogen content. The growth of the fungus appears to be most frequently associated with soil enriched by excreta of bats, chickens and other birds. This provides high nitrogen content. The organism has been isolated from bat caves, bird roosts, chicken houses and similar environments. Bat and bird excreta provide an excellent medium for enrichment of *H. capsulatum*.

Chickens are not susceptible to disseminated, progressive histoplasmosis under natural conditions. The apparent immunity of birds to systemic histoplasmosis may be dependent directly upon their body temperature which is higher than the temperature at which the fungus can grow. Examination of autopsy and culture of many bats have demonstrated that histoplasmosis occurs in bats and the fungus is excreted in bat droppings from intestinal lesions.

Pathogenesis

In addition to humans, many animals (both wild and domestic) are susceptible to histoplasmosis. Some animals including bats, may act as vectors to disseminate the organism in nature. From the soil, the conidia of *H. capsulatum* are airborne and these are inhaled leading to infection. Outbreaks or epidemics of histoplasmosis result from simultaneous exposure of a large number of people. No direct spread from man to man or animal to man has been reported.

Histoplasmosis is ordinarily an asymptomatic or relatively mild, self-limiting pulmonary infection, although chronic or acute disseminated disease with poor prognosis may occur. In addition, it may also involve lymph nodes (Fig. 33.5), spleen, liver, adrenals, kidneys, skin, CNS and other organs of the body. Granulomatous and ulcerative lesions may

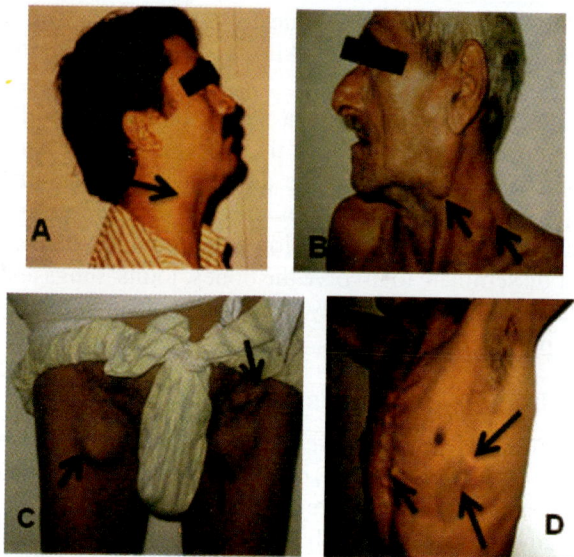

Fig. 33.5. Cervical (A and B), inguinal (C) lymphadenitis, and papulonodular skin nodules (D) caused by *H. capsulatum*.

develop on the skin and mucosa. **In addition, histo-plasmosis is an important complicating infection in patients with AIDS.**

Histopathology

In tissues, *H. capsulatum* is present inside phagocytic cells in yeast phase. They are round or oval, yeast-like cells, 2–5 μm in diameter with budding on a narrow base. All phagocytic cells of the reticulo-endothelial system are involved including those in the liver, spleen, lymph nodes and bone marrow, so that the cytoplasm is filled with masses of fungal cells. Many cells of *H. capsulatum* are also found extracellularly because of the degeneration of the phagocytic cells. With Giemsa or Wright stain, the cell wall and the cell protoplasm stain light blue and dark blue respectively. A clear space is usually seen between the protoplasmic mass and the cell wall.

With H & E staining, only a central protoplasmic mass surrounded by a halo is seen (Fig. 33.6). Only a dark staining can outline the cell wall. In the PAS stain, the wall is stained pink to purplish red with pallor coloured protoplasm filling the cell. In the Gomori methenamine silver stain the cell wall stains intense black (Fig. 33.7). The so called 'capsule'

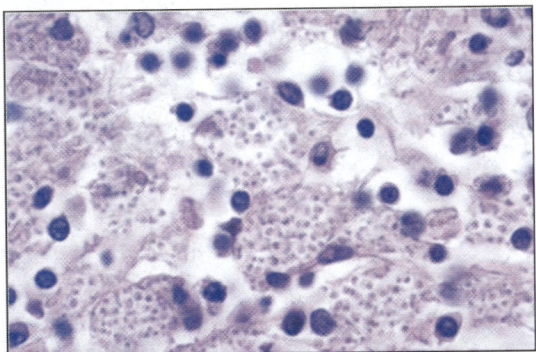

Fig. 33.6. Section of lymph node stained with haematoxylin and eosin showing *Histoplasma capsulatum* surrounded by clear halo filling the cytoplasm of phagocytes.

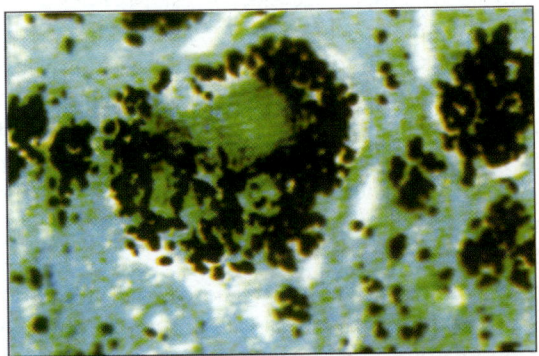

Fig. 33.7. Section similar to that demonstrated in Fig. 33.6 but stained with Gomori methanamine silver staining. It shows black budding yeast cells.

(halo) of *H. capsulatum* is considered to be an artifact resulting from the shrinkage of the protoplasm within the cell wall.

Culture

Body fluids or tissues are inoculated on Sabouraud dextrose agar and incubated at 25–30°C. Growth is slow. Mycelial forms usually mature within 15–20 days but may take up to 8 weeks. Colony is white to brown, or pinkish, with a fine, dense cottony texture. The reverse is white, sometimes yellow or orange. In young cultures, septate hyphae are seen. They bear round to pear-shaped smooth or occasionally spiny microconidia (2–5 μm in diameter). They are sessile or stalked. After several weeks, large, thick-walled, round macroconidia (8–14 μm in diameter) form.

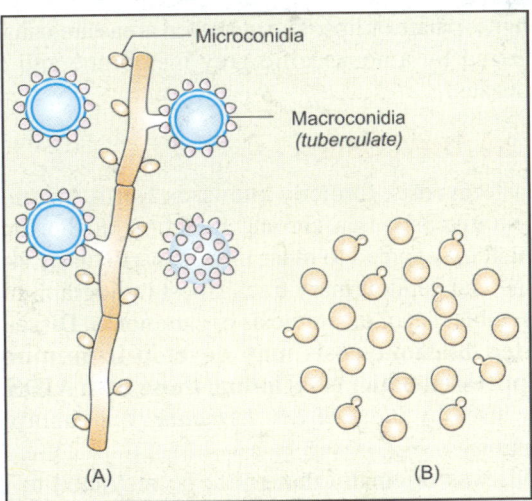

Fig. 33.8. *Histoplasma capsulatum*: (A) mycelial phase; and (B) yeast phase.

They are tuberculate, knobby, or have short cylindrical projections. Occasionally they may be smooth (Fig. 33.8).

At 35–37°C on brain-heart-infusion agar, moist, white, yeast-like colonies may eventually form. These may require many generations. Yeast phase is inhibited by cycloheximide. Microscopically, small, round or oval budding cells (2–3 × 4–5 μm) (Fig. 37.8B) and occasionally abortive hyphae may be seen.

Laboratory diagnosis

Diagnosis may be made by:

- Microscopic examination of stained smears of sputum, bone marrow, peripheral blood, scrapings from dermal or mucosal ulcers and biopsies of lymph nodes and other organs and by culture of the fungus from these materials.
- Serological tests like latex agglutination, precipitation and complement fixation become positive two weeks after infection.
- Delayed hypersensitivity to the fungus can be demonstrated by histoplasmin skin test.

Oral manifestations

The oral lesions appear as nodular, ulcerative or vegetative lesions on the buccal mucosa, gingiva, tongue, palate or lips. The ulcerated areas are usually covered by a nonspecific grey membrane and are indurated.

BLASTOMYCOSIS

Blastomycosis, formerly known as North American blastomycosis, is a chronic infection of the lungs which may spread to other tissues, particularly skin, bone and genitourinary tract. Chest radiograph may resemble that of tuberculosis or carcinoma. **Disseminated blastomycosis may develop in immunosuppressed patients including those with AIDS.** It is caused by *Blastomyces dermatitidis*, a dimorphic fungus.

It was originally thought to be restricted to the North American continent. It is now known to be widely distributed in Africa, and cases have been reported from the Middle East, Poland and India.

Pathogenesis

B. dermatitidis has been isolated from soil. Soil contact has been associated with outbreaks of infection. The infectious particles of *B. dermatitidis* are its mycelial fragments and conidia. The respiratory tract is the portal of entry for all forms of blastomycosis except direct transcutaneous inoculation. There are three clinical types of blastomycosis – pulmonary disease, disseminated extrapulmonary disease, and cutaneous disease.

Laboratory diagnosis

In culture at 25–30°C, it grows as a mold with septate hyphae 1–2 μm in width and smooth, single-celled oval or pyriform conidia, 2–4 μm in diameter borne singly at the tips of long or short conidiophores or directly on the hyphae (Fig. 33.9A).

In tissue or culture at 37°C, the fungus appears as round or oval yeast cells, 8–15 μm in diameter. The cell wall is thick and refractile. The cells characteristically produce only one bud. This is attached to the mother cell by a broad base (Fig. 33.9B). The buds remain attached until they are almost of the size of the mother cell.

Diagnosis can be made by direct microscopy and culture of sputum, pus and scrapings from skin lesions.

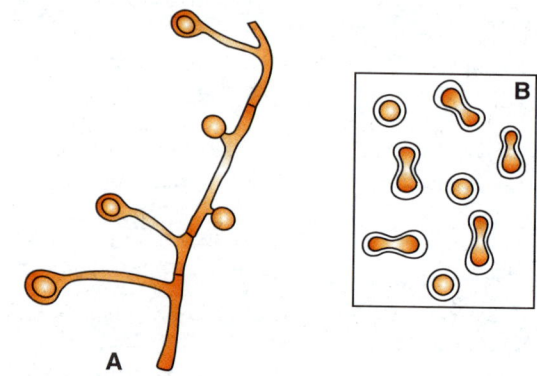

Fig. 33.9. *Blastomyces dermatitidis*: (A) mycelial phase; and (B) yeast phase.

Oral manifestations

Oral lesions may resemble those of actinomycosis, although abscess formation is not usually as prominent. Tiny ulcers may be the chief feature. The oral lesion may be the primary lesion or secondary to lesions elsewhere in the body.

PARACOCCIDIOIDOMYCOSIS

Paracoccidioidomycosis, formerly known as South American blastomycosis, is a chronic progressive granulomatous infection caused by *Paracoccidioides brasiliensis*, a dimorphic fungus. It is characterized by primary pulmonary infection that spreads, by haematogenous route to mucosa of the nose, mouth and the gastrointestinal tract, skin, lymphatic system, and the internal organs producing chronic granulomatous reaction. It occurs most frequently in humid mountain forests of South and Central America. Infection is acquired usually via respiratory route by inhalation of spores from environmental sources. The fungus has been isolated from soil.

Microscopic examination of KOH wet mount of pus, crusts, sputum and biopsies from granulomatous lesions usually shows numerous yeast cells (10–60 μm) with multiple buds. The buds are attached to the mother cell by a narrow base and may almost completely surround the cell, giving the characteristic "ship's wheel" appearance (Fig. 33.10A). Tissue sections should be stained with H & E, PAS and GMS.

The tissue form (yeast phase) may be obtained *in vitro* by inoculation of clinical material on enriched

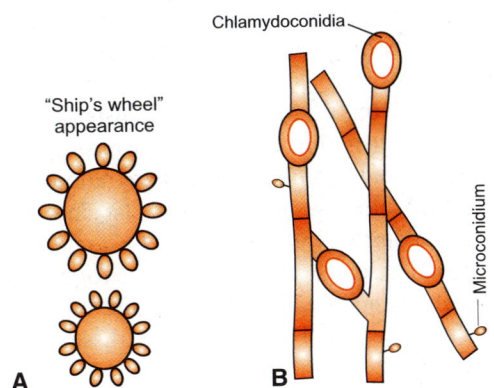

Fig. 33.10. *Paracoccidioides brasiliensis*: (A) yeast phase; and (B) mycelial phase.

media such as brain-heart-infusion agar and incubating at 37°C. Mycelial (mold) phase of the fungus develops on SDA incubated at 25–30°C. It shows septate hyphae bearing intercalary or terminal chlamydoconidia. A few microconidia are sometimes observed along the hyphae (Fig. 33.10B).

Oral manifestations

The organisms may enter through the periodontal tissues and subsequently reach the regional lymph nodes, producing a severe lymphadenopathy. The organisms have also been shown to penetrate the tissues producing papillary lesions of the oral mucosa. Widespread oral ulceration is also a common finding.

COCCIDIOIDOMYCOSIS

Coccidioidomycosis is primarily an infection of the lungs caused by *Coccidioides immitis*, a dimorphic fungus. It is endemic in the southwestern United States, northern Mexico, and scattered areas of Central and South America.

C. immitis exists as a saprophyte in the soil. The arthroconidia of the saprophytic phase are carried by the wind and are inhaled by man and animals. **A few arthroconidia may be sufficient to produce a naturally-acquired respiratory infection.** Patients with *C. immitis* infection may have chronic pneumonia, fungaemia, and extrapulmonary dissemination to skin, bones, meninges, and other body sites.

In the lungs, the arthroconidia form **spherules** (30–60 µm diameter). These contain numerous endoconidia, 2–5 µm diameter (Fig. 33.11A). The mature spherules have double wall measuring 2 µm in thickness. At maturity, the spherules rupture and their endoconidia are released which develop to form new spherules in adjacent tissue or following dissemination, in other organs of the body.

In soil and in culture (both at room temperature and at 37°C), *C. immitis* grows as a mold. The hyphae develop barrel-shaped arthroconidia measuring 2.5–4 × 3–6 µm. They characteristically alternate with smaller intervening empty cells (Fig. 33.11B). The hyphae fragment easily and release the arthroconidia. The latter are highly infectious and are readily airborne, therefore, the handling of a well developed culture is hazardous.

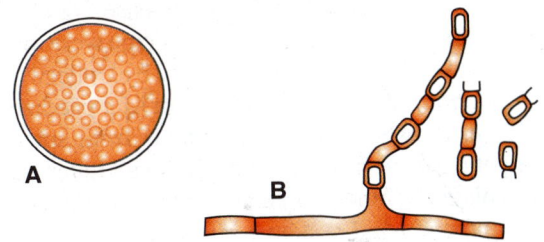

Fig. 33.11. *Coccidioides immitis*: tissue phase (A); and mycelial phase (B) .

Laboratory diagnosis

Diagnosis may be made by microscopic examination of sputum, pus and biopsy material and culture on SDA incubated at 25–30°C. *Since arthroconidia are highly infectious and readily airborne, therefore, petri dish should not be used for isolation of C. immitis and all procedures should be carried out in a safety cabinet.*

Oral manifestations

The lesions of the oral mucosa and skin are proliferative granulomatous and ulcerated that are non-specific in their clinical appearance. The lesions tend to heal by hyalinization and scar formation. Marked chronicity is often a feature of these lesions. Lytic lesions of the jaws may also occur.

CANDIDIASIS

The genus *Candida* comprises about 200 species, of which about 20 have been associated with pathology in humans and animals. The major pathogenic species include *C. albicans*, *C. dubliniensis*, *C. glabrata*, *C. guilliermondii*, *C. kefyr*, *C. krusei*, *C. lusitaniae*, *C. parapsilosis* and *C. tropicalis*. *C. albicans* is round to oval yeast 3–6 μm in diameter. It produces budding cells, pseudohyphae, and true hyphae. This ability to simultaneously display several morphological forms is known as **polymorphism**. Although hyphae are likely to be produced during the process of tissue invasion, yeasts without hyphae may also occur in invasive disease, particularly in infections caused by non-*albicans Candida* species.

The history of candidiasis dates back to the fourth century B.C. when Hippocrates, in his book, *Epidemics*, described oral aphtha (thrush) in two patients with severe underlying disease. The first descriptions of thrush in modern medicine were made by Rosen von Rosenstein in 1771 and by Underwood in 1784, who identified the infection as a paediatric problem. Bennett isolated the fungus from sputum of a patient suffering from tuberculosis. Later on it was isolated by other workers from vaginal infection, brain infection and systemic infection.

Pathogenesis

Candida is a human commensal, so that the infectious source is mostly endogenous. *Candida* spp. reside primarily in the gastrointestinal tract, but they are also commensals in the vagina, urethra, on the skin and under fingernails. *Candida* can be introduced from exogenous sources as well. These include introduction through various catheters and lines, or other indwelling prosthetic medical devices. This route leads to the development of deep-seated and systemic candidiasis as most of these therapeutic modalities are used primarily in compromised hosts whose defence systems are unable to combat the introduced pathogen.

- *C. albicans*, the species most often associated with human disease, is also recovered from fresh water, sea water and soil. Oral carriage rate may be higher in certain settings such as in HIV-infected patients with low CD4 counts, denture users with denture stomatitis, patients suffering from diabetes, patients receiving anticancer chemotherapy, and children.

Predisposing factors for candidiasis are AIDS, diabetes, iatrogenic immunosuppression, intravenous catheters, prolonged administration of antimicrobial agents, neutropenia, haematologic malignant diseases and burns. After *Candida* enters the blood stream, whether from exogenous or endogenous source, it adheres to the endothelial surface of the blood vessels, before dissemination into tissues.

Person-to-person transmission is not a predominant mechanism of pathogenesis in candidiasis. It occurs primarily in oral thrush of newborns acquired during birth from their mothers affected by vaginal infections, and rarely in sexual transmission from vaginitis patients to their male partners.

- *C. dubliniensis* is primarily associated with recurrent erythematous oral candidiasis in HIV-infected patients. It is also known, to a far lesser extent, to cause oral disease in non-HIV-infected individuals.

- *C. glabrata* causes infections usually occurring in the blood stream or urogenital tract and occasionally in the lungs and other sites.

- *C. parapsilosis* is a relatively frequent cause of endocarditis second only to *C. albicans* as a cause of *Candida* endocarditis..

- *C. lucitaniae* is an opportunistic pathogen in immunocompromised patients.

- *C. tropicalis*, *C. kefyr*, *C. guilliermondii*, and *C. krusei* are opportunistic pathogens, causing disease in patients:
  - with a breakdown in the body's immune system;
  - on prolonged treatment with antibiotics, corticosteroids, or cytotoxic drugs;
  - with intravenous catheters;
  - with diabetes mellitus; or
  - who are intravenous drug users.

Virulence factors

Numerous virulence factors exist and may play different roles with differing sites and stages of a given infection. These include adhesin, enzymes, fungal surface hydrophobicity and phenotype switching.

Adhesin

For colonization and tissue invasion adherence of *Candida* spp. to a wide range of tissue types and inanimate surfaces is essential. This is achieved by a combination of specific (ligand-receptor interaction) and non-specific (electrostatic charge) mechanisms. Mutants with reduced adherence exhibit decreased pathogenicity *in vivo*. Following attachment, *Candida* spp., particularly *C. albicans* grow in colonial communities and produce '**biofilms**'. The biofilms contain extracellular materials composed of proteins, carbohydrates, and other substances. Biofilms lead to poorer response of the pathogen in the biofilm to antimicrobials and the difficulties of the hosts' defence system to cope with the microbe, resulting in difficulties of eradication of infection.

Enzymes

Candida spp. produce extracellular proteinases, phospholipases, lipases and hydrolytic enzymes. These are important virulence factors.

Fungal surface hydrophobicity

Hydrophobicity of the cell surface of *C. albicans* plays an important role in the adhesion of the organism to eukaryotic cells and inert surfaces. Blastoconidia of *C. albicans* are hydrophilic, but the germ tube formation is associated with a significant rise in the cell surface hydrophobicity.

Phenotype switching

Phenotype switching is the ability of organisms of a single strain to switch to different colony phenotype. Due to this ability, *C. albicans* can grow in variety of morphological forms, ranging **from budding yeast to filamentous pseudohyphae and true hyphae**. Such switching enables adaptation to different or changing conditions in the host facilitating its ability to survive, invade tissues and escape host defences.

Transformation into the hyphal form is observed during an active infection. It is believed that phospholipase concentrated at the hyphal tip may be related to the greater invasiveness of this form as compared to the yeast. In addition, the hyphae, being larger than the yeast form, are more resistant to phagocytosis. Thus morphological change contributes to the increased pathogenic potential of the fungus.

Clinical features

Candida species can cause a range of clinical forms, from superficial manifestations involving skin, nails, and mucosal surfaces to deep-seated infections involving various internal organs and to disseminated disease (Table 33.2).

Table 33.2. Clinical forms of candidiasis

1. **SUPERFICIAL INFECTIONS**
   I. **Cutaneous infections**
      - Candidal intertrigo
      - Interdigital candidiasis
      - Perianal (diaper) rash
      - Candids
      - Chronic mucocutaneous candidiasis
   II. **Nail infections**
      - Paronychia
      - Onychomycosis
   III. **Mucosal infections**
      - Oral candidiasis
        - Acute pseudomembranous and acute atrophic candidiasis (oral thrush)
        - Chronic atrophic and hyperplastic candidiasis (denture stomatitis)
        - Angular cheilitis
      - Vaginal candidiasis
2. **DEEP INFECTIONS**
   - Candidiasis of gastrointestinal tract
     - Esophagitis
     - Gastrointestinal candidiasis
   - Candidiasis of liver, spleen and other organs
   - Candidiasis of respiratory system
   - Candidiasis of cardiovascular system
   - Renal and urinary tract candidiasis
     - Lower urinary tract infection
     - Renal infection
   - Central nervous system candidiasis
   - Ocular *Candida* infection
3. **DISSEMINATED CANDIDIASIS AND CANDIDEMIA**

SUPERFICIAL INFECTIONS

Superficial infections result from invasion of the superficial layers of skin and/or mucosae by the microorganism. These infections are characterized by the formation of a grayish plaque, surrounded by edema, which on histopathological examination consists of the infecting microorganisms, neutrophils, and cell debris.

Cutaneous infections

The major symptoms discussed under this head are:

- Candidal intertrigo
- Interdigital candidiasis
- Perianal (diaper) rash
- Candids
- Chronic mucocutaneous candidiasis.

Candidal intertrigo

It is the most common clinical form of the cutaneous infection, as *Candida* spp. readily colonize skin folds, particularly in moist and macerated sites. These may include groin, perineum, gluteal folds, umbilicus, axillae, inframammary folds or interdigital spaces. Lesions may be erythematous, with vesicles and pustules, in combination with pruritis. Obesity, diabetes mellitus, various endocrine disturbances, HIV infection and steroid therapy are predisposing factors.

Interdigital candidiasis

In this form the skin folds between the fingers of the hand are macerated and itching. This condition is associated with excessive exposure to moisture, and thus seen particularly among dishwashers.

Perianal (diaper) rash

This occurs in infants wearing diapers. It causes rash in the perianal area and on the buttocks.

Candids

Sterile, grouped, vesicular lesions resembling dermatophytids may be found beyond the limits of infected lesions. They probably represent allergic responses to circulating fungal antigens.

Chronic mucocutaneous candidiasis (CMC)

It is a rare condition in which susceptible individuals develop superficial *Candida* infections as a result of variable defects in T lymphocyte responsiveness to the fungus. It is characterized by the presence of persistent lesions, with high rate of recurrence, starting in early childhood and possibly persisting throughout the individual's lifetime. Lesions can be seen on various skin sites. CMC may appear in a generalized form or may be localized and assume a form of hyperkeratotic lesions – *Candida* granuloma.

Nail infections

The syndromes discussed under this head are:
- Paronychia
- Onychomycosis

Paronychia

It is chronic swelling and inflammation of the nail fold usually affecting the nails of the hands and less frequently those of the feet.

Onychomycosis

It is an invasive infection of the fingernails. As in paronychia, it is more often seen in nails of the hands. Infected nails may become discoloured, eroded, brittle, detached from the nail bed, and painful.

Mucosal infections

Involvement of mucosal surfaces by *Candida* is the most frequent clinical manifestation of candidiasis. The syndromes discussed under this head are:
- Oral candidiasis
- Vaginal candidiasis

Oral candidiasis

Candidiasis of oral mucosa is a disease recognized since antiquity. Very old, very young and very ill persons are more susceptible to oral candidiasis. In the mouth, carbohydrate levels are important; food debris, likely to be present in the mouth of severely ill patients with inadequate oral hygiene may be as significant as diabetic saliva. It has gained renewed significance more recently as an infection frequently seen in AIDS patients and in other conditions. *C. albicans* is the most frequently isolated etiological agent of oral candidiasis. Additional *Candida* spp., such as *C. glabrata*, *C. tropicalis*, *C. parapsilosis* and *C. guilliermondii* are also implicated in oral candidiasis. Oral candidiasis can be clinically classified into:

- acute pseudomembranous and atrophic candidiasis (oral thrush);
- chronic atrophic and hyperplastic candidiasis (denture stomatitis); and
- angular cheilitis.

Acute pseudomembranous and acute atrophic candidiasis

It is also known as **oral thrush**. It occurs predominantly in patients with systemic or local immunosuppression. Immunosuppressed individuals at risk include newborns with birth asphyxia, malnourished or diabetic patients, patients with HIV infections, and those receiving corticosteroid or cytotoxic chemotherapy.

The tongue, soft palate, buccal mucosa and other oral surfaces are characteristically covered with discrete or confluent patches of a cream-white to gray pseudomembrane (Fig. 33.12) composed of hyphae and yeasts of *C. albicans*. The lesions, particularly when covering larger areas, may be painful. They may spread to the mucosa of esophagus (Fig. 33.13), as seen in significant number of AIDS patients, and

cause dysphagia. **Oropharyngeal and oesophageal candidiasis is the commonest opportunistic fungal disease in HIV-infected patients worldwide.** The occurrence of oropharyngeal or oesophageal candidiasis is recognized as an indicator of immune suppression and is most often observed in patients with CD4+ cell count < 200/µl. Antiretroviral treatment has led to a dramatic decline in the prevalence of mucosal candidiasis.

Acute atrophic candidiasis is characterized by painful erythematous mucosa, particularly on the tongue, which can be associated with loss of the tongue papillae, affecting food intake. It may follow the acute pseudomembranous form with the disappearance of the pseudomembranous lesions.

Chronic atrophic and hyperplastic candidiasis

It is frequently seen in elderly patients, particularly those who wear denture. It is characterized by erythema and/or oedema of the mucosa under the dentures. The chronic hyperplastic form is a rare condition. It presents with white plaques, which can appear on various sites of the buccal mucosa. It may transform into a malignant state.

Angular cheilitis

Candida may cause red fissured lesions that crack and crust at the folds of the corners of the mouth. It may accompany other clinical forms of oral candidiasis, such as denture stomatitis or oral thrush.

Vaginal candidiasis

Candidal vulvovaginitis is a common genital complaint in women. This affects primarily young and middle-aged females, particularly during their active reproductive life. Around 75% experience at least one episode of this condition during their lifetime. Severe forms of vaginal candidiasis may be associated with use of oral contraceptives, corticosteroids or antibiotics, diabetes and pregnancy. Besides *C. albicans*, *C. glabrata* and *C. tropicalis* are the most frequently isolated *Candida* spp. both from vulvovaginitis patients and from healthy carriers.

Patient complains of vulvovaginal pruritis, discharge which can be thick and curd-like or thin, and dyspareunia. The lesions on the mucosal surface

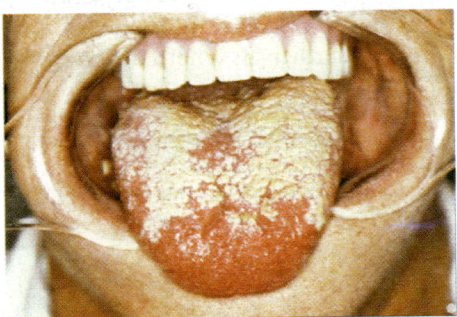

Fig. 33.12. Oral candidiasis (oral thrush).

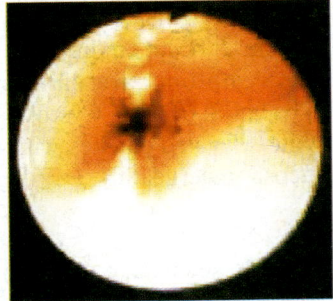

Fig. 33.13. Oesophageal candidiasis.

are basically adherent plaques. Sexual transmission to a male partner is known. In the male, infection presents as a balanitis with lesions and erythema on the penis.

DEEP INFECTIONS

Candida spp. may cause deep infections of several parenchymatous organs. These infections are characterized by microabscesses. Microscopically, these reveal blastoconidia, pseudohyphae, true hyphae (in case of *C. albicans*), neutrophils and mononuclear cells, and a necrotic centre. In chronic infections granulomata with giant cells and lymphocytes may be formed.

Candidiasis of gastrointestinal tract

The syndromes discussed under this head are:
- Esophagitis
- Gastrointestinal candidiasis

Esophagitis

Patient complains of painful dysphagia with nausea and/or vomiting. Endoscopy of esophageal mucosa shows white patches which resemble those of oral candidiasis (Fig. 33.13). Esophagitis may be associated with presence of oral candidiasis. However, it may also present as a separate clinical entity without oral involvement. **Esophageal candidiasis remains one of the most common AIDS-defining illnesses.**

Gastrointestinal candidiasis

Candidiasis can involve any site of gut. These lesions may progress to haematogenous infection, obstruction or even perforation. The pathology of candidal infection of the lower gut ranges from mucosal ulceration with or without pseudomembrane to exophytic lesions. Pseudomembranes are composed of a mixture of yeasts and pseudohyphae embedded in necrotic debris and fibrin. Pseudohyphae may extend beyond the muscular layer and reach the serosa.

Candidiasis of the liver, spleen and other organs

C. albicans and other species may cause candidiasis of liver, spleen, gall bladder, pancreas and peri-toneum. Hepatosplenic candidiasis is seen primarily in leukemics. Fungal elements can be seen in the biopsied tissues from liver and spleen.

Candidiasis of respiratory system

C. albicans may cause pneumonia. It is commonly seen in patients with haematogenous candidiasis. *Candida* empyema occurs among patients with severe underlying diseases, particularly cancer. Diagnosis requires the isolation of *Candida* spp. from an exudative pleural effusion. *C. albicans* may also cause laryngitis, epiglottitis and mediastinitis.

Candidiasis of cardiovascular system

Candida spp. can cause clinical manifestations in pericardium, myocardium or endocardium with endocarditis being the best known clinical entity. It can be caused by *C. albicans* and other species, such as *C. parapsilosis* and *C. tropicalis*. *Candida* endocarditis resembles bacterial endocarditis. It may, however, have a more prolonged onset; e.g., in post-surgery patients it may become apparent months later. Patient presents with fever, heart murmur, splenomegaly, congestive heart failure and anaemia. *Candida* endocarditis is characterized by large vegetations from which emboli may be released.

Renal and urinary tract candidiasis

This syndrome is discussed under following heads:
- Lower urinary tract infection
- Renal infection

Lower urinary tract infection

Candidal infection of lower urinary tract (cystitis) is frequently seen in association with indwelling catheters. They may originate from gastrointestinal tract or genital flora. It occurs more often in females and diabetics. Symptoms are similar to those observed with bacterial cystitis. Cystoscopy reveals soft, pearly white, elevated patches with hyperemic and friable mucosa underneath.

Renal infection

Renal candidiasis is secondary to haematogenous candidiasis. It is characterized by microabscess formation, mostly evident in the cortex of the kidneys.

Central nervous system candidiasis

Central nervous system infections by *Candida* spp. are rare, and present as meningitis or abscesses. Most susceptible individuals are AIDS patients and premature infants.

Ocular Candida infection

Candida spp. can affect both the outer and inner eye. Infection may originate from haematogenous dissemination or from direct fungal introduction, the former, generally results in inner eye infection, and the latter in clinical manifestations of the outer parts of the eye. Both categories of eye involvement are cased by *C. albicans* and some other *Candida* spp., such as *C. parapsilosis*, *C. krusei* and *C. glabrata*.

Outer eye infections include conjunctivitis, keratitis, blepharitis and lacrimal canaliculitis. Such infections follow some ocular trauma, surgery or even the use of contact lenses. Endophthalmitis is generally a result of haematogenous fungal spread, although it may also result from an exogenous source.

DISSEMINATED CANDIDIASIS AND CANDIDEMIA

Disseminated candidiasis may be defined as multi-organ infection with possible candidemia. *Candida* infection may involve central nervous system, liver, spleen, kidneys, heart, eyes or other organs and systems. It occurs mainly in cancer patients, particularly those with acute leukemia, in patients post-surgery, particularly gastrointestinal and cardiac surgery, transplant patients, particularly bone marrow transplants and burn patients.

Laboratory diagnosis

Specimens

Scrapings from mucosal, dermal or nail lesions, sputum, bronchial aspirate, pus, swabs, etc.

Direct examination

Place the specimen in a drop of 10% KOH, warm gently over a small flame and examine under microscope. All species of *Candida* form round to oval budding yeast cells, 3–6 μm in diameter.

They occur singly, in chains, or in small loose clusters. Most species, when invading tissue, form pseudohyphae and true hyphae. Pseudohyphae are actually chains of blastoconidia that have elongated and have not separated from one another. They can be recognized by distinct constrictions at the septa. True hyphae have no, or only slight constrictions at the septa. Blastoconidia develop along the sides of both types of hyphae (Figs. 33.14 and 33.15). *C. glabrata* is unique in that it is slightly smaller (2–5 μm in diameter) than the other species of *Candida*, and it does not produce hyphal forms. For species identification culture is required.

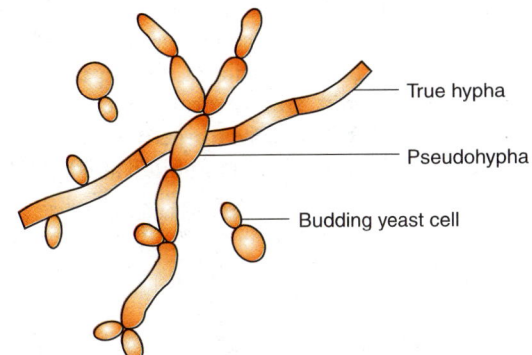

Fig. 33.14. Budding yeast cells, pseudohyphae and true hyphae of *Candida albicans*.

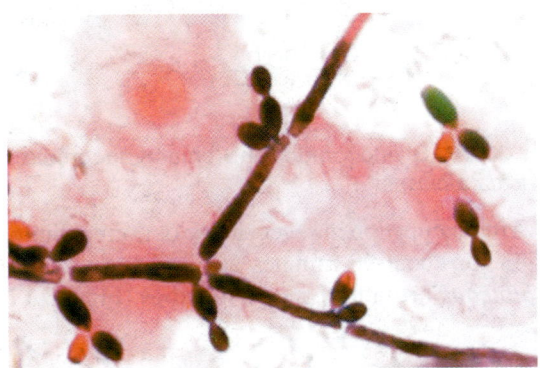

Fig. 33.15. Vaginal smear showing budding yeast cells, true hyphae and epithelial cells.

Histopathology

In systemic infections, *Candida* spp. most commonly elicit an acute suppurative inflammation composed of polymorphonuclear as well as mononuclear cells. Granulomas only rarely occur. *Candida* spp. are also known to invade blood vessels and produce infarcts.

Culture

Candida albicans: For isolation in culture spread pathological material on slants of SDA with chloramphenicol and incubate at 30°C. It grows rapidly. Growth matures in 3 days. Colonies are cream-coloured, pasty and smooth. On enriched media (e.g., blood agar or chocolate agar), extensions commonly called "feet" develop at the border of the colony. Lactophenol cotton blue preparation and Gram-stained smears show round to oval budding yeast cells (3.5–7 × 4–8 μm) and pseudohyphae. Rarely true hyphae may also be seen. On cornmeal-Tween 80 agar at 25°C for 72 hours, pseudohyphae form with clusters of round blastoconidia at the septa. Large thick-walled, usually single terminal chlamydoconidia are characteristically formed (Fig. 33.16). Chlamydoconidia formation is inhibited at 30–37°C.

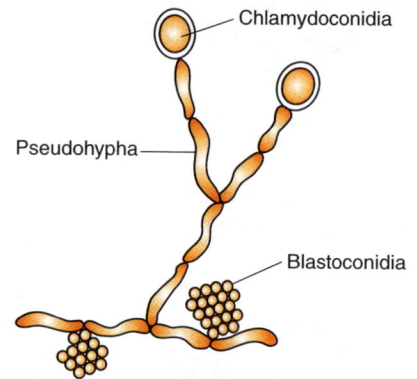

Fig. 33.16. Blastoconidia and chlamydoconidia of *Candida albicans.*

After incubation in sheep, horse or normal human serum for about 90 minutes at 37°C yeast cells of *C. albicans* begin to form **germ tubes** (Fig. 33.17).

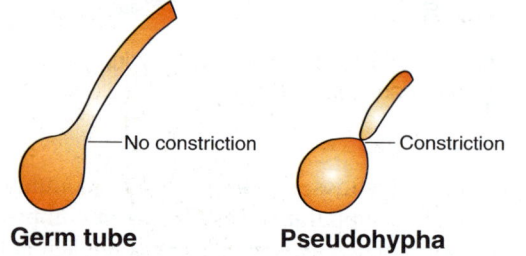

Fig. 33.17. Germ tube and pseudohypha of *Candida albicans.*

Germ tube test is also positive in *C. dubliniensis.* All other species are negative for this test. **Germ tubes are the beginning of true hyphae and appear as filaments that are not constricted at their points of origin on the parent cell.** If the filaments are constricted and septate at their points of origin, they are pseudohyphae, not germ tubes (Fig. 33.16).

GEOTRICHOSIS

Geotrichosis is an infection caused by *Geotrichum candidum*, a fungus found saprophytically in nature and as a commensal in the mouth, bronchi, lungs, gastrointestinal tract and genitourinary tract. The clinical forms of the infection are pulmonary geotrichosis that mimic tuberculosis in its manifestations and superficial infections of the skin, oral mucosa and gastrointestinal tract. The disease occurs more frequently in debilitated persons or as a secondary type of infection.

Oral manifestations

The oral lesions are identical to those of candidiasis or thrush, being white, velvety, patch-like covering the oral mucosa, isolated or diffuse in distribution. The tissue reaction is of a nonspecific, acute inflammatory type. The fungus in tissue appears as septate hyphae with arthroconidia. It produces a rapidly growing, white to cream, and smooth or hairy colony on Sabouraud's dextrose agar at 25°C. The main hyphae are 7–12 μm in diameter and are often dichotomously branched at the colony margin. Hyphae fragment into cylindrical, barrel-shaped, or elliptical arthroconidia (3–5 × 5–10 μm).

KEY FACTS

- Fungi are **eukaryotic** microorganisms, as opposed to bacteria, which are **prokaryotes**
- Fungi exhibit two basic structural forms – the **yeast form** and the **mold form**. The yeasts are unicellular with spherical/ovoid bodies while molds are multicellular with a variety of specialized structures
- The vast majority of medically important fungi grow aerobically on **Sabouraud's dextrose agar**
- *Human infections caused by fungi can be broadly classified as **superficial**, **subcutaneous**, **systemic** and **opportunistic** mycoses*

- *When fungi (such as Candida albicans) that are generally innocuous in healthy humans cause disease in compromised patients they are called **opportunistic infections***
- **Sporotrichosis** may lead to nonspecific ulceration of the oral, nasal and pharyngeal mucosa. It is usually associated with regional lymphadenopathy
- In **histoplasmosis** oral lesions appear as nodular, ulcerative or vegetative lesions on the buccal mucosa, gingiva, tongue or lips. The ulcerated areas are usually covered by a nonspecific grey membrane and are indurated
- Oral lesions of **blastomycosis** may resemble those of actinomycosis, although abscess formation is not usually prominent
- In **paracoccidioidomycosis** the organisms may enter through the periodontal tissues and subsequently reach the regional lymph nodes, producing a severe **lymphadenopathy**
- In **coccidioidomycosis** the lesions of oral mucosa and skin are proliferative granulomatous and ulcerated lesions that are nonspecific in their clinical appearance
- *Candida a common yeast which lives in the oral cavity of 50–60% of the population, can cause either **superficial** (mucosal, cutaneous or mucocutaneous) or **systemic** candidiasis*
- Species of the genus *Candida* found in humans include *C. albicans, C. glabrata, C. dubliniensis, C. krusei, C. parapsilosis, C. guilliermondii* and *C. tropicalis. C. albicans* is responsible for the vast majority of infections (>90%)
- *C. albicans* is indigenous to the oral cavity, gastrointestinal tract, female genital tract and sometimes the skin; hence the infection is usually **endogenous**
- *Candida* species rarely cause oral disease in the absence of predisposing factors, such as intraoral environmental changes (e.g., unhygienic prostheses) and/or systemic factors such as diabetes and immunodeficiency
- *C. albicans* and *C. dubliniensis* may be differentiated from other *Candida* species by their ability to produce **germ tubes** and **chlamydoconidia**
- *Demonstration of yeasts in **Gram-stained smear**, positive culture on Sabouraud's dextrose agar and subsequent confirmation by biochemical reactions constitute a mycological diagnosis of candidiasis*
- The oral lesions of geotrichosis are similar to those of candidiasis or thrush

IMPORTANT QUESTION

Write short notes on:
(a) Classification of fungi
(b) Classification of mycoses
(c) Rhinosporidiosis
(d) Sporotrichosis
(e) Histoplasmosis
(f) Candidiasis
(g) Blastomycosis
(h) Coccidioidomycosis
(i) Paracoccidioidomycosis
(j) Geotrichosis

SECTION F
Parasitology

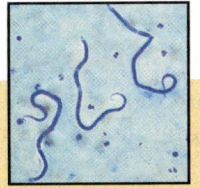

Chapter 34

Commonly Seen Protozoans and Helminths

Parasitology is the area of biology concerned with the phenomenon of dependance of one living organism on another. Medical parasitology is the science that deals with organisms living in the human body (the host) and the medical significance of the host-parasite relationship.

Parasite

It is defined as an animal or plant which lives in or upon another organism and derives its nutrient directly from it.

Host

It is defined as an organism which harbours the parasite and provides the nourishment and shelter to the latter. It is of following types:

1. Definitive host

The host which harbours the adult parasite, the most highly developed form of a parasite or where the parasite replicates sexually. When the most highly developed form is not obvious, the definitive host is the mammalian host.

2. Intermediate host

This is the host which alternates with the definitive host and harbours the larval or asexual stages of a parasite. Some parasites require two intermediate hosts for completion of their life cycle.

3. Reservoir host

It is the host that harbours the parasite and serves as an important source of infection to other susceptible hosts.

4. Vector

It is the insect host which transmits parasites to man and animals.

HOST-PARASITE RELATIONSHIPS

Host-parasite relationship is of following types:

1. Symbiosis

An association in which both host and parasite are so dependent upon each other that one cannot live without the help of the other. Neither of the partners suffers from any harm from this association.

2. Commensalism

An association in which only parasite derives benefit without causing any injury to the host. A commensal lives on food residues or waste products of the body and is capable of leading an independent life.

3. Parasitism

An association in which the parasite derives benefit and host gets nothing in return and always suffers from some injury. The parasite is so adapted to this association that it cannot live an independent life.

CLASSIFICATION OF PARASITES

Parasites are classified into protozoa (unicellular organisms) and helminths (multicellular organisms).

PROTOZOA

Principal protozoan pathogens of man are given in Table 34.1.

Table 34.1. Principal protozoan pathogens of man

Group	Species
1. Amoebae	*Entamoeba histolytica, Naeglaria fowleri, Acanthamoeba* spp.
2. Flagellates	*Giardia lamblia, Trichomonas vaginalis, Trypanosoma brucei gambiense, T. brucei rhodesiense, T. cruzi, Leishmania* spp.
3. Sporozoa	*Plasmodium falciparum, P. vivax, P. malariae, P. ovale, Toxoplasma gondii, Cryptosporidium parvum, Isospora belli*
4. Others	*Balantidium coli, Babesia microti, B. divergens, Pneumocystis jiroveci*

ENTAMOEBA HISTOLYTICA

This is the most important amoebic parasite of humans. It is worldwide with higher incidence in developing countries. In India, the problem of amoebiasis is widespread and the disease is prevalent in all parts of the country. It resides in mucosa and submucosa of large intestine of man.

Morphology

The parasite exists in three morphological forms – trophozoite, precyst and cyst (Fig. 34.1).

1. Trophozoite

It measures 10–60 μm (average 20–30 μm) in diameter.

Cytoplasm

The cytoplasm of the trophozoite can be divided into a **clear outer ectoplasm and an inner finely granular endoplasm in which red blood cells, leucocytes and tissue debris are found within the**

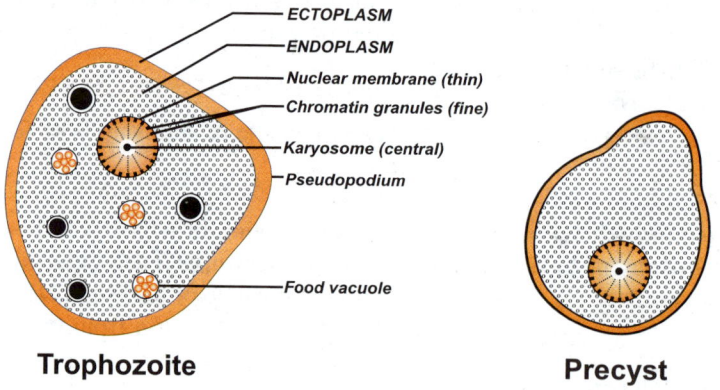

Trophozoite · Precyst

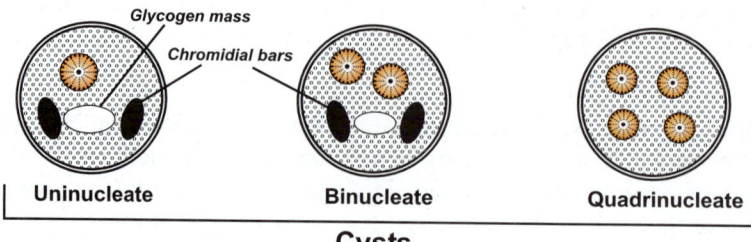

Cysts

Fig. 34.1. Various morphological forms of *Entamoeba histolytica*.

food vacuoles. Red blood cells may, however, be absent if infection is confined to the gut lumen. Trophozoites are motile with active, unidirectional and purposeful motility. Movement results from long finger-like pseudopodial extensions of ectoplasm into which endoplasm flows.

Nucleus

It is spherical in shape varying in size from 4–6 μm in diameter. In stained preparations it shows **a central dot-like karyosome which is surrounded by a clear halo**. The nuclear membrane is delicate and is lined by a single layer of **fine chromatin granules**. The space between the karyosome and the nuclear membrane is traversed by linin network (achromatic fibrils) having spoke-like radial arrangement.

2. Precyst

It is smaller in size, varying from 10–20 μm in diameter. It is oval with a blunt pseudopodium projecting from the periphery. Food vacuoles

disappear. There is no change in the nucleus which shows characteristics of that of the trophozoite.

3. Cyst

It is spherical, 10–15 μm in diameter. It is surrounded by a thick chitinous wall which makes it highly resistant to the gastric acid, adverse environmental conditions and the chlorine concentration found in potable water. It starts as a uninucleate body, but later the nucleus divides to form two and then four nuclei. Uninucleate and binucleate cysts in addition also possess a glycogen mass, which stains brown with iodine, and 1–4 chromidial or chromatoid bars. These do not stain with iodine but appear as refractile oblong bars with rounded ends in normal saline preparations. With iron-haematoxylin stain they stain black in colour.

Life cycle

It passes its life cycle in only one host (Fig. 34.2). Man acquires the infection by ingestion of water and

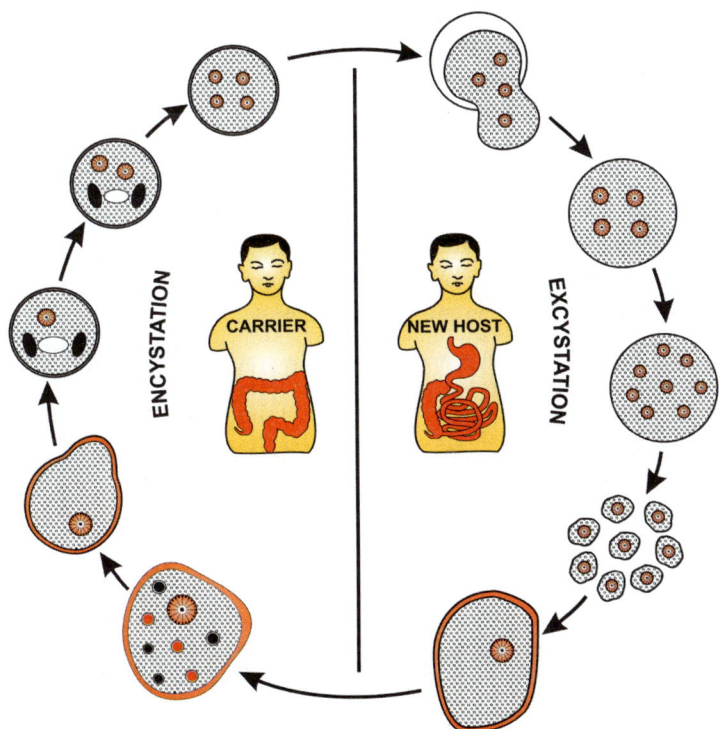

Fig. 34.2. Life cycle of *Entamoeba histolytica*.

food contaminated with mature quadrinucleate cysts. Infection may also be acquired by anal-oral sexual practices in male homosexuals. In the small intestine the cyst wall is lysed by trypsin and a single tetranucleate amoeba (**metacyst**) is liberated. Each nucleus divides by binary fission giving rise to eight nuclei. Almost immediately the cytoplasm becomes separated into as many parts as there are nuclei, thus from each mature cyst eight small amoebulae (**metacystic trophozoites**) are produced. This process is known as **excystation**. Metacystic trophozoites are carried in the faecal stream into the caecum. They invade the mucosa and ultimately lodge in the submucous tissue of large intestine. Here they grow and multiply by binary fission.

During growth, *E. histolytica* secretes a **proteolytic enzyme of the nature of histolysin** which brings about destruction and necrosis of tissue and produces flask-shaped ulcers (Fig. 34.3). The amoebae are mostly present at the periphery of the lesion. At this stage, a large number of trophozoites are excreted along with blood and mucus in the stool leading to amoebic dysentery. In a few cases, erosion of the large intestine may be so extensive that **trophozoites gain entrance into the radicals of portal vein** and are carried away to the liver where they multiply leading to amoebic hepatitis and amoebic liver abscess.

After some time, when the effect of the parasite on the host is toned down and patient has developed resistance, the lesions start healing and patient starts passing normal (formed) stools. The trophozoites, in the lumen of the large intestine, discharge undigested food particle and transform into precysts and then into mature quadrinucleate cysts. **These are the infective forms of the parasite.** This process is known as **encystation**. Cyst formation occurs only within the intestinal tract; once the stool has left the body, cyst formation does not occur.

Pathogenicity

E. histolytica causes intestinal and extraintestinal amoebiasis.

Intestinal amoebiasis

After an incubation period of 1–4 weeks, the amoebae invade the colonic mucosa, producing characteristic ulcerative lesions and a profuse bloody diarrhoea (**amoebic dysentery**). The ulcers may be generalized involving the whole length of the large intestine or they may be localized in the ileocaecal (caecum, ascending colon, ileocaecal valve and appendix) or sigmoidorectal (sigmoid colon and rectum) region. Ulcers are discrete with intervening normal mucosa. They vary in size from pin-head size to more than 2.5 cm in diameter (Fig. 34.4). They may be deep or superficial. Base of the deep ulcers is generally formed by muscular coat. However, superficial ulcers do not extend beyond muscularis mucosae (Fig. 34.3).

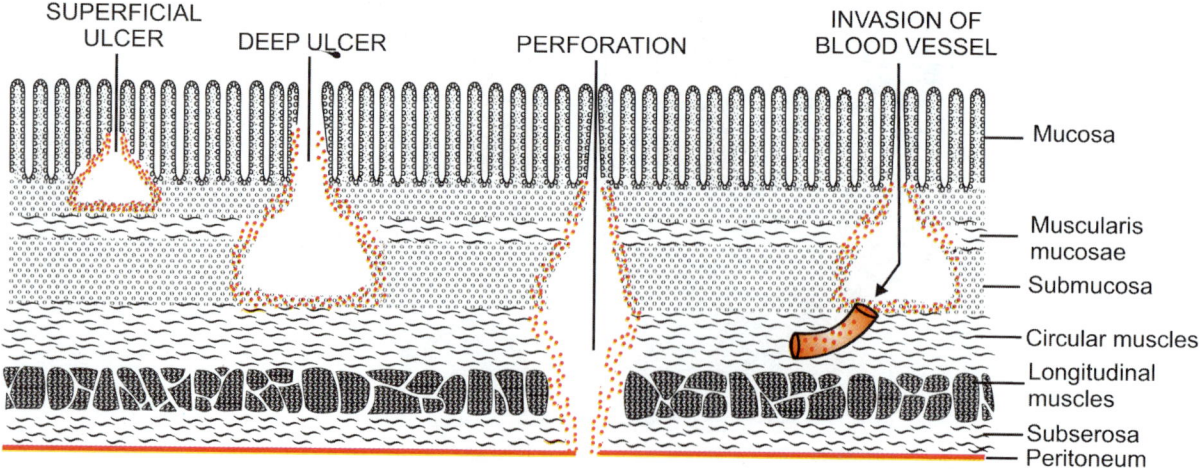

Fig. 34.3. Pathogenesis of intestinal amoebiasis.

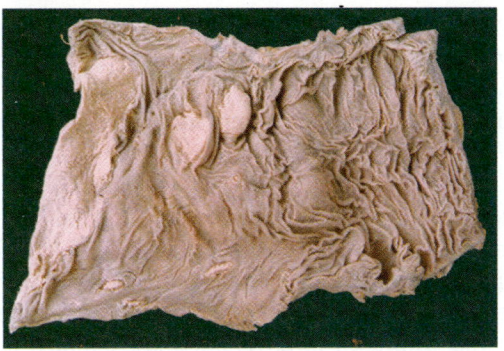

Fig. 34.4. Amoebic ulcers large intestine.

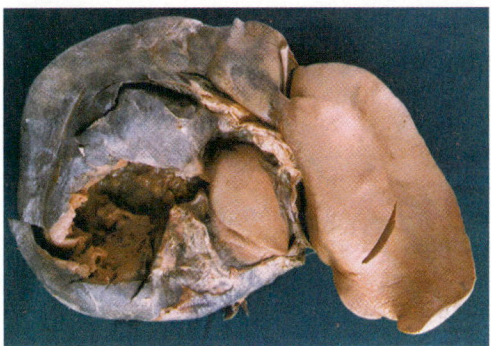

Fig. 34.6. Amoebic liver abscess.

Extraintestinal amoebiasis

About 5% individuals with intestinal amoebiasis, 1–3 months after the disappearance of the dysenteric attack, develop hepatic amoebiasis. Trophozoites of *E. histolytica* are carried as emboli by the radicles of the portal vein from the base of the amoebic ulcer in the large intestine (Fig. 34.3). The capillary system of the liver acts as an excellent filter and holds these parasites. They multiply in the liver and lead to cytolytic action (Fig. 34.5). The amoebae cause obstruction of the portal venules resulting in anaemic necrosis of hepatic cells. The destruction starts here and continues in concentric layers. Necrosis is followed by cytolysis. Small miliary abscesses coalesce to form big liver abscess (Fig. 34.6).

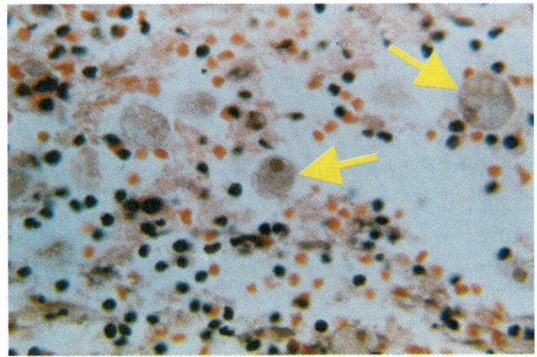

Fig. 34.5. Trophozoites of *Entamoeba histolytica* in liver aspirate showing cytolysis of liver cells (haematoxylin and eosin stain).

Amoebic liver abscess

It varies greatly in size. It has been reported in patients of all ages, but predominate in adults between 20–60 years. It has a marked preference for the right lobe of the liver and it is at least three times more frequent in males than in females. The wall of the abscess cavity is ragged with shreds of connective tissue running across the abscess cavity. A section through the margin of the liver abscess can be differentiated into three zones:

1. A necrotic centre filled with thick pus with no amoebae.
2. An intermediate zone consisting of degenerated liver cells, a few red blood cells, leucocytes and occasional trophozoites of *E. histolytica*.
3. An outer zone of nearly normal hepatic tissue just being invaded by amoebae.

Pus of liver abscess

The centre of an amoebic liver abscess contains a viscous red-brown (anchovy sauce appearance) or grey-yellow fluid consisting of cytolysed liver cells, red blood cells and leucocytes. It is referred to as 'pus' but contains very few pus cells. Since the amoebae actively multiply in the walls of the abscess, the last few drops of pus obtained from the lesion are most likely to yield recognizable trophozoites of the parasite.

From the liver, *E. histolytica* may enter into general circulation involving other organs of the body like lungs, brain, spleen, skin, etc. Both faecal and sigmoidoscopic examinations for the parasite are negative in approximately half of the patients in extra-intestinal disease.

Laboratory diagnosis

I. Intestinal amoebiasis

1. Stool examination

In acute amoebiasis, stool or colonic scrapings from ulcerated areas are examined by macroscopic and microscopic examination. It should be carefully differentiated from bacillary dysentery (Table 34.2). For microscopic examination stool is picked up with a matchstick or a platinum loop and emulsified in a drop of normal saline on a clean glass slide. A clean

Table 34.2. Differences between amoebic and bacillary dysentery

Character	Amoebic dysentery	Bacillary dysentery
Macroscopic		
Number	6–8 motions a day	Over 10 motions a day
Amount	Copious	Small
Odour	Offensive	Odourless
Colour	Dark red	Bright red
Reaction	Acidic	Alkaline
Consistency	Not adherent to the container	Adherent to the container
Microscopic		
RBCs	In clumps	Discrete, sometimes in clumps due to rouleaux formation
Pus cells	Few	Numerous
Macrophages	Few	Numerous, many of them contain RBCs; hence may be mistaken for *E. histolytica*
Eosinophils	Present	Scarce
Charcot-Leyden crystals	Present	Absent
Pyknotic bodies	Present	Absent
Ghost cells	Absent	Present
Parasites	Trophozoites of *E. histolytica*	Absent
Bacteria	Many motile bacteria	Few or absent

coverslip is placed over it and examined under microscope first under low power and then under high power. This method is specially useful for the demonstration of the actively motile trophozoites of *E. histolytica*.

For the demonstration of cysts or dead trophozoites, stained preparation may be required for the study of the nuclear character. For this purpose iodine stained preparation is commonly employed. Stool is emulsified in a drop of five times diluted solution of Lugol's iodine, covered with a clean coverslip and examined under microscope. Both saline and iodine preparations may be prepared on the same slide. Since excretion of cysts in the stool is often intermittent, at least three consecutive specimens should be examined.

DNA probe has been used recently to identify *E. histolytica* in the stool specimen and specific sequences can be amplified by **polymerase chain reaction** (**PCR**).

2. Blood examination

It shows moderate leucocytosis.

3. Serological tests

These are negative in early cases. However, in later stages of invasive intestinal amoebiasis antibodies appear and serological tests become positive. These tests include:

- indirect haemagglutination (IHA),
- indirect fluorescent antibody test (IFA), and
- enzyme-linked immunosorbent assay (ELISA).

II. Hepatic amoebiasis

1. Diagnostic aspiration

Trophozoites of *E. histolytica* can be demonstrated by microscopy of the pus aspirated by exploratory puncture of amoebic liver abscess. Trophozoites can be demonstrated in the pus in less than 15% cases of amoebic liver abscess.

2. Liver biopsy

Trophozoites of *E. histolytica* can be demonstrated in the specimens of liver biopsy from cases of amoebic hepatitis or the wall of the liver abscess.

3. Blood examination

It shows leucocytosis with total leucocyte count of

15,000–30,000/µl, of which 70–75% are polymorphonuclear leucocytes.

4. Stool examination

In about 15% cases of amoebic hepatitis cysts of *E. histolytica* can be demonstrated in the stool. This indicates persistence of intestinal infection.

5. Serological tests

Serological tests like IHA, IFA and ELISA are of immense value in the diagnosis of hepatic amoebiasis. IHA and IFA tests have been reported positive with titres of $\geq 1 : 256$ and $\geq 1 : 200$ respectively in almost 100% cases of amoebic liver abscess. ELISA is now replacing the IHA and is available commercially. Amoebic antibodies persist for months to years even after clinical cure.

Amoebic antigen can be detected in the patient serum by ELISA and a simple and economical slide agglutination test, the coagglutination test. It is present in serum only in active infection and disappears when the patient is cured of active amoebic disease.

6. Molecular methods

DNA probes and PCR are the recent molecular methods of promise for the detection of *E. histolytica* in stool and liver aspirates. The sensitivity is estimated at 87%.

7. Histology

A histological diagnosis of amoebiasis can be made when the trophozoites within the tissue are identified. Organisms must be differentiated from host cells particularly histiocytes. Periodic acid-Schiff is often used to help locate the organisms. The organisms appear bright pink with a green-blue background (depending upon the counterstain used). Haematoxylin and eosin staining also allows the typical morphology to be seen, thus allowing accurate identification (Fig. 34.5). As a result of sectioning, some organisms exhibit evenly arranged nuclear chromatin with central karyosome and some no longer contain nucleus.

ENTAMOEBA COLI

It is a worldwide parasite. It lives freely in the lumen of large intestine of man and is non-pathogenic. Like *E. histolytica* it exists in three stages – trophozoite, precyst and cyst (Table 34.3). Life cycle of *E. coli* is similar to that of *E. histolytica*.

Table 34.3. Trophozoites and cysts of *E. histolytica* and *E. coli*

	E. histolytica	*E. coli*
Trophozoite		
Size	20–30 µm	20–50 µm
Motility	Active	Sluggish
Cytoplasm	Clearly defined into ectoplasm and endoplasm.	Not defined.
Cytoplasmic inclusions	Red blood cells, leucocytes and tissue debris but no bacteria.	Bacteria and cellular debris but never red blood cells.
Nucleus	Central karyosome, the nuclear membrane is delicate and is lined by fine chromatin granules. It is not visible in unstained preparations.	Eccentric karyosome, the nuclear membrane is thick and is lined by coarse chromatin granules. It is visible in unstained preparations.
Precyst	Oval with a blunt pseudopodium, 10–20 µm in diameter. Nucleus shows characteristics of that of its trophozoite.	20 µm in diameter, resembles in shape with that of *E. histolytica*. Nucleus shows characteristics of that of its trophozoite.
Cyst		
Size	Spherical, 10–15 µm in diameter.	Spherical, 15–20 µm in diameter.
Number of nuclei	1–4	1–8
Chromatoid bars	Rounded	Filamentous

ENTAMOEBA GINGIVALIS

E. gingivalis is the **first parasitic amoeba to be recognized**. It was described by Gros in 1849 in the soft tartar between the teeth. *E. gingivalis* is unusual among the *Entamoeba* in two respects:

- it inhabits the mouth rather than the large bowel, and
- no cyst of *E. gingivalis* has ever been found.

Trophozoite

It measures 10–25 µm in diameter and is actively motile by multiple pseudopodia.

Cytoplasm

The cytoplasm is differentiated into clear ectoplasm and granular endoplasm in which digested leucocytes and epithelial cells are found within food vacuoles. At times bacteria and rarely red blood cells are also seen.

Nucleus

It is spherical, 2–4 µm in diameter. It has a central karyosome and nuclear membrane is lined with closely packed chromatin granules (Fig. 34.7).

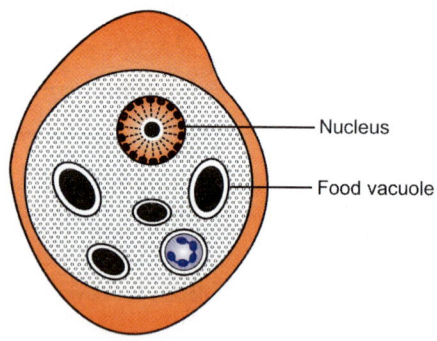

Fig. 34.7. Trophozoite of *Entamoeba gingivalis*.

Since morphologically *E. gingivalis* is very similar to the trophozoite of *E. histolytica,* it is important to make the correct identification from a sputum specimen, that is, *E. gingivalis,* which is considered to be a nonpathogen, rather than *E. histolytica* from a pulmonary abscess.

Habitat

E. gingivalis occurs as a commensal in the gingival tissue around the teeth, particularly if there is suppuration, as in pyorrhoea alveolaris, but it also occurs in apparently hygienic mouths and on dental plates if they are not kept clean. It has also been seen in the crypts and histologic sections of diseased tonsils and in vaginal and cervical smears from women using intrauterine devices. It is transmitted from person to person by close contact like kissing or from contaminated drinking utensils.

Laboratory diagnosis

It can be established by demonstration of trophozoites of *E. gingivalis* in the material removed from gingival margin of the gums, from between teeth or from denture.

GIARDIA LAMBLIA

Giardia lamblia is worldwide. This lives attached to the mucosal surface of the small intestine, notably in duodenum and upper part of jejunum of man. It exists in two stages – trophozoite and cyst.

Trophozoite

It is pear-shaped with rounded anterior and pointed posterior end (Fig. 34.8). It measures 14 µm in length and 7 µm in maximum width. The dorsal surface is convex while on the ventral surface it has a shallow posteriorly notched concavity (sucking disc) that embraces anterior half of the organism. It acts as an organelle of attachment.

It is bilaterally symmetrical and has **one pair of nuclei**, one on each side of the midline, one pair of axostyles, one pair of parabasal bodies present on the axostyles and four pairs of flagella and probably four pairs of blepharoblasts from which the flagella arise.

The **cytoplasm** is finely granular. The **nuclei** are rounded and possess a central karyosome. The nuclear membrane is delicate and is not lined by chromatin material. By rapid movement of flagella, the trophozoites move from place to place.

Cyst

Mature cyst is oval in shape and measures 12×7 µm in size. It has **two pairs of nuclei** which may remain clustered at one end or lie in pairs at opposite

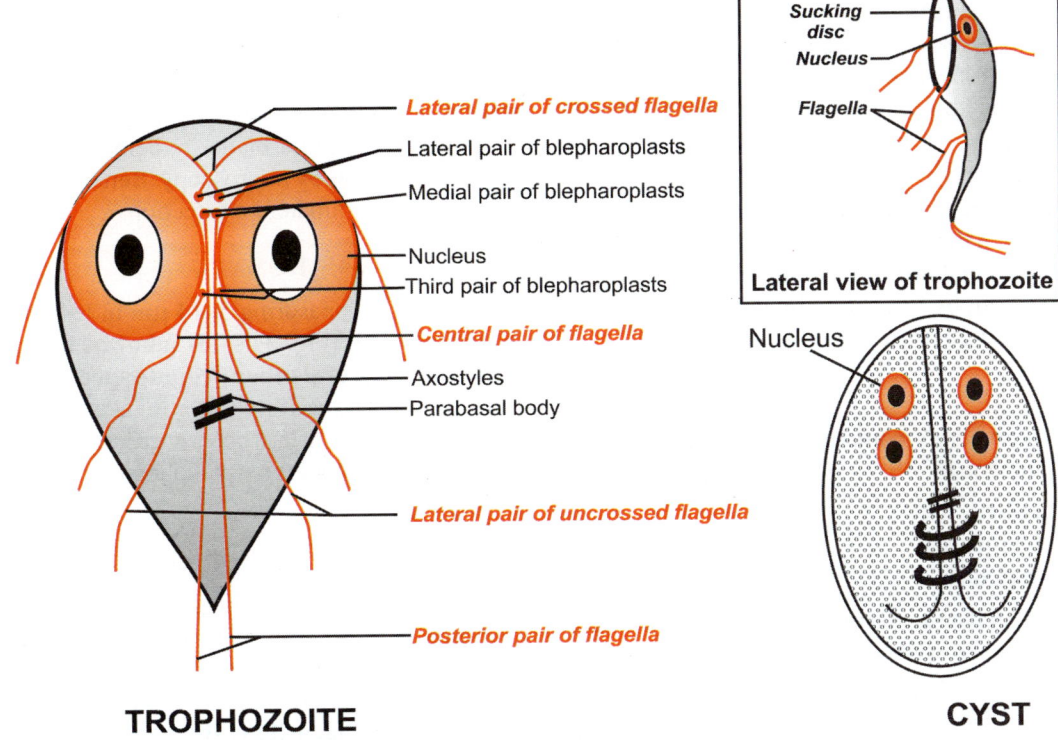

TROPHOZOITE   **CYST**

Fig. 34.8. Morphological forms of *Giardia lamblia*.

ends. The remains of the flagella and margins of the sucking disc may be seen inside the cytoplasm of the cyst (Fig. 34.8).

Life cycle

It passes its life cycle in one host. Mature cyst is the infective form of the parasite. **Man acquires infection by ingestion of water and food contaminated with the cysts.** Infection may also be acquired by anal-oral sexual practices. Within 30 minutes of ingestion **excystation** occurs in the duodenum. The cyst hatches out two trophozoites, which then multiply to form enormous numbers and colonize in the duodenum and upper part of jejunum. To avoid acidity of duodenum, it may localize in biliary tract.

By means of the concavity on its ventral surface the trophozoite attaches to the mucosal surface of the duodenum and jejunum. In frankly diarrhoeic stools, it is usual to find only the trophozoites. **Encystation** occurs commonly in transit down the colon where the intestinal contents lose moisture and patient starts passing formed stools. The trophozoites retract their flagella and secrete a thin, tough and hyaline cyst wall. As cyst matures, the internal structures are doubled, so that when **excystation** occurs, the cytoplasm divides, thus producing two trophozoites.

Pathogenicity

The presence of *G. lamblia* in the glandular crypts of duodenal-jejunal mucosa ordinarily causes no irritation. These flagellates do not invade the tissues, but feed on mucous secretions. With the help of sucking disc the parasite attaches itself to the surface of the epithelial cells in the duodenum and jejunum and may cause duodenal and jejunal irritation leading to duodenitis and jejunitis. Patient may complain of dull epigastric pain, flatulence and **chronic diarrhoea of steatorrhoea type**. The stool is voluminous, foul smelling and contains large amount of mucus and fat but no blood. This is due to malabsorption since the parasites are coated on the mucosa, thus absorption suffers. Patient loses weight. When *Giardia* localizes in the biliary tract, it may lead to chronic cholecystitis and jaundice.

Laboratory diagnosis

Giardiasis can be diagnosed by identification of cysts of *G. lamblia* in the formed stools or the trophozoites of the parasite in diarrhoeal stools and bile aspirated from duodenum by intubation by normal saline and iodine preparation as in case of *E. histolytica*.

TRICHOMONAS

Genus *Trichomonas* contains three species which occur in humans:

1. *T. tenax*
2. *T. hominis*,
3. *T. vaginalis*

These flagellates exist **only in trophozoite stage**. Cystic stage is absent. They have four anterior flagella and one lateral flagellum which is attached to the surface of the parasite to form undulating membrane. The undulating membrane is supported at the base by a rod-like structure known as costa. The axostyle runs down the middle of the body and ends in the pointed tail-like extremity. A round nucleus is located in the anterior portion.

TRICHOMONAS TENAX

It is a pyriform flagellate. It measures 5–12 µm in length and 5–10 µm in width (Fig. 34.9). It is a **harm-less commensal of the human mouth**, living in the tartar around the teeth, in cavities of carious teeth, in necrotic mucosal cells in the gingival margins of gums and in pus pockets in tonsillar follicles. It is transmitted by kissing, salivary droplets and fomites.

Diagnosis can be made by demonstration of *T. tenax* in the tartar by microscopy. Better oral hygiene will rapidly eliminate the infection.

TRICHOMONAS HOMINIS

It is pyriform, measuring 5–14 µm in length and 7–10 µm in width (Fig. 34.9). **It inhabits the caecum of man and several other primate species** and feeds on enteric bacteria. It does not invade the intestinal mucosa. Though it has been occasionally found in the diarrhoeic stools, its pathogenicity is yet to be established.

TRICHOMONAS VAGINALIS

Morphologically it resembles *T. tenax* but it is larger than this. It measures 7–23 µm in length and 5–15 µm in width (Fig. 34.9). In a wet mount the tropho-zoite has a characteristic jerky motility. **The normal habitat of the parasite is the vagina and urethra of women and the urethra, seminal vesicles and prostate of man.** It may also be found in the Bartholin's glands and urinary bladder in female.

Pathogenicity

The parasite lives on the mucosa feeding on bacteria and leucocytes. *T. vaginalis* is an **obligate parasite**. It cannot live without close association with the vaginal, urethral or prostatic tissues.

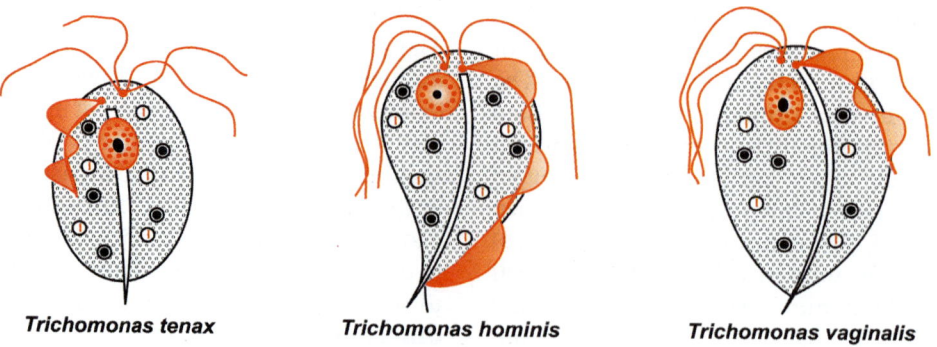

Trichomonas tenax   *Trichomonas hominis*   *Trichomonas vaginalis*

Fig. 34.9. Trophozoites of *Trichomonas* spp.

The organism is responsible for a mild **vaginitis with discharge**. Vaginal discharge contains a large number of parasites and leucocytes and is liquid, greenish or yellow. It covers the mucosa down to the urethral orifice, vestibular glands and clitoris. Male patients usually have mild or asymptomatic infections. They may develop itching and discomfort inside penile urethra, especially during urination. The parasite is transmitted by sexual intercourse.

Laboratory diagnosis

The diagnosis can be made by demonstration of trophozoites of *T. vaginalis* in wet mounts of the sedimented urine, vaginal secretions or vaginal scrapings. In males it may be found in urine or prostatic secretions. Fixed smears may be stained with Papanicolaou (Fig. 34.10), Giemsa, Leishman and periodic acid-Schiff stain, and seen under light microscope.

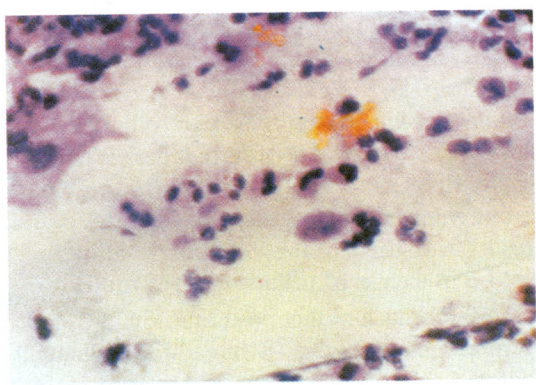

Fig. 34.10. Trophozoites of *Trichomonas vaginalis* in vaginal smear (Papanicolaou stain).

PLASMODIUM

Genus *Plasmodium* has approximately 172 named species which infect various species of vertebrates. Four are known to infect humans – *P. vivax*, *P. falciparum*, *P. malariae* and *P. ovale*. They cause the most important life-threatening protozoan disease called malaria. It continues to be an important vector-borne disease with an annual morbidity of 4–5 million cases. The incidence of malaria is increasing due to resistance of vectors to insecticides and drug-resistant parasites. In India, *P. vivax* and *P. falciparum* are very

common, a few cases of *P. malariae* and *P. ovale* have also been reported.

Life cycle

Malaria parasites exhibit a complex life cycle (Figs. 34.11 and 34.12) involving alternating cycles of asexual division (schizogony) occurring in man (intermediate host) and sexual development (sporogony) occurring in female anopheles mosquito (definitive host). Therefore, **malaria parasites exhibit alternation of generations and alternation of hosts**.

Human cycle

The sporozoites are the infective form of the parasite. They are present in the salivary glands of female anopheles mosquito. Man gets infection by the bite of infected mosquito. It usually bites at night or during the twilight hours, either right after sunset or before sunrise. During the act of biting, the proboscis of the mosquito pierces the skin and saliva containing sporozoites is injected directly into the blood stream. The cycle in man comprises of following stages:

1. Primary exo-erythrocytic or pre-erythrocytic schizogony
2. Erythrocytic schizogony
3. Gametogony
4. Secondary exo-erythrocytic or dormant schizogony

1. Primary exo-erythrocytic or pre-erythrocytic schizogony

Within one hour all the **sporozoites** leave the blood stream and enter into liver parenchyma cells. The sporozoites which are elongated, spindle-shaped bodies become rounded inside the liver cells. They undergo a process of multiple nuclear division, followed by cytoplasmic division and develop into **schizont**. In different species it varies in size from 24–60 µm in diameter and contains 2,000–30,000 merozoites. Primary exoerythrocytic schizogony consists of only one generation. The duration of this cycle of *P. falciparum*, *P. vivax*, *P. ovale* and *P. malariae* is 6, 8, 9 and 13–16 days, respectively. When primary exoerythrocytic schizogony is complete, the liver cell ruptures and releases merozoites into blood stream.

2. Erythrocytic schizogony

The **merozoites** liberated from primary exo-erythrocytic schizogony penetrate red blood cells where they multiply at the expense of the host cells. Here they pass through the stages of trophozoites, schizonts and merozoites (Table 34.4 and Figs. 34.11 and 34.12). Depending on the species about 6–24 nuclei are produced before cytoplasmic division occurs, and the red cell ruptures to release the individual merozoites, which then infect fresh red blood cells.

The parasitic multiplication during the erythrocytic phase is responsible for bringing on a clinical attack of malaria. Erythrocytic schizogony may be continued for a considerable period, but in the course of time the infection tends to die out. *P. falciparum* differs from the other forms of malaria parasites in that developing erythrocytic schizonts aggregate in the capillaries of the brain and other internal organs, so that only young ring forms are found in peripheral blood.

3. Gametogony

After malaria parasites have undergone erythrocytic schizogony for certain period, some merozoites develop within red cells into male and female gametocytes known as **microgametocytes** and **macrogametocytes**, respectively. They develop in the red blood cells of the capillaries of internal organs like spleen and bone marrow. Only mature gametocytes are found in the peripheral blood. They do not cause any febrile condition in human host. These are produced for the propagation and continuance of the species. The host carrying gametocytes is known as **carrier**. The microgametocytes of all the four species of *Plasmodium* are smaller in size, cytoplasm stains light blue and the nucleus (chromatin) is diffuse and large. On the other hand the macrogametocytes are larger, the cytoplasm stains deep blue and the nucleus is compact and small (Table 34.4).

4. Secondary exo-erythrocytic or dormant schizogony

In case of *P. vivax* and *P. ovale*, some sporozoites on entering into hepatocytes enter into a resting (dormant) stage before undergoing asexual multiplication while others undergo multiplication without delay. The resting stage of the parasite is rounded, 4–6 μm in diameter, uninucleate and is known as **hypnozoite** or **sleeping form**. After a period of weeks, months or years (usually up to 2 years) hypnozoites are reactivated to become schizonts and release merozoites which infect red blood cells producing **relapse** of malaria. Hypnozoites are not formed in case of *P. falciparum* and *P. malariae*, therefore, relapses do not occur in disease caused by these species.

Mosquito (sexual) cycle

Sexual cycle actually starts in the human host itself by the formation of gametocytes which are present in the peripheral blood. Both asexual and sexual forms of the parasite are ingested by female anopheles mosquito during its blood meal from the patient. *Female anopheles mosquito has a stout proboscis which can pierce the human skin like a needle. On the other hand the proboscis of the male is not stout, it is flexible, hence it cannot pierce through the skin.* In the mosquito, only the mature sexual forms are capable of further development and rest die. In order to infect a mosquito, **the blood of human carrier must contain at least 12 gametocytes/μl and the number of female gametocytes must be in excess of the number of males**.

In the stomach of the mosquito (Fig. 34.11) from one microgametocyte 5–8 thread-like filamentous structures called **microgametes** are formed by the process of exflagellation. The macrogametocyte does not show any exflagellation. It develops into a **macrogamete**, its nucleus shifts to the surface, where a projection is formed. **Fertilization** occurs when a microgamete penetrates this projection. The fertilized macrogamete is known as **zygote**. This occurs in 20 minutes to 2 hours. In next 24 hours, the zygote lengthens and matures into **ookinete**, a motile vermiculate stage. It penetrates the epithelial lining of the stomach of the mosquito and comes to lie between the external border of the epithelial cell and peritrophic membrane.

Here it develops into **oocyst**. It is rounded, 6–12 μm in diameter with a single vesicular nucleus. It

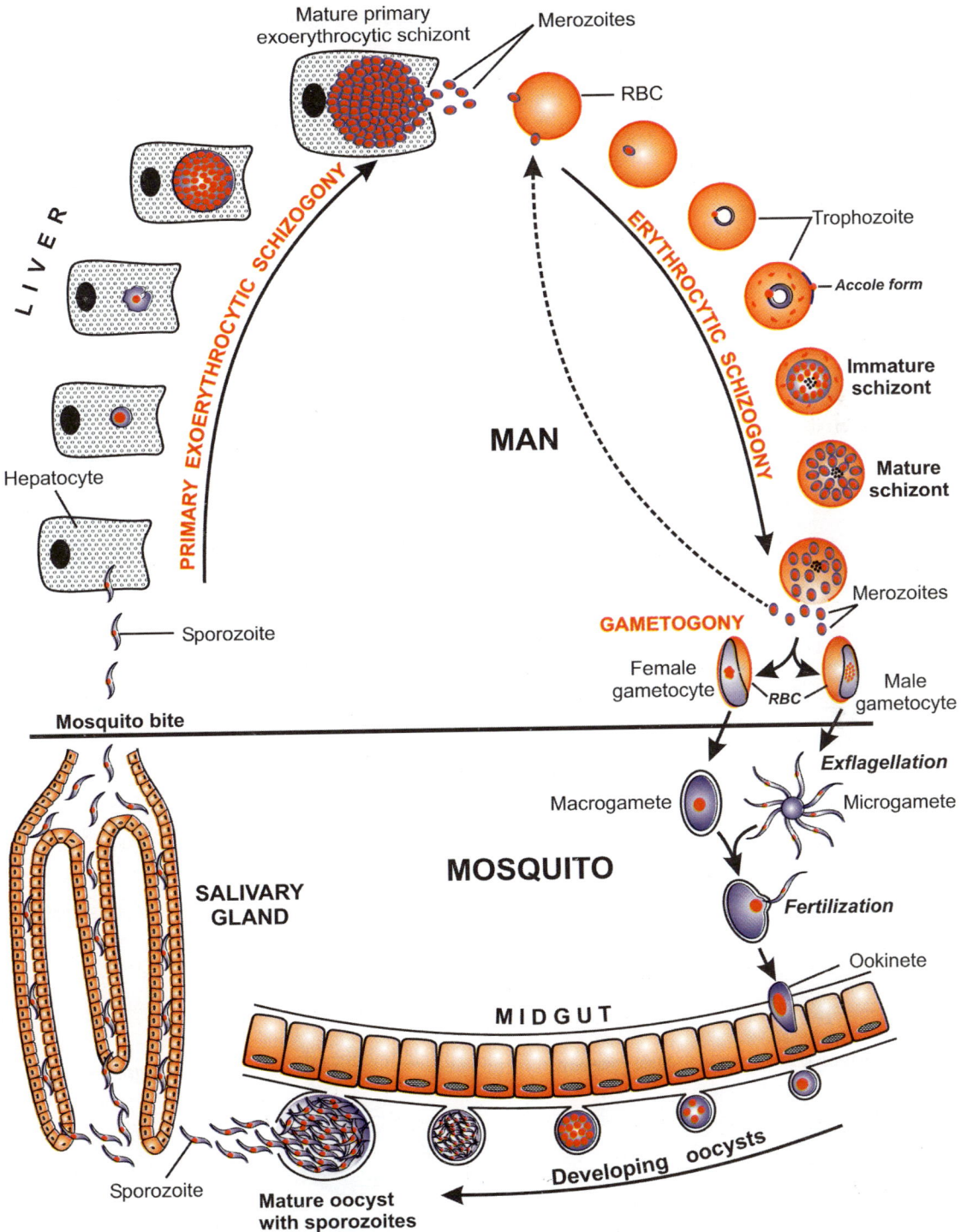

Fig. 34.11. Life cycle of malaria parasite.

Plasmodium vivax

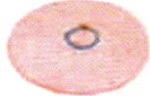

Early trophozoite
(Ring stage)

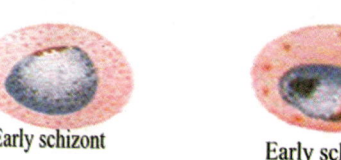

Late trophozoite with
Schuffner's dots

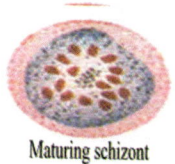

Amoeboid form with
Schuffner's dots

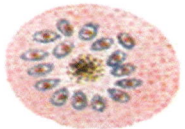

Early schizont

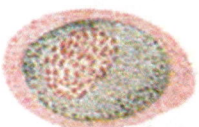

Maturing schizont

Mature schizont

Male gametocyte

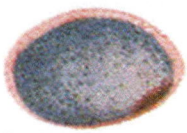

Fenale gametocyte

Plasmodium falciparum

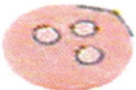

Early trophozoite
(Ring stage)

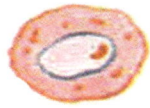

Multiple infections
with accolé form

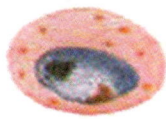

Ring with Maurer's dots

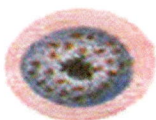

Early schizont

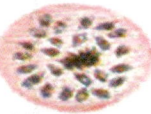

Maturing schizont

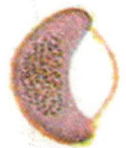

Mature schizont

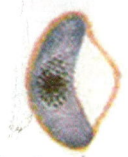

Male gametocyte

Female gametocyte

Plasmodium malariae

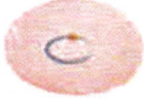

Early trophozoite
(Ring stage)

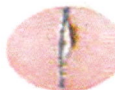

Band form

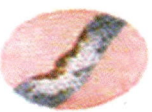

Band form

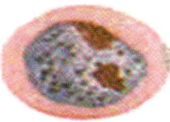

Early schizont

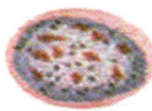

Maturing schizont

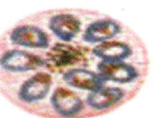

Mature schizont

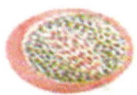

Male gametocyte

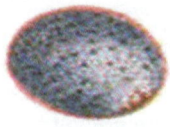

Female gametocyte

Plasmodium ovale

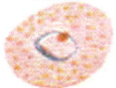

Early trophozoite (Ring stage)
with Schuffner's dots

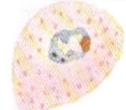

Early trophozoite
(enlarged RBC)

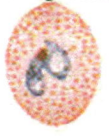

Slightly amoeboid

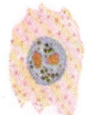

Early schizont

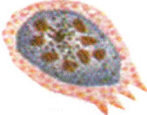

Maturing schizont

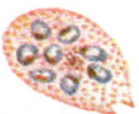

Mature schizont

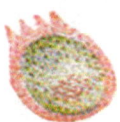

Male gametocyte

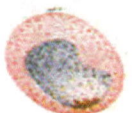

Female gametocyte

Fig. 34.12. Morphological forms of malaria parasites.

Table 34.4. Differential characters of erythrocytic phase of plasmodia of man

	P. vivax	P. falciparum	P. malariae	P. ovale
1. Forms in peripheral blood	Trophozoites, schizonts and gametocytes.	Rings and crescents (gametocytes).	Trophozoites, schizonts and gametocytes.	Trophozoites, schizonts and gametocytes.
2. Early trophozoite or ring stage	Large, 2.5 μm in diameter, usually one prominent chromatin dot, sometimes two, cytoplasm opposite the chromatin dot thicker, usually one and occasionally two rings in one red blood cell.	Small, delicate, 1.25–1.5 μm in diameter, often with two chromatin dots, two rings in one red blood cell are common. Some parasites lie along the red cell membrane. These are known as accolé forms.	Similar to that of *P. vivax*.	Similar to that of *P. vivax*.
3. Late trophozoite	Large, markedly amoeboid, prominent vacuole.	Medium-sized, compact and rounded.	Small, compact, band-shaped, slightly amoeboid, vacuole disappears early.	Slightly amoeboid.
4. Schizont	Large, 9–10 μm in diameter, almost fills an enlarged red cell.	Small, 4.5–5.0 μm in diameter, fills two-thirds of normal-sized red blood cell which is not enlarged.	Small, 6.5–7.0 μm in diameter, almost fills a normal-sized red blood cell.	Small, 6.2 μm in diameter, fills about three quarters of slightly enlarged red blood cell.
5. Number of merozoites	14–24	14–32	6–12	6–12
6. Microgametocytes	Spherical, 9–10 μm in diameter, compact, no vacuole, diffuse chromatin, cytoplasm stains light blue or reddish.	Crescent-shaped (banana-shaped), 8–10 μm × 2–3 μm, chromatin diffuse.	Similar to that of *P. vivax* but smaller.	Similar to that of *P. vivax* but smaller.
7. Macrogametocytes	Spherical, 10–12 μm in diameter, compact, larger than microgametocyte, compact chromatin, cytoplasm stains dark blue.	Crescent-shaped, longer and more slender, 10–12 μm × 2–3 μm, chromatin compact, cytoplasm stains dark blue.	Similar to that of *P. vivax* but smaller.	Similar to that of *P. vivax* but smaller.
8. Malaria pigment	Yellowish-brown; fine granules	Dark brown; one or two solid blocks	Dark brown coarse granules	Dark yellowish-brown, coarser than those of *P. vivax*
9. Age of red blood cells invaded	Young	All ages (young and old)	Old	Young
10. Alterations in infected red cell	Enlarged, pale and the portion of the cytoplasm not occupied by the parasite shows a dotted or stippled appearance, called Schuffner's dots. With Leishman stain they appear as fine pink granules.	Normal size and possesses 6–12 Maurer's dots which stain brick-red with Leishman stain.	Normal size and occasionally show fine stippling (Ziemann's dots) on prolonged staining.	Enlarged, pale, James' dots resembling Schuffner's dots appear early and infected cell may be oval.
11. Duration of erythrocytic schizogony	48 hours	36–48 hours	72 hours	48 hours
12. Presence of secondary exoerythrocytic cycle	Yes	No	No	Yes

increases in size from 6 to 60 μm in diameter. Inside this develop sporozoites. The number of sporozoites in each oocyst varies from a few hundreds to a few thousands and number of oocysts in the stomach wall varies from a few to more than a hundred. On about 10th day the oocyst is fully mature, ruptures and releases sporozoites in the body cavity of the mosquito. Through the body fluid the sporozoites are distributed to various organs of the body except the ovaries. They have special predilection for salivary glands and ultimately reach in maximum numbers in the salivary ducts. At this stage the mosquito is capable of transmitting infection to man.

Pathogenicity

Man develops infection by the bite of infected female anopheles mosquito. However, infection may also be transmitted by:

1. Transfusion of blood from a patient of malaria. This is known as **transfusion malaria**. Plasmodia can remain viable in refrigerated blood for up to 10 days.
2. Transmission of infection to foetus in utero through some placental defect. This is known as **congenital malaria**.
3. By the use of contaminated syringes particularly in drug addicts. This is known as **"mainline" malaria**.

The above conditions are also known as **trophozoite-induced malaria**. In this condition there is no primary and secondary exoerythrocytic schizogony, incubation period is short and there is no relapse.

After an incubation period of 12 days for *P. falciparum*, 13–17 days for *P. vivax* and *P. ovale*, and 28–30 days for *P. malariae* patient develops malaria. The typical picture of malaria consists of febrile paroxysm, anaemia and splenomegaly.

1. Febrile paroxysm

It generally begins in the early afternoon and comprises of three successive stages – cold stage, hot stage and sweating stage. In the cold stage, lasting for 15–60 minutes, the patient experiences intense cold and shivering. This is followed by hot stage, lasting for 2–6 hours, when the patient feels intense hot. Patient develops high fever (40.0–40.6°C), severe headache, nausea and vomiting. Thereafter, fever ends by crisis accompanied by profuse sweating.

The periodicity of the attack varies with the species of the infecting parasite. The periodicity is 48 hours in *P. vivax* (**benign tertian**) and *P. ovale* (**ovale tertian**), and 72 hour in *P. malariae* (**quartan**). However, with *P. falciparum*, the cycles of different broods of parasite do not become synchronized as they do in other species. Therefore, typical tertian fever is not usual in falciparum (**malignant tertian**) malaria. **Quotidian periodicity** with the fever occurring at 24 hour intervals may be due to two broods of tertian parasites maturing on successive days or due to mixed infection.

Mixed infection with more than one species of *Plasmodium* is more common than previously suspected. Febrile paroxysms follow the completion of erythrocytic schizogony when the mature schizont ruptures releasing merozoites, malaria pigment and other parasitic debris. Macrophages and polymorphs phagocytose these and release endogenous pyrogens leading to pyrexia. Exoerythrocytic schizogony and gametogony do not contribute to clinical illness.

2. Anaemia

After a few paroxysms, anaemia of a microcytic or a normocytic hypochromic type develops as a result of:

- Direct RBC lysis as a result of life cycle of the parasite.
- Splenic removal of both infected and uninfected RBCs (coated with immune complexes).
- Autoimmune lysis of coated infected and uninfected RBCs.
- Decreased incorporation of iron into haem.
- Increased fragility of RBCs.
- Decreased RBC production from bone marrow suppression.

3. Splenomegaly

After some paroxysms spleen gets enlarged and becomes palpable. Splenomegaly is due to massive proliferation of macrophages which phagocytose both parasitized and non-parasitized red blood cells.

P. falciparum **is the most pathogenic of the human *Plasmodium* species.** It causes a high level of parasitaemia with parasite density exceeding 250,000–300,000/μl of blood. Nearly 30–40% of the red blood cells may be parasitized. In contrast to other *Plasmodium* species, it invades erythrocytes of all ages (young and old).

Erythrocytic schizogony in *P. falciparum* takes place in the capillaries of the internal organs (spleen, bone marrow, brain, kidney, intestine, heart and placenta). **Membrane protuberances (knobs)** appear on the surface of the infected red blood cells. These mediate attachment of parasitized red blood cells to one another and to the lining of capillaries and venules as the parasites (except gametocytes) grow older. Therefore, only young rings and gameto-cytes are typically found in the peripheral blood film of the patient with falciparum malaria.

The characteristic lesions of falciparum malaria are due to blockade of small vessels by **sticky para-sitized erythrocytes**. This leads to tissue hypoxia.

Pernicious malaria

Pernicious malaria is a complex of **life-threatening complications** that sometimes supervene in acute falciparum malaria. It is due to heavy parasitization and is of three types:

1. Cerebral malaria

Cerebral malaria is a severe complication of falci-parum malaria and frequently leads to death, even when appropriate therapy has been given. It is characterized by hyperpyrexia, coma and paralysis. Brain is congested. Capillaries of the brain are plugged with parasitized red blood cells, each cell containing malaria pigment.

2. Algid malaria

It resembles surgical shock with cold clammy skin, peripheral circulatory failure and profound shock. Patient may also develop vomiting and diarrhoea or dysentery.

3. Septicaemic malaria

It is characterized by a high degree of prostration, there is high continuous fever with involvement of various organs.

Blackwater fever

It is a manifestation of repeated infections with *P. falciparum* which were inadequately treated with quinine. Sometimes resumption of quinine therapy for new attack is followed by massive destruction of RBCs, fever, haemoglobinuria and renal failure.

The exact mechanism of haemolysis in black-water fever is not known. An **autoimmune mechanism** has been suggested. Parasitized and quininized red blood cells, during previous infection, act as antigen against which antibodies are formed. With subsequent infection and treatment with quinine, there is massive destruction of both infected and uninfected red blood cells. As other antimalarials have replaced quinine, blackwater fever has now become rare.

Host immunity

Immunity in malaria is of two types:

1. Innate immunity

This refers to inherent, non-immune mechanisms of host defence against malaria. This is due to age of red blood cells, nature of haemoglobin, enzyme content of red blood cells and presence or absence of certain factors:

Age of red blood cells

P. falciparum infects both young and old red blood cells while *P. vivax* and *P. ovale* infect only young erythrocytes, and *P. malariae* only old erythrocytes.

Nature of haemoglobin

Presence of abnormal haemoglobin like thalassaemia haemoglobin and foetal haemoglobin confers resistance against all *Plasmodium* spp., while sickle cell anaemia trait and haemoglobin E protect against *P. falciparum* and *P. vivax*, respectively.

Enzyme content of red blood cells

A genetic deficiency known as glucose-6-phosphate dehydrogenase (G6PD) trait confers some protection against *P. falciparum* infection. This enzyme is essential for respiratory process of the parasite.

Presence or absence of certain factors

The presence of the Duffy factor increases the

susceptibility to malaria. It is believed that Duffy factor present on the surface of erythrocytes act as receptors for attachment of malaria parasite.

2. Acquired immunity

Acquired immunity in malaria involves both humoral and cellular immunity. Antibodies against sporozoites and asexual and sexual blood stages develop in malaria patients. Antibodies (IgM, IgG and IgA) against asexual blood stages may protect by inhibiting red cell invasion and antibodies against sexual stages are believed to reduce malaria transmission.

A variety of cellular mechanisms may play a role in conferring protection against malaria. These include natural killer activity and activated macrophages. The latter phagocytose and induce extracellular killing of target cells. T cells are crucial for malaria immunity. Their major function seems to be to provide help for the production of antibodies and to activate macrophages.

Immunity produced following infection with malaria parasites is species-specific, stage-specific and strain-specific and the immunity lasts only till original infection remains active. This is known as **concomitant immunity** (previously called **premunition** or **infection immunity**).

Malaria parasites like many other microorganisms, are capable of periodically changing the expression of their antigens. This provides the parasite with a powerful means for evading host immunity. The ability of *P. falciparum* to remain sequestrated by cytoadherence to the capillary lining of certain tissues is regarded as a selective advantage as such parasites can avoid frequent passage through spleen and thus exposure to immune effector mechanisms. Sequestration does not exist in other human malaria parasites and this is considered the main reason for the difference in disease severity.

Laboratory diagnosis

Malaria is one of the few parasitic infections considered to be **immediately life-threatening**, and a patient with diagnosis of *P. falciparum* malaria should be considered a medical emergency because the disease can be rapidly fatal.

1. Microscopy

Diagnosis of malaria can be established by demonstration of malaria parasites in the blood. Thick and thin smears of the blood are prepared on the same or different slides. Blood is taken by pricking a finger or ear lobule before starting treatment with antimalarials. For preparation of thick smear take a large drop of blood on the slide. Spread it in an area of 1 cm square. Dehaemoglobinization of thick smear is done by keeping the slide in distilled water in Koplin's jar in vertical position for 5–10 minutes till the slide becomes white and then it is dried in air. Both thick and thin smears are stained with Leishman stain. The smears are then examined under oil-immersion lens.

The parasites are most abundant in peripheral blood late in the febrile paroxysm (a few hours after the height of paroxysm). Therefore, blood for smear should be collected at this period. All asexual erythrocytic stages, as well as gametocytes can be seen in peripheral blood in infection with *P. vivax*, *P. malariae* and *P. ovale*, but in *P. falciparum* infection, only the ring forms and crescent-shaped gametocytes can be seen. Late trophozoite and schizont stages of *P. falciparum* are usually confined to the internal organs and appear in peripheral blood only in severe or pernicious malaria.

The occurrence of **multiple rings** in an individual red blood cell with **accolé forms** is diagnostic of *P. falciparum* infection. Malaria pigments may be demonstrated inside the monocytes and polymorphonuclear leucocytes. The presence of malaria pigments only, in the absence of malaria parasites, suggests *P. falciparum* infection. Schuffner's dots, in the red blood cells, can be seen in case of *P. vivax* and *P. ovale* infection, while Maurer's dots and Ziemann's dots are seen in case of *P. falciparum* and *P. malariae* infection, respectively. Red blood cells are enlarged in *P. vivax* infection.

Thin film is examined first and if parasites are found, there is no need for examining the thick film. If parasites are not seen in thin film in a few minutes the thick film should be examined. If parasites are seen in thick film but identity is not clear, the thin film is re-examined more thoroughly to determine the identity of the species. **The parasites are more** along the upper and lower margins of the "tail" of the film. Examination of thin film usually takes 15–20 minutes (≥ 300 oil-immersion fields), and examination of thick film usually requires 5–10 minutes (approximately 100 oil-immersion fields), before the smears are considered negative.

2. Other techniques

Malaria parasites in the peripheral blood may also be identified by quantitative buffy coat test, detection of antigens in lysed blood and polymerase chain reaction.

Treatment

Chloroquine was the standard treatment for acute malaria for many years. However, **resistance to this drug in *P. falciparum* is widespread**. Less commonly *P. vivax* may also be chloroquine-resistant. **Quinine is the most reliable alternative to chloroquine** for the treatment of malaria caused by chloroquine-resistant strains. Tetracycline and clindamycin exhibit some antimalarial activity and are used as an adjunct to quinine therapy. **Mefloquine** and **halofantrine** are also active against chloroquine-resistant strains, but resistance to these drugs has also been reported.

   Chloroquine and quinine do not eliminate exo-erythrocytic parasites in the liver. For this **primaquine** (8-aminoquinoline drug) should be used. However, this drug may precipitate haemolysis in individuals who are deficient in the enzyme glucose-6-phosphate dehydrogenase.

HELMINTHS

Medical helminthology deals with the study of helminths (parasitic worms). Most helminths are truly parasitic because they have no independent existence outside the host. Pathogenic manifestations of helminthic disease are due to the location of the worms, their size and life style. Helminths are divided into two major groups – nematodes or round worms and platyhelminths or flat worms. The latter are further divided into trematodes (flukes) and cestodes (tapeworms). Common helminths of man are given in Table 34.5.

Table 34.5. Common helminths of man

Species	Common name
Nematodes	
• *Enterobius vermicularis*	Threadworm
• *Ascaris lumbricoides*	Common roundworm
• *Ancylostoma duodenale*	Old world hookworm
• *Necator americanus*	New world hookworm
• *Wuchereria bancrofti*	Bancroft's filaria
Cestodes	
• *Echinococcus granulosus*	Dog tapeworm
• *Taenia solium*	Pork tapeworm
• *Taenia saginata*	Beef tapeworm

ENTEROBIUS VERMICULARIS

Enterobius vermicularis infects children throughout the world. The adult worms live in caecum, vermiform appendix and adjacent portions of ascending colon.

Morphology

Adult worms

These are small, white, spindle-shaped and resemble short pieces of thread. At the anterior end, both male and female worms possess a pair of wing-like expansions, known as **cervical alae**. The male measures 2–4 mm in length and 0.1–0.2 mm in breadth. The posterior one third of the body is curved. The female is longer, 8–12 mm in length and 0.3–0.5 mm in width. Its posterior one third is straight and drawn out into a thin pointed pin-like tail (Fig. 34.13).

Eggs

The eggs are colourless, non-bile stained and flattened on one side (planoconvex). They measure 60 μm in length and 30 μm in width. They are surrounded by a transparent shell and usually contain fully developed larvae (Figs. 34.13 and 34.14). **They float in saturated solution of common salt.**

Life cycle

Of all the intestinal worms, it has the simplest life cycle (Fig. 34.13). It is completed in a **single host**. The adult worms live in caecum, appendix and adjacent portions of ascending colon. Male fertilizes

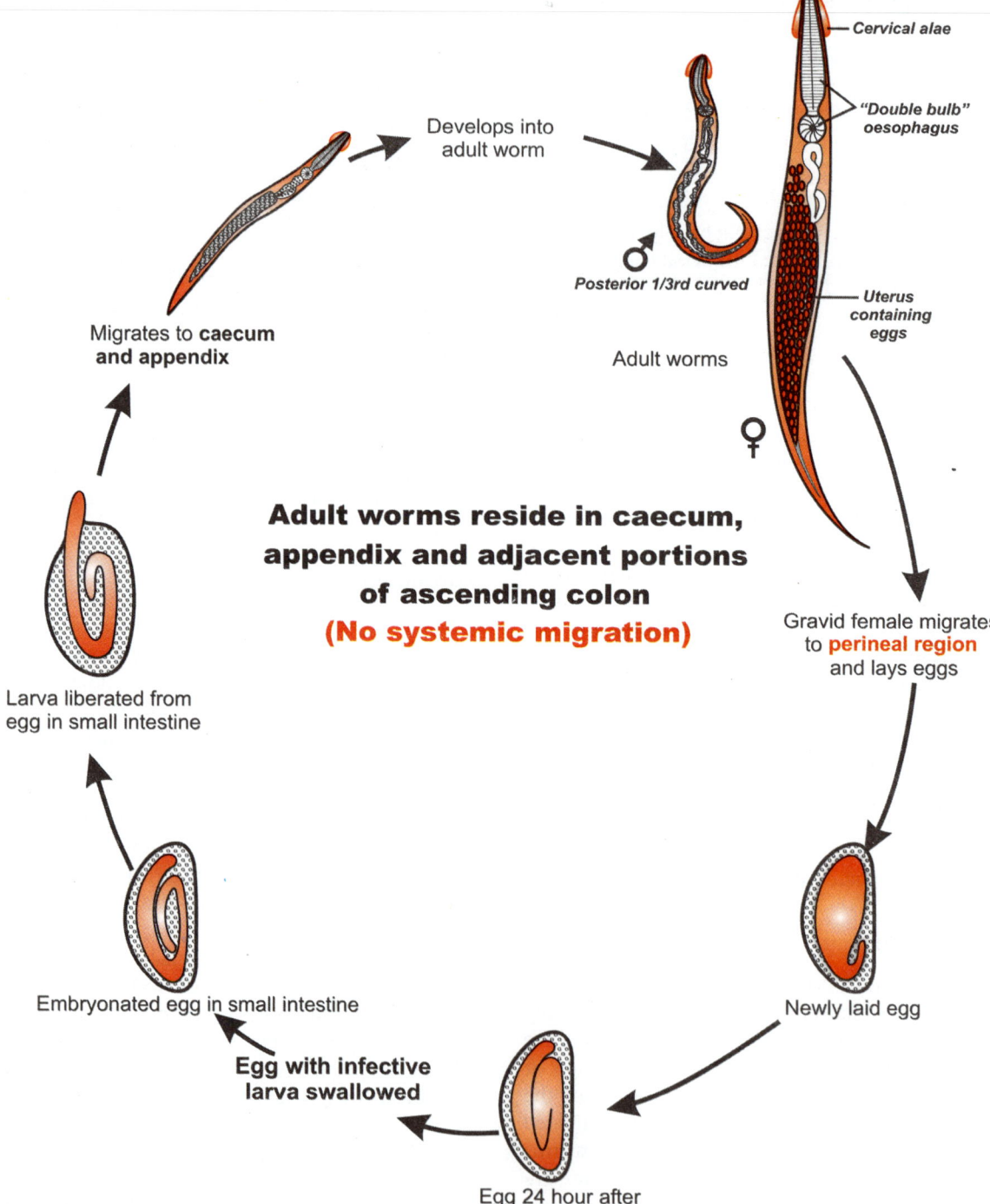

Develops into
adult worm

Cervical alae

"Double bulb"
oesophagus

Posterior 1/3rd curved

♂

Adult worms

Uterus
containing
eggs

Migrates to **caecum
and appendix**

♀

**Adult worms reside in caecum,
appendix and adjacent portions
of ascending colon
(No systemic migration)**

Gravid female migrates
to **perineal region**
and lays eggs

Larva liberated from
egg in small intestine

Embryonated egg in small intestine

Newly laid egg

**Egg with infective
larva swallowed**

Egg 24 hour after

Fig. 34.13. Life cycle of *Enterobius vermicularis*.

female and dies, and is excreted in faeces. The gravid female migrates down the colon to the rectum. At night, when the host is in bed, it comes out of the anus. It then crawls on the perianal and perineal skin and deposits the eggs. Crawling of the gravid female worm leads to intense pruritis and the patient scratches the affected part.

Such patients have eggs of *E. vermicularis* on the fingers and under the nails. These individuals may develop autoinfection by direct anus-to-mouth transfer by finger contamination. Persons handling night clothes and bed linen of infected patients can also contract infection. Infection may also be acquired from contaminated objects like door knobs, table tops, etc. Airborne eggs that are dislodged from bed linens and clothes may get into mouth and swallowed.

The larvae, from embryonated eggs, hatch out in the small intestine. They then migrate to the caecum and vermiform appendix and develop into adult worms. Eggs laid on perianal skin may immediately hatch into infective-stage larvae and may ascend through anus to develop into adolescent worms in the caecum and vermiform appendix.

After laying eggs on the perianal and perineal skin the worm may retreat into the anal canal and come out again to lay more eggs. The worm may also wander into the vulva, vagina, uterus, fallopian tubes and peritoneum.

Pathogenicity

It causes nocturnal perianal and perineal pruritis. It may also lead to appendicitis, vulvovaginitis and salpingitis.

Laboratory diagnosis

Detection of adult worms

The adult worms may be noticed by the patient or by the parents of the patient at the time of commencement of pruritis. They may be recovered in the stools after administration of a purgative or in the vermiform appendix during appendicectomy.

Demonstration of eggs

Since eggs are not discharged by the worm into faeces, therefore, faecal examination is not useful in the laboratory diagnosis of threadworm infection.

However, in a small proportion of patients stool examination may show the presence of eggs of *E. vermicularis* (Fig. 34.14).

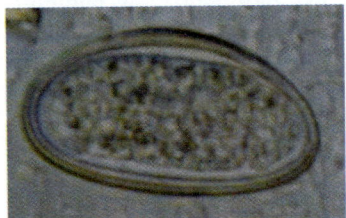

Fig. 34.14. Egg of *Enterobius vermicularis*.

Eggs which are deposited in large numbers on the perianal and perineal skin at night can be demonstrated by scraping these areas with NIH (National Institute of Health) swab (Fig. 34.15) in the morning before the child goes to toilet and takes bath. NIH swab consists of a glass rod at one end of which a piece of transparent cellophane (with sticky surface out) is wrapped and held in place with a rubber band. The other end of the glass rod is fixed in a rubber stopper and kept in a test tube. The cellophane part is used for swabbing by rolling over the perianal and perineal area. Then the cellophane is detached, spread over glass slide and examined microscopically. This procedure should be repeated on three successive days. Eggs may also be recovered from under the fingernails and the washings from garments.

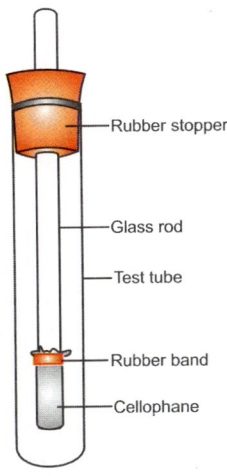

Fig. 34.15. NIH swab

ASCARIS LUMBRICOIDES

Ascaris lumbricoides, the common roundworm, has worldwide distribution. Adult worm resides in the small intestine, particularly the jejunum of man. It resembles an ordinary earthworm and is **the largest intestinal nematode parasitizing man**.

Morphology

Adult worm

It is elongated and cylindrical in shape with both ends tapering. The mouth opens at the anterior end. It possesses three finely toothed lips – one dorsal and two ventral. The digestive and respiratory organs of the worm float inside the body cavity possessing a **toxic fluid known as ascaron**. Allergic reactions seen in infected individuals are due to this toxin.

Male worm

It measures 15–30 cm in length and 3–4 mm in diameter. The posterior end is curved ventrally to form a hook. The ejaculatory duct along with the anus open into the cloaca from which arise a pair of copulatory spicules of equal size (Fig. 34.16).

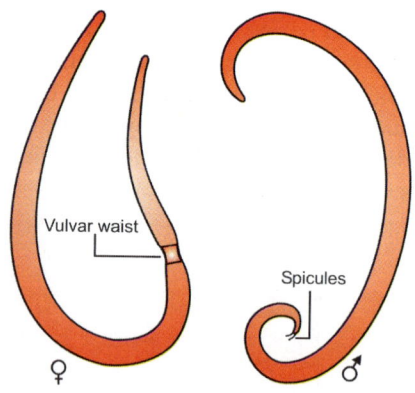

Fig. 34.16. Adult worms of *Ascaris lumbricoides*.

Female worm

It is longer and stouter than the male worm and measure 25–40 cm in length and 5 mm in diameter. The tail is straight and conical. The anus is sub-terminal and opens on the ventral surface in the form of a transverse slit. The vulva opens at the junction of anterior and middle one third of the body on the midventral part of the worm. This part of the worm

is narrow and is known as **vulvar waist** (Fig. 34.16). A mature female *A. lumbricoides* lays enormous number of eggs (nearly 200,000 eggs daily) which are passed in the faeces. Eggs are of two types:

Fertilized eggs

The fertilized eggs are round or oval in shape and measure 60–75 µm in length and 40–50 µm in breadth (Fig. 34.17). They are bile-stained and brown in colour. They are surrounded by a thick, transparent shell, consisting of a relatively nonpermeable innermost lipoidal vitelline membrane, a thick transparent middle layer and an outermost coarsely mammillated albuminoid layer. Outer mammillated coat is sometimes lost. Such eggs are called **decorticated eggs**. They contain a large conspicuous unsegmented ovum with **a clear crescentic area at each pole. Fertilized eggs float in saturated solution of common salt.**

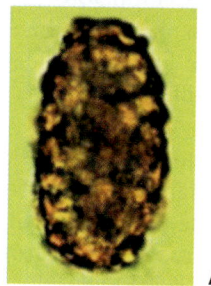 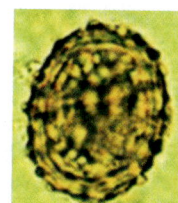

Fig. 34.17. Unfertilized (A) and fertilized (B) eggs of *Ascaris lumbricoides*.

Unfertilized eggs

In the absence of a male worm, the female produces unfertilized (infertile) eggs. These are narrower and longer and measure 90 µm in length and 55 µm in breadth (Fig. 34.17). They are bile-stained and brown in colour. They have a small atrophied ovum and a thin shell within an irregular coating of albumin. The innermost lipoidal vitelline membrane of the shell is absent. The unfertilized eggs are heaviest of all the helminthic eggs, therefore, they **do not float in saturated solution of common salt**.

Life cycle (Fig. 34.18)

The life cycle of *A. lumbricoides* is passed **in only one host, man**. No intermediate host is required.

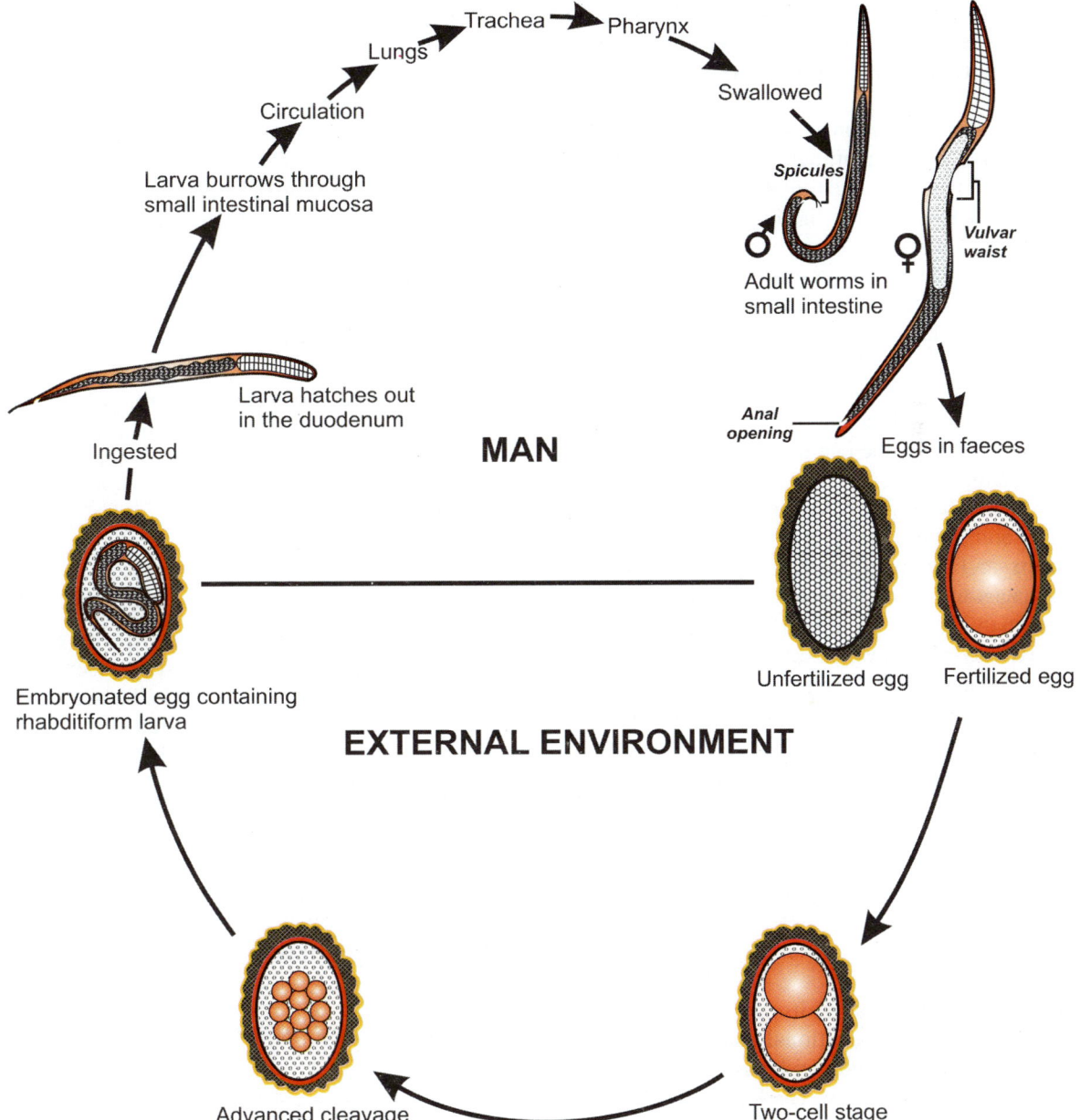

Fig. 34.18. Life cycle of *Ascaris lumbricoides*.

Adult worms reside in the small intestine, particularly the jejunum of man. Fertilized eggs containing unsegmented ova are passed in the faeces. However, they are not immediately infective to man. They have to undergo a period of incubation in soil before acquiring infectivity. Depending on the temperature and humidity, a **rhabditiform larva** develops from the unsegmented ovum and undergoes first moulting within the egg shell in 10–40 days. The optimum temperature and humidity for the development of the larva within the egg shell is 20–40°C and more than 40%, respectively. **The embryonated eggs containing rhabditiform larvae are pathogenic to man.**

Man acquires infection by ingestion of food, water or raw vegetable contaminated with embryonated eggs. In the small intestine (duodenum) rhabditiform larvae are hatched out of the ingested eggs. These larvae then burrow their way through the mucous membrane of the small intestine and are carried by the portal circulation to the liver, where they reside for 3–4 days. They then pass via hepatic vein, inferior vena cava, right heart and pulmonary artery and reach the lungs. Here they grow in size and moult twice (first on 5th day and second on 10th day). The larvae then break through the capillary wall and reach the lung alveoli.

From the alveoli, the larvae migrate up the bronchi, trachea and larynx, crawl over the epiglottis to the pharynx and are swallowed. They pass down the oesophagus and stomach and localize in the upper part of the small intestine, their normal abode. On twenty-fifth to twenty-ninth day of infection, the larvae undergo another moulting and transform into **adult worms**. In about 6–10 weeks they become sexually mature and by 12 weeks the gravid females begin to discharge eggs in the stool and the cycle is repeated.

Pathogenicity

Disease produced by *A. lumbricoides* is known as **ascariasis** and is caused by both adult worms and migrating larvae.

Pathogenicity of adult worms

1. By robbing the host of its nutrition, the adult worms affect the nutritional status of the host leading to **malnutrition and night blindness** due to vitamin A deficiency. The long-term effect of the malnutrition caused by ascariasis is **retardation of growth.**
2. The presence of adult worms in the intestine may also lead to intermittent colicky cramps and loss of appetite. In heavy infection, adult worms may cause **obstruction of the intestinal tract.**
3. **The worms are restless wanders.** They tend to probe and insinuate themselves into any aperture

they find on the way. They may crawl out of mouth or may enter the nasal meatus via nasopharynx and pass out of a naris. From the oropharynx, the worm may enter a eustachian tube and penetrate to the middle ear and through the tympanic membrane to external auditory meatus. The worm may also enter into the trachea leading to **respiratory obstruction**. The worms may migrate downwards and lodge in appendix, bile duct and pancreatic duct leading to appendicitis, obstructive jaundice and acute haemorrhagic pancreatitis, respectively. They may perforate the intestinal wall weakened by ulcers or gangrene.

4. Release of toxic body fluid (ascaron) of the adult worm in the body of the patient may lead to various **allergic manifestations** such as fever, urticaria, angioneurotic oedema, wheezing and conjunctivitis.

Pathogenicity of migrating larvae

In persons repeatedly infected with *Ascaris* and sensitized to the parasite antigens, the migrating larvae may lead to inflammatory and hypersensitivity reactions in the lungs. There is formation of granuloma and eosinophilic infiltrates. It leads to fever, cough, dyspnoea, urticarial rash and eosinophilia. The sputum may be blood-tinged and may contain *Ascaris* larvae and Charcot-Leyden crystals. This condition is known as **Loeffler's syndrome.** Allergic inflammatory reaction to migrating larvae may involve other organs such as liver and kidneys.

Laboratory diagnosis

Parasitic diagnosis

Diagnosis of *A. lumbricoides* infection can be made by:

1. Demonstration of adult worms

Worm may be passed through anus, mouth, nose and rarely through ear. Barium meal may occasionally reveal the presence of adult worms in the small intestine.

2. Demonstration of larvae

Ascaris larvae may be detected in the sputum during the stage of migration.

3. Demonstration of both fertilized and unfertilized eggs

These may be detected by direct microscopy or concentration of the faeces by salt floatation or formol-ether concentration method. However, eggs may not be seen if only male worms are present.

Serodiagnosis

Ascaris antibody can be detected by indirect haem-agglutination (IHA) and immunofluorescence antibody (IFA) test. These tests are useful for the diagnosis of extra-intestinal ascariasis like Loeffler's syndrome.

Visceral larva migrans

Visceral larva migrans (VLM) is a syndrome caused by ingestion of embryonated eggs of nematodes of animals like *Toxocara canis* (dog roundworm) and *T. cati* (cat roundworm). These eggs are usually found in soil contaminated by dog or cat faeces. Larvae hatch in the small intestine and immediately penetrate the intestinal wall and migrate to liver. They may move onto the lungs or to other parts of the body or remain in the liver. Occasionally, the larvae reach the eye and cause serious retinal lesions. Several other roundworms, including *Angiostrongylus*, *Gnathostoma* and *Anisakis* species are occasionally implicated in visceral larva migrans.

Wherever the larvae settle, they are attacked by phagocytic cells, consisting mainly of eosinophils, histiocytes and occasionally giant cells leading to the formation of a granulomatous lesion and their progress is arrested. From lungs, like *A. lumbricoides*, they may even migrate through trachea and oesophagus and reach small intestine but, in the human body, they do not convert into adult worms.

Visceral larva migrans is characterized by hyper-eosinophilia (15–80%) together with hepatomegaly or pneumonitis or both, hypergammaglobulinaemia and fever. The larvae may invade the eye producing an **eosinophilic granulomatous reaction**, usually in the retina, and lead to **endophthalmitis**.

Visceral larva migrans can be diagnosed by IHA and IFA test, and by identification of larvae in biopsy or autopsy specimens.

HUMAN HOOKWORMS

Human hookworms, *Ancylostoma duodenale* and *Necator americanus*, are common throughout the tropics and subtropics. Adult worms reside in small intestine mostly in jejunum, sometimes in duodenum and rarely in ileum.

ANCYLOSTOMA DUODENALE

Morphology

Adult worms

They are small, pinkish and fusiform in shape (Fig. 34.19). The anterior end is curved dorsally, hence the name hookworm. This curve is in the same direction as the general body curvature. The oral cavity is provided with four hook-like teeth on ventral surface and two knob-like teeth on dorsal surface (Fig. 34.20). The differences between male and female *A. duodenale* are given in Table 34.6. Owing to the position of genital openings of male and female worms they assume a Y-shaped figure during copulation.

Table 34.6. Differences between male and female *A. duodenale*

	Male	Female
Size	8 mm	12.5 mm
Posterior end	Expanded in an umbrella-like fashion. This is known as copulatory bursa.	Tapering
Genital opening	Opens posteriorly with cloaca.	Opens at the junction of posterior and middle third of the body.

Copulatory bursa

Copulatory bursa is present in the male worm for attachment with the female during copulation. This consists of three lobes. These lobes are supported by 13 chitinous rays, five each in lateral lobes and three in dorsal lobe (Fig. 34.20).

Eggs

Eggs are oval measuring 60 µm in length and 40 µm in width. They are colourless (not bile-stained) and

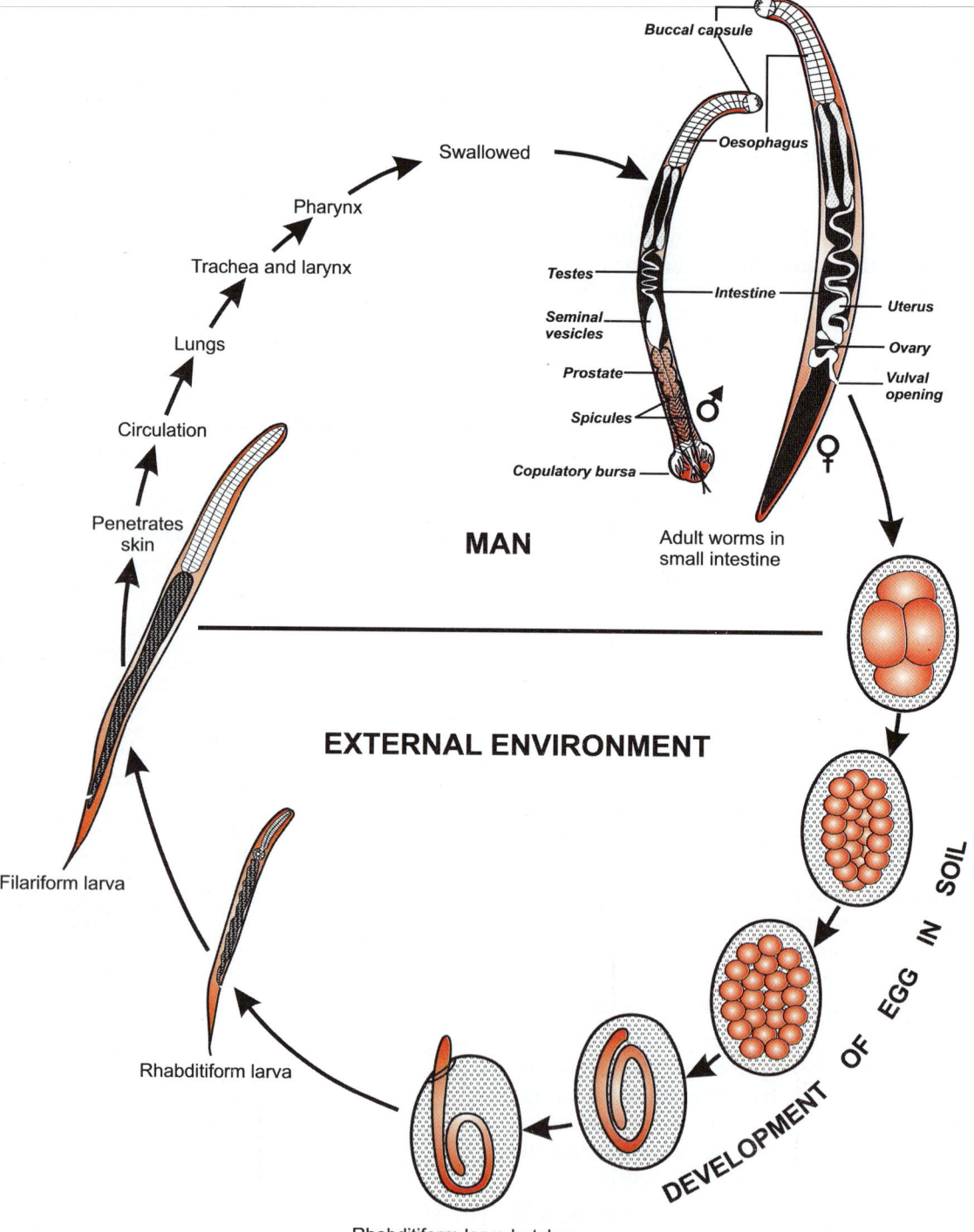

Fig. 34.19. Life cycle of *Ancyclostoma duodenale*.

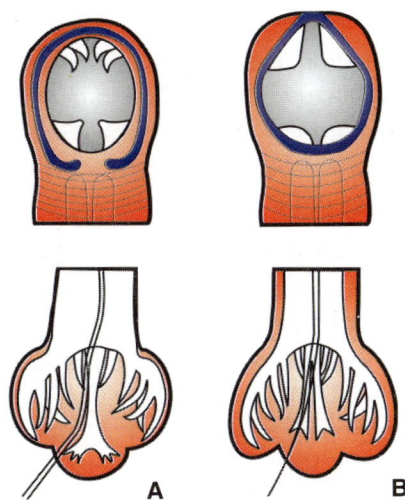

Fig. 34.20. Buccal capsule and copulatory bursa of (A) *Ancylostoma duodenale*, and (B) *Necator americanus*.

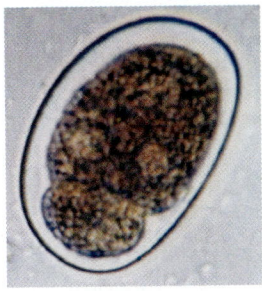

Fig. 34.21. Egg of *Ancylostoma duodenale*.

are surrounded by a thin transparent hyaline shell. They possess a segmented ovum with usually four blastomeres. **There is a clear space between the segmented ovum and the egg shell** (Figs. 34.19 and 34.21). **The eggs float in saturated salt solution.**

Life cycle (Fig. 34.19)

Man is the only host. No intermediate host is required. Adult worms inhabit the small intestine of man attaching themselves to the mucous membrane by means of their mouthparts. The eggs containing segmented ova are passed out in the faeces of infected person. In the warm and moist soil, **rhabditiform larva** hatches out from the egg in 24–48 hours. The rhabditiform larva moults twice on the third and fifth day and develops into a **filariform larva**. This is

capable of penetrating unbroken skin and is the **infective stage of the parasite**.

When a person walks barefooted on soil containing the filariform larvae they penetrate the skin, particularly the skin between the toes, the dorsum of the foot and the medial aspect of the sole. In farm workers the larvae may penetrate the skin of the hands. On reaching the subcutaneous tissue the larvae enter into the lymphatics or small venules and begin a migratory phase similar to that of *Ascaris*. Through lymph-vascular system they enter into venous circulation and are carried via the right heart into the pulmonary capillaries. Here they break through the capillary walls and enter into the alveolar spaces. From alveoli, the larvae migrate up the bronchi, trachea and larynx, crawl over the epiglottis to the pharynx and are swallowed.

During migration or on reaching oesophagus they undergo third moulting. Thereafter they reach small intestine, undergo fourth moulting and develop into **adult worms**. They attach themselves to the mucous membrane of small intestine by means of their mouthparts. In about six weeks, from the time of infection, adult worms become sexually mature. Male fertilizes female and the latter lays eggs which are passed in faeces and the cycle is repeated.

Pathogenicity

Clinical disease in *A. duodenale* infection may be caused by the migrating larvae or adult worms.

Pathogenicity of migrating larvae

Migrating larvae of *A. duodenale* may cause two types of lesions:

1. Ancylostoma dermatitis or ground itch

When filariform larvae enter the skin they may lead to dermatitis. This causes intense itching and burning followed by erythema and oedema of the area which soon develops into papular and vesicular eruptions. This condition is more common with *N. americanus* than with *A. duodenale* infection. It disappears in 1–2 weeks.

2. Pulmonary lesions

When the filariform larvae break through the pulmonary capillaries and enter the alveoli, they may lead to bronchitis and bronchopneumonia. A **marked eosinophilia** occurs at this stage.

Pathogenicity of adult worms

The disease caused by adult worms is responsible for the syndrome commonly referred to as **hookworm disease**. The maturing and adult worms attach themselves to the mucosa of small intestine by means of their mouthparts. Hookworms ingest blood. One adult worm of *A. duodenale* and *N. americanus* sucks 0.2 ml and 0.03 ml of blood daily, respectively. In addition, the worms frequently leave one site and attach themselves to another site leaving behind small bleeding lesions.

As the secretions of the worms contain anticoagulant activity, the bleeding from abandoned sites may continue for some time. These two facts are responsible for microcytic, hypochromic type of iron deficiency anaemia. The degree of anaemia depends on the number of worms, body iron store and dietary iron.

Patient develops epigastric pain, dyspepsia, vomiting and diarrhoea, the stool being reddish or black. Tongue, conjunctiva and skin become pale. Skin, in addition, becomes cold and dry. Hair become dry and lustreless and there is oedema of feet and ankles.

Laboratory diagnosis

Diagnosis of hookworm infection can be established by:

1. Direct methods

- Demonstration of characteristic eggs in the faeces by direct microscopy or by concentration methods.
- Adult worms may also be detected in the stool.
- Aspiration of duodenal contents by Ryle's tube may reveal eggs or the adult worms.

2. Indirect methods

- Blood examination may reveal microcytic, hypochromic anaemia and eosinophilia.
- In many cases of hookworm disease stool examination may show occult blood and Charcot-Leyden crystals.

NECATOR AMERICANUS

Necator americanus adult worms are slightly smaller and thinner than those of *A. duodenale*. Differences between the adult worms of these two human hookworms are given in Table 34.7. The eggs of *N. americanus* are indistinguishable from those of *A. duodenale* and the life cycle, pathogenicity and diagnosis of the former is also similar to that of the latter.

Cutaneous larva migrans

Cutaneous larva migrans (CLM) is a parasitic skin infection caused by hookworm larvae that usually infect cats, dogs and other animals. Humans can be infected with the larvae by walking barefoot on moist soft soil that has been contaminated with animal faeces. It is also known as **creeping eruption** as once

Table 34.7. Differences between the adult worms of *A. duodenale* and *N. americanus*

	A. duodenale	*N. americanus*
Size	Large and thicker	Smaller and thinner
Anterior end	Bends in the same direction as the body curvature	Bends in the opposite direction of the body curvature
Buccal capsule	Six teeth, four hook-like on ventral surface and two knob-like on dorsal surface	Four chitinous plates, two each on ventral and dorsal surface
Number of rays in copulatory bursa	Thirteen	Fourteen
Posterior end of female	A posterior spine is present	No posterior spine is present
Vulval opening	Situated behind the middle of the body	Situated in front of the middle of the body
Pathogenicity	More pathogenic	Less pathogenic

infected, the larvae migrate under the skin's surface and cause itchy red lines or tracks. Many types of hookworm can cause cutaneous larva migrans. It is caused by:

- *Ankylostoma braziliense*: hookworm of wild and domestic dogs and cats
- *Ankylostoma caninum*: dog hookworm found in Australia
- *Uncinaria stenocephala*: dog hookworm found in Europe
- *Bunostomum phlebotomum*: cattle hookworm
- *Gnathostoma* sp.

Occasionally *Ancylostoma duodenale*, *Necator americanus* and *Strongyloides stercoralis* may also cause cutaneous larva migrans.

People of all ages and races, and of both sexes can be affected if they have been exposed to the larvae. It is most commonly found in tropical and subtropical geographic locations. Groups at risk include those with occupations or hobbies that bring them into contact with warm, moist, sandy soil.

Parasite eggs are passed in the faeces of infected animals on warm, moist soil, where the larvae hatch. On contact with human skin, the larvae can penetrate through hair follicles, cracks or even intact skin to infect the human host. Between a few days and a few months after the initial infection, the larvae migrate beneath the skin.

In an animal host the larvae are able to penetrate the deeper layers of the skin (the dermis) and infect the blood and lymphatic system. Once in the intestine they mature sexually and lay more eggs that are then excreted to start the cycle again. However, in a human host, the larvae are unable to penetrate the basement membrane to invade the dermis so the disease remains confined to the outer layers of the skin.

At the site of penetration a non-specific eruption occurs. There may be a tingling or prickling sensation within 30 minutes of the larvae penetrating. The larvae can then either lie dormant for weeks or months or immediately begin creeping activity that create 2–3 mm wide, snake-like tracks stretching 3–4 cm from the penetration site. These are slightly raised, flesh-coloured or pink and cause intense itching. Tracks advance a few millimetres to a few centimetres daily and if many larvae are involved a disorganised series of loops and tortuous tracks may form. Biopsy shows larvae with round cells, particularly eosinophil infiltration.

Sites most commonly affected are the feet, spaces between the toes, hands, knees and buttocks.

The disease is self-limiting. Humans are an accidental and "dead-end" host so the larvae eventually die. The natural duration of the disease varies considerably depending on the species of larvae involved. In most cases, lesions will resolve without treatment within 4–8 weeks.

However, effective treatment is available to shorten the course of the disease. Anthelmintics such as thiabendazole, albendazole, mebendazole and ivermectin are used. Topical thiabendazole is considered the treatment of choice for early, localised lesions. Oral treatment is given when the lesions are widespread or topical treatment has failed. Itching is considerably reduced within 24–48 hours of starting treatment and within 1 week most lesions/tracts resolved.

Any secondary skin infections may require treatment with appropriate antibiotics.

WUCHERERIA BANCROFTI

Wuchereria bancrofti occurs in tropical and subtropical countries. In India, it is distributed along the sea coast and along the banks of big rivers. Adult worms inhabit lymph nodes and lymphatic vessels of man. The microfilariae (embryonic forms) are found in peripheral blood.

Morphology

Adult worms

Adult worms (Fig. 34.22) are transparent, creamy white, long, hair-like structures. They are filiform in shape with both ends tapering. The male and female worms measure 2.5–4 cm × 0.1 mm and 8–10 cm × 0.2–0.3 mm, respectively. The posterior end of the female worm is straight, while that of the male is curved ventrally and contains two spicules of unequal length. Both male and female worms remain coiled together and it is difficult to separate them. The female is viviparous and liberates sheathed embryos (microfilariae) into lymph from where they find their way into blood.

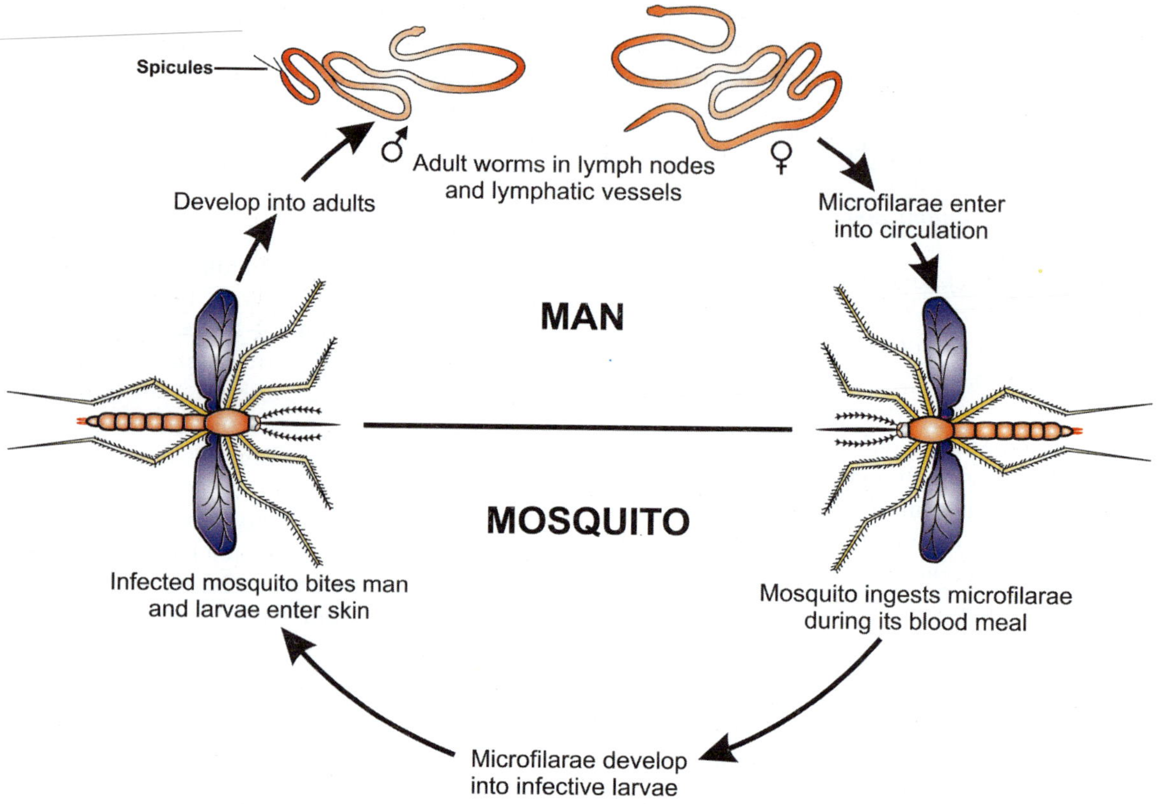

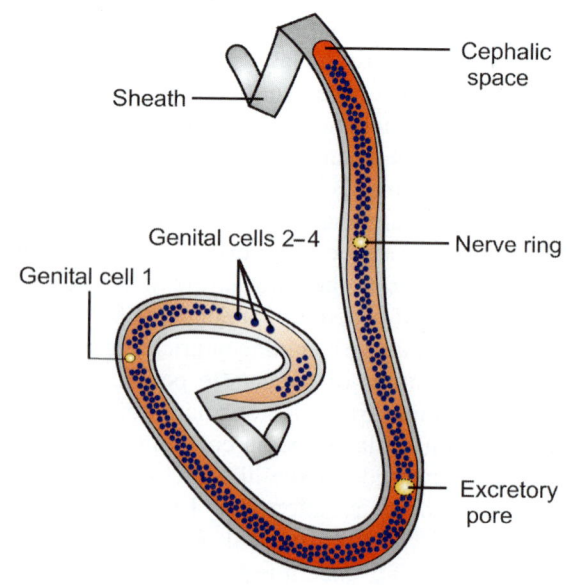

Spicules

♂

Adult worms in lymph nodes and lymphatic vessels

♀

Develop into adults

Microfilarae enter into circulation

MAN

MOSQUITO

Infected mosquito bites man and larvae enter skin

Mosquito ingests microfilarae during its blood meal

Microfilarae develop into infective larvae

Fig. 34.22. Life cycle of *Wuchereria bancrofti.*

Microfilaria

It is transparent and colourless with blunt head and pointed tail. It measures 290×6–7 µm in size and is covered by a hyaline sheath which is much longer (359 µm) than the microfilaria. It can move forwards and backwards within the sheath. The somatic cells appear as granules in the central axis of the microfilaria. At places, these granules are absent. These form the landmarks for recognition of various microfilariae. The tail-tip is free from nuclei (Figs. 34.23 and 34.24).

Life cycle

W. bancrofti passes its life cycle in two hosts (Fig. 34.22). Man is the definitive host and the female mosquitoes belonging to the genera *Culex, Aedes* and *Anopheles* act as intermediate host. Adult worms reside in lymph nodes and lymphatics (usually inguinal, scrotal and abdominal) of man. The lymph

Cephalic space

Sheath

Genital cells 2–4

Nerve ring

Genital cell 1

Excretory pore

Fig. 34.23. *Microfilaria bancrofti.*

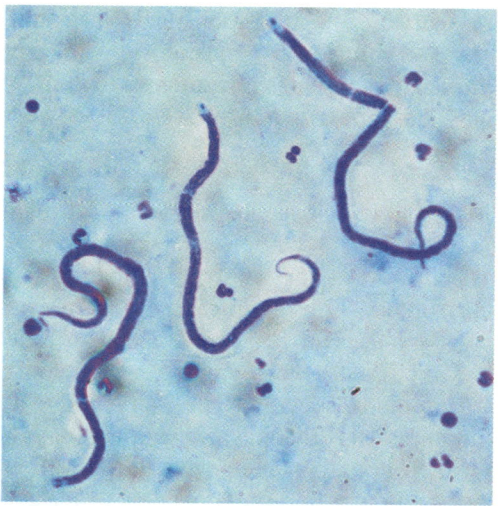

Fig. 34.24. *Microfilaria bancrofti* in peripheral blood (Giemsa stain).

provides nutrition to the adult worms. The male fertilizes female and the gravid female gives birth to microfilariae. Through lymphatics, they find their way into general circulation. The microfilariae appear in large numbers in peripheral blood at night, between 10 pm and 2 am This correlates with the nocturnal biting habit of the insect vector. The periodicity may also be related to the sleeping habits of the hosts. It has been reported that if the sleeping habits of the hosts are reversed, over a period of time, the micro-filariae change their periodicity from night to day.

Sheathed microfilariae are ingested by the mosquito during its blood-meal and reach the stomach of the mosquito. They cast off their sheaths, penetrate the stomach wall and reach thoracic muscles. Here they develop into infective stage of the larvae. These larvae then migrate from thoracic muscles to the proboscis sheath of the mosquito. When the infected mosquito bites a human being, the larvae, in its proboscis, are deposited on the skin near the site of puncture. They then either enter through the puncture wound or penetrate through the skin on their own. Thereafter, they enter into lymphatics and settle down usually in inguinal, scrotal and abdominal lymph nodes, where they develop into adult worms. They become sexually mature. Male fertilizes female, the gravid female gives birth to microfilariae and the cycle is repeated.

Pathogenicity

Infection caused by *W. bancrofti* is known as **wuchereriasis** or **filariasis.** The disease is mainly caused by adult worms (classical filariasis) and sometimes by larvae (occult filariasis).

Classical filariasis

Presence of the adult worms in the lymph nodes and lymphatics leads to lymphangitis, lymphadenitis, lymphangiovarix, gross lymphoedema with hyper-trophy of the affected part (elephantiasis), hydrocele and chyluria.

Occult filariasis

This is a **hypersensitivity reaction to microfilarial antigens**. Patient develops massive eosinophilia (30–80%; absolute count >3000/µl), generalized lymph node enlargement, hepatosplenomegaly and pulmonary symptoms. Microfilariae are not found in the peripheral blood and classical features of lymphatic filariasis are absent.

Laboratory diagnosis

I. Direct evidence

1. Demonstration of microfilariae in peripheral blood film (Fig. 34.24), chylous urine and hydrocele fluid.
2. Demonstration of adult worm in biopsied lymph nodes (Fig. 34.25) and calcified worm can be seen on X-ray.

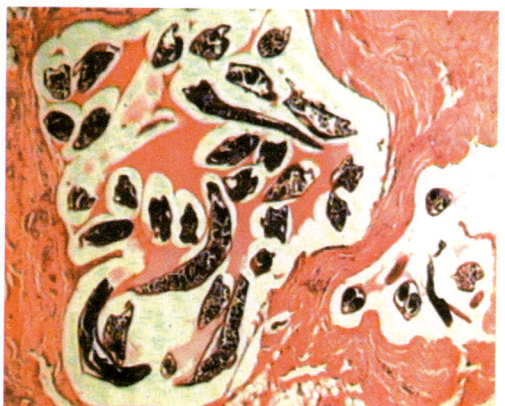

Fig. 34.25. *Wuchereria bancrofti* in lymph node (haematoxylin and eosin stain).

II. Indirect evidence

Filarial antigen may be detected in the patient serum by enzyme immunoassay using monoclonal antibodies against microfilarial surface antigens.

TAENIA SAGINATA AND TAENIA SOLIUM

T. saginata (beef tapeworm) and *T. solium* (pork tapeworm) are worldwide, however the former is much more prevalent than the latter.

Adult worms

Adult worms live in small intestine (upper jejunum) of man. The adult worms consist of scolex (head), neck and strobila which is made up of a large number of proglottids (segments). The differentiating features of *T. saginata* and *T. solium* are given in Table 34.8.

Eggs

Eggs (Figs. 34.26 and 34.27) of both species are indistinguishable. They are spherical, brown in colour (bile-stained) and measure 31–43 μm in diameter. They are surrounded by embryophore which is brown, thick-walled and radially striated. Outside this may be present thin transparent shell which represents the remnant of yolk mass. Inside the embryophore is present hexacanth embryo (onco-

sphere) with three pairs of hooklets. **It does not float in saturated solution of common salt. The eggs of *T. solium* are infective to pig and also to man, while those of *T. saginata* are infective only to cattle.**

Life cycle of T. saginata (Fig. 34.26)

It is passed in two hosts. Definitive host is man and intermediate host is cattle (cow and buffalo). The adult worm lives in the small intestine (upper jejunum) of man. Eggs or gravid segments are passed out with the faeces on the ground. These are ingested by cows or buffaloes while grazing in the field. When they reach the duodenum, the embryophore of the eggs ruptures and liberates **oncospheres**. With the help of their hooklets they penetrate the wall of the intestine and enter into portal vessels or mesenteric lymphatics. Then they reach general circulation via liver, right side of the heart, lungs and left side of the heart. From general circulation, they are filtered out in striated muscles where in 60–75 days, they develop into bladder worm – **cysticercus bovis**.

The mature cysticerci are ovoid in shape, milky-white, opalescent and measure 7.5–10 mm in breadth and 4–6 mm in length. They have unarmed scolices (scolices without hooklets) invaginated in them. These can live in flesh of cattle for about 8 months,

Table 34.8. Differentiating features of *T. saginata* and *T. solium*

	T. saginata	*T. solium*
Length	5–10 metres	2–3 metres
Scolex	Large, quadrate without rostellum and hooklets. Possesses four suckers which may be pigmented.	Small, globular, armed with a double row of alternating large and small hooklets. Possesses four suckers which are not pigmented.
Neck	Long	Short
Proglottids:		
• Measurement of gravid segment	20 mm in length and 5 mm in breadth	12 mm in length and 4 mm in breadth
• Number	1000–2000	800–1000
• Expulsion	Expelled singly	Expelled in chains of 5 or 6
• Number of lateral branches of uterus	15–30	5–10
• Vaginal sphincter	Present	Absent
• Ovaries	Two without any accessory lobe	Two with an accessory lobe
• Testes	300–400 follicles	150–200 follicles
Larva	Cysticercus bovis, present in cow and not in man	Cysticercus cellulosae, present in pig and may also develop in man

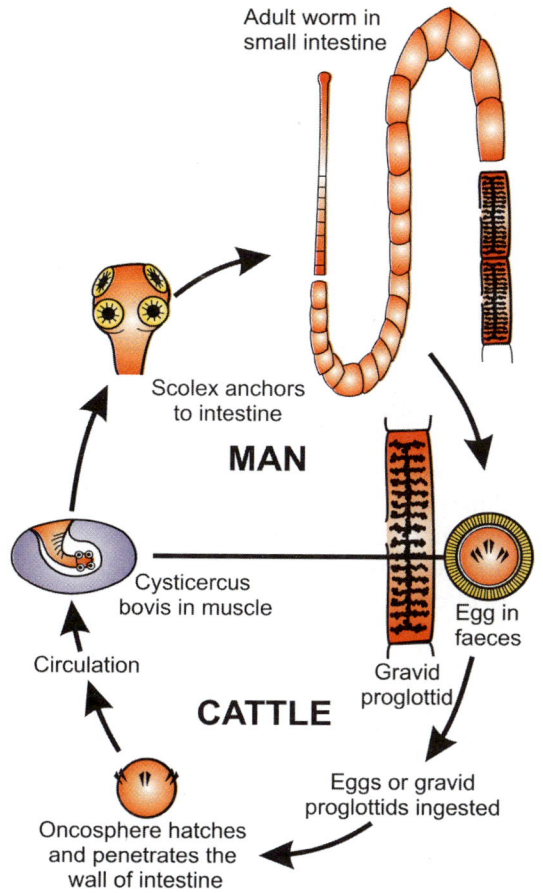

Fig. 34.26. Life cycle of *Taenia saginata*.

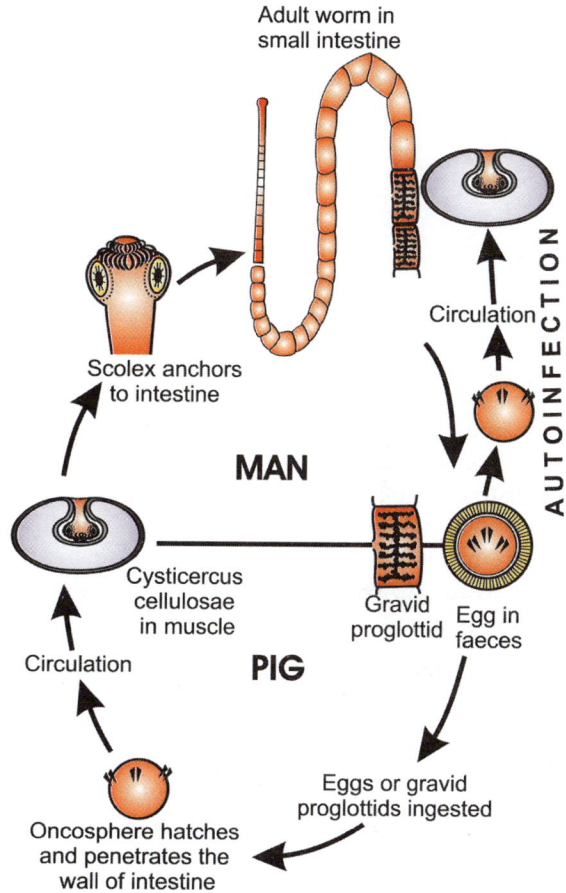

Fig. 34.27. Life cycle of *Taenia solium*.

but can develop further only when ingested by man, its definitive host. **Cysticercus bovis is unknown in humans.**

Man acquires infection by eating raw or undercooked beef containing encysted larval stage (cysticercus bovis). The larvae hatch out in the small intestine, the scolices exvaginate and anchor to the mucosal surface by means of their suckers and develop into adult worms. They grow to sexual maturity in 2–3 months, lay eggs which are passed out in faeces along with the gravid segments and the cycle is repeated.

Life cycle of T. solium (Fig. 34.27)

It is similar to that of *T. saginata*. However, the intermediate host for *T. solium* is pig and its larval form

is known as **cysticercus cellulosae**. Man acquires infection by eating raw or undercooked pork containing the encysted larval stage. Mature cysticercus cellulosae (Figs. 34.28 and 34.29) is an opalescent, ellipsoidal body and measures 8–10 mm in breadth and 5 mm in length. Its long axis lies parallel

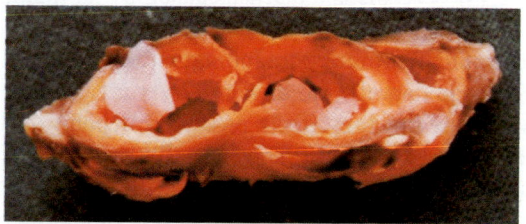

Fig. 34.28. Cysticerci (three in number) in tongue muscle.

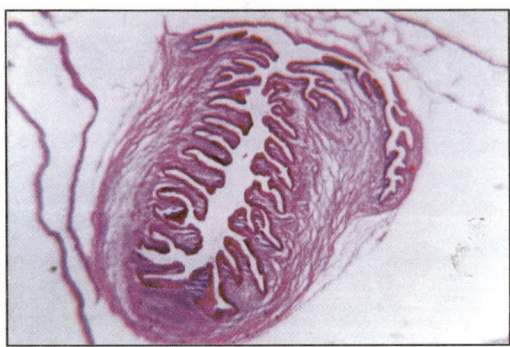

Fig. 34.29. Cysticercus cellulosae in tongue muscle.

to the muscle fibres. It has an invaginated scolex with its four suckers and a rostellum with a double row of alternating large and small hooklets.

Cysticercus bovis and cysticercus cellulosae occur in cattle and pig (intermediate hosts), respectively. However, **the latter can also develop in man as follows:**

1. By ingesting the eggs with contaminated water and food.
2. A man harbouring adult worms may autoinfect oneself either by unhygienic personal habits or by reverse peristaltic movements of the intestine whereby the gravid segments are thrown into the stomach, equivalent to the swallowing of thousands of eggs. Further development to cysticercus cellulosae in man is similar to that in pig.

Pathogenicity

Adult worms in the small intestine usually produce no symptoms. But at times, they may cause vague abdominal discomfort, indigestion, persistent diarrhoea or diarrhoea alternating with constipation and loss of appetite.

Cysticercosis is a disease caused by larval stage of *T. solium* an important public health problem of the tropical countries including India. Cysticercus cellulosae (larval form of *T. solium*) may develop in any organ and the effects produced depend on the location of cysticerci. They usually occur in large numbers (Fig. 34.28), sometimes they may occur singly. They usually develop in the subcutaneous tissues and muscles forming visible nodules. It may also develop in brain leading to epileptic attacks and

in anterior and vitreous chamber of the eye. *In India, it is regarded as second most important cause of intracranial space-occupying lesion following tuberculosis and the most common cause of epilepsy. It is estimated that 5–20% of all cases with epilepsy in India have neurocysticercosis.*

Laboratory diagnosis

1. The diagnosis of *T. saginata* and *T. solium* adult worm infection can be carried out by:
   • **Demonstration of characteristic eggs** in the stool by direct and concentration method by sedimentation technique (formol-ether technique). **They do not float in saturated solution of common salt.**
   • Since eggs of both *T. saginata* and *T. solium* are similar, therefore for the species diagnosis, the **demonstration of gravid proglottids and scolices** is essential (Table 34.8).
2. The diagnosis of cysticercosis can be carried out by:
   • *Biopsy of subcutaneous nodule:*
     It may reveal cysticerci (Figs. 34.28 & 34.29).
   • *X-ray of skull and soft tissue:*
     It may reveal calcified cysticerci.
   • *CT scan of the brain:*
     It can accurately locate the lesion in the brain.
   • *Differential leucocyte count:*
     It reveals eosinophilia.
   • *Serological tests:*
     Serological tests such as indirect haemagglutination (IHA), indirect fluorescent antibody (IFA) and enzyme-linked immunosorbent assay (ELISA) can be used for demonstration of specific antibodies in the serum.

ECHINOCOCCUS GRANULOSUS

Echinococcus granulosus or dog tapeworm is worldwide, but it is more common in sheep and cattle-raising countries. Adult worm resides in the small intestine of dog and other canine animals (wolf, fox and jackal). Larval form is seen in man and other intermediate hosts (sheep, goat, cattle, pig and horse). **The dog and sheep are the optimum definitive and intermediate hosts, respectively** and the cycle of transmission is maintained between them.

Morphology

Adult worm

It is a very small tapeworm measuring 3–6 mm in length. It consists of a scolex, neck and strobila (Fig. 34.30).

Scolex

It is piriform in shape and measures about 300 μm in diameter. It possesses four suckers and a protrusible rostellum with two circular rows of hooklets.

Neck

It is short and thick.

Strobila

It consists of three segments (occasionally four). The first segment is immature, the second is mature and the third (and the fourth when present) is gravid.

Eggs

These are indistinguishable from those of other *Taenia* species. These measure 31–43 μm in diameter and contain hexacanth embryos with three pairs of hooklets.

Larval form

This is found within the hydatid cyst which develops in the intermediate host (see pathogenicity).

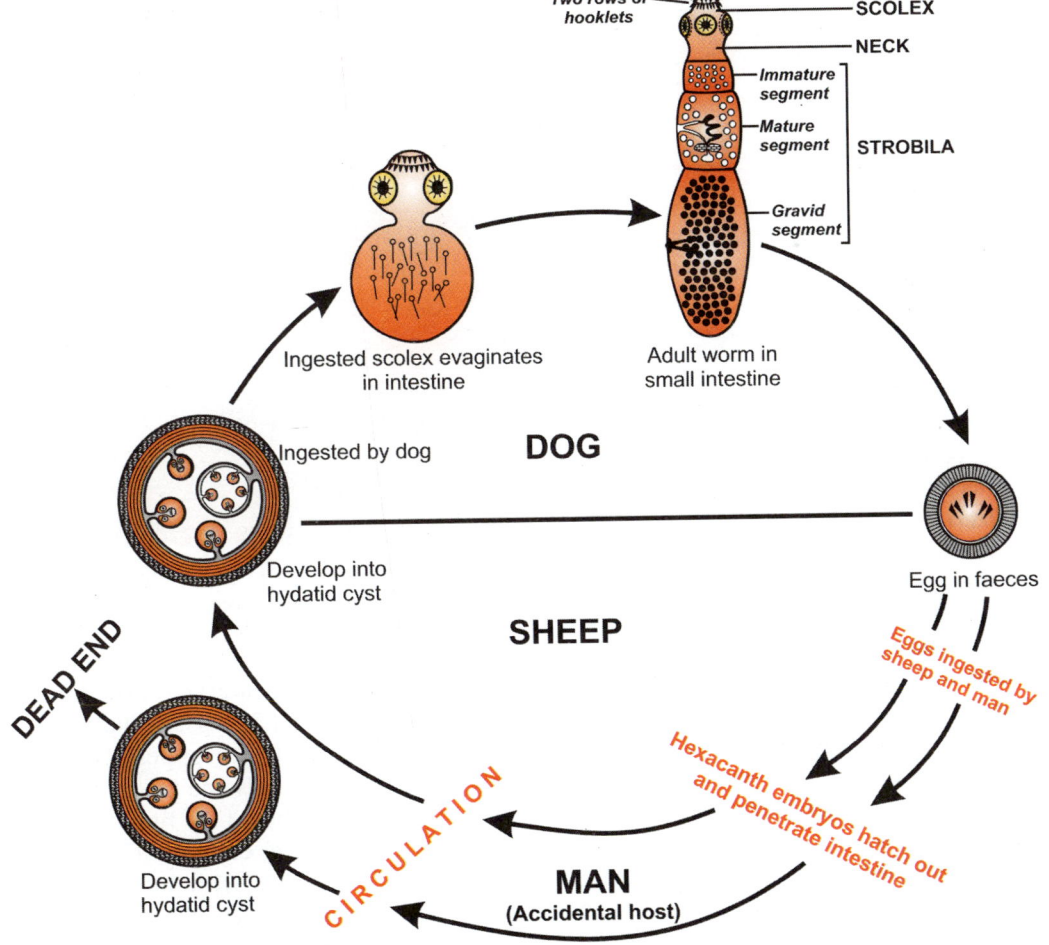

Fig. 34.30. Life cycle of *Echinococcus granulosus*.

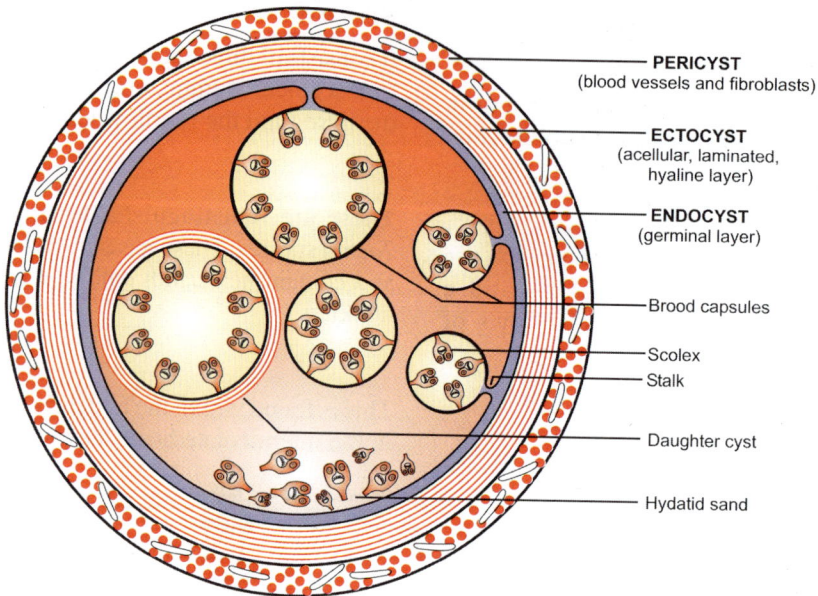

PERICYST
(blood vessels and fibroblasts)

ECTOCYST
(acellular, laminated,
hyaline layer)

ENDOCYST
(germinal layer)

Brood capsules

Scolex

Stalk

Daughter cyst

Hydatid sand

Fig. 34.31. Hydatid cyst.

Life cycle

E. granulosus passes its life cycle in two hosts (Fig. 34.30). The adult worm lives attached to the mucosa of small intestine of dog and other canine animals. The eggs are discharged in the faeces. These are swallowed by the intermediate hosts while grazing in the fields. Man acquires infection by a direct contact with infected dog or by allowing the dog to feed from the same dish or by ingesting water and food contaminated with dog's faeces containing eggs of *E. granulosus*.

In the duodenum the hexacanth embryos hatch out. These penetrate the intestinal wall and enter into the radicals of portal vein and are carried to the liver. The liver acts as the first filter where about 70% of human infections are located. Some embryos may pass through the hepatic capillaries and enter the pulmonary circulation. Lungs act as the second filter. A few of these embryos may pass pulmonary circulation too and enter general circulation and may lodge in various organs.

Wherever the embryos settle an active cellular reaction consisting of monocytes, giant cells and eosinophils takes place around the parasite. A large number of the parasites may thus be destroyed by

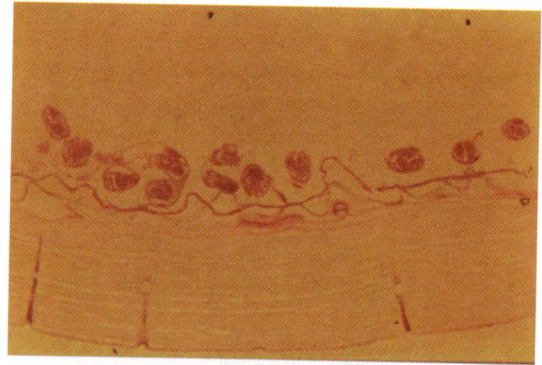

Fig. 34.32. Hydatid cyst showing laminated hyaline ecto-cyst and endocyst with scolices.

host defence mechanism. Some of the embryos, however, escape destruction and develop into hydatid cysts (Figs. 34.30–34.32). The cellular reaction in these cases gradually disappears, followed by appearance of fibroblasts and the formation of new blood vessels. Fibroblasts lay fibrous tissue, which envelops the growing embryo. This is known as **pericyst**. This merges with surrounding normal tissue. The parasite derives its nutrition through this layer. In old cysts the pericyst may become sclerosed or calcified and parasite within it may die.

Inside the pericyst, the embryo develops into a fluid-filled bladder known as **hydatid cyst**. From inner side of the cyst, **brood capsules** with a number of **scolices** are developed. The mature hydatid cyst when ingested by dog and other canine animals develop into a number of adult worms. These lay eggs which are passed in the faeces of infected animals and the cycle is repeated. Since dog has no access to the hydatid cysts developed in viscera of man, therefore, the life cycle of the parasite comes to a dead end.

Pathogenicity

E. granulosus causes **echinococcosis** or hydatid disease or **hydatid cyst** in man. It represents larval form of the parasite. The disease is generally acquired during childhood though it does not manifest before adult life. The cyst wall secreted by the embryo consists of two layers (Figs. 34.30 to 34.32):

1. Ectocyst

It is outer layer. It is laminated hyaline membrane about 1 mm in thickness. It resembles white of a hard-boiled egg. It is elastic, therefore, when excised or ruptured, it curls on itself thus exposing the inner layer containing brood capsules, scolices and daughter cysts.

2. Endocyst

It is inner or germinal layer. It consists of a number of nuclei embedded in a protoplasmic mass. It measures 22–25 µm in thickness. It gives rise to ecto-cyst on outside and brood capsules and scolices on inside. It also secretes hydatid fluid.

Hydatid fluid

It is clear, colourless or pale yellow. It has specific gravity of 1.005–1.010. It is slightly acidic (pH 6.7) and contains sodium chloride, sodium sulphate, sodium phosphate and sodium and calcium salts of succinic acid. It is antigenic, therefore, it is used for **Casoni's test** and when absorbed it leads to anaphylactic shock. Centrifuged deposit of the hydatid fluid shows **hydatid sand** which consists of brood capsules, free scolices and hooklets.

Acephalocysts

Sometimes brood capsules and/or scolices are not formed. These types of hydatid cysts are known as acephalocysts. These are sterile and if ingested by definitive host do not lead to infection.

Endogenous daughter cyst

Sometimes a fragment of the germinal layer may detach and develop daughter cyst inside the mother cyst. This is known as endogenous daughter cyst (Fig. 34.31). It also has both ectocyst and endocyst with brood capsules and scolices. Granddaughter cysts may also be formed.

Exogenous cyst

In case of hydatid disease of bone, because of high intracystic pressure, herniation or rupture of germinal and laminated layer may occur through some weaker part of the bone resulting in formation of exogenous cyst.

Organs involved

Hydatid cyst may involve liver, lung, central nervous system, heart, spleen, kidneys, bone, muscles, female genital tract, eye, etc. It may lead to visible swelling and pressure effects.

Laboratory diagnosis

It can be carried out by the following tests:

1. Casoni's test

It is an immediate hypersensitivity skin test which was introduced by Casoni in 1911. Antigen for the Casoni's test is sterile hydatid fluid drawn from **unilocular hydatid cysts** from sheep, pigs, cattle or man. The fluid is filtered, tested for sterility and stored in sealed ampoules under refrigeration. For the test, 0.2 ml of the antigen is injected intradermally in one arm. For control, an equal amount of sterile normal saline is injected intradermally on the other arm. The control fades almost immediately, while the tested site in positive cases develops a large wheal measuring 5 cm or more in diameter with multiple pseudopodia within 30 minutes. This test has a low sensitivity (55–70%) and gives false positive reactions in patients suffering from other cestode infections.

2. Differential leucocyte count

Differential leucocyte count may reveal eosinophilia (20–25%).

3. Serological tests

Serodiagnosis of hydatid cyst may be carried out by enzyme-linked immunosorbent assay (ELISA), radioimmunoassay (RIA), complement fixation, indirect haemagglutination (IHA), bentonite floculation and latex agglutination tests.

4. Examination of cyst fluid

Examination of cyst fluid reveals scolices, brood capsules and hooklets. Because leakage of fluid in the adjoining tissue may lead to anaphylactic shock, therefore, the fluid aspirated from surgically removed cyst should be examined and diagnostic puncture of cyst is not recommended.

5. Histological examination

Histological examination of surgically removed cyst reveals different layers of the hydatid cyst, i.e., pericyst, ectocyst and endocyst (Fig. 34.32).

6. Radiodiagnosis

X-ray, ultrasound and CT scan are also helpful in the diagnosis of hydatid cyst.

KEY FACTS

- The symptoms of amoebic dysentery, caused by *Entamoeba histolytica* vary from fulminating colitis to absence of symptoms
- About 5% individuals of amoebic dysentery, 1–3 months after the disappearance of the dysenteric attack, develop **hepatic amoebiasis**
- *E. gingivalis* occurs as a **commensal** in the gingival tissue around the teeth; its role, if any, in **periodontal disease** is unclear
- *Trichomonas tenax* is a **harmless commensal** of the human mouth, living in the tartar around the teeth, in cavities of carious teeth, and in necrotic mucosal cells in the gingival margin of gums. Its role in disease is unclear
- The parasites of the genus *Plasmodium* cause the most important **life-threatening protozoan disease called malaria**
- Immunity produced following infection with malaria parasites lasts only till original infection remains active. This is known as **concomitant immunity**

- *Enterobius vermicularis* causes nocturnal perianal and perineal pruritis
- Disease produced by *Ascaris lumbricoides* is known as **ascariasis** and is caused by both adult worms and migrating larvae
- **Visceral larva migrans** is a syndrome caused by ingestion of embryonated eggs of nematodes of animals like *Toxocara canis* and *Toxocara cati*
- *Ancylostoma duodenale* and *Necator Americanus* cause epigastric pain, dyspepsia, vomiting, diarrhoea, and **microcytic, hypochromic anaemia**
- **Cutaneous larva migrans** is caused by exposure of human skin to filariform larvae of animal (canine and feline) hookworms
- **Cysticercus cellulosae** and **hydatid cysts** are the larval forms of *Taenia solium* and *Echinococcus granulosus* respectively

IMPORTANT QUESTIONS

1. Describe morphology, life cycle, pathogenicity and laboratory diagnosis of:
   (a) *Entamoeba histolytica*
   (b) *Giardia lamblia*
   (c) Malaria parasites
   (d) *Enterobius vermicularis*
   (e) *Ascaris lumbricoides*
   (f) *Ancylostoma duodenale*
   (g) *Wuchereria bancrofti*
   (h) *Taenia solium*
   (i) *Echinococcus granulosus*
2. Tabulate differences between:
   (a) Amoebic and bacillary dysentery
   (b) *Entamoeba histolytica* and *Entamoeba coli*
   (c) Four species of *Plasmodium*
   (d) *Ancylostoma duodenale* and *Necator americanus*
   (e) *Taenia saginata* and *Taenia solium*
3. Write short notes on
   (a) Extraintestinal amoebiasis
   (b) *Entamoeba gingivalis*
   (c) Blackwater fever
   (d) *Trichomonas tenax*
4. Draw labelled diagrams of:
   (a) Life cycle of *Plasmodium* vivax
   (b) Microfilaria of *Wuchereria bancrofti*
   (c) Hydatid cyst

SECTION G
Oral Microbiology

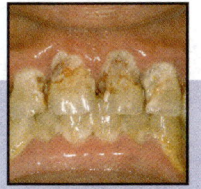

Normal Flora, Dental Plaque, Dental Caries, Periodontal Diseases and Dentoalveolar Abscess

NORMAL FLORA

Natural, indigenous, resident or normal flora or the microbiota refers to the population of microorganisms that inhabit skin and mucous membranes of normal healthy persons. The number of these microorganisms greatly outnumbers the host cells. A healthy foetus in utero is free from microorganisms. During birth the infant is exposed to vaginal flora and after birth to the environmental microorganisms. Within a few hours after birth, there develops oral and nasopharyngeal flora and in a day or two resident flora of the lower intestine appears. The normal flora at each site on the body varies in composition and complexity within the same animal species and for the same anatomical site in different animal species. It can be divided into two groups:

1. Resident flora

It consists of organisms which are regularly present in a given area at a given age and when disturbed, it promptly re-establishes itself. For example, *Escherichia coli* is a normal inhabitant of the intestine of man and many other animal species in all parts of the world. Similarly α-haemolytic streptococci and lactobacilli are regularly present in the nasopharynx and other sites in man and animals.

2. Transient flora

It consists of both pathogens and non-pathogens that inhabit the skin or mucous membrane for a limited period. If the resident flora is intact, there is very little significance of the transient flora. However, if the normal flora is disturbed, the transient flora may colonize, proliferate and produce disease. Pathogens such as pneumococcus, meningococcus and *Haemophilus influenzae* may be found among nasopharyngeal microbiota of man from time to time.

Role of resident flora

A. Beneficial role

1. They prevent or suppress the colonization/invasion of the body by pathogens by bacterial interference.
2. Members of the resident flora in the intestinal tract synthesize vitamins, especially vitamin K and several B vitamins.
3. Antibodies produced in response to commensals cross-react with pathogens thus raising the overall immune status of the host.
4. Bacteriocins produced by some organisms of normal flora have harmful effect on pathogens.
5. The endotoxins liberated by them may help the defence mechanism of the body by triggering the alternative complement pathway.

B. Disease production

1. Most members of the normal microbiota are generally non-pathogenic, some, however, may assume a pathogenic role when resistance of the host is lowered as in cases of diabetes, leukaemia and AIDS, and in patients on cytotoxic and immunosuppressive drugs (**opportunistic pathogens**). Debilitated tissues (e.g., in burns) may become similarly infected.

2. Normal oral flora may cause **dental caries**.

3. Viridans streptococci may be introduced into the blood stream through wounds created by dental treatment. When this occurs in a patient with heart valves damaged by congenital defect or rheumatic heart disease, these organisms may adhere to the valves and multiply, leading to **infective endo-carditis**.

4. *Escherichia coli* and *Enterococcus faecalis* which are normal flora of the intestine, may cause **urinary tract infection** particularly when there is some abnormality of the urinary tract like congenital malformation and urinary calculi.

5. **Peritonitis** may follow the accidental introduction of gut organisms into the peritoneum during surgery on the bowel or by leakage of intestinal contents.

6. Use of broad spectrum antibiotics affects the gut microbiota by inhibiting or killing sensitive bacteria and thereby allowing overgrowth of resistant bacteria as well as pathogenic bacteria.

Normal flora of the mouth

The normal microbial flora of the oral cavity is complex and consists of a large number of species of bacteria, fungi and protozoa (Tables 35.1 and 35.2). This is because of the fact that the mouth has many distinct habitats including:

- saliva and crevicular fluids,
- the surfaces of soft tissues such as lips, palate, cheek, tongue and gums, and
- hard surfaces of teeth.

Microbial flora varies qualitatively and quanti-tatively after tooth eruption, tooth extraction, artificial dentures, dental treatments (scaling, polishing, filling), the frequency and type of food ingested and antibiotic treatment.

The oral cavity may be considered as an ideal microbial incubator. It possesses:

- an abundance of moisture,
- an excellent supply of various types of foods, and
- differences in oxygen tension.

Many aerobic, facultative and anaerobic organisms find conditions favourable for growth.

At birth the mouth of the newborn is usually sterile. Within a few hours of the birth streptococci, of which *Streptococcus salivarius* is dominant, establish themselves in the mouth. During the first month of life, other species of streptococci, staphylococci, neisseriae, veillonellae, lactobacilli,

Table 35.1. Normal bacterial flora of the oral cavity

Gram-positive cocci	Gram-negative cocci	Gram-positive bacilli	Gram-negative bacilli
• **Viridans streptococci**	• *Neisseria* spp.	• *Actinomyces israelii*	• *Bacteroides* spp.
Streptococcus salivarius	• *Veillonella* spp.	• *A. viscosus*	• *Borrelia vincentii*
S. sanguis		• *A. naeslundii*	• *T. denticola*
S. mutans		• Lactobacilli	• *T. refringens*
S. sorbinus			• *Porphyromonas gingivalis*
S. cricetus			• *Actinobacillus*
S. rattus			*actinomycetemcomitans*
S. gordonii			• *Fusobacterium* spp.
S. mitis			• *Prevotella* spp.
S. milleri			• *Capnocytophaga* spp.
• *Staphylococcus aureus*			
• *S. epidermidis*			
• *Micrococcus* spp.			
• *Peptostreptococcus* spp.			

Table 35.2. Fungi and protozoa normally present in the oral cavity

Fungi	Protozoa
• *Candida albicans*	• *Entamoeba gingivalis*
• *C. dubliniensis*	• *Trichomonas tenax*
• *C. glabrata*	
• *C. tropicalis*	
• *C. krusei*	
• *C. guilliermondii*	
• *C. parapsilosis*	
• *C. kefyr*	

Actinomyces and fusobacteria also colonize. Eruption of teeth provides hard surfaces in the oral cavity. These are colonized by *S. mutans*, *S. sanguis* and *Actinomyces viscosus*. By the first year of life, the oral microbial flora of the child resembles that of adult.

Normal flora of the respiratory tract

The respiratory tract can be divided into upper part (anterior and posterior naris and the nasopharynx), an intermediate zone (the oropharynx and the tonsils) and a lower part (the larynx, trachea, bronchi, and lungs). The normal flora of nose and nasopharynx is given in Table 35.3.

Table 35.3. Normal flora of nose and nasopharynx

- *Staphylococcus aureus*
- *S. epidermidis*
- Viridans streptococci
- β-haemolytic streptococci
- *Streptococcus pneumoniae*
- Diphtheroids
- *Neisseria* spp. including *N. meningitidis*
- *Peptostreptococcus* spp.
- *Fusobacterium* spp.
- *Haemophilus influenzae*
- *Candida* spp.

Staphylococcus aureus, *S. epidermidis* and diphtheroids are far more frequent in the nose than in the nasopharynx. On the other hand, viridans streptococci and Gram-negative cocci of *N. subflava* type are far less frequent in nasopharynx than in the nose. *S. pneumoniae*, β-haemolytic streptococci and *H. influenzae* are less frequent in nose than in the

nasopharynx. *N. meningitidis* is carried in the nasopharynx and the nose of 5–20% and 0–4% healthy individuals, respectively.

DENTAL PLAQUE

Dental plaque may be defined as the soft deposits that form the biofilm adhering to the tooth surface or other hard surfaces in the oral cavity, including removable restorations. It consists of dense masses of a variety of microorganisms from the normal flora, proteins from the saliva, and desquamated epithelial cells. More than 200 different bacterial species and some fungi may be found in the plaque.

Many oral bacteria produce extracellular polysaccharides like glucans, dextrans and fructans from carbohydrates. These enable bacteria to adhere to a pellicle on the tooth surface. The pellicle consists of components of saliva and crevicular fluid, and bacterial and host tissue cell products adsorbed to the enamel mineral to form a membranous film. It is rather insoluble, as well as adherent, and thus resists removal by water spray or mouth rinsing. Only more aggressive means such as tooth brushing and flossing between the teeth remove it.

Initially *Actinomyces viscosus*, *S. sanguis* and *S. mutans* colonize the dental pellicle through specific molecules termed adhesins. This is followed by colonization by *Prevotella intermedia*, *P. loescheii*, *Fusobacterium nucleatum* and *Porphyromonas gingivalis*. These microorganisms adhere to cells of bacteria already in the plaque mass by a process known as **coaggregation** or **coadhesion**. Other microorganisms which may also be found in the plaque include *Mycoplasma* spp., yeasts, protozoa and viruses. **One gram of plaque contains approximately 2×10^{11} bacteria.** In addition, plaque may also contain host cells such as epithelial cells, macrophages and leucocytes.

Based on its position on the tooth surface, dental plaque is classified as supragingival, marginal and subgingival plaque.

Supragingival plaque

It is found at or above the gingival margin.

Marginal plaque

The supragingival plaque that is in direct contact with the gingival margin is known as marginal plaque.

Subgingival plaque

The plaque below the gingival margin, between the tooth and gingival sulcular tissue is known as subgingival plaque.

If the plaque is left undisturbed then the calcium and phosphate ions derived from saliva may become deposited within deeper layers of dental plaque (as saliva is supersaturated with respect to these ions). This process is accelerated by bacterial phosphatases and proteases that degrade some of the calcification inhibitors in saliva. These processes lead to the formation of insoluble calcium phosphate crystals which coalesce to form a calcified mass of plaque, termed **calculus**. Calculus, therefore, consists of mineralized bacterial plaque. It can form extensive deposits around the teeth. Calculus per se is not directly implicated in disease but acts as a nidus for further plaque accumulation. Many toothpastes now contain pyrophosphate compounds which adsorb excess calcium ions, thus reducing intraplaque mineral deposition.

DENTAL CARIES

Dental caries is a chronic endogenous infection caused by the normal oral flora. The carious lesion is the result of demineralization of enamel and later of dentine by acids produced by plaque micro-organisms as they metabolize dietary carbohydrates. However, the initial process of enamel demineralization is usually followed by remineralization, and cavitation occurs when the former process overtakes the latter. When the surface layer of enamel has been lost, the infection invariably progresses to dentine, with the pulp becoming firstly inflamed and then necrotic. Dental caries is the most common cause of tooth loss before the age of 35.

Traditionally, the rate of caries has been higher in industrialized countries, where there is ready access to processed foods containing large amounts of carbohydrates. However, global trends may change these demographics. First of all, the rate of caries has dramatically dropped in countries such as the United States, where improved oral hygiene and fluoridation of the drinking water has become a standard practice. Fluoride incorporates into the crystalline structure of enamel, forming fluoropatite, and contributes to resistance to degradation by bacterial acids. Secondly, with globalization of world's economy, increased amounts of processed foods with high carbohydrate content are being imported into developing nations. With these trends, one can expect the rate of caries to dramatically increase in the less developed world over the next several decades.

Aetiology

Four factors host, diet, time and commensal microbes in plaque have been documented to interact in a specific manner to produce dental caries:

1. Host factors

Structure of enamel and mineral content of the teeth and the nature of saliva play an important role in dental caries. The continuous flow and mechanical washing action of saliva are very effective mechanisms in the removal of food debris and unattached oral microorganisms. By its buffering effects saliva neutralizes the acid produced by bacteria and its high calcium and phosphorus contents are important for remineralization during early stage of the disease.

2. Diet

Microorganisms in the oral cavity ferment carbohydrates with the production of acid which destroys the dental tissue. All carbohydrates are cariogenic but some like sucrose have high cariogenicity. Sucrose is highly soluble and diffuses easily into dental plaque, acting as a substrate for the production of extracellular polysaccharides and acids. Sticky, solid carbohydrates are more caries-producing than those consumed as liquids. Polysaccharides are less easily fermented by plaque bacteria than monosaccharides and disaccharides. Carbohydrates which are rapidly cleared from the oral cavity by saliva and swallowing are less cariogenic.

3. Time

Prior to ingestion of carbohydrates the pH of the oral cavity is slightly acidic or alkaline. After ingestion of carbohydrates it drops by 2 or more. If pH remains sufficiently low for long time acid damages the enamel. Therefore, the chances of development of caries are more in those individuals who repeatedly ingest carbohydrates at short intervals.

4. Commensal microbes in plaque

Many species of viridans streptococci inhabiting the oral cavity have emerged as significant pathogens associated predominantly with the initiation and pathogenesis of dental caries. **Cariogenic streptococci** (*Streptococcus mutans*, *S. sorbinus*, *S. cricetus* and *S. rattus*) produce water-insoluble **glucan** from sucrose, which in addition to facilitating initial adhesion of the organism to the tooth surface serve as a nutritional source and a matrix for further plaque development.

Attachment of *S. mutans* and other organisms to the insoluble, adherent glucans and subsequent formation of acid leads to **demineralization** of the tooth enamel and the initiation of carious lesions. *S. sanguis*, *S. salivarius*, *S. gordonii*, *S. milleri*, *Prevotella*, *Lactobacillus casei*, *L. fermentum*, *L. acidophilus*, *L. salivarius*, *Actinomyces viscosus*, *A. naeslundii* and *A. israelii* have also been incriminated in the pathogenesis of dental caries.

For dental caries to develop from a plaque, the appropriate microorganisms need to be present on susceptible tooth surface, with access to suitable substrates (such as trapped food, salivary glyco-proteins) for an adequate time. Initially, cocci predominate in the plaque and produce **extracellular matrix**. This matrix is then colonized by other bacteria including filamentous bacteria and anaerobes. Organic acids and enzymes produced by the microorganisms cause decalcification, proteo-lysis, and slow, progressive decay of the tooth, starting with the covering enamel.

The earliest change in dental caries is the appearance of a small, chalky-white spot on the enamel which subsequently enlarges and often becomes yellow to brown and breaks down to form cavity. If unchecked, the infection penetrates the dentin and destroys the pulp.

Several factors influence the production of dental caries:

1. Microorganisms are essential for the development of caries.
2. Regular brushing and flossing prevent accumu-lation of food debris, reducing the incidence of caries and their sequelae.

3. Since bacteria metabolize carbohydrate, therefore, sugar promotes dental caries. The stickiness of the dental plaque is caused by dextran, which is a product of sucrose fermentation by *S. mutans*.
4. Adherent plaque cannot be removed by brushing, but periodic mechanical removal of the plaque (scaling) by the dentist or dental hygienist decreases the incidence of caries.
5. Fluoride ingested or locally applied to tooth surfaces is an effective preventive agent because it has bactericidal action and, it makes enamel more resistant to bacterial degradation.
6. Saliva has a mechanical action and contains bactericidal substances such as lysozyme and IgA.

Prevention of dental caries

1. Stopping or reducing between meal consumption of carbohydrates or substituting non-cariogenic artificial sweeteners (**sugar substitutes**), e.g., sorbital, xylitol or lycasin.
2. Making the tooth structure less soluble to acid attack by using **fluorides**. Fluoride can be delivered in domestic water supply, tablets, topical application of fluoridated gel or fluoridated toothpaste may be used.
3. Using **sealants** to protect susceptible areas of the tooth (e.g., pits and fissures) that cannot easily be kept plaque-free by routine oral hygiene measures.
4. **Reducing cariogenic flora** so that even in the presence of sucrose, acid production will be minimal. This can be carried out by mechanical cleansing, antimicrobial therapy and immunization.
5. **Replacement** of cariogenic bacteria by genetically engineered mutans streptococci which have low or no cariogenic potential.

PERIODONTAL DISEASES

Periodontal diseases can be defined as disorders of supporting structures of the teeth, including the gingival, periodontal ligament and supporting alveolar bone. Periodontal disease can be broadly categorized into **gingivitis** and **periodontitis** (Fig. 35.1). The former includes acute necrotizing ulcerative gingivitis and chronic gingivitis, and the latter includes chronic periodontitis, and localized and generalized aggressive periodontitis.

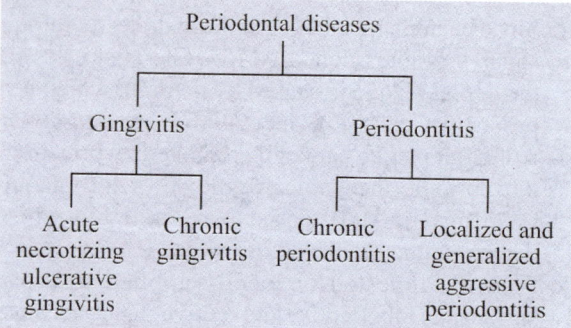

Fig. 35.1. Classification of periodontal diseases.

Acute necrotizing ulcerative gingivitis

It is commonly associated with poor and neglected oral hygiene, malnutrition, heavy smoking, emotional stress, primary herpetic gingivostomatitis and infection with human immunodeficiency virus.

The disease is a specific, anaerobic, polymicrobial infection mainly due to the combined activity of fuso-bacteria (*Fusobacterium nucleatum*) and oral spirochaetes (*Treponema* spp.). It may also be caused by *Prevotella intermedia, Veillonella* and strepto-cocci.

It is characterized by acutely inflamed, red, shiny and bleeding gingivae with irregularly shaped ulcers which initially appear on the tips of interdental papillae. If untreated the ulcers enlarge and spread to involve the marginal, and rarely, the attached gingivae. The lesions are extremely painful and are covered by a pseudomembrane or slough which can be wiped from the surface. The slough consists of leucocytes, erythrocytes, fibrin, necrotic tissue debris and microorganisms. If the disease is inadequately treated, tissue destruction slows down and the disease may enter a chronic phase with pronounced loss of supporting tissues.

Microscopic examination of a Gram-stained, deep gingival smear of the ulcerated lesion shows pre-dominance of three components – fusobacteria, spiro-chaetes and leucocytes.

Chronic gingivitis

Chronic gingivitis is characterized by gingival redness, oedema, bleeding, changes in contour, and loss of tissue adaptation to the teeth.

It is caused by the prolonged exposure of host tissues to a non-specific mixture of gingival plaque organisms. These include *streptococcus sanguis, S. milleri, Actinomyces israelii, A. naeslundii, Prevotella intermedia, Capnocytophaga* spp., *Fusobacterium nucleatum* and *Veillonella* spp.

Chronic periodontitis (formerly adult periodontitis)

Periodontitis refers to an inflammatory process that affects the supporting structures of the teeth – periodontal ligaments, alveolar bone, and cementum. With progression, periodontitis can lead to serious sequelae, including the loss of attachment caused by complete destruction of the periodontal ligament and alveolar bone. Loosening and eventual loss of teeth are possible.

Microorganisms implicated in chronic peri-odontitis are *Actinobacillus actinomycetemcomitans, Porphyromonas gingivalis, Prevotella intermedia, Fusobacterium nucleatum, Bacteroides forsythus, Selenomonas* spp., *Capnocytophaga* spp. and *Treponema* spp.

Although the histologic picture is well defined, the mechanism by which the microorganisms cause the destruction remain controversial. Microorganisms in the plaque produce a variety of factors that damage the periodontium either directly or indirectly by initiating the inflammatory response. Among these factors are exotoxins, endotoxins, enzymes (such as collagenase, hyaluronidase and protease), lipo-teichoic acid, and peptidoglycan. Immunologic mediators that have been implicated include prosta-glandins, interleukin-1, and tumour necrosis factor.

Localized and generalized aggressive periodontitis

The disease is more common in West Africans and Asians. It appears around puberty. It has rapid progress with active and quiscent periods. It is relatively common in girls and case clusters are usually seen in families.

In the localized variant the incisors and/or first permanent molars in both jaws are affected for unknown reason. Later other teeth may be involved, producing the appearance of generalized alveolar bone loss. In generalized variant of the disease many areas may be involved in a similar manner.

Aggressive periodontitis is caused by *Actinobacillus actinomycetemcomitans, Capnocytophaga* spp., *Porphyromonas gingivalis* and *Prevotella intermedia*. This disease may be associated with cellular immune or genetic defects.

DENTOALVEOLAR ABSCESS

Dentoalveolar infection may be defined as pyogenic (pus-producing) infections associated with the teeth and surrounding supporting structures, such as the peridontium and the alveolar bone. A dentoalveolar abscess usually develops by the extension of the initial carious lesion into dentine, and spread of bacteria to the pulp via the dentinal tubules. Once pus formation occurs, it may remain localized at the root apex and develop into either an acute or chronic abscess, or spread into surrounding tissues.

Dentoalveolar abscess may be caused by obligate anaerobes and facultative anaerobes (Table 35.4).

Table 35.4. Causative agents of dentoalveolar abscess.

Obligate anaerobes
- *Prevotella intermedia*
- *P. melaninogenica*
- *Porphyromonas gingivalis*
- *Fusobacterium nucleatum*
- *Peptostreptococcus* spp.

Facultative anaerobes
- *Streptococcus milleri*
- *Actinomyces* spp.

Pus should be collected by needle aspiration, or in a sterile container after external incision. Both anaerobic and aerobic cultures are done using conventional methods and isolates identified.

KEY FACTS

- The oral flora comprise a diverse group of organisms and includes bacteria, fungi, mycoplasmas, protozoa and possibly viruses
- There are probably some 350 different **cultivable species** and a further proportion of **uncultivable flora**

- Streptococci are the predominant supragingival bacteria; they are *Streptococcus salivarius, S. mutans, S. mitis, S. sanguis* and *S. milleri*
- The predominant cultivable species in sublingual plaque are **Actinomyces**, **Prevotella**, **Porphyromonas**, **Fusobacterium** and **Veillonella spp.**
- **Adherence** of a microbe to an oral surface is a prerequisite for colonization and is the initial step in the path leading to subsequent infection or invasion of tissues
- Saliva modulates bacterial growth by (a) providing a **pellicle** for bacterial adhesion, (b) acting as a **nutrient source**, (c) **coaggregating bacteria**, (d) providing non-specific (e.g., lysozyme, lactoferrin and histatins) and specific (e.g., mainly IgA) **defence factors**, and (e) maintaining **pH**
- Large masses of bacteria and their products accumulate on tooth surfaces to produce **dental plaque**, present both in health and disease; plaque is an example of a natural **biofilm**
- *Dental plaque may be defined as a tenacious, complex microbial community, found on tooth surfaces, comprising living, dead and dying bacteria and their products, embedded in a matrix of polymers mainly derived from saliva*
- **Dental caries** may be defined as localized destruction of the tissues of the tooth by bacterial fermentation of dietary carbohydrates
- Key factors in the development of tooth caries are the **host** (susceptible tooth surface and saliva), **plaque bacteria**, and **diet** (mainly fermentable carbohydrates)
- The **initial caries lesion** is the 'white spot' created by the demineralization of enamel; this is reversible and can be remineralized; cavitation represents irreversible disease
- The **specific plaque hypothesis** postulates that mutans streptococci are important in caries initiation, while heterogenous groups of bacteria are implicated in the **non-specific plaque hypothesis**
- Lactobacilli are implicated in the **progression of caries**, especially in the advancing front of the carious lesions

- The properties of cariogenic flora that correlate with their pathogenicity are the ability to metabolize sugars to acids, survive and grow under low pH conditions, and ability to synthesize extracellular and intracellular polysaccharides
- *Strategies to prevent caries include sugar substitutes, fluoridation (to increase enamel hardness), fissure sealants and control of cariogenic flora (by antimicrobials, vaccination or replacement therapy)*
- High salivary or plaque counts of mutans streptococci ($>10^6$/ml) and lactobacilli ($>10,000$/ml) indicate high risk of disease
- Periodontal disease can be broadly categorized into **gingivitis** and **periodontitis**
- Periodontitis can be classified into two main groups – chronic, and localized and generalized aggressive. The chronic form is by far the most prevalent globally
- **Localized and generalized aggressive periodontitis** is strongly associated with *Actinobacillus actinomycetemcomitans*, either alone or synergistically with *Capnocytophaga* spp. and *Porphyromonas gingivalis*
- **Acute necrotizing ulcerative gingivitis** is a specific polymicrobial infection due to the combined activity of *Fusobacterium nucleatum* and oral spirochaetes (*Treponema* spp.) – the fusospirochaetal complex
- **Dentoalveolar infections** are usually **polymicrobial** in nature and **endogenous** in origin, with a predominance of strict anaerobes

IMPORTANT QUESTION

Write short notes on:
(a) Normal flora of the mouth
(b) Dental plaque
(c) Dental caries
(d) Gingivitis
(e) Chronic periodontitis
(f) Dentoalveolar abscess

36. **Infective Syndromes**

Chapter 36

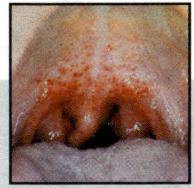

Infective Syndromes

In this chapter important infective syndromes, caused by different microorganisms, have been discussed briefly, and the reader should refer back to the corresponding chapters for details including laboratory diagnosis.

Sore throat

It is essentially an acute tonsillitis or pharyngitis. It is characterized by redness and oedema of mucosa, exudation of tonsils, pseudomembrane formation, oedema of uvula, grey coating of tongue and enlargement of cervical lymph nodes. Causative agents of sore throat are given in Table 36.1. Of these, *Corynebacterium diphtheriae*, *Candida albicans*, β-haemolytic group A *Streptococcus*, *Borrelia vincentii* and *Leptotrichia buccalis* may lead to pseudomembrane formation.

For laboratory diagnosis, refer to corresponding chapters.

Urinary tract infection

Urinary tract infection (UTI) may be defined as the presence of bacteria undergoing multiplication in urine within the urinary drainage system. Kass (1956), gave a criterion of active bacterial infection of urinary tract according to which a count exceeding 10^5 organisms/ml denotes significant bacteriuria and

Table 36.1. Causative agents of sore throat

BACTERIA
- *Streptococcus*, β-haemolytic group A and occasionally groups C and G
- *Corynebacterium diphtheriae*
- *Haemophilus influenzae*
- *Bordetella pertussis*
- *Neisseria gonorrhoeae*
- *Borrelia vincentii*
- *Leptotrichia buccalis*

FUNGI
- *Candida albicans*

VIRUSES
- Epstein-Barr virus
- Adenoviruses
- Coxsackievirus A

indicates active UTI. Contamination accounts for less than 10^4 organisms/ml and usually less than 10^3/ml. UTI is generally caused by one species, while contaminants are generally of mixed species. However, in case of obstructive uropathy (bladder stones, prostate hypertrophy, spinal paralysis), it may be caused by more than one species of bacteria.

UTI is caused by *Escherichia coli* (70–80%), *Proteus mirabilis* and other spp. (10%), *Staphylo-*

381

coccus saprophyticus (10–15%), *S. epidermidis* (1–5%), *S. aureus* (1–5%), *Enterococcus* spp. (1–5%), *Klebsiella* spp. (1–5%) and *Pseudomonas aeruginosa* (1–2%). Other organisms which may occasionally cause UTI include *Mycobacterium tuberculosis*, *Enterobacter*, *Citrobacter*, salmonellae, *Streptococcus pyogenes*, *S. agalactiae* and *Gardnerella vaginalis*. *Candida albicans* may cause UTI in diabetics and immunocompromised patients. *Ureaplasma urealyticum* accounts for some cases of urethritis and cystitis. *Mycoplasma pneumoniae* has been isolated from renal tissues of patients with acute pyelonephritis. Adenovirus causes acute haemorrhagic cystitis in children and in some young adults.

Sexually transmitted diseases

The sexually transmitted diseases (STD) are a group of communicable diseases that are transmitted predominantly by sexual contact and caused by a wide range of bacterial, viral, protozoal and fungal agents. STD may cause genital ulcers, genital discharge, or no genital lesion but only systemic manifestations. The organisms causing these infections are given in Table 36.2.

For laboratory diagnosis of these infections, refer to corresponding chapters.

Meningitis

Meningitis is an inflammation of the membranes of the brain or spinal cord. It is of two types, purulent meningitis and aseptic meningitis. The causative agents of these types are given in Table 36.3.

Purulent meningitis

In purulent meningitis, the CSF is turbid due to the presence of a large number of leucocytes (from 100 to several thousands/ml) most of which are polymorphs.

Aseptic meningitis

In aseptic meningitis CSF is slightly turbid. It contains lesser number of leucocytes (10–500/µl), most of which are lymphocytes. Most of these cases are caused by viruses and a few cases are caused by bacteria, fungi and protozoa. In tuberculous meningitis also, cell count is usually 100–500 leuco-

Table 36.2. Organisms causing sexually transmitted diseases

Disease	Causative agents
GENITAL ULCERS	
Painless ulcers	
• Syphilis	*Treponema pallidum*
• Lymphogranuloma venereum	*Chlamydia trachomatis*
• Donovanosis	*Klebsiella* (*Calymmatobacterium*) *granulomatis*
Painful ulcers	
• Chancroid	*Haemophilus ducreyi*
• Herpes genitalis	Herpes simplex virus types 2 and 1
GENITAL DISCHARGE	
• Gonorrhoea	*Neisseria gonorrhoeae*
• *Trichomonas vaginitis*	*Trichomonas vaginalis*
• Non-gonococcal urethritis	*Chlamydia trachomatis* *Ureaplasma urealyticum* *Mycoplasma genitalium* *M. hominis* *Acinetobacter lwoffii* *Bacteroides urealyticus* *Candida albicans* *Torulopsis glabrata*
• Bacterial vaginosis	*Mobiluncus curtisii* *M. mulieris* *Mycoplasma hominis* *Gardnerella vaginalis* *Bacteroides* spp.
NO GENITAL LESIONS BUT ONLY SYSTEMIC MANIFESTATIONS	
• AIDS	HIV-1 and HIV-2
• Hepatitis B	HBV
• Hepatitis C	HCV

cytes/µl most of which are lymphocytes. When CSF is allowed to stand, a fibrin web (cobweb) often develops. In immunocompromised hosts, aseptic meningitis may be caused by *Listeria monocytogenes* and *Cryptococcus neoformans*. The latter is particularly seen in AIDS cases.

For laboratory diagnosis of meningitis, CSF is collected by lumbar puncture in three separate sterile

Table 36.3. Causative agents of purulent and aseptic meningitis

PURULENT MENINGITIS

- *Haemophilus influenzae*
- *Streptococcus pneumoniae*
- *Neisseria meningitidis*
- *Escherichia coli*
- Group B streptococci
- *Pseudomonas*
- Salmonellae
- *Staphylococcus aureus*
- *S. epidermidis*
- *Listeria monocytogenes*
- *Klebsiella*
- Anaerobic cocci
- *Bacteroides*

(Contd.)

Table 36.3. (*Contd.*)

ASEPTIC MENINGITIS

Viruses

- Enteroviruses (echoviruses, polioviruses, coxsackieviruses)
- Mumps
- Herpes simplex
- Varicella-zoster
- Measles
- Adenoviruses
- Arboviruses

Bacteria

- *Leptospira interrogans* serovars *icterohaemorrhagiae* and *canicola*
- *Treponema pallidum*
- *Mycobacterium tuberculosis*

Protozoa

- *Acanthamoeba*
- *Naegleria*
- *Toxoplasma gondii*

Fungi

- *Cryptococcus neoformans*

vials, one each for cell count, chemical examination and culture. Differentiating features in CSF in purulent and aseptic meningitis are given in Table 36.4. For culture and identification of the causative agent refer to the corresponding chapters.

Pyrexia of unknown origin (PUO)

PUO may be defined as any febrile illness (body temperature greater than 38°C) lasting more than a few days, without an obvious cause. The causes of

PUO are given in Table 36.5. Urinary tract infection, tuberculosis, infective endocarditis, osteomyelitis, and biliary tract infection are the commonest infectious causes of PUO. For diagnosis, refer to the chapters dealing with specific causative agents.

Table 36.4. Differentiating features in CSF in purulent and aseptic meningitis

Features	CSF values in		
	Normal	**Purulent meningitis**	**Aseptic meningitis**
Pressure	90–180 mm H_2O	Highly increased	Slightly to moderately increased
Total proteins	30–45 mg%	Highly increased (100–600 mg%)	Slightly increased (60–120 mg%)
Sugar	40–80 mg%	Diminished (10–20 mg%) or absent	Normal
Cell count	1–3/µl	100 to several thousands/µl	10–500/µl
Type of cells	Lymphocytes	Neutrophils 98% Lymphocytes 2%	Lymphocytes
Smear from the centrifuged deposits			
Gram staining	—	Gram-negative or positve, cocci or bacilli depending on the causative agent	—
Ziehl-Neelsen staining	—	—	Acid-fast bacilli in case of tuberculous meningitis

Table 36.5. Causes of PUO

BACTERIAL

- Urinary tract infection
- Lung, subphrenic, appendix and other deep abscesses
- Septicaemia associated with pneumonia, pyelo-nephritis, biliary tract infection, infective endocarditis, osteomyelitis, etc.
- Enteric fever
- Tuberculosis
- Brucellosis
- Syphilis
- Relapsing fever
- Rheumatic fever
- Leptospirosis without jaundice or meningitis
- Typhus fever
- Non-meningitic meningococcal infection
- Q fever

PARASITIC

- Malaria
- Hepatic amoebiasis
- Leishmaniasis
- Trypanosomiasis
- Toxoplasmosis
- Filariasis

VIRAL

- EBV infection
- CMV infection
- HIV infection
- Rubella and other infectious fevers without typical rash

Table 36.6. Causative agents of infective endocarditis

Causative agent	Incidence
BACTERIA	
• Viridans group of streptococci	70%
– *Streptococcus sanguis*	
– *S. mutans*	
– *S. intermedius*	
– *S. mitis*	
• Groups F and G streptococci	10%
• *Staphylococcus epidermidis*	10%
• *Enterococcus faecalis*	5%
• *S. aureus*	5%
• Diphtheroids	Rare
• *Haemophilus* spp.	Rare
• Coliforms	Rare
• *Pseudomonas*	Rare
• *Coxiella burnetii*	Rare
• *Chlamydia psittaci*	Rare
FUNGI	
• *Candida* spp.	Rare
• *Aspergillus* spp.	Rare

Infective endocarditis

Normal healthy endocardium of an immuno-competent host is generally not at risk when challenged transiently by a small number of organisms in the circulation. However, the heavy challenges that accompany intravenous drug use or the use of intravascular catheters in debilitated host or damage to the natural heart valve by rheumatic fever or atheroma and cardiac surgery, in particular prosthetic valve replacement may lead to infections of the endocardium. The important causative agents of infective endocarditis are given in Table 36.6.

Diagnosis of infective endocarditis can be established by isolation of the causative agent from the blood. Three to six samples of blood, 10 ml each should be collected from antecubital vein over 24 hours. Each sample should be inoculated into 50–100 ml of glucose broth. Large amount of blood is required because the number of organisms in the blood may be very few. In addition, blood provides nutrition for the growth of organisms. Repeated blood cultures are made because the bacteraemia is inter-mittent.

The blood is inoculated into large amount (50–100 ml) of culture medium so that bactericidal substances present in the blood are diluted. Cultures are incubated at 37°C for at least 3 weeks. Subcultures are made on blood agar and MacConkey agar after 24 hours, 48 hours and once a week thereafter. *Coxiella burnetii* and *Chlamydia* spp. cannot grow on cell free media. For the diagnosis of these agents, refer to corresponding chapters.

Index